# Neuroscience

## FUNDAMENTALS for REHABILITATION

### *FOURTH EDITION*

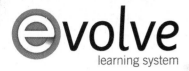
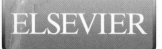

LAURIE LUNDY-EKMAN, PT, PhD

Professor of Physical Therapy
Pacific University
Hillsboro, Oregon

# Neuroscience

## FUNDAMENTALS
## for REHABILITATION

*FOURTH EDITION*

3251 Riverport Lane
St. Louis, Missouri 63043

Neuroscience: Fundamentals for Rehabilitation, Fourth Edition    ISBN: 978-1-4557-0643-3

---

**Notices**

Knowledge and best practice in this field are constantly changing. As new research and experience broaden our understanding, changes in research methods, professional practices, or medical treatment may become necessary. Practitioners and researchers must always rely on their own experience and knowledge in evaluating and using any information, methods, compounds, or experiments described herein. In using such information or methods they should be mindful of their own safety and the safety of others, including parties for whom they have a professional responsibility. With respect to any drug or pharmaceutical products identified, readers are advised to check the most current information provided (i) on procedures featured or (ii) by the manufacturer of each product to be administered, to verify the recommended dose or formula, the method and duration of administration, and contraindications. It is the responsibility of practitioners, relying on their own experience and knowledge of their patients, to make diagnoses, to determine dosages and the best treatment for each individual patient, and to take all appropriate safety precautions. To the fullest extent of the law, neither the Publisher nor the authors, contributors, or editors, assume any liability for any injury and/or damage to persons or property as a matter of products liability, negligence or otherwise, or from any use or operation of any methods, products, instructions, or ideas contained in the material herein.

---

Previous editions copyright ©2007, 2002, 1998

**Library of Congress Cataloging-in-Publication Data**

Lundy-Ekman, Laurie.
  Neuroscience : fundamentals for rehabilitation / Laurie Lundy-Ekman.—4th ed.
    p. ; cm.
  Includes bibliographical references and index.
  ISBN 978-1-4557-0643-3 (pbk.)
  I. Title.
  [DNLM: 1. Nervous System—anatomy & histology.  2. Nervous System Physiological
Phenomena.  3. Nervous System—physiopathology.  4. Nervous System Diseases—rehabilitation.  WL 102]
  616.8—dc23
                                                              2012007427

*Acquisitions Editor:* Kathy Falk
*Developmental Editor:* Megan Fennell
*Publishing Services Manager:* Julie Eddy and Hemamailini Rajendrababu
*Senior Project Manager:* Andrea Campbell
*Project Manager:* Saravanan Thavamani
*Design Direction:* Jessica Williams
*Cover Designer:* Jessica Williams

Printed in the United States of America

Last digit is the print number:   9   8   7   6   5   4   3

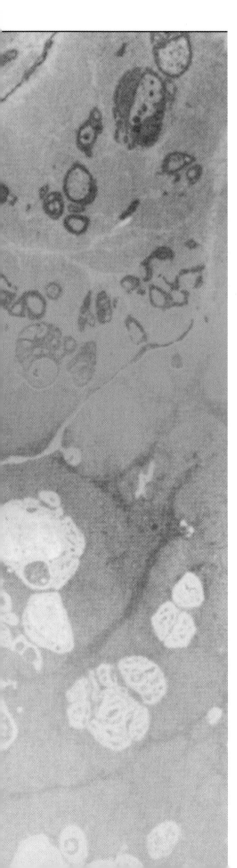

# Contributors

**Catherine Siengsukon, PT, PhD**
Assistant Professor
University of Kansas Medical Center
Physical Therapy and Rehab Science
Kansas City, Kansas

*Chapter 4—Neuroplasticity*

**Lisa Stehno-Bittel, PT, PhD**
Associate Professor
Department of Physical Therapy Education
University of Kansas Medical Center
Kansas City, Kansas

*Chapter 2—Physical and Electrical Properties of Cells in the
        Nervous System*
*Chapter 3—Synapses and Synaptic Transmissions*

**Contributor to the First and Second Editions**

**Anne Burleigh Jacobs, PhD, PT**
SensoMotor Neurological Rehab
Los Altos, California

*Chapters 2, 3, and 4*

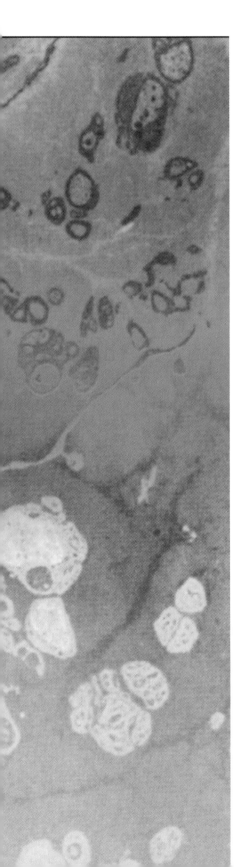

# Preface

How do we perceive, feel emotions, move, learn, and remember? And what are the common neural disorders that affect these processes? Neuroscience is the attempt to answer these questions. However, the answers in neuroscience are not static; knowledge progresses rapidly. This third edition of *Neuroscience: Fundamentals for Rehabilitation* reflects updated concepts and recent research. Yet the original purpose of the book remains unaltered: to present carefully selected, clinically important information essential for understanding the neurologic disorders encountered by therapists. Feedback from students, clinicians, and educators indicates that they find the book exceptionally useful both as an introduction to neuroscience and as a reference during clinical practice.

This text is unique in addressing neuroscience issues critical for the practice of physical rehabilitation. Clinical issues including abnormal muscle tone, chronic pain, and control of movement are emphasized, whereas topics often discussed extensively in neuroscience texts, such as the function of neurons in the visual cortex, are omitted.

The text has five sections: Cellular Level, Development, Systems, Regions, and Support Systems. The **Cellular Level** discusses the variety of neural cells, neuron ion channels, membrane potentials, synapses, and mechanisms of learning/memory (Chapters 2–4). **Development** covers embryology of the nervous system and developmental disorders (Chapter 5). Three systems comprise the **Systems** section: somatosensory, autonomic, and motor (Chapters 6–11). The somatosensory system transmits information from the skin and the musculoskeletal system to the brain. The autonomic system conveys information between the brain and smooth muscles, viscera, and glands. The motor system transmits information from the brain to the skeletal muscles. Disorders that affect these three systems are presented. **Regions** covers the peripheral nervous system, spinal region, brainstem and cerebellar region, and the cerebrum (Chapters 12–18). The final section, **Support Systems**, discusses the blood supply and the cerebrospinal fluid system (Chapter 19). This organization provides the student the opportunity to learn how neural cells operate first, and then apply that knowledge while developing an understanding of systems neuroscience. In learning systems neuroscience, the student develops familiarity with landmarks throughout the nervous system that are revisited in the regions section. The final chapter integrates much of the information from previous chapters in the discussion of the effects of strokes. Thus the text is structured so that subsequent chapters build on the information in earlier chapters, and earlier information is developed more fully and applied to new clinical disorders later in the text. This structure provides a framework for neurologic examination and evaluation: first the systems involved are identified and then the region(s) implicated are identified.

**Distinctive features of this text include:**
- *Personal stories written by people with neurologic disorders.* These stories give the information immediacy and a connection with reality that is sometimes missing from textbook presentations.
- *Clinical notes containing case examples to challenge students to apply the information to clinical practice*
- *Disease profiles that provide a quick summary of the features of common neurologic disorders:* pathology, etiology, signs and symptoms, region affected, demographics, and prognosis
- *Brief introductions to clinical examination techniques*

**Topics that are new or extensively revised in this edition include:**
- Neural stem cells
- Neuroplasticity
- Effects of rehabilitation on plasticity
- Differential diagnosis of dizziness
- Neuropathic pain
- Pain matrix malfunction
- Phantom pain

- Small fiber neuropathy
- Medications for neuropathic pain, fibromyalgia, and low back pain
- Spasticity
- Basal ganglia function
- Decision making and somatic marker dysfunction
- Memory
- Attention
- Behavioral and cognitive effects of cerebral lesions
- The reward pathway and motivational disorders
- Autism spectrum disorders
- Psychological disorders, signs, and symptoms

**Learning Aids**

- **Chapter Outlines, Introductions, and Summaries** clarify the organization of each chapter and reinforce important topics.
- **Terms in bold** highlight important terminology. These terms are defined when first used and are also collected as a glossary at the end of the book.
- **Clinical Notes** are opportunities for the students to test their ability to apply neuroscience information to a specific case. Answers to the Clinical Notes are available on the Evolve website (see Supplementary Learning Resources).
- **Review Questions** focus student attention on significant topics. Answers to the review questions are available at the back of the book.

- **References** are provided as guides into the research literature.
- **Term definitions** are available in the glossary of this textbook.
- Hundreds of original **full-color illustrations** complement the content.

**Supplementary Learning Resources**

Online learning resources to complement this textbook are available at the Elsevier Evolve website (*http://evolve.elsevier.com/ Lundy/\*\*\**). At this website, students will find:

- Workbook
- Content updates
- Weblinks to facilitate further exploration
- Atlas of photographs of normal sections of the human brain, accompanied by labeled line drawings
- Author contact information

The workbook provides multiple-choice and short-answer questions, matching exercises, drawings to label, and terms to define for each chapter. Correct answers are available online for all of the exercises except the term definitions. In addition to the student resources, instructors using this textbook have access to an online course management system and an image collection of the textbook illustrations. The course management system provides tools for online discussion, a calendar, the ability to upload and download documents, and quiz capability. The images can be downloaded for use in presentations.

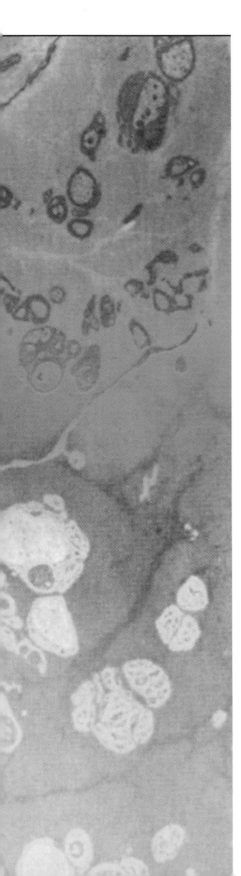

# Acknowledgments

This edition has been significantly improved by the contributions of several key people. Lisa Ekman served as my research assistant. Lisa Stehno-Bittel updated and revised Chapters 2 and 3. Catherine Siengsukon updated and revised Chapter 4. Megan Fennell, Developmental Editor, and Andrea Campbell, Senior Project Manager, were consistently helpful throughout the process. Jeanne Robertson created the new illustrations. David A. Brown, Carmen Cirstea, and Catherine Siengsukon made major contributions to the significant improvements in the motor neuron/spasticity section. Their suggestions both enriched and clarified the topic. The authors of the personal stories willingly shared their experiences and are each credited at the end of their contribution. My husband Andy and my daughter Lisa have, as always, been patient, good humored, and supportive during the writing of this book.

My thanks to Anne Burleigh-Jacobs, who wrote Chapters 2, 3, and 4 in the first edition, coauthored the same chapters in the second edition, and wrote the third edition of the workbook. Students who provided guidance on previous editions include Christopher Boor, Nancy Heinley, Mike Hmura, and Susan Hendrickson. Clinicians and faculty who reviewed previous manuscripts include Anne Burleigh-Jacobs, Erin Jobst, Renate Powell, Mike Studer, Robert Rosenow, and Daiva Banaitis. The Digital Anatomist images are from the "Digital Anatomist Interactive Atlases" by Drs. John W. Sundsten and Kathleen A. Mulligan, Department of Biological Structure, University Washington, Seattle, Washington, U.S.A.

# Contents

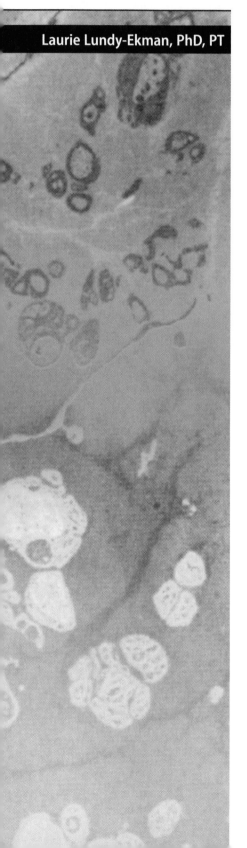

# 1 Introduction to Neuroscience

**Laurie Lundy-Ekman, PhD, PT**

Many people live with functional limitations related to nervous system damage or disease. People who have experienced brain damage, spinal cord injury, birth defects, or neurologic diseases must cope with the effects. Tasks as seemingly simple as sitting, standing, walking, getting dressed, and remembering a name may become incredible challenges. Physical and occupational therapy play a crucial role in helping people regain the ability to function as independently as possible. The design of physical and occupational therapy treatments and the management of each individual case are dependent on an understanding of the nervous system and on continued research.

## WHAT IS NEUROSCIENCE?

The quest to understand the nervous system is called *neuroscience*. Neuroscience is a relatively new science concerned with the development, chemistry, structure, function, and pathology of the nervous system. Rigorous scientific research on neural function has a relatively short history, beginning in the late 1800s. At that time, physiologists Fritsch and Hitzig reported that electrical stimulation of specific areas of an animal's cerebral cortex elicited movement, and physicians Broca and Wernicke separately confirmed, by autopsy, localized brain damage in people who had language deficits after stroke. About the same time, Hughlings Jackson proposed that multiple brain areas are essential for complex functions such as perception, action, and language.

About 1890, Cajal, a neuroanatomist, established that each nerve cell (neuron) is a distinct, individual cell, not directly continuous with other nerve cells. Sherrington, a physiologist studying involuntary reactions that occur in response to stimuli, proposed that nerve cells communicated at special sites he named *synapses*. The next major advances in understanding the nervous system did not occur until the 1950s, when both the electron microscope and the microelectrode were developed. The electron microscope allows visualization of cellular organelles, and the microelectrode can record the activity of a single nerve cell.

Beginning in the 1970s, new imaging techniques were developed that create clear images of the living spinal cord and brain, unobscured by the surrounding skull and vertebrae. These imaging techniques provide physiologic and pathologic information never before available. Computed tomography (CT), positron emission tomography (PET), and magnetic resonance imaging (MRI) all use computerized analysis to create an image of the nervous system. Figure 1-1 shows CT and PET scans. Magnetic resonance imaging has three variants: blood oxygen level dependent (BOLD), diffusion tensor imaging (DTI), and functional MRI (fMRI; Figure 1-2). Table 1-1 compares medical imaging techniques.

In 1985, the development of transcranial magnetic stimulation (TMS) enabled researchers to stimulate brain activity without opening the skull. An electrical current in a coil near the scalp generates a magnetic field that passes through the skull. The magnetic field induces an electrical current in a small area of the brain (Figure 1-3). The electrical current activates local neurons. For example, if a specific part of the motor cortex is stimulated, the hand moves without the intent of the person receiving the stimulation. TMS is usually painless. After TMS, the stimulated brain area is temporarily inactive. Thus TMS allows researchers to (1) investigate the effects of stimulating a part of the brain and (2) study the effects of briefly inactivating part of the brain without damaging the area or using invasive techniques.

All of these techniques used historically to examine neural function are still used today, although with many refinements. Current approaches to understanding the nervous system include multiple levels of analysis:
- Molecular
- Cellular
- Systems
- Behavioral
- Cognitive

## TABLE 1-1    MEDICAL IMAGING TECHNIQUES

| | Positron Emission Tomography (PET) | Computed Tomography (CT) | MAGNETIC RESONANCE IMAGING (MRI) | | |
|---|---|---|---|---|---|
| | | | Blood Oxygen Level Dependent (BOLD) Changes MRI | Diffusion Tensor Imaging (DTI) | Functional MRI (fMRI) |
| Mechanism | Emissions from radioactive compounds injected into blood | X-rays pass through body to detector; computer generates image. | Magnetic fields and radio waves detect hydrogen ions. | Magnetic fields and radio waves measure water diffusion in axons. | Magnetic fields and radio waves measure changes in blood oxygenation. |
| Use | Assess blood flow (over a time span of minutes), oxygen or glucose metabolism, receptor location | Suspected strokes or increased intracranial pressure; detailed images of bone, fractures | Detailed images of soft tissues; detects tumors, infection, multiple sclerosis | Detailed images of white matter tracts; useful for traumatic brain injury, best of scans for detecting ischemic stroke | Information about changes in blood flow that occur in a second or less |
| Time to complete scan | 15–75 minutes | 5 minutes | 30 minutes | 30 minutes | 15–60 minutes |
| Cost | $2,000–$5,000 | $1,200–$3,200 | $1,200–$4,000 | Same as other MRI | Same as other MRI |
| Risks | Radiation exposure | Radiation exposure | None reported | None reported | None reported |

PET

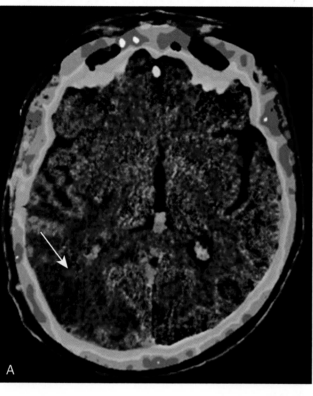

CT

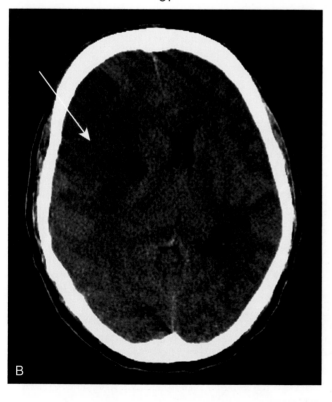

## Analysis of the Nervous System

*Molecular neuroscience* investigates the chemistry and physics involved in neural function. Studies of the ionic exchanges required for a nerve cell to conduct information from one part of the nervous system to another and the chemical transfer of information between nerve cells are molecular-level neuroscience. Reduced to their most fundamental level, sensation, moving, understanding, planning, relating, speaking, and most other human functions depend on chemical and electrical changes in nervous system cells.

*Cellular neuroscience* considers distinctions between different types of cells in the nervous system and how each cell type functions. Inquiries into how an individual neuron processes and conveys information, how information is transferred among neurons, and the roles of non-neural cells in the nervous system are cellular-level questions.

*Systems neuroscience* investigates groups of neurons that perform a common function. Systems-level analysis studies the connections, or circuitry, of the nervous system. Examples are the proprioceptive system, which conveys position and movement information from the musculoskeletal system to the central nervous system, and the motor system, which controls movement.

*Behavioral neuroscience* looks at the interactions among systems that influence behavior. For example, studies of postural control investigate the relative influence of visual, vestibular, and proprioceptive sensations on balance under different conditions.

*Cognitive neuroscience* covers the fields of thinking, learning, and memory. Studies focused on planning, using language, and identifying the differences between memory for remembering specific events and memory for performing motor skills are examples of cognitive-level analysis.

## What Do We Learn From These Studies?

From a multitude of investigations at all levels of analysis in neuroscience, we have begun to be able to answer questions such as the following:

* How do ions influence nerve cell function?
* How does a nerve cell convey information from one location in the nervous system to another?

**Fig. 1-1 Brain scans that use radiation to generate an image. A,** Positron emission tomography (PET) scans are used to assess blood flow, oxygen or glucose metabolism, or receptor location. This PET scan reveals a tumor (indicated by white arrow). **B,** Computed tomography (CT) brain scans are typically used to investigate suspected strokes or increases in intracranial pressure. In this horizontal section, the white arrow points to a dark area indicating tissue death from lack of blood supply. *(A, reproduced with permission from Miletich RS: Positron emission tomography for neurologists, Neurol Clin 27(1):71, 2009. B, reproduced with permission from Biller J, Love BB, Schneck MJ: from Bradley neurology in clinical practice, ed 5, Philadelphia, 2008 Butterworth-Heinemann, p 1214.)*

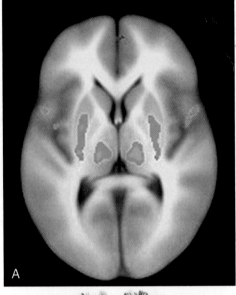

A

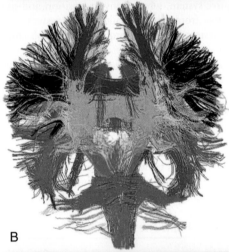

B

**Fig. 1-2 Computed scans of the brain using magnetic resonance imaging (MRI; no radiation).** MRI produces the best resolution of various soft tissues. **A,** Blood oxygen level dependent (BOLD) MRI. Average brain activation during a complex finger-tapping task in a group of neurologically normal subjects. **B,** Diffusion tensor imaging (DTI) measures the movement of water and generates an image of tracts that connect parts of the nervous system. This scan provides a three-dimensional view of fibers connecting areas of the brain, looking directly at the front of the brain. **C,** Functional MRI (fMRI) of brain activity comparing pain reduction effects of expectation versus acupuncture. *(A. From Fox RJ: Advanced MRI in multiple sclerosis: current status and future challenges, Neurol Clin 29(2):369, 2011. B, From Wang X, Grimson WE, Westin CF: Tractography segmentation using a hierarchical Dirichlet processes mixture model, Neuroimage 54(1):290–302, 2011. C, From Kong J, Kaptchuk TJ, Polich G, et al: Expectancy and treatment interactions: a dissociation between acupuncture analgesia and expectancy evoked placebo analgesia, Neuroimage 45(3): 940–949, 2009.)*

L          R

L          R

A          P

z = −6

y = −15

x = −54

0          20

C

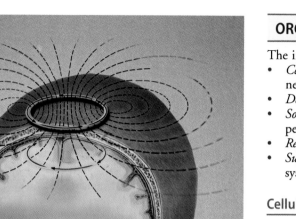

**Fig. 1-3** During transcranial magnetic stimulation, an electromagnetic coil is held against a person's scalp. The coil emits magnetic pulses that pass though the skull and induce an electrical current in the brain. This electrical current alters the activity of neurons. *(Courtesy L. Kibiuk/Society for Neuroscience.)*

- How is language formed and understood?
- How does information about a hot stove encountered by a fingertip reach conscious awareness?
- How are the abilities to stand and walk developed and controlled?
- How can modern medicine contribute to the recovery of neural function?
- How can physical therapy and occupational therapy assist a patient in regaining maximal independence after neurologic injury?

The answers to these questions are explored in this text. The purpose of this text is to present information that is essential for understanding the neurologic disorders encountered by therapists. Therapists who specialize in neurologic rehabilitation typically treat clients with brain and spinal cord disorders. However, clients with neurologic disorders are not confined to neurologic rehabilitation; therapists specializing in orthopedics frequently treat clients with chronic neck or low back pain, nerve compression syndromes, and other nervous system problems. Regardless of the area of specialty, a thorough knowledge of basic neuroscience is important for every therapist.

## ORGANIZATION OF THIS BOOK

The information in this text is presented in six parts:
- *Cellular level:* structure and functions of the cells in the nervous system
- *Development:* how the nervous system forms
- *Somatic and autonomic systems:* groups of neurons that perform a common function
- *Regions:* areas of the nervous system
- *Support systems:* blood supply and cerebrospinal fluid systems

### Cellular Level

Cells in the nervous system are neurons and glia. A *neuron* is the functional unit of the nervous system, consisting of a nerve cell body and the processes that extend outward from the cell body: dendrites and the axon.
- Neurons that convey information into the central nervous system are afferent.
- Neurons that transmit information from the central nervous system to peripheral structures are efferent.
- Neurons that connect only with other neurons are interneurons.

**Glia** are non-neuronal cells that provide services for neurons. Some specialized glial cells form myelin sheaths, the coverings that surround and insulate axons in the nervous system and aid in the transmission of electrical signals. Other types of glia nourish, support, and protect neurons.

### Development of the Human Nervous System

The development of the human nervous system in utero and through infancy is considered in this section. Common developmental disorders are also described.

### Somatic and Autonomic Systems

The nervous system is composed of many smaller systems, each with distinct functions. Many systems are discussed in the context of an appropriate region of the nervous system; for example, the cognitive system is discussed in the chapter on the cerebrum. However, three systems extend through all regions of the nervous system: the somatosensory, autonomic, and somatic motor systems. The somatosensory system conveys information from the skin and the musculoskeletal system to areas of the brain. The autonomic system provides bidirectional communication between the brain and smooth muscle, cardiac muscle, and gland cells. The somatic motor system transmits information from the brain to skeletal muscles. Because much of the nervous system is devoted to somatosensory, autonomic, and motor functions, being familiar with these three systems allows one to assign meaning to many of the terms encountered in studying the regions of the nervous system.

### Regions of the Nervous System

The nervous system can be divided into four regions: peripheral, spinal, brainstem and cerebellar, and cerebral regions (Figure 1-4).

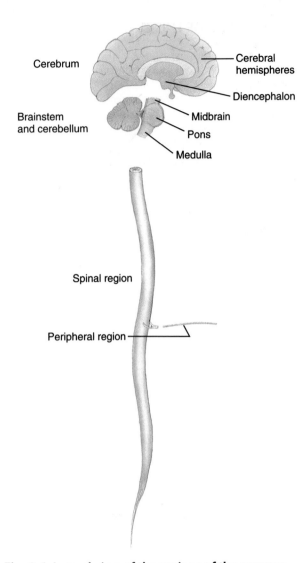

**Fig. 1-4 Lateral view of the regions of the nervous system.** Regions are listed on the left, and subdivisions are listed on the right.

## Peripheral Nervous System

The peripheral nervous system consists of all parts of the nervous system that are not encased in the vertebral column or skull. Peripheral nerves, including the median, ulnar, sciatic, and cranial nerves, are groups of axons.

## Spinal Region

The spinal region includes all parts of the nervous system encased in the vertebral column. In addition to the spinal cord, axons attached to the cord are within the spinal region until the axons exit the intervertebral foramen.

## Brainstem and Cerebellar Region

The brainstem connects the spinal cord with the cerebral region. The major divisions of the brainstem are the medulla,

pons, and midbrain (see Figure 1-4). Although cranial nerve receptors and axons are part of the peripheral nervous system, because most cranial nerves are functionally and structurally closely related to the brainstem, the cranial nerves are discussed with the brainstem/cerebellar region in this text. Connected to the posterior brainstem is the cerebellum.

## Cerebral Region

The most massive part of the brain, the cerebrum, consists of the diencephalon and cerebral hemispheres (see Figure 1-4). The diencephalon, in the center of the cerebrum, is almost completely surrounded by the cerebral hemispheres. The thalamus and the hypothalamus are major structures of the diencephalon. Cerebral hemispheres consist of the cerebral cortex, axons connecting the cortex with other parts of the nervous system, and deep nuclei.

## Support Systems

The cerebrospinal fluid and vascular systems provide essential support to the nervous system. Cerebrospinal fluid fills the ventricles, four continuous cavities within the brain, and then circulates on the surface of the central nervous system. Membranous coverings of the central nervous system, the meninges, are part of the cerebrospinal fluid system. The blood supply of the brain is delivered by the internal carotid and vertebral arteries.

## INTRODUCTION TO NEUROANATOMY

A general knowledge of basic neuroanatomy is required before one proceeds in this text. As noted earlier, the nervous system is divided into four regions: peripheral, spinal, brainstem and cerebellar, and cerebral regions. The peripheral nervous system consists of all nervous system structures not encased in bone. The central nervous system, encased in the vertebral column and skull, includes the spinal cord, brainstem and cerebellum, and cerebral regions.

Parts of the nervous system are classified according to the types of non-neural structures they innervate. Thus, the somatic nervous system connects with cutaneous and musculoskeletal structures, the autonomic nervous system connects with viscera, and the special sensory systems connect with visual, auditory, vestibular, olfactory, and gustatory (taste) structures.

Planes are imaginary lines through the nervous system (Figure 1-5). There are three planes:
- Sagittal
- Horizontal
- Coronal

A sagittal plane divides a structure into right and left portions. A midsagittal plane divides a structure into right and left halves, and a parallel cut produces parasagittal sections. A horizontal plane cuts across a structure at right angles to the long axis of the structure, creating a horizontal section, or a cross-section. A coronal plane divides a structure into anterior and posterior portions. The plane of an actual cut is used to name the cut surface, for example, a cut through the brain along the coronal plane is called a *coronal section*.

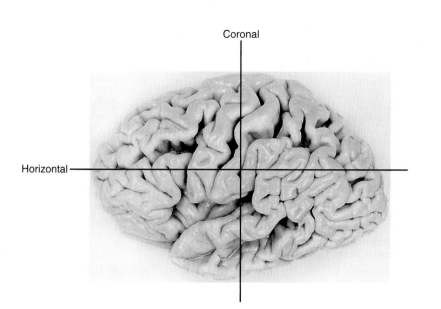

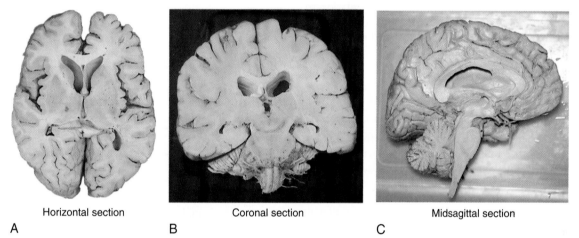

Horizontal section

A

Coronal section

B

Midsagittal section

C

**Fig. 1-5** Planes and sections of the brain. *(Lateral view courtesy Dr. Melvin J. Ball.)*

## Cellular-Level Neuroanatomy

Differences in cellular constituents produce an obvious feature—the difference between white and gray matter—in sections of the central nervous system (Figure 1-6). White matter is composed of axons, projections of nerve cells that usually convey information away from the cell body, and myelin, an insulating layer of cells that wraps around the axons. Areas with a large proportion of myelin appear white because of the high fat content of myelin. A bundle of myelinated axons that travel together in the central nervous system is called a *tract, lemniscus, fasciculus, column, peduncle,* or *capsule*.

Areas of the central nervous system that appear gray contain primarily neuron cell bodies. These areas are called *gray matter*. Groups of cell bodies in the peripheral nervous system are called *ganglia*. In the central nervous system, groups of cell bodies are most frequently called *nuclei*, although gray matter on the surface of the brain is called *cortex*.

The axons in white matter convey information among parts of the nervous system. Information is integrated in gray matter.

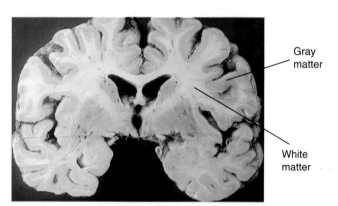

Gray matter

White matter

**Fig. 1-6** Coronal section of the cerebrum, revealing white and gray matter. White matter is composed of axons surrounded by large quantities of myelin. Gray matter is composed mainly of neuron cell bodies. *(Courtesy Jeanette Townsend.)*

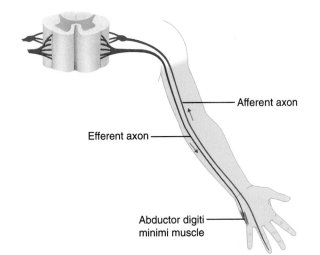

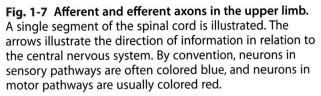

**Fig. 1-7  Afferent and efferent axons in the upper limb.** A single segment of the spinal cord is illustrated. The arrows illustrate the direction of information in relation to the central nervous system. By convention, neurons in sensory pathways are often colored blue, and neurons in motor pathways are usually colored red.

## Peripheral Nervous System

Within a peripheral nerve are afferent and efferent axons. Afferent axons carry information from peripheral receptors toward the central nervous system, for example, an afferent axon transmits information to the central nervous system when the hand touches an object. Efferent axons carry information away from the central nervous system, for example, efferent axons carry motor commands from the central nervous system to skeletal muscles (Figure 1-7). Peripheral components of the somatic nervous system include axons, sensory nerve endings, and glial cells. In the autonomic nervous system, entire neurons, sensory endings, synapses, ganglia, and glia are found in the periphery.

These components enable peripheral nerves to convey information from sensory receptors into the central nervous system, and to transmit signals from the central nervous system to skeletal and smooth muscle and glands.

## Spinal Region

Within the vertebral column, the spinal cord extends from the foramen magnum (the opening at the inferoposterior aspect of the skull) to the level of the first lumbar vertebra. Distally, the spinal cord ends in the conus medullaris. The spinal cord has 31 segments, and a pair of spinal nerves arises from each segment.

Each spinal nerve is connected to the cord by a dorsal root and a ventral root (Figure 1-8, *A*). An enlargement of the dorsal root, the dorsal root ganglion, contains the cell bodies of sensory neurons. Cell bodies of neurons forming the ventral root are located within the spinal cord. The union of the dorsal and ventral roots forms the spinal nerve. The spinal nerve exits the vertebral column via openings between vertebrae, then divides into dorsal and ventral rami that communicate with the

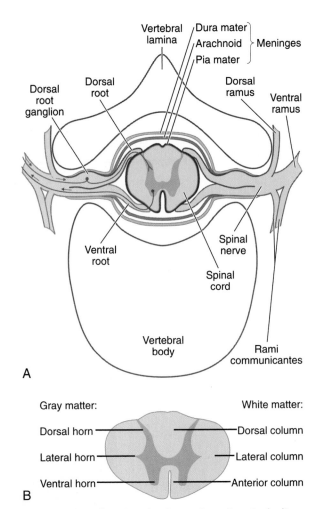

**Fig. 1-8  A,** Spinal region: horizontal section, including vertebra, spinal cord and roots, the spinal nerve, and rami. Afferent and efferent neurons are illustrated on the left side. The spinal nerve is formed of axons from the dorsal and ventral roots. The bifurcation of the spinal nerve into dorsal and ventral rami marks the transition from the spinal to the peripheral region. **B,** Cross-section of the spinal cord. The central gray matter is divided into horns and a commissure. The white matter is divided into columns.

periphery. The rami communicantes conduct signals between the spinal cord and the sympathetic ganglia.

Cross-sections of the spinal cord reveal centrally located gray matter forming a shape similar to the letter "H" surrounded by white matter (Figure 1-8, *B*). Each side of the gray matter is subdivided into ventral, lateral, and dorsal horns. These horns contain cell bodies of motor neurons, interneurons, and the endings of sensory neurons. The gray matter commissure connects the lateral areas of gray matter. The white matter is divided into three areas (funiculi):

- Anterior column
- Lateral column
- Dorsal column

The meninges, connective tissue surrounding the spinal cord and brain, are discussed later in this chapter.

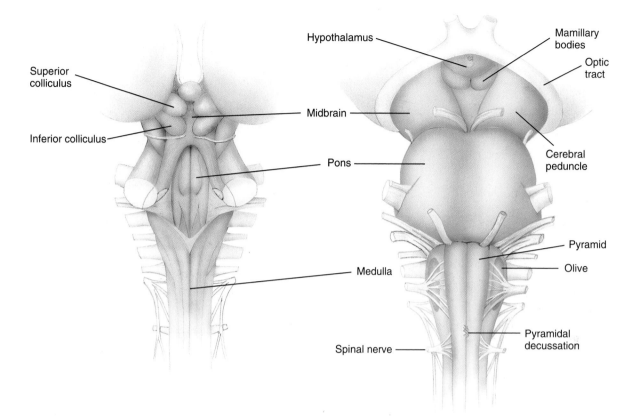

**Fig. 1-9** Brainstem: posterior and anterior views.

The spinal cord has two main functions:
- To convey information between neurons innervating peripheral structures and the brain
- To process information

The cord conveys somatosensory information to the brain and conveys signals from the brain to neurons that directly control movement. An example of spinal cord processing of information is the reflexive movement of a limb away from a painful stimulus. Within the cord are the necessary circuits to orchestrate the movement.

## Brainstem and Cerebellar Region

Many fiber tracts carrying motor and sensory information travel through the brainstem; other fiber tracts begin or end within the brainstem. In addition, the brainstem contains important groups of neurons that control equilibrium (sensations of head movement, orienting to vertical, postural adjustments), cardiovascular activity, respiration, and other functions. External features of the brainstem are illustrated in Figure 1-9. The parts of the brainstem are the medulla, pons, and midbrain.

## Medulla

The medulla is continuous with the spinal cord. Features of the anterior surface of the medulla include the olive, the pyramid, and the roots of four cranial nerves. The olive is an oval bump on the superior anterolateral surface of the medulla. The pyramids are axons projecting from the cerebral cortex to the spinal cord. As these fibers cross the midline, they form the pyramidal decussation.

## Pons

Superior to the medulla is the pons. The junction of the medulla and the pons is marked by a transverse line. The ventral part of the pons forms a large bulge anteriorly, containing fiber tracts and interspersed nuclei. Four cranial nerves attach to the pons.

## Midbrain

The superior section of the brainstem is the midbrain. The anterior portion of the midbrain is formed by two cerebral peduncles consisting of fibers that descend from the cerebral cortex. Dorsally, the tectum of the midbrain consists of four small rounded bodies—two superior colliculi and two inferior colliculi. The colliculi are important for orientation to auditory and visual stimuli. Two cranial nerves arise from the midbrain.

> ◎ **Clinical Pearl**
>
> The brainstem conveys information between the cerebrum and the spinal cord, integrates information, and regulates vital functions (e.g., respiration, heart rate, temperature).

## Cranial Nerves

Twelve pairs of cranial nerves emerge from the surface of the brain (Figure 1-10). Each cranial nerve is designated by a name and by a Roman numeral. Numbering is assigned according to

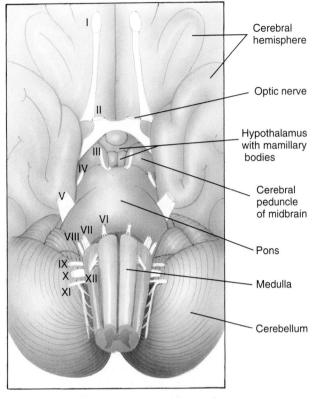

**Fig. 1-10** Inferior surface of the brain showing attachments of cranial nerves, except the attachment of cranial nerve IV. Cranial nerve IV attaches to the posterior brainstem (see Figure 1-9).

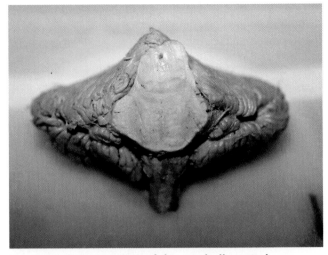

**Fig. 1-11 Anterior view of the cerebellum and brainstem.** The midbrain and the pons have been partially dissected to show the fiber tracts.

| TABLE 1-2 | CRANIAL NERVES | |
|---|---|---|
| Number | Name | Related Function |
| I | Olfactory | Smell |
| II | Optic | Vision |
| III | Oculomotor | Moves pupil of the eye up, down, medially; raises upper eyelid; constricts pupil |
| IV | Trochlear | Moves pupil of the eye medially and down |
| V | Trigeminal | Facial sensation, chewing, sensation from temporomandibular joint |
| VI | Abducens | Abducts pupil of the eye |
| VII | Facial | Facial expression, closes eyes, tears, salivation, and taste |
| VIII | Vestibulocochlear | Sensation of head position relative to gravity and head movement; hearing |
| IX | Glossopharyngeal | Swallowing, salivation, and taste |
| X | Vagus | Regulates viscera, swallowing, speech, and taste |
| XI | Accessory | Elevates shoulders, turns head |
| XII | Hypoglossal | Moves tongue |

the site of attachment to the brain, from anterior to posterior. Most cranial nerves innervate structures in the head, face, and neck. The exception is the vagus nerve, which innervates thoracic and abdominal viscera, in addition to structures in the head and neck.

Some cranial nerves are purely sensory. Purely sensory cranial nerves are the olfactory (I), optic (II), and vestibulocochlear (VIII) nerves. Other cranial nerves are principally motor but contain some sensory fibers that respond to muscle and tendon movement. They include the oculomotor (III), trochlear (IV), abducens (VI), accessory (XI), and hypoglossal (XII) nerves. The remaining cranial nerves are mixed nerves, containing both motor and sensory fibers. Table 1-2 lists the cranial nerves and their functions.

## Cerebellum

The cerebellum consists of two large cerebellar hemispheres and a midline vermis (Figure 1-11). *Vermis* means "worm," a fitting description for the appearance of the cerebellar midline. Internally, the cerebellar hemispheres are composed of the cerebellar cortex on the surface, underlying white matter, and centrally located deep nuclei. The cerebellum is connected to the posterior brainstem by large bundles of fibers called *peduncles*. The superior, middle, and inferior peduncles join the midbrain, pons, and medulla with the cerebellum. The function of the cerebellum is to coordinate movements.

## Cerebrum

### Diencephalon

The diencephalon consists of four structures (Figure 1-12):
- Thalamus
- Hypothalamus
- Epithalamus
- Subthalamus

The thalamus is a large, egg-shaped collection of nuclei in the center of the cerebrum. The other three structures are

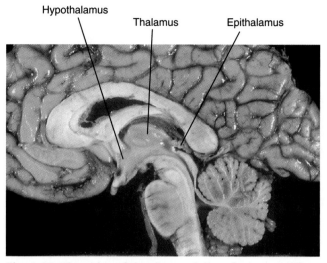

Hypothalamus Thalamus Epithalamus

**Fig. 1-12** The parts of the diencephalon that are visible in a midsagittal section are the thalamus, hypothalamus, and epithalamus. The subthalamus is lateral to the plane of section. *(Courtesy Jeanette Townsend.)*

named for their anatomic relationship to the thalamus: the hypothalamus is inferior to the thalamus, the epithalamus is located posterosuperior to the thalamus, and the subthalamus is inferolateral to the thalamus. The epithalamus consists primarily of the pineal gland.

Thalamic nuclei relay information to the cerebral cortex, process emotional and some memory information, integrate different types of sensations (i.e., touch and visual information), or regulate consciousness, arousal, and attention. The hypothalamus maintains body temperature, metabolic rate, and the chemical composition of tissues and fluids within an optimal functional range. The hypothalamus also regulates eating, reproductive, and defensive behaviors, expression of emotions, growth, and the function of reproductive organs. The pineal gland influences the secretion of other endocrine glands, including the pituitary and adrenal glands. The subthalamus is part of a neural circuit that controls movement.

## Cerebral Hemispheres

The longitudinal fissure divides the two cerebral hemispheres. The surfaces of the cerebral hemispheres are marked by rounded elevations called *gyri* (singular: gyrus) and grooves called *sulci* (singular: sulcus). Each cerebral hemisphere is subdivided into six lobes (Figure 1-13):
• Frontal
• Parietal
• Temporal
• Occipital
• Limbic
• Insular
The first four lobes are named for the overlying bones of the skull. The limbic lobe is on the medial aspect of the cerebral hemisphere. The insula is a section of the hemisphere buried within the lateral sulcus. The insula is revealed by separating the temporal and frontal lobes.

Distinctions among the lobes are clearly marked in only a few cases; in the remainder, boundaries between lobes are approximate. Clear distinctions include the following:
• The boundary between the frontal lobe and the parietal lobe, marked by the central sulcus
• The boundary between the parietal lobe and the occipital lobe, clearly marked only on the medial hemisphere by the parieto-occipital sulcus
• The division of the temporal lobe and the frontal lobe, marked by the lateral sulcus
• The limbic lobe, on the medial surface of the hemisphere, bounded by the cingulate sulcus and by the margin of the parahippocampal gyrus
The entire surface of the cerebral hemispheres is composed of gray matter, called the *cerebral cortex*. The cerebral cortex processes sensory, motor, and memory information and is the site for reasoning, language, nonverbal communication, intelligence, and personality. Deep to the cortex is white matter, composed of axons connecting the cerebral cortex with other central nervous system areas. Several collections of these fibers are of particular interest: the commissures and the internal capsule. The commissures are bundles of axons that convey information between the cortices of the left and right cerebral hemispheres. The corpus callosum is a huge commissure that connects most areas of the cerebral cortex. The much smaller anterior commissure connects the temporal lobe cerebral cortices. The internal capsule consists of axons that project from the cerebral cortex to subcortical structures and from subcortical structures to the cerebral cortex. The internal capsule is subdivided into anterior and posterior limbs, with a genu (bend) between them (Figure 1-14, *A*).

Within the white matter of the hemispheres are additional areas of gray matter; the most prominent is the basal ganglia. Basal ganglia nuclei in the cerebral hemispheres include the caudate, the putamen, and the globus pallidus (see Figure 1-14). The putamen and the globus pallidus together are called the *lenticular nucleus*. The caudate and the putamen together are called the *corpus striatum*. Two additional nuclei, the subthalamic nuclei (in the diencephalon) and the substantia nigra (in the midbrain), are part of the basal ganglia neural circuit. The basal ganglia circuit helps to control movement.

Another functional group of structures within the cerebrum is the limbic system, located in the diencephalon and the cerebral hemispheres. The limbic system includes parts of the hypothalamus, thalamus, and cerebral cortex; several deep cerebral nuclei, the most prominent being the amygdala and the ventral striatum; and the hippocampus, a region of the temporal lobe (Figure 1-15). The limbic system is involved with emotions and the processing of some types of memory.

## Support Systems

### Cerebrospinal Fluid System

Cerebrospinal fluid, a modified filtrate of plasma, circulates from cavities inside the brain to the surface of the central nervous system and is reabsorbed into the venous blood system. The cavities inside the brain are the four ventricles: paired lateral ventricles in the cerebral hemispheres; the third ventricle, a midline slit in the diencephalon; and the fourth ventricle,

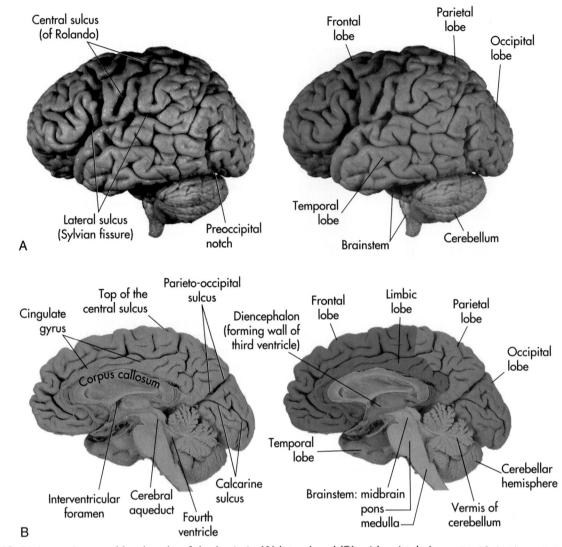

**Fig. 1-13** Major regions and landmarks of the brain in **(A)** lateral and **(B)** midsagittal views. *(Modified with permission from Nolte J. The human brain: an introduction to its functional anatomy, ed 4, St Louis, Mo, 1999, Mosby.)*

located posterior to the pons and medulla and anterior to the cerebellum (Figure 1-16). The ventricular system continues through the medulla and spinal cord as the central canal and ends blindly in the caudal spinal cord. Within the ventricles, cerebrospinal fluid is secreted by the choroid plexus. The lateral ventricles are connected to the third ventricle by the interventricular foramina. The third and fourth ventricles are connected by the cerebral aqueduct. Cerebrospinal fluid leaves the fourth ventricle through the lateral foramina and the medial foramen to circulate around the central nervous system.

The meninges, membranous coverings of the brain and spinal cord, are part of the cerebrospinal fluid system. From internal to external, the meninges consist of the pia, the arachnoid, and the dura. Only the second two can be observed in gross specimens. The pia is a very delicate membrane adherent to the surface of the central nervous system. The arachnoid, also a delicate membrane, is named for its resemblance to a spider's web. The dura, named for its toughness, has two

projections that separate parts of the brain: the falx cerebri separates the cerebral hemispheres, and the tentorium cerebelli separates the posterior cerebral hemispheres from the cerebellum (Figure 1-17). Within these dural projections are spaces called *dural sinuses,* which return cerebrospinal fluid and venous blood to the jugular veins. The cerebrospinal fluid system regulates the contents of the extracellular fluid and provides buoyancy to the central nervous system by suspending the brain and the spinal cord within fluid and membranous coverings.

## Vascular Anatomy

This section is presented regionally, beginning with blood supply to peripheral nerves, then to the spinal cord, followed by the vasculature of the brain.

Peripheral nerves are accompanied by blood vessels. Branches from the blood vessels pierce the epineurium surrounding the peripheral nerves. Arterioles and venules travel parallel to

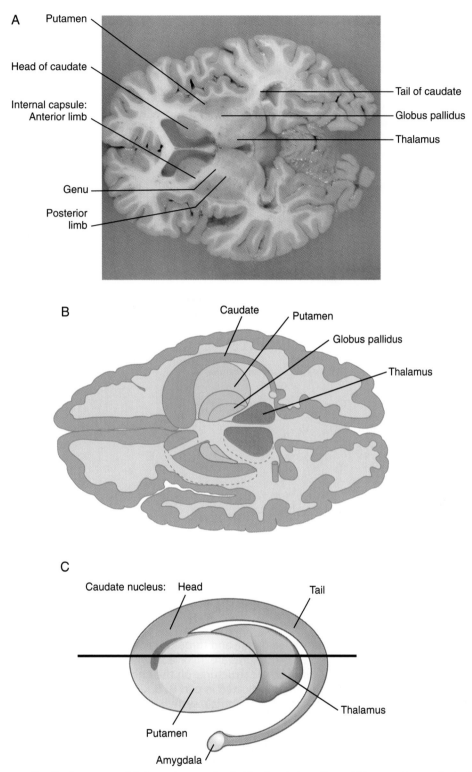

**A** Putamen

Head of caudate

Internal capsule:
Anterior limb

Genu

Posterior
limb

Tail of caudate

Globus pallidus

Thalamus

**B** Caudate  Putamen

Globus pallidus

Thalamus

**C** Caudate nucleus:  Head    Tail

Thalamus

Putamen

Amygdala

**Fig. 1-14 Basal ganglia, thalamus, and internal capsule. A,** Horizontal section of the cerebrum. Anterior is to the left. The internal capsule is the white matter bordered by the head of the caudate and the thalamus medially and by the lenticular nucleus (putamen and globus pallidus) laterally. **B,** Horizontal section of the cerebrum. Anterior is to the left. The location of the basal ganglia and thalamus within the white matter of the cerebral hemispheres is illustrated. The basal ganglia are shown in three dimensions on the right side of the brain. **C,** View from the side of the left caudate, putamen, thalamus, and amygdala. The line indicates the level of the section in **B.** *(Photograph in A is Copyright 1994, University of Washington. All rights reserved. Digital Anatomist Interactive Brain Atlas and the Structural Informatics Group, Department of Biological Structure. No re-use, re-distribution or commercial use without prior written permission of the author Dr. John W. Sundsten and the University of Washington, Seattle, Washington, U.S.A.)*

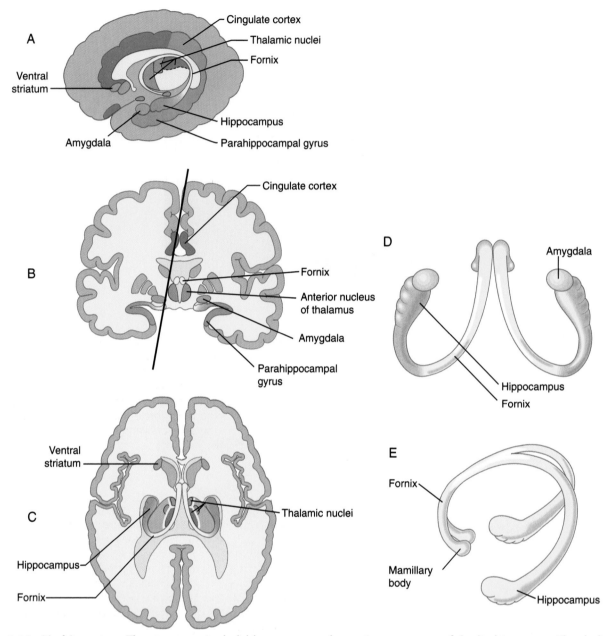

**Fig. 1-15. Limbic system.** The structures in dark blue, green, and turquiose are parts of the limbic system. The dark blue structures are involved in emotions, the green structures are involved in memory, and the turquoise structures are involved in both emotions and memory. **A,** View of limbic structures on the right side of the brain. Anterior is to the left. The plane of the section is at approximately the angle indicated in part **B. B,** Coronal section of the brain. The pale blue area is a fluid-filled space in the brain, which is part of the ventricle system (see Fig. 1-16). **C,** Horizontal section. Anterior is at the top. View from above shows the hippocampus and the fornix in three dimensions. The hippocampus is below the plane of the section, and the fornix is above the plane of the section. The amygdala is within the white matter and thus is not visible in this section. **D,** The hippocampus, fornix, and amygdala from above. Anterior is at the top. **E,** The mammillary body, fornix, and hippocampus. View is from above and laterally. Anterior is toward the left.

fascicles of neurons (Figure 1-18) to provide ionic exchange and nourishment.

Blood is supplied to the spinal cord by three spinal arteries running vertically along the cord: one is in the anterior midline and two are posterior, on either side of midline but medial to the dorsal roots (Figure 1-19). The anterior spinal artery supplies the anterior two thirds of the cord. The posterior spinal arteries supply the posterior third of the cord. The spinal arteries receive blood via the vertebral and medullary arteries. The medullary arteries are branches of vertebral, cervical, thoracic, and lumbar arteries. There are seven to ten medullary arteries. The vertebral arteries, which supply blood to the upper spinal cord, enter the skull through the foramen magnum to supply part of the brain.

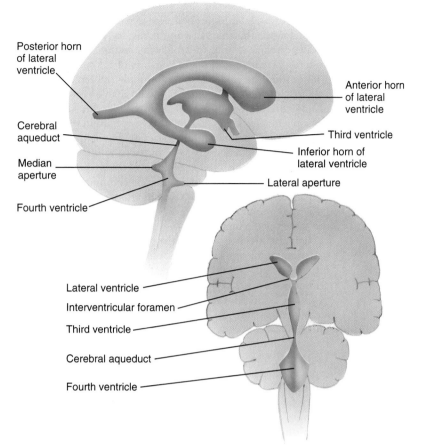

Fourth ventricle

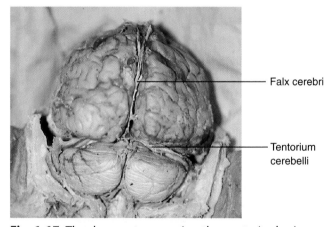

**Fig. 1-16** The four ventricles: two lateral ventricles, the third ventricle, and the fourth ventricle. Each lateral ventricle is within a cerebral hemisphere. The third ventricle is between the left and right thalamus, and the fourth ventricle is between the midbrain and the pons anteriorly and the cerebellum posteriorly.

**Fig. 1-17** The dura mater covering the posterior brain has been removed to reveal the dural projections: the falx cerebri and the tentorium cerebelli.

Two pairs of arteries supply blood to the brain (Figure 1-20, *A*):
- Two internal carotid arteries
- Two vertebral arteries

The internal carotid arteries provide blood to most of the cerebrum; the vertebral arteries provide blood to the occipital and inferior temporal lobes and to the brainstem/cerebellar region. The paired internal carotid arteries supply the anterior, superior, and lateral cerebral hemispheres. The paired vertebral arteries supply the brainstem, cerebellum, and posteroinferior cerebrum. The arterial branches discussed in the following sections are only the major arteries. Each artery has many branches, an elaborate capillary bed, and multiple arteriovenous junctions.

### Vascular Supply to the Brainstem and Cerebellum

The brainstem and the cerebellum are supplied by branches of the vertebral arteries and branches of the basilar artery (Figure 1-20, *B*). The basilar artery is formed by the union of the vertebral arteries. Each **vertebral artery** has three main branches: the anterior and posterior spinal arteries and the posterior inferior cerebellar artery. The medulla receives blood from all three branches of the vertebral arteries. The posterior inferior cerebellar artery also supplies the inferior cerebellum.

Near the pontomedullary junction, the vertebral arteries join to form the *basilar artery.* The basilar artery and its branches (anterior inferior cerebellar, superior cerebellar) supply the pons and most of the cerebellum. At the junction of the pons and the midbrain, the basilar artery divides to become the *posterior cerebral arteries.* The posterior cerebral artery is the primary source of blood supply to the midbrain.

*Vascular Supply to Cerebral Hemispheres*

**Internal Carotid and Posterior Cerebral Arteries.** The cerebrum is entirely supplied by the internal carotid and posterior cerebral arteries. The internal carotid arteries enter the skull through the temporal bones; small branches from each internal carotid become posterior communicating arteries that join the internal carotid with the posterior cerebral artery. Near the optic chiasm, the internal carotid divides into anterior and middle cerebral arteries (see following sections). Together, the posterior cerebral arteries and branches of the internal carotid arteries form the circle of Willis to supply the cerebrum.

**Circle of Willis.** The circle of Willis is an anastomotic ring of nine arteries, which supply all of the blood to the cerebral hemispheres (see Figure 1-20, *A*). Six large arteries anastomose via three small communicating arteries. The large arteries are the anterior cerebral artery (a branch of the internal carotid), the internal carotid artery, and the posterior cerebral artery (branches of the basilar). The anterior communicating artery (unpaired) joins the anterior cerebral arteries together, and the posterior communicating artery links the internal carotid with the posterior cerebral artery.

**Cerebral Arteries.** Each of the three major cerebral arteries (anterior, middle, posterior) has both cortical branches (supplying the cortex and outer white matter) and deep branches (to central gray matter and adjacent white matter).

From its origin, the *anterior cerebral artery* moves medially and anteriorly into the longitudinal fissure. The artery sweeps up and back above the corpus callosum, its branches supplying the medial surface of the frontal and parietal lobes (Figure 1-21, *A*). The *middle cerebral artery* supplies the internal capsule, globus pallidus, putamen, and caudate, then passes through the lateral sulcus. The branches of the middle cerebral artery fan out to supply most of the lateral hemisphere. The *posterior cerebral artery* wraps around and supplies the midbrain and then supplies the occipital lobe and parts of the medial and inferior temporal lobes. The major cerebral arteries connect at their beginning (via the circle of Willis) and at their ends (watershed area [see Figure 1-21, *A*]). The *watershed area* is an area of marginal blood flow on the surface of the lateral hemispheres, where small anastomoses link the ends of cerebral arteries.

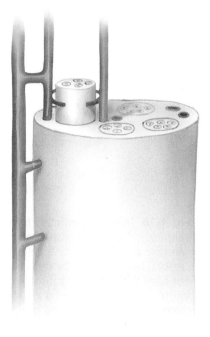

**Fig. 1-18** Arterial supply to a group of axons within a peripheral nerve.

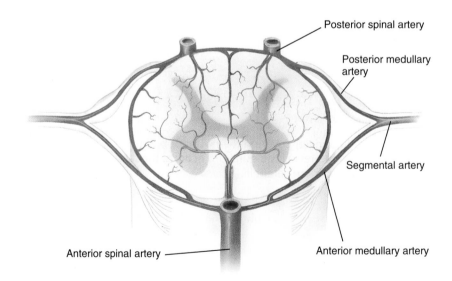

Posterior spinal artery

Posterior medullary artery

Segmental artery

Anterior spinal artery

Anterior medullary artery

**Fig. 1-19** Blood supply of the spinal cord.

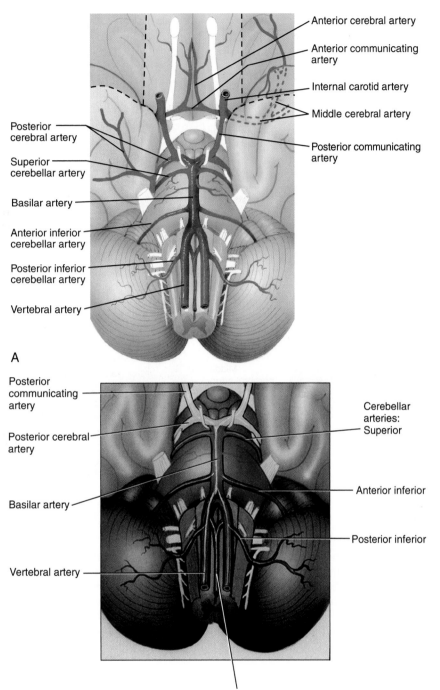

**Fig. 1-20  Arterial supply to the brain. A,** The posterior circulation, supplied by the vertebral arteries, is labeled on the left. The anterior circulation, supplied by the internal carotid arteries, is labeled on the right. The area supplied by the posterior cerebral artery is indicated in yellow; the middle cerebral artery territory is blue, and the anterior cerebral artery territory is green. The watershed area, supplied by small anastomoses at the ends of the large cerebral arteries, is indicated by dotted black lines. **B,** Blood supply of the brainstem and cerebellum. Each artery is color coded to match the territory it supplies.

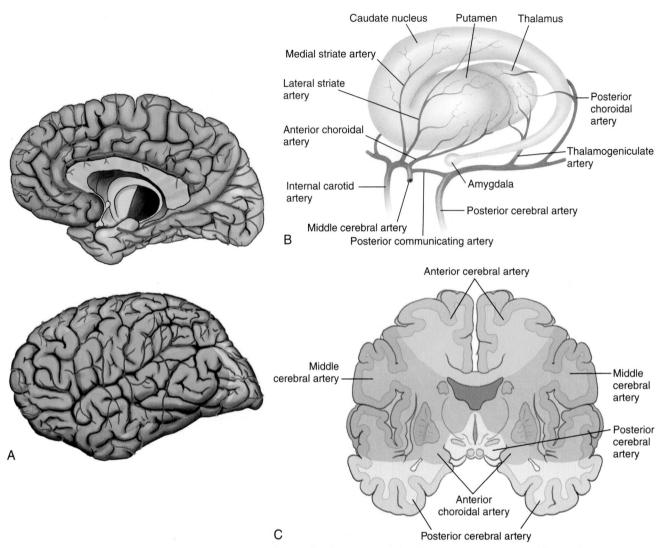

**Fig. 1-21  Arterial supply to the cerebral hemispheres. A,** The large cerebral arteries: anterior, middle, and posterior. Green indicates the area supplied by the anterior cerebral artery; blue indicates the area supplied by the middle cerebral artery, and yellow indicates the area supplied by the posterior cerebral artery. **B,** Branches of the internal carotid artery supply parts of the caudate and putamen. The supply to the putamen is via the anterior choroidal artery. The posterior choroidal artery, a branch of the posterior cerebral artery, supplies the choroid plexus of the third ventricle and parts of the thalamus and hippocampus. **C,** Coronal section illustrating the arterial supply of the cerebrum.

---

### ◎ Clinical Pearl

The anterior cerebral artery supplies the anterosuperior parts of the medial cerebral hemisphere. The middle cerebral artery supplies most of the lateral cerebral hemisphere, the caudate, and parts of the putamen and internal capsule. The posterior cerebral artery supplies the midbrain, the occipital lobe, and parts of the medial and inferior temporal lobe.

---

In addition to the branches of major cerebral arteries supplying deep structures, two other arteries supply only deep structures: the *anterior and posterior choroidal arteries.* The anterior choroidal (a branch of the internal carotid) supplies the choroid plexus in the lateral ventricles, as well as parts of the

visual pathway (optic tract and optic radiations; see Chapter 16), putamen, thalamus, internal capsule, and hippocampus. The posterior choroidal (a branch of the posterior cerebral artery) supplies the choroid plexus of the third ventricle and parts of the thalamus and hippocampus (Figure 1-21, *B*). Figure 1-21, *C*, illustrates the arterial supply of the cerebrum in coronal section.

In contrast to other parts of the body that have major veins corresponding to the major arteries, venous blood from the cerebrum drains into dural (venous) sinuses. Dural sinuses are canals between layers of dura mater. In turn, the dural sinuses drain into the jugular veins. The vascular system provides oxygen, ionic exchange, and nourishment for the cells of the nervous system. Table 1-3 reviews the arterial supply of the central nervous system.

**TABLE 1-3    ARTERIAL SUPPLY OF THE CENTRAL NERVOUS SYSTEM**

| Artery | Branches | Area Supplied |
|---|---|---|
| Vertebral artery | Anterior and posterior spinal arteries | Spinal cord and medulla |
| | Posterior inferior cerebellar artery | Medulla and cerebellum |
| Basilar artery | Anterior inferior cerebellar and superior cerebellar arteries | Pons and cerebellum |
| | Posterior cerebral artery | Midbrain, occipital lobe, and inferomedial temporal lobe |
| | Branch of posterior cerebral artery: posterior choroidal | Choroid plexus of third ventricle; parts of thalamus and hypothalamus |
| Internal carotid | Anterior choroidal | Choroid plexus in lateral ventricles, parts of the visual pathway (optic tract and optic radiation), parts of the putamen, thalamus, internal capsule, and hippocampus |
| | Anterior cerebral artery | Medial frontal and parietal lobes |
| | Middle cerebral artery | Globus pallidus, putamen, most of lateral hemisphere, part of internal capsule and caudate |

## INCIDENCE AND PREVALENCE OF DISORDERS

*Incidence* is the proportion of a population that develops a **new** case of the disorder within a defined time period. Incidence is typically reported per 100,000 people. For example, when I asked 40 adults who developed a new dental cavity in the past year, only one new case was reported, indicating an incidence of 2500 per 100,000. *Prevalence* is the current proportion of the population with the condition, including both old and new cases. The prevalence rate is typically reported per 1000 people. The prevalence of dental cavities in the same group of people was 39/40, indicating a prevalence of 975 per 1000.

Migraine headache has a low incidence and a high prevalence, because prevalence is the cumulative sum of past year incidence rates. The incidence of migraine is 3800/100,000 people per year (3.8% of the population develops a new case during a given year[1]). The migraine prevalence for women is 17.5% and for men is 8.6%, for a prevalence overall of 13.2%.[2] In contrast, the motor neuron disease called *amyotrophic lateral sclerosis (ALS)* is fatal. Only 50% of people with ALS survive longer than 30 months after onset of the first symptom.[3] The annual incidence of ALS is 1.5/100,000, and the prevalence is 5.5/100,000.[4] Figure 1-22 indicates the incidence of selected neurologic disorders.[3-26]

## CLINICAL APPLICATION OF LEARNING NEUROSCIENCE

For therapists, the main purpose in studying the nervous system is to understand the effects of nervous system lesions. A *lesion* is an area of damage or dysfunction. Signs and symptoms following a lesion of the nervous system depend on the location of the lesion. For example, complete destruction of a specific area of cerebral cortex severely interferes with hand function. The cause of the damage could be blood supply interruption, a tumor, or local inflammation, but regardless of the cause, damage to that area of the cerebral cortex compromises the dexterity of the hand. Depending on their distribution in the nervous system, lesions can be categorized as follows:

- Focal: limited to a single location
- Multifocal: limited to several nonsymmetric locations
- Diffuse: affects bilaterally symmetric structures but does not cross the midline as a single lesion

A tumor in the spinal cord is an example of a focal lesion. A tumor that has metastasized to several locations is multifocal. Alzheimer's disease, a memory and cognitive disorder, is diffuse because it affects cerebral structures bilaterally but does not cross the midline as a single lesion.

> **Ⓞ *Clinical Pearl***
>
> Regardless of the cause of nervous system dysfunction, resulting signs and symptoms depend on the site and size of the lesion(s).

### Neurologic Evaluation

The neurologic evaluation has two parts:
- History
- Examination

The purpose of the neurologic evaluation is to determine the probable cause of neurologic problems so that appropriate care can be provided. Events that may affect the nervous system include the following:
- Trauma
- Vascular disorders
- Inflammation
- Degenerative disorders
- Neoplasms
- Immunologic disorders
- Toxic or metabolic disorders

### History

A history is essentially a structured interview conducted to identify the symptoms that led the person to seek physical or occupational therapy. Knowing the typical speed of onset and the expected pattern of progression for each category of

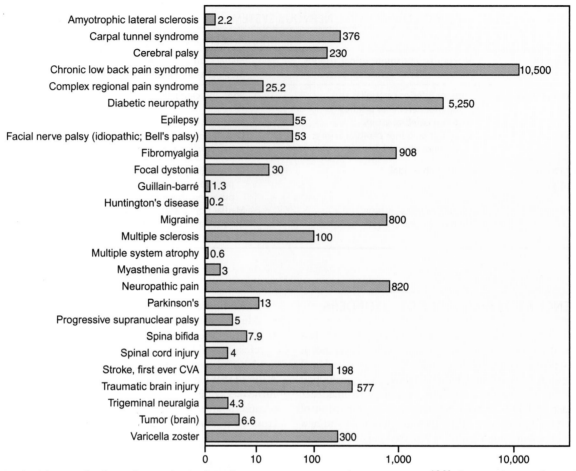

**Fig. 1-22** Incidence of selected neurologic disorders per 100,000 population in 1 year.[1,3-26] The number to the right of each bar indicates the precise incidence of the disorder. Note that the y-axis uses a logarithmic scale.

pathology is critical for recognizing when a specific client's signs and symptoms necessitate referral to a medical practitioner.

The speed of onset and the pattern of progression provide important clues to the origin, or cause, of nervous system dysfunction. Speed of onset is classified as follows:

- Acute, indicating minutes or hours to maximal signs and symptoms
- Subacute, progressing to maximal signs and symptoms over a few days
- Chronic, gradual worsening of signs and symptoms continuing for weeks or years

Acute onset usually indicates a vascular problem, subacute onset frequently indicates an inflammatory process, and chronic onset often suggests a tumor or degenerative disease. In cases of trauma, the cause is usually obvious, and in cases of immune, toxic, or metabolic disorders, the speed of onset varies according to the specific cause. The pattern of progression can be stable, improving, worsening, or fluctuating.

While discussing the person's history, the therapist can often obtain adequate information about the person's mental status:

- Is the person awake?
- Is the person aware?
- Is the person able to respond appropriately to questions?

## Examination

Specific tests are performed to assess the function of the sensory, autonomic, and motor systems. These tests are described in subsequent chapters. If indicated, additional tests that assess function within specific regions of the nervous system may be performed.

## Diagnosis

By synthesizing information obtained from the history and the physical examination, the therapist begins to answer the following questions:

- Is the lesion in the peripheral or central nervous system?
- Are the signs symmetric on the right and left sides of the body?
- Is the lesion focal, multifocal, or diffuse?
- Does the pattern of signs and symptoms indicate a syndrome?
- What region or regions of the nervous system are involved?
- What is the probable cause?
- What is the diagnosis?

Figure 1-23 shows, in the form of flowcharts, how information is integrated in reaching a diagnosis. In many cases, the

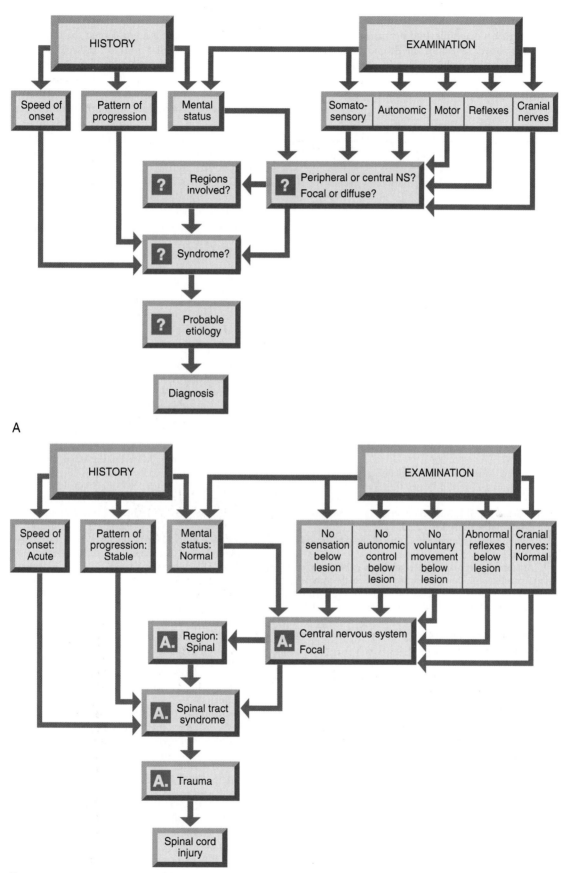

**Fig. 1-23 Flowcharts illustrating the process of neurologic evaluation. A,** The generalized process. A "?" indicates a question that can be answered by analyzing the information that flows into that box. **B,** Application of the neurologic evaluation process. Findings on the history and physical examination are indicated, as are the subsequent steps to reach a diagnosis. "A" indicates an answer to a question in **A.** In this case, the diagnosis is spinal cord injury.

therapist is able to reach a diagnosis. In other cases, the therapist may not be able to answer several of the diagnostic questions, or the diagnosis may be beyond the scope of physical therapy practice. In such cases, the person must be referred to the appropriate medical practitioner.

## SUMMARY

To gain an understanding of the nervous system, each level of analysis is essential. As noted by Joaquin Fuster (1994),[27] a brain researcher and psychiatrist, "the problem with the molecular approach to higher neurophysiology is that it proceeds at the wrong (i.e., impractical) level of discourse and analysis (like trying to understand the written message by studying the chemistry of the ink)." To extend Fuster's analogy, if there is a problem with the ink, then studying the chemistry of the ink

is appropriate. If there is a problem at the molecular level, with the supply of particular ions or molecules required by the nervous system, then the molecular level is the appropriate level of analysis. However, a molecular-level approach to understanding language is not practical; a cognitive-level analysis is appropriate. Some types of dysfunction in the nervous system interfere with cellular-level processes, other types of dysfunction interfere with the processing of one type of information, and still other types interfere with all functions processed in a specific area. To enhance understanding of each type of dysfunction, appropriate levels of analysis must be applied.

Scientific investigations at each level of analysis have revealed many details of neural function. These details have promoted an improved understanding of function and have provided new insight into the treatment of neurologic disorders. Continued neuroscience research and ongoing development of new treatment regimens can only bring us closer to a full understanding of nervous system function in health, disease, and recovery.

## References

1. Gopen Q, Viirre E, Anderson J: Epidemiologic study to explore links between Ménière syndrome and migraine headache. *Ear Nose Throat J* 88:1200–1204, 2009.

2. Victor TW, Hu X, Campbell JC, et al: Migraine prevalence by age and sex in the United States: a life-span study. *Cephalalgia* 30:1065–1072, 2010.

3. Kiernan MC, Vucic S, Cheah BC, et al: Amyotrophic lateral sclerosis. *Lancet* 377:942–955, 2011.

4. Chen A, Montes J, Mitsumoto J: The role of exercise in amyotrophic lateral sclerosis. *Phys Med Rehabil Clin N Am* 19:545–557, 2008.

5. Gelfman R, Melton LJ, 3rd, Yawn B, et al: Long-term trends in carpal tunnel syndrome. *Neurology* 72:33–41, 2009.

6. Jan MM: Cerebral palsy: comprehensive review and update. *Ann Saudi Med* 26:123–132, 2006.

7. El Sissi W, Arnaout A, Chaarani MW: Prevalence of neuropathic pain among patients with chronic low-back pain in the Arabian Gulf Region assessed using the LEEDs assessment of neuropathic symptoms and signs pain scale. *J Int Med Res* 38:2135–2145, 2010.

8. de Mos M, de Bruijn AG, Huygen FJ, et al: The incidence of complex regional pain syndrome: a population-based study. *Pain* 129:12–20, 2007.

9. Dreher T, Hagmann S, Wenz W: Reconstruction of multiplanar deformity of the hindfoot and midfoot with internal fixation techniques. *Foot Ankle Clin* 14:489–531, 2009.

10. Hesdorffer DC, Logroscino G, Benn E, et al: Estimating risk for developing epilepsy: a population-based study in Rochester, Minnesota. *Neurology* 76:23–27, 2011.

11. Monini S, Lazzarino AI, Iacolucci C, et al: Epidemiology of Bell's palsy in an Italian Health District: incidence and case-control study. *Acta Otorhinolaryngol Ital* 30:198, 2010.

12. Dieleman JP, Kerklaan J, Huygen FJ, et al: Incidence rates and treatment of neuropathic pain conditions in the general population. *Pain* 137:681–688, 2008.

13. Adler CH: Strategies for controlling dystonia: overview of therapies that may alleviate symptoms. *Postgrad Med* 108:151–152, 155–156, 159–160, 2000.

14. Poropatich KO, Walker CL, Black RE, et al: Quantifying the association between *Campylobacter* infection and Guillain-Barré syndrome: a systematic review. *J Health Popul Nutr* 28:545–552, 2010.

15. Courtney AM, Treadaway K, Remington G, et al: Multiple sclerosis. *Med Clin North Am* 93:451–476, 2009.

16. Stefanova N, Bücke P, Duerr S: Multiple system atrophy: an update. *Lancet Neurol* 8:1172–1178, 2009.

17. McGrogan A, Sneddon S, de Vries CS: The incidence of myasthenia gravis: a systematic literature review. *Neuroepidemiology* 34:171–183, 2010.

18. de Lau LM, Breteler MM: Epidemiology of Parkinson's disease. *Lancet Neurol* 5:525–535, 2006.

19. Bower JH, Maraganore DM, McDonnell SK, et al: Incidence of progressive supranuclear palsy and multiple system atrophy in Olmsted County, Minnesota, 1976 to 1990. *Neurology* 49:1284–1288, 1997.

20. Canale ST, Beaty JH: Meningomyelocele. In *Campbell's operative orthopaedics*, ed 11, Philadelphia, 2007, Mosby.

21. Jackson AB, Dijkers M, Devivo MJ, et al: A demographic profile of new traumatic spinal cord injuries: change and stability over 30 years. *Arch Phys Med Rehabil* 85:1740–1748, 2004.

22. Ovbiagele B: National sex-specific trends in hospital-based stroke rates. *J Stroke Cerebrovasc Dis* 2010 Aug 17 [Epub ahead of print].

23. Faul M, Xu L, Wald MM, et al: *Traumatic brain injury in the United States: emergency department visits, hospitalizations and deaths 2002–2006*, Atlanta, Ga, 2010, Centers for Disease Control and Prevention, National Center for Injury Prevention and Control.

24. Obermann M: Treatment options in trigeminal neuralgia. *Ther Adv Neurol Disord* 3:107–115, 2010.

25. Howlader N, Noone AM, Krapcho M, et al, editors: *SEER cancer statistics review*, Bethesda, Maryland, 1975–2008, National Cancer Institute. Available at: http://seer.cancer.gov/csr/1975_2008/ (based on November 2010 SEER data submission). Posted on the SEER Web site, 2011.

26. Thakur R, Kent JL, Dworkin RH: Herpes zoster and postherpetic neuralgia. In Ballantyne JC, Fishman SM, Rathmell JP, editors: *Bonica's management of pain*, ed 4, Baltimore, Md, 2010, Lippincott Williams & Wilkins.

27. Fuster JM: Brain systems have a way of reconciling "opposite" views of neural processing; the motor system is no exception. In *Movement control*, Cambridge, 1994, Cambridge University Press, p 139.

# 2 Physical and Electrical Properties of Cells in the Nervous System

Lisa Stehno-Bittel

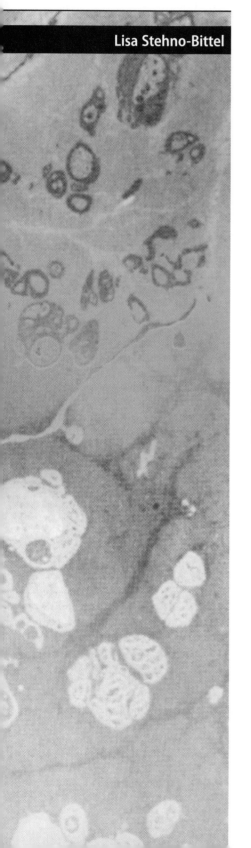

## Chapter Outline

This chapter includes content from a previous contribution to the first and second edition by Anne Burleigh Jacobs, PhD, PT.

I am a 37-year-old female college professor and physical therapist living with multiple sclerosis (MS). Prior to teaching, I was a full-time physical therapist for 6 years, working with neurologically impaired adults in rehabilitation settings. I began teaching physical therapy when I was 29 years old.

When I was 28 years old, I experienced early symptoms of MS. My right arm felt numb for about 3 days. A few weeks after the numbness subsided, I experienced a right foot drop. This progressed over 24 hours, and I was seen in an emergency room. Initial tests included a lumbar puncture and myelogram, evoked potentials, and a CT scan, all of which produced normal results. I continued to have mildly slurred speech and weakness on my right side. These symptoms resolved in about 10 days. I underwent an MRI, which confirmed the diagnosis of MS secondary to the discovery of a lesion in the cortex. About 6 weeks later, I suffered rapid-onset (about 2 hours) symptoms of left-sided weakness, inability to swallow, unclear speech, and sensory deficits on the left side. I experienced Lhermitte's sign* and had (and continue to have) a perfect midline cut (up to but not including the face) in which the right side of my body feels as if it is on fire, every minute of every day.

In the 9 years that I have had MS, I have experienced nine attacks (although none in the past 27 months). Each attack has been different. I have had two that were purely sensory involving both lower limbs, two that were purely autonomic in which I vomited for hours, and one that was a visual field cut only. The others had elements of sensory, motor, visual, and vestibular problems. I have not experienced any bowel or bladder dysfunction.

I have had nearly full return of function following every attack, with the only remaining symptoms being persistent sensory hypersensitivity on my right side (greater in the limbs than in the trunk), mild visual disturbances including hypersensitivity to light and diminished night-driving ability, impaired vibratory sensation, and minor balance deficits. None of the unresolved symptoms has changed my life in a major way. I am active and have only made some minor accommodative changes. I do not suffer from increased levels of fatigue or have difficulty with heat, unlike many people with MS. I consider my condition to be fairly static. I maintain my fitness with aerobic and anaerobic activities.

I have not had any type of therapy except as a participant in research studies. As a regular participant in research studies in the Portland, Oregon, area, I have been involved in a cell-cloning study and a study using the drug Betaseron. I am currently midway through a 2-year study of Avonex, an interferon treatment. Before the Avonex study, I would typically have one attack per year, including during the 2-year period of the Betaseron study, in which I received a placebo. I have not had an attack in 27 months. Part of that time I received Betaseron treatments via subcutaneous injection, and part incorporates the period since I initiated the Avonex interferon study protocol of weekly intramuscular injections. Because the course of MS is unpredictable and the Avonex study is incomplete, conclusions cannot be drawn regarding the effectiveness of the treatment. I also attribute my continued health to other practices, including diet, exercise, stress management, and purpose in my life. I believe all these factors play positive roles in maintaining health and preventing or minimizing the disease state.

—*Lori Avedisian*

*Lhermitte's sign *is characterized by abrupt electric-like shocks traveling down the spine upon flexion of the head. Cross-talk between neurons when the spinal cord moves causes the shock-like sensation. In MS, loss of insulation between neurons in the cervical cord allows the cross-talk. Although Lhermitte's sign frequently occurs in MS, it also occurs with traumatic, radiation, or other injury to the cervical spinal cord.*[1]

**Professor Avedisian's story is typical for relapsing/remitting MS, the most common type of the disease. In relapsing/remitting MS, signs and symptoms appear, then resolve completely. Because the disease randomly attacks cells that provide insulation in the central nervous system, and thus the lesions can occur anywhere in the white matter of the spinal cord or brain, MS can create problems with any neurologic function. Most frequently, MS interferes with somatosensation, vision, movement, and autonomic and cognitive functions. Medications can delay or even prevent new attacks in this type of MS.[2] MS is discussed in greater detail later in this chapter.**

## INTRODUCTION

With an average of 21 billion cerebral cortical neurons and 150,000 kilometers of myelinated (insulated) nerve fibers[3] controlling sensation, movement, and autonomic and mental processes, the human nervous system is incredibly complex. This vast network of cells constantly develops new interactions and modifies output based on input into the system. The functions of the human body require chemical and electrical interactions among neural cells. Sensory information from peripheral receptors is conveyed to the spinal cord and brain, where it is analyzed as perception of the environment. On the basis of this sensory information, a motor command may be issued for coordinated movement of muscles. Chemical and electrical interactions within the brain are also responsible for memory of experiences and movements.

This chapter, which will introduce the basic physical, electrical, and chemical properties of the nervous system, is divided into three sections: The first covers *neurons* (nerve cells), the second describes *glia* (cells that support neurons), and the third covers *stem cells* (precursors to neurons and glial cells).

## STRUCTURE OF NEURONS

Neurons receive information, process it, and generate output (Figure 2-1). The organelles of a neuron include a nucleus, Golgi bodies, mitochondria, lysosomes, and endoplasmic reticulum. The nucleus, Golgi apparatus, and rough endoplasmic reticulum are restricted to the *soma*, or cell body, of the neuron. Other organelles, such as mitochondria and smooth

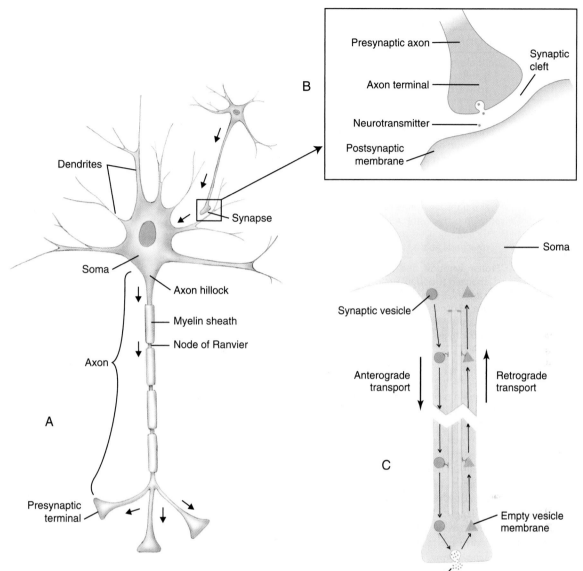

**Fig. 2-1 Parts of a neuron. A,** The cell body (soma), the input units (dendrites), and the output unit (axon) with its presynaptic terminals. The axon hillock and nodes of Ranvier contribute to electrical signaling within the neuron. Also shown is a synapse, where a presynaptic terminal of one neuron communicates with a dendrite of a postsynaptic neuron. Arrows indicate the direction of information transfer. **B,** A synapse, the site of communication between neurons or between a neuron and a muscle or gland. The components of a synapse are the axon terminal of the presynaptic neuron, the synaptic cleft, and the postsynaptic membrane. **C,** Axoplasmic transport. Substances required by the axon are delivered from the soma via anterograde transport. Retrograde transport moves substances from the axon to the soma. The proteins that "walk" the vesicles along the microtubules are shown in red.

endoplasmic reticulum, are distributed throughout the neuron. A plasma membrane surrounds the cell, separating the extracellular environment from its contents. Table 2-1 lists information about each organelle.

Neurons are easily identified under a microscope because of their unique shape. Long protein strands called *microtubules, microfilaments,* and *neurofilaments* make up the cytoskeleton inside the cell and are responsible for maintaining the unique neuronal shape.

## Components of Neurons

A typical neuron has four main components (Figure 2-1, *A*):
- Soma
- Dendrites
- Axon
- Presynaptic terminals

The soma synthesizes a large quantity and variety of proteins used as neurotransmitters. *Dendrites,* branch-like

**TABLE 2-1    FUNCTION OF CELLULAR ORGANELLES**

| Organelle | Function |
|---|---|
| Nucleus | Control center, contains the neuron's genetic material, directs the metabolic activity of the neuron |
| Golgi apparatus | Packages neurotransmitter |
| Mitochondria | Convert nutrients into an energy source the neuron can use (e.g., synthesizes adenosine triphosphate) |
| Endoplasmic reticulum | Rough endoplasmic reticulum (called *Nissl substance* in neurons): synthesizes and transports proteins<br>Smooth endoplasmic reticulum: releases $Ca^{2+}$ for signaling, and synthesizes and transports lipids |
| Ribosomes | Protein synthesis: free ribosomes (not attached to endoplasmic reticulum) synthesize proteins for the neuron's use; ribosomes attached to rough endoplasmic reticulum synthesize neurotransmitters |

extensions that serve as the main input sites for the cell, project from the soma. They are specialized to receive information from other cells.

Another process that extends from the soma is the *axon*, which reaches from the cell body to target cells. The axon is the output unit of the cell, specialized to send information to other neurons, muscle cells, or glands. Most neurons have a single axon that arises from a specialized region of the cell, called the *axon hillock.* Axons vary in length. The shortest axons are less than 1 mm in length,[4] whereas axons that transmit motor information from the spinal cord to the foot may be up to 1 meter long. Axons end in *presynaptic terminals,* or finger-like projections that are the transmitting elements of the neuron. Neurons transmit information about their activity via the release of chemicals called *neurotransmitters* from presynaptic terminals into the *synaptic cleft.* The synaptic cleft, the space between neurons, serves as the site for interneuronal communication (Figure 2-1, *B*). Communication across the synaptic cleft will be described fully in Chapter 3. Briefly, the presynaptic neuron releases a neurotransmitter into the synaptic cleft, the neurotransmitter diffuses from one side of the cleft to the other, and then the neurotransmitter binds to receptors on the postsynaptic neuron, muscle cell, or gland.

◎ *Clinical Pearl*

The basic functions of a neuron are reception, integration, transmission, and transfer of information.

## Axoplasmic Transport

The cellular mechanism that transports substances along an axon is *axoplasmic transport* (Figure 2-1, *C*). Axoplasmic transport occurs in two directions: anterograde and retrograde.

*Anterograde transport* moves neurotransmitters and other substances from the soma down the axon toward the presynaptic terminal. *Retrograde transport* moves substances from the synapse back to the soma. Axonal transport can occur at a wide variety of speeds and appears to slow with the aging process[5] and in several neurodegenerative diseases, including Alzheimer's disease, Huntington's disease, and amyotrophic lateral sclerosis (ALS; both Huntington's disease and ALS disrupt the control of movement).[6]

◎ *Clinical Pearl*

Neurons are electrically active cells with unique specializations, including dendrites, axons, and synaptic terminals. Cellular organelles within neurons make and transport neurotransmitters for cell-to-cell interaction.

## Types of Neurons

Although the four general components of the neuron remain the same—soma, dendrites, axon, and presynaptic terminal—the organization of these parts varies with the type of neuron. Vertebrate neurons are classified into two groups:
- Bipolar cells
- Multipolar cells

### Bipolar Cells

This classification is based on the number of processes that directly arise from the cell body (Figure 2-2, *A*). *Bipolar cells* have two primary processes that extend from the cell body:
- Dendritic root
- Axon

The dendritic root divides into multiple dendritic branches, and the axon projects to form its presynaptic terminals. The retinal bipolar cell in the eye is an example of this type of cell.

*Pseudounipolar cells,* a subclass of bipolar cells, appear to have a single projection from the cell body that divides into two axonal roots. Pseudounipolar cells have two axons and no true dendrites. The most common pseudounipolar cells are sensory neurons, which bring information from the body into the spinal cord (Figure 2-2, *B*). The peripheral axon conducts sensory information from the periphery to the cell body, while the central axon conducts information from the cell body to the spinal cord.

### Multipolar Cells

*Multipolar cells* have multiple dendrites arising from many regions of the cell body and a single axon. They are the most common cells in the vertebrate nervous system, with a variety of different shapes and dendritic organizations. Multipolar cells are specialized to receive and accommodate huge amounts of synaptic input to their dendrites. An example of a multipolar cell is the spinal motor neuron, which projects from the spinal cord to innervate skeletal muscle fibers. A typical spinal motor cell receives approximately 8000 synapses on its dendrites and 2000 synapses on the cell body itself. Multipolar cells in the cerebellum, called *Purkinje cells,* receive as many as 150,000 synapses on their expansive dendritic trees.

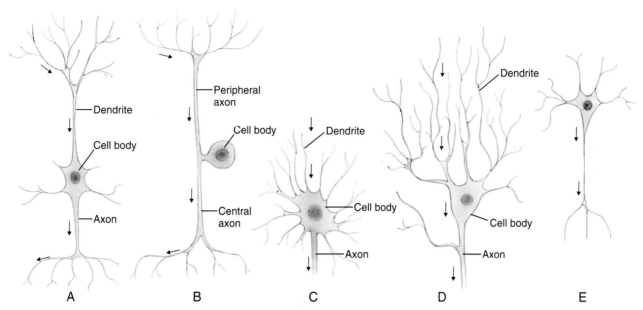

**Fig. 2-2 Morphology of neurons.** Cells are not drawn to the same scale. Arrows indicate the direction of information flow. **A,** Bipolar cell of the retina. **B,** Pseudounipolar cell, a neuron that transmits information from the periphery into the central nervous system. These cells are unique in having two axons: a peripheral axon that conducts signals from the periphery to the cell body, and a central axon that conducts signals into the spinal cord. **C,** Multipolar cell. Multipolar cells have many dendrites and a single axon. The cell represented transmits information from the spinal cord to skeletal muscle. **D,** Multipolar cell typical of cerebellum. **E,** Interneuron. This type of cell is distributed throughout the central nervous system.

## TRANSMISSION OF INFORMATION BY NEURONS

Neurons function by undergoing rapid changes in electrical potential across the cell membrane. An electrical potential across a membrane exists when the distribution of ions creates a difference in electrical charge on each side of the cell membrane. Four types of membrane channels allow ions to flow across the membrane:

- Leak channels
- Modality-gated channels
- Ligand-gated channels
- Voltage-gated channels

### Membrane Channels

All channels serve as openings through the membrane. When channels are open, ions including $Na^+$, $K^+$, $Cl^-$, and $Ca^{2+}$ diffuse through the openings. *Leak channels* allow diffusion of a small number of ions through the membrane at a slow continuous rate. The other channels are termed *gated* because they open in response to a stimulus and close when the stimulus is removed. Leak channels can be important in maintaining osmotic gradients.

*Modality-gated channels,* specific to sensory neurons, open in response to mechanical forces (i.e., stretch, touch, and pressure), temperature changes, or chemicals. *Ligand-gated channels* open in response to a neurotransmitter binding to the surface of a channel receptor on a postsynaptic cell membrane. When open, these channels allow the flow of electrically charged ions between extracellular and intracellular environments of the cell,

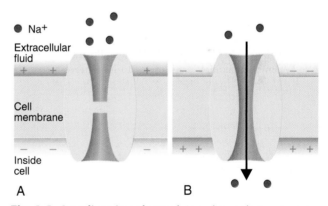

**Fig. 2-3 A sodium ion channel.** Ion channels are proteins that span the cell membrane. **A,** When the ion channel is closed, ions cannot pass through the channel. **B,** Application of voltage to the cell membrane causes the channel to change configuration, allowing ions to pass through the gate. Because the concentration of $Na^+$ is greater outside the neuron than inside, opening the $Na^+$ channels produces an influx of $Na^+$ into the neuron.

resulting in the generation of local potentials. *Voltage-gated channels* open in response to changes in electrical potential across the cell membrane (Figure 2-3). Voltage-gated channels open almost instantaneously and close as quickly. Voltage-gated channels are important in the release of neurotransmitters (see Chapter 3) and the formation of action potentials, as will be discussed later in this chapter.

## Electrical Potentials

A rapid change in electrical charge across the cell membrane transmits information along the length of an axon and elicits the release of chemical transmitters to other neurons or to the electrically excitable membrane of a muscle. The difference in electrical charge, carried by ions, is referred to as the membrane's *electrical potential*. Three types of electrical potentials in neurons are essential for transmission of information:

- Resting membrane potential
- Local potential
- Action potential

## RESTING MEMBRANE POTENTIAL

When a neuron is not transmitting information, the value of the electrical potential across the membrane is called the *resting membrane potential*. The resting membrane potential is a steady-state condition with no net flow of ions across the membrane. Although some individual ions may continually move across the membrane through leak channels, when the cell is at its resting membrane potential, there is no net change in the total distribution of ions across the two sides.

When the neuron is resting, the cell membrane serves as a capacitor, separating the electrical charges on either side of the plasma membrane. An unequal distribution of ionic charge across the membrane is essential for neurons to be excitable. Two forces act on ions to determine their distribution across the plasma membrane: the *concentration gradient* and the *electrical gradient*.

In a simplified example, consider what happens if only sodium chloride (NaCl) ions are outside the cell and membrane channels allow only Na⁺ to pass through, as illustrated in Figure 2-4. When the channels are closed, no ions move across the membrane (Figure 2-4, *A*) and the membrane potential is constant. When the channels open, Na⁺ flows from the region of high Na⁺ concentration to low Na⁺ concentration, in this case from outside to inside the cell (Figure 2-4, *B*). Only a certain amount of Na⁺ enters the cell because an electrical force (electrical gradient) across the membrane is produced as Na⁺ ions move into the cell. Because only Na⁺ passes through the membrane, Cl⁻ remains outside with its negative charge (Figure 2-4, *C*). The negative charge attracts Na⁺ out of the cell, and an electrical-chemical equilibrium is achieved. Once Na⁺ equilibrium is achieved, even if Na⁺ channels remain open, no net movement of Na⁺ ions occurs across the membrane.

These chemical and electrical forces control the movement of ions. Equilibrium of the distribution of a specific ion is reached when there is no net movement of that ion across the membrane. Individual ions continue to diffuse through the membrane, but equal quantities of the ion enter and leave the cell.

In a resting neuron, the membrane potential is the difference in voltage between the interior and exterior of the neuron. Typically, the resting membrane potential of a neuron is approximately −70 mV, indicating that the inside of the neuron contains more negative charges than the outside (Figure 2-5).

In neurons, the proper electrochemical gradient and the resulting membrane resting potential are maintained by the following:

- Negatively charged molecules (anions) trapped inside the neuron, because they are too large to diffuse through the channels
- Passive diffusion of ions through leak channels in the cell membrane
- The Na⁺-K⁺ pump

The Na⁺-K⁺ pump uses energy from adenosine triphosphate (ATP) to actively move ions across the membrane against their electrochemical gradient. The Na⁺-K⁺ pump carries two K⁺ ions

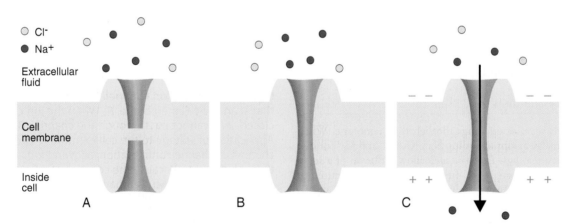

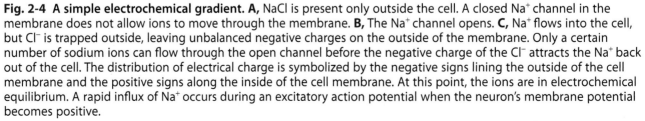

**Fig. 2-4 A simple electrochemical gradient. A,** NaCl is present only outside the cell. A closed Na⁺ channel in the membrane does not allow ions to move through the membrane. **B,** The Na⁺ channel opens. **C,** Na⁺ flows into the cell, but Cl⁻ is trapped outside, leaving unbalanced negative charges on the outside of the membrane. Only a certain number of sodium ions can flow through the open channel before the negative charge of the Cl⁻ attracts the Na⁺ back out of the cell. The distribution of electrical charge is symbolized by the negative signs lining the outside of the cell membrane and the positive signs along the inside of the cell membrane. At this point, the ions are in electrochemical equilibrium. A rapid influx of Na⁺ occurs during an excitatory action potential when the neuron's membrane potential becomes positive.

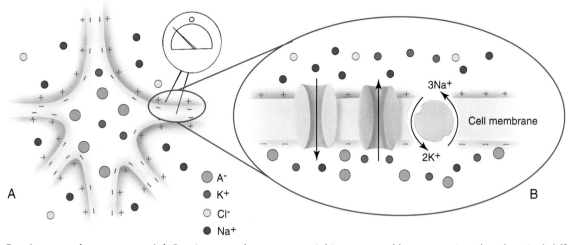

**Fig. 2-5 Resting membrane potential.** Resting membrane potential is measured by comparing the electrical difference between the inside and the outside of the cell membrane. At rest, the inside of the cell membrane is approximately 70 mV more negative than the outside of the cell membrane. *A⁻*, anion. *Inset,* The resting membrane potential is maintained via passive diffusion of ions across the cell membrane and via active transport of Na⁺ and K⁺ by Na⁺-K⁺ pumps. The concentrations of Na⁺ and Cl⁻ are kept higher on the outside compared with the inside of the cell, while the concentration of K⁺ is kept higher on the inside compared with the outside of the cell. High concentrations of unneutralized negative charged molecules (anions) inside the cell also contribute to the negative resting membrane potential.

into the cell and three Na⁺ ions out of the cell with each cycle. Thus, as long as the cell has ATP, an unequal distribution of K⁺ and Na⁺ will exist across the membrane.

> **◎ Clinical Pearl**
>
> The unequal distribution of ions creates an electrical charge across the membrane of the neuron known as the *membrane potential.* The distribution of a specific ion depends on (1) the concentration gradient of the ion, and (2) the electrical forces acting on the ion.

## CHANGES FROM RESTING MEMBRANE POTENTIAL

The resting membrane potential is significant because it prepares the membrane for changes in electrical potential. Sudden changes in membrane potential result from the flow of electrically charged ions through voltage-gated channels spanning the cell membrane (see Figure 2-3). The membrane is *depolarized* when the potential becomes less negative than the resting potential. Depolarization increases the likelihood that the neuron will generate a transmittable electrical signal and is excitatory. Conversely, when the membrane is hyperpolarized, the potential becomes more negative than the resting potential. Hyperpolarization decreases the ability of the neuron to generate an electrical signal, and is inhibitory.

These sudden, brief changes last only milliseconds. Gradual and longer-lasting changes in membrane potential are referred

to as *modulation.* Modulation, which involves small changes in the electrical potential of the membrane that alter the flow of ions across a cell membrane, is discussed in greater detail later in Chapter 3.

> **◎ Clinical Pearl**
>
> Alteration in membrane potential occurs when ion channels open to selectively allow the passage of specific ions.

### Local Potentials and Action Potentials

Electrical potentials within each neuron conduct information in a predictable and consistent direction. Conduction originates with local potentials at the receiving sites of the neuron: in sensory neurons, the receiving sites are the sensory receptors; in motor neurons and interneurons, receiving sites are on the postsynaptic membrane. The initial change in membrane potential is called a *local potential* because it spreads only a short distance along the membrane.

If the change in local potential results in sufficient depolarization of the cell membrane, then an action potential is generated. An action potential is a brief, large depolarization in electrical potential that is repeatedly regenerated along the length of an axon. Regeneration allows an action potential to actively spread long distances, transmitting information down the axon to presynaptic chemical release sites of the presynaptic terminal.

Figure 2-6 illustrates the events that transmit sensory information along an axon, starting with a local potential change

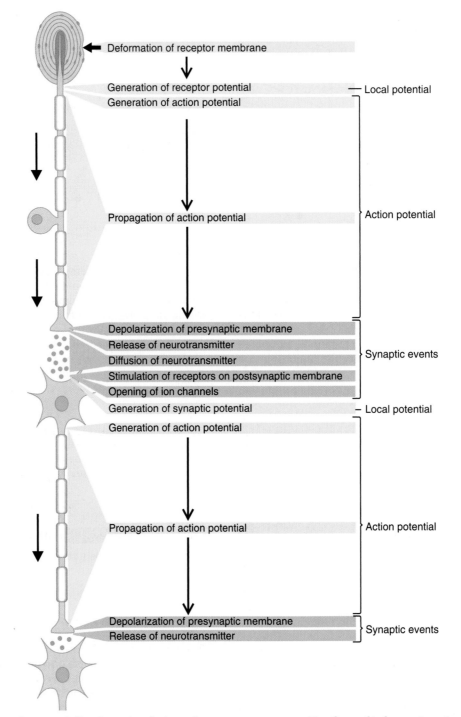

**Fig. 2-6  Sequence of events following stimulation of a sensory receptor.** The flow of information via the interaction among receptor potentials, action potentials, and synaptic potentials is shown. A receptor potential is generated by mechanical change (pressure) of the end-receptor. An action potential propagates along the axon of the sensory neuron from the periphery to the spinal cord. Release of chemical transmitters at the synapse with the second neuron generates a synaptic potential in the second neuron. If sufficient stimuli are received by the second neuron, an action potential is generated in this neuron. The action potential propagates along the axon. When the action potential reaches the axon terminal, a chemical transmitter is released from the terminal. The transmitter then binds to receptors on the membrane of the third neuron, and opening of membrane channels generates synaptic potentials.

**TABLE 2-2**   FEATURES OF LOCAL AND ACTION POTENTIALS

| | Amplitude | Effect on Membrane | Propagation | Ion Channels Responsible for the Change in Membrane Potential |
|---|---|---|---|---|
| Local potential | Small, graded | Either depolarizing or hyperpolarizing | Passive | Sensory neuron end-receptor: modality-gated channel<br>Postsynaptic membrane: ligand-gated channel |
| Action potential | Large, all-or-none | Depolarizing | Active and passive | Voltage-gated channels |

and developing into an action potential. This sequence is as follows:

1. Deformation of a peripheral pressure receptor
2. Change in local membrane potential of the sensory ending
3. Development of an action potential in the sensory axon
4. Release of transmitter from the sensory neuron presynaptic terminal
5. Binding of transmitter to the ligand-gated channel on the postsynaptic cell membrane
6. Activation of synaptic potential in the postsynaptic membrane

The specific features of local and action potentials are summarized in Table 2-2 and are discussed in the following sections.

## Local Potentials

Local potentials are categorized as *receptor potentials* or *synaptic potentials,* depending on whether they are generated at a peripheral receptor of a sensory neuron or at a postsynaptic membrane. These local potentials can spread only passively and so are confined to a small area of the membrane.

Peripheral receptors have modality-gated channels. Local receptor potentials are generated when the peripheral receptors of a sensory neuron are stretched, compressed, deformed, or exposed to thermal or chemical agents. These changes in protein structure of the membrane cause modality-gated ion channels to open, encoding the sensory information into a flow of ionic current. For example, stretching a muscle opens ion channels in the membrane of sensory receptors embedded in the muscle. Opening the channels allows ionic flow, generating receptor potentials that are graded in both amplitude and duration. If the stimulus is larger or longer-lasting, the resulting receptor potential will be larger or longer-lasting. Most receptor potentials are depolarizing (and therefore excitatory). However, sensory stimulation can also cause a receptor potential that is hyperpolarizing (and therefore inhibitory).

Local synaptic potentials are generated in motor neurons and interneurons when they are stimulated by input from other neurons. When a presynaptic neuron releases its neurotransmitter, the chemical travels across the synaptic cleft and interacts with chemical receptor sites on the membrane of the postsynaptic cell (see Figure 2-6). Binding of the neurotransmitter to receptors on the postsynaptic cell opens ligand-gated ion channels, locally changing the resting membrane potential of the cell. The action of the neurotransmitter on the

membrane channel determines whether the synaptic potential will be depolarizing (excitatory) or hyperpolarizing (inhibitory). Similar to receptor potentials, synaptic potentials are graded in both amplitude and duration: if the neurotransmitter is available in larger amounts for a longer time, the resulting synaptic potential will be larger and longer-lasting.

Because local potentials can spread only passively along their receptors or synaptic membranes, they generally travel only 1 to 2 mm, and the amplitude decreases with the distance traveled. The strength of local potentials can be increased and multiple potentials integrated via the processes of temporal and spatial summation (Figure 2-7). *Temporal summation* is the combined effect of a series of small potential changes that occur within milliseconds of each other. *Spatial summation* is the process by which receptor or synaptic potentials generated in different regions of the neuron are added together. Via summation, a sufficient number of potentials occurring within a short period cause significant changes in the membrane potential and promote or inhibit the generation of an action potential. The neuronal membrane integrates depolarizing and hyperpolarizing local potentials that sometimes occur simultaneously. The net change in potential determines what happens to the neuron.

---

**◉ Clinical Pearl**

Neurons undergo rapid changes in the electrical potential of the membrane to conduct electrical signals. Receptor and synaptic potentials are graded in amplitude and duration and conduct local electrical information in the neuron.

---

## Action Potentials

Because receptor and synaptic potentials spread only short distances, another cellular mechanism, the action potential, is essential for rapid movement of information over long distances. An *action potential* is a large depolarizing signal that is actively propagated along an axon by repeated generation of a signal. Because they are actively propagated, action potentials transmit information over longer distances than receptor or synaptic potentials. The meaning of the signal is determined not by the signal itself but by the neural pathway along which

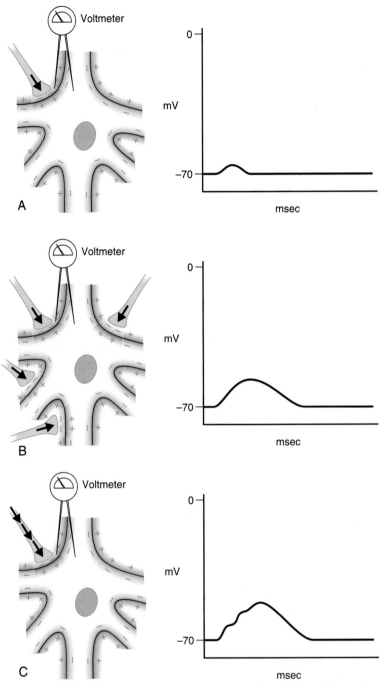

**Fig. 2-7  Integration of local signals. A,** A single weak input to a cell results in only slight depolarization of the membrane. **B,** Spatial summation of several different inputs results in significant depolarization of the membrane. **C,** Temporal summation of several inputs in rapid succession results in significant depolarization of the membrane.

it is conducted. Unlike local input signals, which vary in amplitude, the action potential is *all-or-none*. This means that every time even minimally sufficient stimuli are provided, an action potential will be produced. Stronger stimuli produce action potentials of the same voltage and duration as are produced by minimally sufficient stimuli.

---

### ◎ Clinical Pearl

Initiation or firing of an action potential is similar to striking of a key on a computer keyboard. Regardless of whether the key is struck gently and slowly or rapidly and hard, the letter will be inscribed when the sufficient amount of pressure is achieved. The shape of the letter is not influenced by how hard the key is pressed.

---

In neurons, the generation of action potentials involves a sudden influx of $Na^+$ through voltage-gated channels. Although voltage-gated $Na^+$ channels are generally absent in the region of the receptor terminal and the synaptic membrane, within approximately 1 mm of the input regions is a dense distribution of $Na^+$ channels. In sensory neurons, the region closest to the receptor with a high density of $Na^+$ channels is called the *trigger zone*. In interneurons and motor neurons, the region closest to the synapse with a high density of $Na^+$ channels is called the *axon hillock*. Receptor or synaptic potentials that have passively traveled a short distance toward the trigger zone or axon hillock are both spatially and temporally summated. If summation of local potentials depolarizes the membrane beyond a voltage threshold level, then the opening of many voltage-dependent $Na^+$ channels generates an action potential. If summation does not result in depolarization exceeding the threshold, then there will be no action potential.

The stimulus intensity that is just sufficient to produce an action potential is called the *threshold stimulus intensity*. Typically, a 15 mV depolarization (a change in membrane potential from −70 mV to −55 mV) is sufficient to trigger an action potential. When the voltage across the membrane reaches −55 mV, many voltage-dependent $Na^+$ channels open. $Na^+$ flows rapidly into the cell, propelled by the high extracellular $Na^+$ concentration and attracted by the negative electrical charge inside the membrane. When $K^+$ channels open later, $K^+$ leaves the cell, repelled by the positive electrical charge inside the membrane (created by the influx of $Na^+$) and by the $K^+$ concentration gradient. With $K^+$ movement, the membrane becomes temporarily more polarized than when at rest—essentially a *hyperpolarization*. Figure 2-8 illustrates the change in membrane potential that occurs during an action potential. The peak occurs at about 35 mV, and then the potential quickly drops back toward the resting membrane potential.

In summary, an action potential is produced by a sequence of three events:
1. Rapid depolarization due to opening of the voltage-gated $Na^+$ channels
2. A decrease in $Na^+$ conduction due to closing of the channels
3. Rapid repolarization due to opening of voltage-gated $K^+$ channels

Owing to continued efflux of $K^+$, repolarization is followed by a period of hyperpolarization, during which the membrane potential is even more negative than during resting. When the membrane is hyperpolarized, it is more difficult to initiate a subsequent action potential. During this time, the membrane is said to be *refractory*. The characteristics of the ion channels define the refractory period. Some channels become inactivated immediately after opening for an action potential and require a specific amount of time before they can be activated again for a subsequent action potential. The refractory period can be divided into two distinct states:
- Absolute refractory period
- Relative refractory period

During the *absolute refractory period*, the membrane is unresponsive to stimuli. This state occurs because the $Na^+$ channels responsible for the upstroke of the action potential cannot be reopened for a specific period of time following their closure. The *relative refractory period* occurs during the latter part of the action potential (Figure 2-9). During this period, the membrane potential is returning toward its resting level and may even be hyperpolarized. A stimulus may activate the $Na^+$ channels at this time, but it must be stronger than normal. The refractory period promotes forward propagation of the action potential while preventing its backward flow. If there were no refractory period, the passive flow of ions associated with an action potential could spread both forward and backward along the length of the axon. Although the flow of $K^+$ out of the cell restores the resting membrane potential, the resting levels of ion concentration must be restored over time by the $Na^+$-$K^+$ pump, which actively moves $Na^+$ out of the neuron and $K^+$ into the neuron.

---

### ◎ Clinical Pearl

When the opening of voltage-gated $Na^+$ channels depolarizes the trigger zone or the axon hillock to the threshold level, an action potential is generated. An action potential is an all-or-none electrical response to local depolarization of a membrane. Action potentials are generated in the axon by the influx of $Na^+$ into the neuron, causing depolarization of the membrane; the efflux of $K^+$ then repolarizes the membrane.

---

### Propagation of Action Potentials

Once an action potential has been generated, the change in electrical potential spreads passively along the axon to the adjacent region of the membrane. The impulse is propagated by flipping of the polarity of the electrical signal, like a line of dominoes being knocked down. When depolarization of the adjacent, inactive region reaches threshold, another action potential is generated. This process, the passive spread of depolarization to the adjacent membrane and the generation of new action potentials, is repeated along the entire length of the axon (Figure 2-10). The process is analogous to lighting a trail of gunpowder: once the trail has been lit, the heat generated ignites the adjacent gunpowder and the process propagates down the trail. Propagation of an action potential is dependent

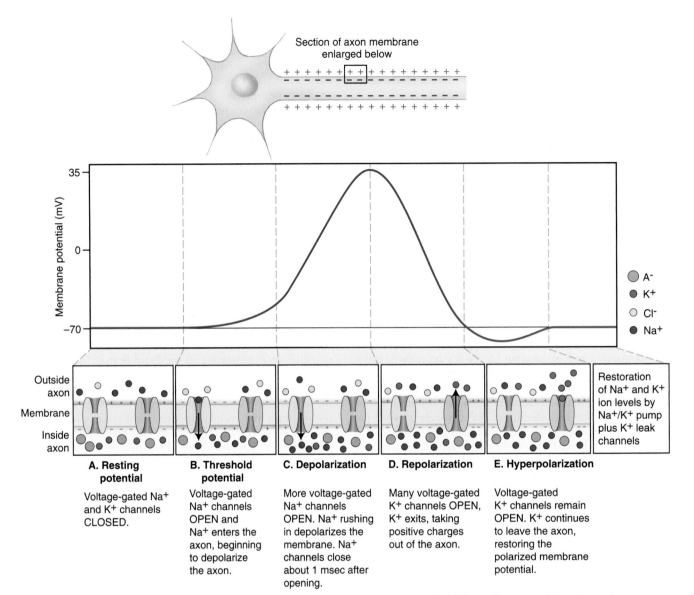

**Fig. 2-8 Action potential. A,** In this example, the resting membrane potential of the cell is −70 mV and membrane channels are closed. **B,** Initiation of the action potential begins with opening of voltage-sensitive Na⁺ channels and rapid influx of Na⁺, causing the cell membrane to become less negative (i.e., depolarized). **C,** The membrane is depolarized. **D,** Closing of Na⁺ channels and opening of K⁺ channels then causes a reversal of membrane potential. **E,** Ultimately, brief hyperpolarization of the membrane results in the potential becoming more negative than the resting potential. Later, the cell membrane returns to resting potential after closure of the membrane channels via the action of the Na⁺-K⁺ pump (not shown).

on both passive properties of the axon and active opening of ion channels distributed along the length of the axon.

Some axons are specialized for faster action potential propagation. These faster-conducting axons have two structural adaptations that improve their passive properties:

• Increased diameter of the axon
• Myelination

The effect of these adaptations on propagation of an electrical signal along an axon is similar to the flow of water through a hose. A wider hose will allow more water through in less time. Similarly, a larger-diameter axon will allow greater current flow, with less time required to change the electrical charge of the adjacent membrane.

**⊚ Clinical Pearl**

Wrapping a leaky hose with tape will prevent water from leaking through the wall of the hose, ensuring that most of the water will travel to the end of the hose. Similarly, myelination prevents the leakage of current across the axon membrane.

Myelination is the presence of a sheath of proteins and fats surrounding an axon. Myelin provides insulation, preventing current flow across the axonal membrane. If ions were allowed to run down their electrochemical gradient during propagation of the action potential, the amplitude of the potential would dissipate as the impulse traveled down the axon. Similarly, when a hose has leaky walls, the flow diminishes as distance from the faucet increases. In an axon, to keep the amplitude of the action potential above threshold, the uneven distribution of ions must be maintained (the membrane

potential cannot be allowed to return to the resting potential). When there is a greater separation of charges across the axon membrane, as provided by myelin, fewer positive ions must be deposited along the inner membrane to depolarize the membrane to a threshold level; therefore, current flow for a shorter period of time can result in membrane depolarization over a greater distance.

Myelination increases the speed of action potential propagation and the distance a current can passively spread. Thicker myelin leads to faster conduction and greater chances for action potential propagation. Myelinated axons have small patches that lack myelin, called *nodes of Ranvier*. These nodes are specialized for active propagation of an action potential by allowing ion flow across the membrane. Nodes of Ranvier are distributed every 1 to 2 mm along the axon and contain high densities of Na⁺ channels and K⁺ channels. An action potential spreads rapidly along a myelinated region, then slows when crossing the high-capacitance, unmyelinated region of the node of Ranvier. High capacitance at the node stores charge, preparing to produce an action potential. As a node becomes depolarized, voltage-gated Na⁺ channels open, generating a new action potential and the spread of ionic current along the axon to the next node (Figure 2-11). Consequently, as the action potential propagates down a myelinated axon, it appears to quickly jump from node to node. This is called *saltatory conduction*. Because Na⁺ channels remain open only a brief time, the generation of a refractory period again plays a critical role in the forward propagation of the action potential by preventing the backward flow of electrical potential. Propagation of the action potential in a myelinated axon requires that a new action potential be generated at each node of Ranvier and passed on down the axon. In this manner, the action potential maintains its size and shape as it travels along the axon.

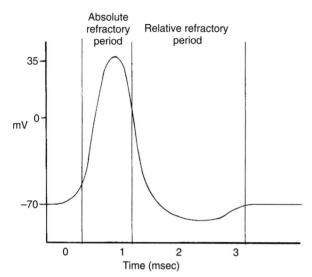

**Fig. 2-9 Refractory periods.** During and immediately following the action potential are two refractory periods. The absolute refractory period corresponds to the time the firing level is reached until repolarization (reversal of potential) is one third complete. The relative refractory period corresponds to the time immediately following the absolute refractory period until the membrane potential returns to the resting level.

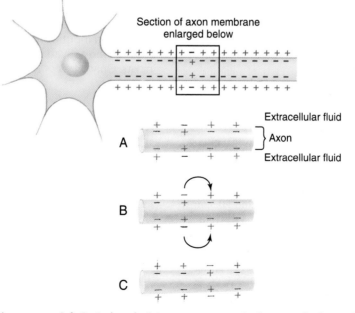

**Fig. 2-10 Propagation of action potential. A,** A depolarizing current passively spreads down the axon, causing the interior of the axon to become more positive than when the membrane is resting. **B,** In the adjacent membrane, when the depolarizing current reaches threshold level, Na⁺ channels open, causing rapid depolarization of the membrane. **C,** An action potential is generated, and the depolarizing current continues to propagate down the axon.

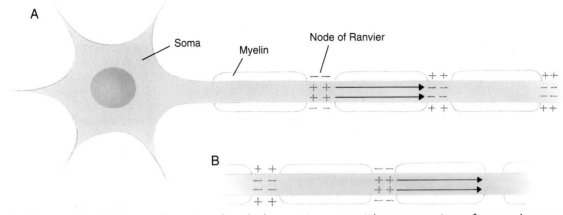

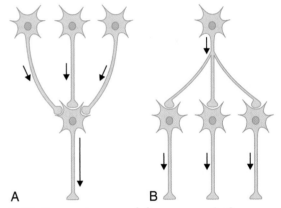

**Fig. 2-11** Saltatory conduction, or the process by which an action potential appears to jump from node to node along an axon. **A,** A depolarizing potential spreads rapidly along the myelinated regions of the axon, then slows when crossing the unmyelinated node of Ranvier. **B,** When an action potential is generated at a node of Ranvier, the depolarizing potential again spreads quickly across myelinated regions, appearing to jump from node to node.

> ◎ **Clinical Pearl**
>
> Action potentials are propagated down the length of an axon via both passive and active membrane properties.

## DIRECTION OF INFORMATION FLOW IN NEURONS

Normally, information within a neuron is transferred in only one direction. Depending on its role in the direction of information transfer, a neuron falls into one of three functional groups:
- Afferent neurons
- Efferent neurons
- Interneurons

*Afferent neurons* carry sensory information from the outer body toward the central nervous system (CNS). *Efferent neurons* relay commands from the CNS to smooth and striated muscles and to glands. *Interneurons,* the largest class of neurons, act throughout the nervous system, processing information locally or conveying information short distances. For example, interneurons in the spinal cord control the activity of local reflex circuits within the spinal cord.

The terms *afferent* and *efferent* can also refer to the direction of information conveyed by a particular group of neurons within the CNS. For example, when thalamocortical neurons convey information from the thalamus to the cerebral cortex, this information is efferent from the thalamus and afferent to the cerebral cortex. Neuronal pathways within the CNS are commonly named by combining the names of efferent (i.e., site of origin) and afferent (i.e., site of termination) regions. For example, corticospinal neurons originate in the cerebral cortex and terminate in the spinal cord.

## INTERACTIONS BETWEEN NEURONS

The specificity and diversity of function within the nervous system can be attributed to neuronal convergence and neuronal

**Fig. 2-12 Convergence and divergence. A,** Convergent input to interneurons and motor neurons in the spinal cord includes afferent input from the musculoskeletal system and input from the brain. **B,** Divergent output includes the activation of several neurons by single inputs. Only a few of the actual connections are shown.

divergence. *Convergence* is the process by which multiple inputs from a variety of cells terminate on a single neuron. *Divergence* is the process whereby a single neuronal axon may have many branches that terminate on a multitude of cells. Via temporal and spatial summation, a sufficient number of convergent inputs occurring within a short period of time cause significant changes in the membrane potential and either promote or inhibit the generation of an action potential.

Through the processes of convergence and divergence (Figure 2-12), a single stimulus may produce a substantial response. An example of convergence is the neural input to sensory association areas in the cerebral cortex, where information from hearing, vision, and touch is integrated. An example of divergence is the signaling of information from a pinprick. The pinprick activates end-receptors of a sensory neuron that transmits information about tissue damage. The message is conveyed to multiple neurons in the spinal cord, eliciting a motor response that moves the body part away from the stimulus, such as flexing the elbow to pull the finger away from the painful stimulus. Other neurons relay information to the brain that leads to conscious awareness of pain.

> ◎ **Clinical Pearl**
>
> Divergence and convergence contribute to the distribution of information throughout the nervous system.

## GLIA: SUPPORTING CELLS

Glial cells form a critical support network for neurons. In early research, glia was thought to be a substance similar to glue, responsible for determining the shape of the nervous system. The term *glia* is derived from the Greek word for glue. Electron microscopy revealed glia as more complex, composed of cells. More recently, studies have shown that glial cells do more than provide the structure for the nervous system; they actually transmit information.[7] Further, glial cells may be actively involved in the pathogenesis of a number of ailments, including the cognitive and memory disorder Alzheimer's disease[8] and the disorders associated with multiple sclerosis (MS).

### Types of Glia

Glial cells are categorized by size and function. Large glial cells are called *macroglia,* and small glial cells are *microglia.*

### Macroglial Cells

*Macroglial cells* are classified into three groups:
* Astrocytes
* Oligodendrocytes
* Schwann cells

*Astrocytes,* star-shaped macroglial cells found throughout the CNS, have a direct role in cell signaling.[9] Astrocytes can be stimulated by signals from adjacent neurons or by mechanical changes (changes in shape or pressure). Stimulated astrocytes spread waves of $Ca^{2+}$ to neighboring astrocytes through openings (called *gap junctions*) from one cell to the next (Figure 2-13). Signaling in gap junctions is bidirectional because $Ca^{2+}$ and other small molecules can diffuse through them in either direction. These $Ca^{2+}$ waves can be regulated by neuronal activity.[10,11] Spontaneous $Ca^{2+}$ waves can also arise from astrocytes without input from other astrocytes or neurons.

Communication between neurons and astrocytes travels in both directions. Stimulation of astrocytes can increase or decrease communication between neurons.[9] Stimulated astrocytes can release glutamate, a gliotransmitter that binds to receptors on the neurons.[12] Even though astrocytes release neurotransmitters, they do not have synapses and do not generate action potentials.

Astrocytes also serve important functions in the maintenance of normal neuronal signaling. They act as scavengers, taking up extra $K^+$ ions in the extracellular environment, removing chemical transmitters from the synaptic cleft between neurons, and cleaning up other debris in the extracellular space. Astrocytes have end-feet that connect neurons and blood capillaries (Figure 2-14), providing a nutritive function for neurons. Specific $Ca^{2+}$ signals in the astrocytes activate $K^+$ efflux that is

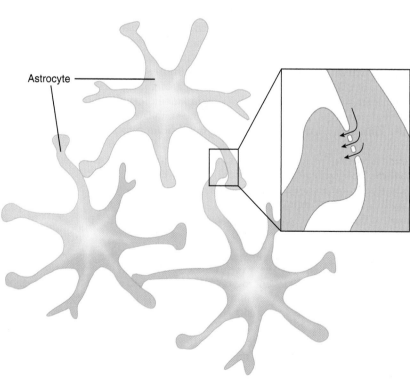

**Fig. 2-13 Communication between astrocytes.** The green color indicates the presence of Ca⁻. The upper astrocyte has been stimulated, producing a wave of Ca⁻ ions passing through the gap junctions from the stimulated cell to the unstimulated cell. The insert shows a magnification of the gap junction.

Astrocyte

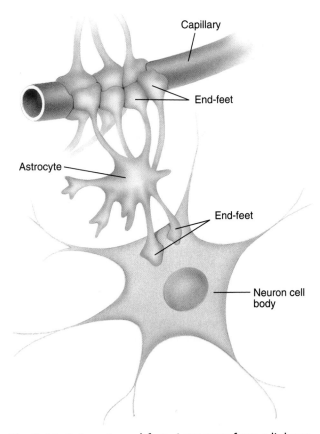

Capillary

End-feet

Astrocyte

End-feet

Neuron cell
body

**Fig. 2-14 Astrocyte end-feet.** Astrocytes form a linkage between neurons and capillaries, providing nutrition.

sensed by the nearby vascular smooth muscle cell, allowing communication with the blood vessel.[13] When neurons are experiencing times of high activity, more blood is needed in the region to nourish the neuron. Astrocytes serve as the liaison, filling the communication gap between the neuron and vascular smooth muscle cells. Astrocytes are also components of the blood-brain barrier, which will be discussed in Chapter 19. Finally, astrocytes play an important role in early CNS development by providing a pathway for migrating neurons. This same pathway may be important during recovery from an injury.

Other types of macroglial cells, *oligodendrocytes* and *Schwann cells,* form a protective covering called the *myelin sheath,* which insulates the axon. The macroglia use lipids and proteins to create this covering. Neurons of the CNS are myelinated by oligodendrocytes, and neurons of the peripheral nervous system are myelinated by Schwann cells. Myelin is an effective insulator for neurons, shielding them from the extracellular environment. Oligodendrocytes in the CNS envelop several axons from different neurons.

In the peripheral nervous system, a Schwann cell may wrap around one axon or several axons (Figure 2-15). An axon is *myelinated* when the sheath wraps completely around the axon, usually several times. If the myelin sheath only partially covers the axon, the neuron is classified as *unmyelinated,* even though the term *partially myelinated* would be more accurate. Schwann cells, the only supporting cells of the peripheral nervous system,

must provide for the peripheral nervous system all of the functions performed by other classes of glial cells in the CNS. When peripheral nerves are inflamed, Schwann cells act as phagocytes—cells that ingest and destroy bacteria and other cells.

### Microglial Cells

*Microglial cells* normally function as phagocytes. Microglia act as the immune system of the CNS and clean the neural environment. In the healthy nervous system, microglia continually sample the extracellular environment for indicators of damage.[14] They are activated during nervous system development and following injury, infection, or disease. During normal development of the nervous system, many neurons that do not make strong synapses die. As neural cells die, whether as part of normal development or from a pathologic process, the dying cells secrete proteins that attract microglia into the site. The microglia clean up and remove debris from the dying cells. This role of the microglia is essential for normal healing following stroke, traumatic brain injury, or CNS infection. However, abnormal microglia activity contributes to neural damage in certain diseases,[15] as explained in the next section.

## NEUROINFLAMMATION: BENEFICIAL AND HARMFUL EFFECTS

*Neuroinflammation* is the response of the CNS to infection, disease, and injury. This response is mediated by reactive microglia and astrocytes (Figure 2-16). Reactive microglia are beneficial when they remove debris, produce neurotrophic factors that support axonal regeneration and remyelination, and mobilize astrocytes to reseal the blood-brain barrier and provide trophic support.[16] However, neuroinflammation can cause death of neurons and oligodendrocytes and inhibit neural regeneration.[16] Thus there is a correlation between abnormal glial activity and neural damage in stroke, Alzheimer's disease, Parkinson's disease, and MS.[15] Microglia and astrocytes can become excessively activated, losing their physiologic buffering function and releasing toxic compounds into the neuronal environment.[16-18] Also, human immunodeficiency virus (HIV), associated with acquired immunodeficiency syndrome (AIDS), can activate microglia and stimulate a cascade of cellular breakdown. Clearly, there is a delicate balance between the normal, protective roles of microglia and the more recently identified destructive roles. As researchers continue to investigate the intricate functions of glial cells, the roles of these cells in health and disease of the nervous system are increasingly appreciated.

○ **Clinical Pearl**

Oligodendrocytes and Schwann cells contribute to the myelination of neurons throughout the nervous system. Astrocytes exchange signals with other astrocytes and with neurons. Astrocytes and microglia contribute to nutritive and cleanup functions throughout the CNS and, when overactive, can contribute to the damage associated with neurodegenerative disease.

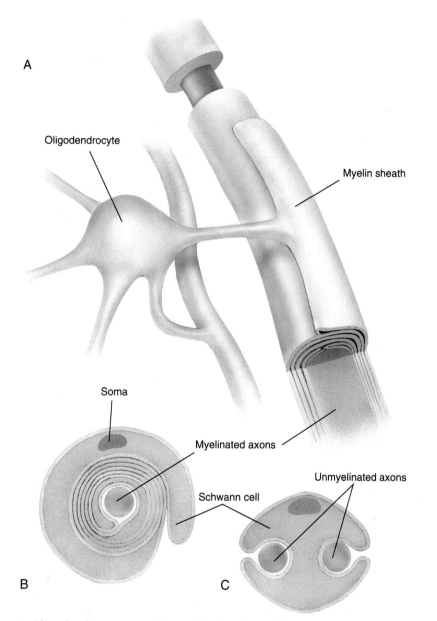

**Fig. 2-15 Myelination. A,** Oligodendrocytes provide myelin sheaths in the central nervous system. **B** and **C,** Schwann cells provide insulation to peripheral axons. Myelinated axons are completely enveloped by Schwann cells. Unmyelinated axons are partially surrounded.

## MYELIN: CLINICAL APPLICATION

Myelin is critical to the conduction of information in the nervous system. As an action potential travels along an axon from a myelinated region to an area where myelin has been damaged, resistance to the electrical signal increases. The propagation of the electrical current slows and eventually may stop before it reaches the next site of conduction. Although most neurons are myelinated, there are types of neurons that normally lack myelin, including the gray matter on the surface of the brain. Why some neurons have myelinated axons and others

are unmyelinated is still a mystery, but clues are starting to come into place. First, there appears to be a size requirement, as short axons are not myelinated. Second, diffusible nerve growth factors appear to regulate the myelination process.[19]

Considerable advances have been made using cell implantation to enhance neuronal regeneration in demyelinating disease and following nerve trauma. For example, in animals, Schwann cell implants result in significant regeneration of axons across a spinal cord transection.[20] This regeneration is often associated with improved motor function and has great potential as a medical intervention for individuals with spinal cord injury.

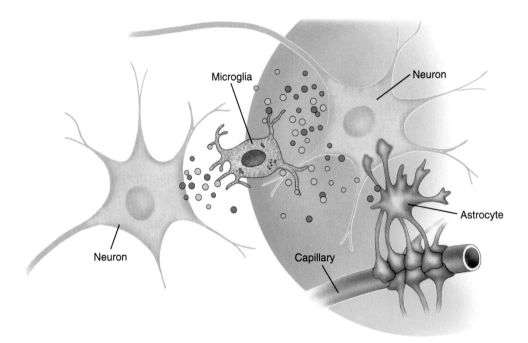

**Fig. 2-16 Neuroinflammatory response after ischemic stroke.** The gray area is ischemic. Reactive microglia release proinflammatory and anti-inflammatory chemicals. Reactive astrocytes stop maintaining neurons and instead release neurotrophic and neurotoxic substances, including glutamate. In the ischemic area, dead neurons further stimulate glial cells. *(Adapted from Ceulemans AG, Zgave T, Kooijman R, et al: The dual role of the neuroinflammatory response after ischemic stroke: Modulatory effects of hypothermia. Journal of Neuroinflammation 7:74, 2010.)*

## Peripheral Nervous System Demyelination

Peripheral neuropathy is any pathologic change involving peripheral nerves. Peripheral neuropathies often involve destruction of the myelin surrounding the largest, most myelinated sensory and motor fibers, resulting in disrupted proprioception (awareness of limb position) and weakness. Autoimmune disorders, metabolic abnormalities, viruses, trauma, and toxic chemicals can cause peripheral demyelination.

*Guillain-Barré syndrome* involves acute inflammation and demyelination of peripheral sensory and motor fibers. The person's immune system generates antibodies that attack Schwann cells. Guillain-Barré syndrome often occurs 2 to 3 weeks after a mild infection. In about two thirds of cases, Guillian-Barré is preceded by an intestinal infection that activates the immune system, causing production of an antibody that mistakenly cross-reacts with the myelin sheath.[21] In severe cases, segmental demyelination is so extreme that axons within the myelin sheath degenerate, resulting in greater residual complications than are seen in people whose axons remain intact (Figure 2-17).

Signs and symptoms of the syndrome include decreased sensation and skeletal muscle paralysis (Pathology 2-1).[22-24] Cranial nerves of the face may be affected, causing difficulty with chewing, swallowing, speaking, and facial expressions. Pain is prominent in some cases. Patients most often report deep aching pain or hypersensitivity to touch. Typically, signs and symptoms have rapid onset followed by a plateau and then gradual recovery. In most cases, a person affected by Guillain-Barré syndrome will experience complete recovery. In severe cases, the nerves of the autonomic nervous system and the

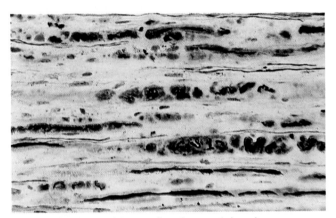

**Fig. 2-17** A nerve biopsy showing peripheral demyelination and axon degeneration, which occur in severe Guillain-Barré syndrome. *(Courtesy Dr. Melvin J. Ball.)*

respiratory system become affected, causing changes in cardiac and respiratory function. Three percent of those with Guillain-Barré syndrome die of cardiac or respiratory failure.

Medical treatment may include *plasmapheresis* and *intravenous immunoglobulin therapy.* Plasmapheresis is the process of filtering the blood plasma to remove the circulating antibodies responsible for attacking the Schwann cells. *Intravenous immunoglobulin therapy* neutralizes specific antibodies and decreases inflammation.[25] Occupational therapy is directed at activities of daily living, including self-care. Physical therapy initially entails stretching and range-of-motion exercises during the

| PATHOLOGY 2-1 | GUILLAIN-BARRÉ SYNDROME |
|---|---|
| Pathology | Demyelination |
| Etiology | Autoimmune |
| Speed of onset | Acute, subacute, or chronic |
| Signs and symptoms | Weakness is typically greater than sensory loss; may have pain or hypersensitivity to touch |
| Consciousness | Normal |
| Cognition, language, and memory | Normal |
| Sensory | Abnormal sensations (tingling, burning); pain |
| Autonomic | Blood pressure fluctuation, irregular cardiac rhythms |
| Motor | Paresis or paralysis; may include respiratory muscles |
| Cranial nerves | Motor cranial nerves most affected (eye and facial movements, chewing, swallowing) |
| Region affected | Peripheral nervous system |
| Demographics | Affects all ages, no gender preference |
| Incidence | 1.3 per 100,000 people per year[23] |
| Lifetime prevalence | 0.2 per 1000[24] |
| Prognosis | Progressively worse for 2–3 weeks, then gradual improvement; 3% mortality rate; 25% require artificial ventilation owing to involvement of respiratory muscles; 20% have permanent severe deficits in ambulation or require ventilator assistance a year post hospital discharge.[25] Complete functional recovery occurs in 75% of patients |

acute phase of the disorder. In the recovery phase, physical therapy is directed toward strengthening and the return of functional mobility. When voluntary movement is present, exercise should be gentle to avoid overwork damage in partially denervated muscles, because exercise of partially denervated muscles interferes with axonal regrowth.[26]

> ### ◎ Clinical Pearl
>
> Destruction of Schwann cells impedes conduction of electrical signals along sensory and motor pathways of the peripheral nervous system.

## Central Nervous System Demyelination

CNS demyelination involves damage to the myelin sheaths in the brain and spinal cord. Multiple sclerosis (MS) occurs when the immune system produces antibodies that attack oligodendrocytes.[27] Destruction of the oligodendrocytes in MS produces patches of demyelination, called *plaques,* in the white matter of the CNS (Figure 2-18). Similar to demyelination of peripheral neurons, demyelination of CNS neurons causes slowed or blocked transmission of signals.[28]

Signs and symptoms of MS include weakness, lack of coordination, impaired vision, double vision, impaired sensation, and slurred speech (Pathology 2-2).[29-31] In addition, disruption of memory and emotions may occur. Diagnosis is difficult because MS usually manifests with one sign that may completely resolve. For example, a person might report double vision, caused by edema or inflammation of cranial nerves that aim the eyes, and then may not experience any signs for months.

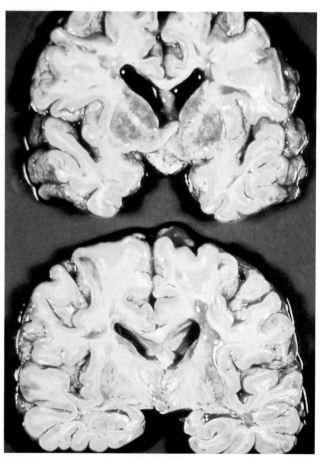

**Fig. 2-18** A coronal section of the cerebrum showing central demyelination. Abnormal areas in the white matter are plaques characteristic of multiple sclerosis. *(Courtesy Dr. Melvin J. Ball.)*

## PATHOLOGY 2-2 MULTIPLE SCLEROSIS

| | |
|---|---|
| Pathology | Demyelination |
| Etiology | Autoimmune, due to a combination of genetic susceptibility with inadequate vitamin D levels and inadequate sunlight exposure or other factors, including Epstein-Barr virus exposure |
| Speed of onset | Can be acute, subacute, or chronic |
| Time course | Exacerbations and remissions |
| Signs and symptoms | |
| Consciousness | Normal |
| Cognition, language, and memory | Infrequently affects cognition and/or memory |
| Sensory | Tingling, numbness, pins and needles |
| Autonomic | Bladder disorders, sexual impotence in men, genital anesthesia in women |
| Motor | Weakness, incoordination, reflex changes |
| Cranial nerves | Partial blindness in one eye, double vision, dim vision, eye movement disorders |
| Region affected | Central nervous system |
| Demographics | Typical age at onset is 20–40 years; affects three times as many women as men |
| Incidence | 100 per 100,000 people per year[1] |
| Lifetime prevalence | 1 per 1000[30] |
| Prognosis | Variable course; very rarely fatal; most people with MS live a near normal life span. Within 10 years after diagnosis, approximately half of people use a cane while walking and 15% use a wheelchair[1] |

Neurologic signs that completely resolve, including this temporary double vision, disappear when swelling and inflammation subside. Diagnosis has improved with the use of imaging techniques and other tests, leading to earlier and more accurate diagnoses. Demyelination and axonal transection produce relatively permanent impairments associated with the progressive stage.[32]

MS onset most commonly occurs between the ages of 20 and 40 years, and women are three times more frequently affected than men. There are four types of MS, all named according to the course of disease progression. *Relapsing/remitting MS* begins with alternating relapses and remissions. During relapses, new signs and symptoms appear and old signs/symptoms recur or worsen. Each relapse is followed by remission, when the person fully or partially recovers from the deficits acquired during the relapse. Relapsing/remitting is the initial disease course in 85% of cases. Without treatment, most people with relapsing/remitting MS transition to *secondary progressive MS*, distinguished by a continuous neurologic decline with fewer or no relapses. The course in *primary progressive MS* is a steady functional decline from time of onset with predominantly spinal cord symptoms; this course occurs in 10% of cases. *Progressive relapsing MS* begins with a steady functional decline with superimposed relapses and partial remissions; function never fully recovers during the remissions. Progressive relapsing MS is the course in 5% of cases.[1]

For quite some time, scientists have looked for the environmental factors that, along with genetics, increase a person's risk for developing MS. When genetically predisposed people are exposed to the Epstein-Barr virus later in life, the risk of MS appears to be increased.[33] But the Epstein-Barr/MS connection is not nearly as strong as the link between MS and inadequate sunlight exposure.[34,35] These conclusions were largely based on population studies that showed a higher incidence of MS in countries at latitudes with less sunlight.[36] Less sunlight reduces vitamin D levels, because vitamin D is manufactured in the skin when exposed to sunlight. Because of much greater global mobility and wider use of sunscreen, the correlation between distance to the equator and MS prevalence has not held up over time. However, vitamin D insufficiency as a risk factor for MS is supported by a significant number of publications.[36] One theory for the molecular mechanism involves the activation of vitamin D receptors on immune regulatory cells. Once these receptors are activated by vitamin D, they decrease the immune activity, potentially decreasing the likelihood of developing an autoimmune disease like MS.[37]

MS has always affected women more than men, but over time, epidemiology studies have shown a significant increase in the percentage of women diagnosed with MS compared with men.[37] Many factors, including obesity, later childbirth, and better health care for women leading to better diagnosis, must be explored to understand the disproportionate increase in female diagnoses. One possibility is a direct effect of XX chromosomes on immune function, which may lead to an increased likelihood that a woman's immune system will become overactive.[38] Related research has shown that vitamin D appears to have a stronger immunomodulatory effect in women than in men.[39]

Physical and occupational therapists work to maintain or improve function where possible. Patients are encouraged to avoid high temperatures and excessive exertion, because increases in body temperature are believed to interfere with the activity of membrane proteins in axons, further disabling action potential conduction. Adequate vitamin $D_3$, stress management, regular exercise, and proper medical management may slow disease progression.[40] Fortunately, medical treatment includes a variety of new drugs, some acting on the immune system, that are making major improvements in patients' quality of life.[2]

> ◎ *Clinical Pearl*
>
> Destruction of oligodendrocytes impedes conduction of electrical signals along pathways of the CNS.

## NEURAL STEM CELLS

The nervous system, unlike many other tissues, has a limited ability to repair itself following injury. Mature neurons cannot reproduce. However, in the past decade, neural stem cells have been discovered in both developing and adult brains. These cells are immature and undifferentiated, the precursors to both neurons and glial cells. Through maturation and differentiation, stem cells can give rise to different types of cells in the CNS.[41] Growth factors have been shown to have an effect on stem cell proliferation.[42] Experimentally, adult neural cells can be derived from these primitive cells. The characteristics of neural stem cells include the ability to:

- Self-renew
- Differentiate into most types of neurons and glial cells
- Populate developing and degenerating regions of the CNS

Two areas of the adult brain produce most of the new neurons: part of the hippocampus, and the cells that line the lateral ventricle wall. Cells from both areas constantly produce new neurons that are important in creating neuronal networks in the brain.[43] Neural stem cells in the healthy mature brain are involved in forming memories and learning new tasks.[44] In addition, there is a great deal of excitement concerning the possible role of stem cells as brain cell implants for rehabilitation after injury or disease. Stem cell transplants in patients with the motor neuron disease ALS, a disease currently without effective treatments, have had conflicting results.[45]

Neurons survive and proliferate after implantation only if they, like stem cells, are immature.[46] The ability of stem cells to differentiate in the brain and make connections with existing neurons has been verified. This ability is greatest in the young, even fetal, brain, but it can also occur in adult animal brains, leading to the possibility of therapies for individuals with degenerative disease or brain injury. One barrier to the use of neuronal stem cells as therapeutic tools will be the difficulty in obtaining them from the brain. Umbilical cord and bone marrow can serve as sources of neural stem cells.[47] Other forms of neurogenesis (creation of new neurons) are being explored. For example, adult fibroblast cells, which are plentiful in the body, can be reprogrammed to form neurons by exposing them to a cocktail of growth factors and other molecules.[48] This process circumvents any ethical conflict because no embryonic tissue is required for the conversion.

Other possibilities for stem cell therapy include the use of neuronal stem cells following spinal cord injury. Embryonic stem cell–derived oligodendrocytes have been used to treat spinal cord injuries in animals. Initial approval for clinical trials using these cells was granted by the Food and Drug Administration, but subsequently studies were put on hold because the early trial showed a higher rate of epithelial cysts in patients receiving stem cells.[49] Stem cell researchers and transplant surgeons who place the cellular grafts in the brain or spinal cord have almost entirely ignored the ability of the nervous system to adapt to stresses and new learning opportunities. The mixed results obtained following stem cell transplantation may be due to lack of controlled rehabilitation therapy after the transplant to stimulate the newly transplanted cells for optimal outcomes.[50] Future rehabilitation may consist of evidence-based therapies to help cellular transplants make new connections in the brain, spinal cord, or peripheral neurons with the potential to return full function to the patient.

## SUMMARY

All nervous system activity relies on the complex physical and electrical properties of cells. Diverse, adaptable, and versatile, these cells affect both normal and abnormal activity. Although physical and occupational therapists work with patients' entire bodies, the basis for rehabilitation lies at the cellular level. A thorough understanding of the roles of these cells—and their contributions to movement, activity, and disease—allows a therapist to more effectively design treatment interventions.

## CLINICAL NOTES

### Case 1

I.D., a 19-year-old man, suffered severe flu symptoms, requiring him to stay home from work for 2 days. Four days after his return to work, I.D. noted tingling and numbness in his fingers. By the end of the day, he noticed his hand movements were clumsy. The following day, I.D. returned to work. Midday he was unable to stand and could not use his hands. At the hospital, he experienced respiratory weakness and was placed on a ventilator. He had nearly total paralysis of voluntary muscles, including facial and swallowing muscles. He was unable to close his eyes and required tube feeding. Nerve conduction studies for both motor and sensory pathways were conducted. (To test peripheral sensory nerve pathways, an electrical stimulus is given to the skin at a distal point over a nerve and is recorded with surface electrodes at a more proximal point over the same nerve. The time required to transmit the signal between the two points indicates the conduction velocity. Peripheral

*Continued*

## CLINICAL NOTES—cont'd

motor conduction studies are similar, except that the electrical stimulus is given proximally over the nerve and is recorded from the skin over an associated muscle.) For I.D., studies indicated that peripheral sensory and motor conduction times were significantly prolonged bilaterally.

I.D. had suffered peripheral nerve demyelination, presumably due to an autoimmune response to viral infection. With loss of myelin, nerve conduction was severely impaired. I.D. had sensory loss and muscular weakness that significantly impaired his ability to move. Occupational therapy trained I.D. to use sip-and-puff switches to control an electric wheelchair, prescribed durable medical equipment, and instructed caregivers on skin care and positioning in the wheelchair and bed and, later, on activities of daily living training. Physical therapy included postural drainage positions for lung hygiene, increasing tolerance to the upright position, range-of-motion exercises, breathing exercises, low-load low-repetition gradual strengthening exercises, and, later, functional mobility training.

### Questions

1. The disease was confirmed to involve the peripheral nervous system. Did the loss of myelin involve oligodendrocytes or Schwann cells?
2. How does loss of myelin along peripheral sensory fibers affect the propagation of action potentials in the affected axons?
3. Would loss of myelin in sensory neuron fibers impair the generation of local receptor potentials or the propagation of action potentials?

### Case 2

J.R. is a 27-year-old woman with MS who was admitted to the hospital twice in the past year with complaints of bilateral lower extremity weakness and blurred vision. Upon examination, she exhibited about 30% of normal muscle strength in the left lower extremity and about 50% of normal strength in the right lower extremity. She exhibited mild left foot drop during the swing phase of gait and slight knee hyperextension during the stance phase. At the hospital, visual evoked potentials were evaluated to assess nerve conduction velocity along the visual tracts. Evoked potentials are extracted from an electroencephalogram (EEG) recorded during repetitive presentation of a flash of light. The time from the stimulus to the appearance of the potential on the EEG indicates the central conduction time. For J.R., decreased visual sensory conduction times were determined. J.R. was referred to physical therapy for strengthening exercises and gait training with an ankle-foot orthosis. The physician's orders specified low-repetition exercises and avoidance of physical overexertion.

### Questions

1. Delayed conduction times for the evoked potentials suggest a problem with sensory conduction within the central nervous system. What nervous system abnormality can explain delayed sensory nerve conduction times?
2. What mechanism related to generation of the action potential may be directly impaired by increases in body temperature associated with overexertion?

## REVIEW QUESTIONS

1. Do dendritic projections function as input units or output units for a neuron?
2. Name one example of a pseudounipolar cell. Why is it called *pseudounipolar*?
3. What is the specialized function of multipolar cells?
4. What are the three major ions that contribute to the electrical potential of a cell membrane in its resting state?
5. Define the terms *depolarization* and *hyperpolarization* with respect to resting membrane potential.
6. If a membrane channel opens when it is bound by a neurotransmitter, what type of membrane channel is it?
7. What does the term *graded* mean with respect to the generation of local receptor and synaptic potentials?
8. How is the resting membrane potential maintained?
9. Why is hyperpolarization of a neuronal membrane considered inhibitory?
10. Peripheral receptors have what types of ion channels?
11. List two types of local potential summation that can result in depolarization of a membrane to the threshold level.
12. The generation of an action potential requires the influx of what ion? Is the influx mediated by a voltage-gated channel?
13. Do large-diameter or small-diameter axons promote faster conduction velocity of an action potential?
14. What are the unique features of the nodes of Ranvier that promote generation of an action potential?
15. Names of tracts in the central nervous system identify the origin and termination of the tract. Where does the spinothalamic tract originate? Where does this tract terminate?
16. Are networks composed of interneuronal convergence and divergence found throughout the central nervous system or only in the spinal cord?
17. List two ways in which glial cells differ from nerve cells.

**18.** What are the four functions of astrocytes in the mature nervous system?
**19.** To what critical function do both oligodendrocytes and Schwann cells contribute in the nervous system?
**20.** What are the differences between oligodendrocytes and Schwann cells?

**21.** Compare and contrast Guillain-Barré syndrome and multiple sclerosis.
**22.** How could naturally occurring stem cells in the brain assist recovery after brain injury?

## References

1. Courtney AM, Treadaway K, Remington G, et al: Multiple sclerosis. *Med Clin North Am* 93:451–476, 2009.
2. Bates D: Treatment effects of immunomodulatory therapies at different stages of multiple sclerosis in short-term trials. *Neurology* 76:S14–S25, 2011.
3. Pakkenberg B, Pelvig D, Marner L, et al: Aging and the human neocortex. *Exp Gerontol* 38:95–99, 2003.
4. Purves D, Augustine GJ, Fitzpatrick D, et al: Neural signaling. In *Neuroscience*, ed 2, Sunderland, Mass, 2001, Sinauer Associates.
5. Li W, Hoffman PN, Stirling W, et al: Axonal transport of human alpha-synuclein slows with aging but is not affected by familial Parkinson's disease-linked mutations. *J Neurochem* 88:401–410, 2004.
6. Morfini GA, Burns M, Binder LI, et al: Axonal transport defects in neurodegenerative diseases. *J Neurosci* 29:12776–12786, 2009.
7. Parpura V, Haydon PG: Physiological astrocytic calcium levels stimulate glutamate release to modulate adjacent neurons. *Proc Natl Acad Sci U S A* 97:8629–8634, 2000.
8. Kadir A, Marutle A, Gonzalez D, et al: Positron emission tomography imaging and clinical progression in relation to molecular pathology in the first Pittsburgh Compound B positron emission tomography patient with Alzheimer's disease. *Brain* 134:301–317, 2011.
9. Araque A, Navarrete M: Glial cells in neuronal network function. *Philos Trans R Soc Lond B Biol Sci* 365:2375–2381, 2010.
10. Halassa MM, Haydon PG: Integrated brain circuits, astrocytic networks modulate neuronal activity and behavior. *Annu Rev Physiol* 72:335–355, 2010.
11. Rouach N, Glowinski J, Giaume C: Activity-dependent neuronal control of gap-junctional communication in astrocytes. *J Cell Biol* 149:1513–1526, 2000.
12. Gourine AV, Kasparov S: Astrocytes as brain interoceptors. *Exp Physiol* 96:411–416, 2011.
13. Dunn KM, Nelson MT: Potassium channels and neurovascular signaling. *Circulation* 4:608–616, 2010.
14. Graeber MB: Changing face of microglia. *Science* 330:783–788, 2010.
15. Amor S, Puentes F, Baker D, van der Valk P: Inflammation in neurodegenerative disease. *Immunology* 129:154–169, 2010.
16. Wee Yong V: Inflammation in neurological disorders: a help or a hindrance? *Neuroscientist* 16:408–420, 2010.
17. Ceulemans AG, Zgavc T, Kooijman R, et al: The dual role of the neuroinflammatory response after ischemic stroke: modulatory effects of hypothermia. *J Neuroinflamm* 7:74, 2010.
18. Philips T, Robberecht W: Neuroinflammation in amyotrophic lateral sclerosis: role of glial activation in motor neuron disease. *Lancet Neurol* 10:253–263, 2011.
19. Sherman DL, Brophy PJ: Mechanisms of axon ensheathment and myelin growth. *Nat Rev Neurosci* 6:683–690, 2005.
20. Deng LX, Hu J, Liu N, et al: GDNF modifies reactive astrogliosis allowing robust axonal regeneration through Schwann cell-seeded guidance channels after spinal cord injury. *Exp Neurol* 229:238–250, 2011.
21. Kuwabara S: Guillain-Barré syndrome. *Curr Neurol Neurosci Rep* 7:57–62, 2007.
22. Poropatich KO, Walker CL, Black RE, et al: Quantifying the association between *Campylobacter* infection and Guillain-Barré syndrome: a systematic review. *J Health Popul Nutr* 28:545–552, 2010.
23. MacDonald BK, Cockerell OC, Sander JW, et al: The incidence and lifetime prevalence of neurological disorders in a prospective community-based study in the UK (see comments). *Brain* 123:665–676, 2000.
24. Khan F, Amatya B, Ng L: Use of the International Classification of Functioning, Disability and Health to describe patient-reported disability: a comparison of Guillain Barré syndrome with multiple sclerosis in a community cohort. *J Rehabil Med* 42(8):708–714, 2010.
25. Kuwabara S: Guillain-Barré syndrome: epidemiology, pathophysiology and management. *Drugs* 64:597–610, 2004.
26. Tam SL, Gordon T: Neuromuscular activity impairs axonal sprouting in partially denervated muscles by inhibiting bridge formation of perisynaptic Schwann cells. *J Neurobiol* 57:221–234, 2003.
27. Tzakos AG, Troganis A, Theorou V, et al: Structure and function of the myelin proteins: current status and perspectives in relation to multiple sclerosis. *Curr Med Chem* 12:1569–1587, 2005.
28. Martino G, Furlan R, Brambilla E, et al: Cytokines and immunity in multiple sclerosis: the dual signal hypothesis. *J Neuroimmunol* 109(1):3–9, 2000.
29. Kumar V, Abbas AK, Fausto N, et al: *Robbins and Cotran pathologic basis of disease, professional edition*, ed 8, Philadelphia, 2009, Elsevier Saunders.
30. Kaufman M, Moyer D, Norton J: The significant change for the Timed 25-Foot Walk in the Multiple Sclerosis Functional Composite. *Mult Scler* 6:286–290, 2000.
31. Vleugels L, Lafosse C, van Nunen A, et al: Visuoperceptual impairment in multiple sclerosis patients diagnosed with neuropsychological tasks. *Mult Scler* 6:241–254, 2000.
32. Motl RW, McAuley E: Association between change in physical activity and short-term disability progression in multiple sclerosis. *J Rehabil Med* 43:305–310, 2011.
33. Ascherio A, Munger KL: Epstein-Barr virus infection and multiple sclerosis: a review. *J Neuroimmune Pharmacol* 5:271–277, 2010.
34. Goodin DS: The causal cascade to multiple sclerosis: a model for MS pathogenesis. *PLoS One* 4:e4565, 2009.
35. Becklund BR, Severson KS, Vang SV, et al: UV radiation suppresses experimental autoimmune encephalomyelitis independent of vitamin D production. *Proc Natl Acad Sci U S A* 107:6418–6423, 2010.
36. Sloka S, Silva C, Pryse-Phillips W, et al: A quantitative analysis of suspected environmental causes of MS. *Can J Neurol Sci* 38:98–105, 2011.
37. Sellner J, Kraus J, Awad A, et al: The increasing incidence and prevalence of female multiple sclerosis—a critical analysis of potential environmental factors. *Autoimmun Rev* 10:495–502, 2011.
38. Smith-Bouvier DL, Divekar AA, Sasidhar M, et al: A role for sex chromosome complement in the female bias in autoimmune disease. *J Exp Med* 205:1099–1108, 2008.

39. Correale J, Ysrraelit MC, Gaitan MI: Gender differences in 1,25-dihydroxyvitamin D3 immunomodulatory effects in multiple sclerosis patients and healthy subjects. *J Immunol* 185:4948–4958, 2010.

40. Jelinek GA, Hassed CS: Managing multiple sclerosis in primary care: are we forgetting something? *Qual Prim Care* 17:55–61, 2009.

41. Lynch WP, Portis JL: Neural stem cells as tools for understanding retroviral neuropathogenesis. *Virology* 271:227–233, 2000.

42. Gage FH: Mammalian neural stem cells. *Science* 287:1433–1438, 2000.

43. Landgren H, Curtis MA: Locating and labeling neural stem cells in the brain. *J Cell Physiol* 226:1–7, 2011.

44. Deng W, Aimorne JB, Gage FH: New neurons and new memories: how does adult hippocampal neurogenesis affect learning and memory? *Nat Rev Neurosci* 11:339–350, 2010.

45. Silani V, Calzarossa C, Cova L, et al: Stem cells in amyotrophic lateral sclerosis: motor neuron protection or replacement? *CNS Neurol Disord Drug Targets* 9:314–324, 2010.

46. Bjorklund A, Lindvall O: Cell replacement therapies for central nervous system disorders. *Nat Neurosci* 3:537–544, 2000.

47. Venkataramana NK, Kumar SK, Balaraju S, et al: Open-labeled study of unilateral autologous bone-marrow-derived mesenchymal stem cell transplantation in Parkinson's disease. *Transl Res* 155:62–70, 2010.

48. Vierbuchen T, Ostermeier A, Pang ZP, et al: Direct conversion of fibroblasts to functional neurons by defined factors. *Nature* 463:10–31, 2010.

49. Schwarz SC, Schwarz J: Translation of stem cell therapy for neurological diseases. *Transl Res* 156:155–160, 2010.

50. Dobrossy M, Busse M, Piroth T, et al: Neurorehabilitation with neural transplantation. *Neurorehabil Neural Repair* 24:692–701, 2010.

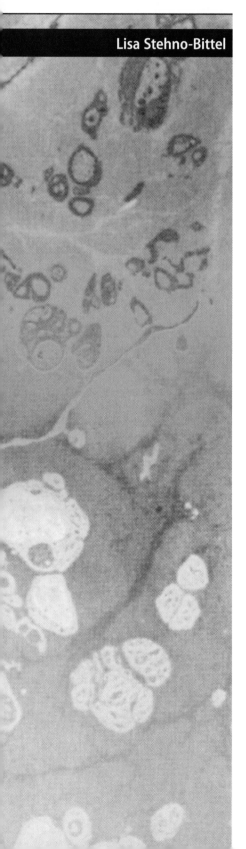

# 3

# Synapses and Synaptic Transmission

Lisa Stehno-Bittel

## Chapter Outline

This chapter includes content from a previous contribution to the first and second edition by Anne Burleigh Jacobs, PhD, PT.

When I was young, I found the story of *Mutiny on the Bounty* fascinating. I thought *mutiny* sounded like a word I should have in my vocabulary. Little did I know I would one day use the word in the context of my own body. Today, my immune system wages a mutiny of sorts: I have myasthenia gravis (MG).

My disease first became apparent a year ago, when I was a 28-year-old college student completing the prerequisites for a graduate program in physical therapy. My vision started behaving strangely. I experienced dizziness and disorientation when I tried to scan from one point to another. It was as though one eye couldn't keep up with the other. I visited my ophthalmologist, who suggested everything from a brain tumor to multiple sclerosis. After a battery of tests, including an MRI, all of his theories had been eliminated. Fortunately, I was then referred to a neuro-ophthalmologist, who knew what I had before he even examined me. He gave me a Tensilon test, which was positive, and officially diagnosed MG, which is a disease that affects muscle receptors, interfering with muscle contraction.

My life has changed significantly over the last year. I am lucky, however, because the disease only affects my eyes at this point. I experience double vision much of the time, and I have difficulty keeping my eyelids open. I have learned that I depended on my eyes in ways I had never realized. I most notice the absence of depth perception, caused by weakness of the muscles that should normally align my eyes.

After quick deterioration at the onset of the disease, my condition stabilized. I take a medication called pyridostigmine bromide (Mestinon), which controls my symptoms to some degree for short periods of time. I also underwent a thymectomy last summer because studies have shown that, for largely unknown reasons, removal of the thymus gland can result in dramatic improvement in patients with MG. These improvements can take up to a year to manifest themselves. I have noticed modest improvements in my condition since the surgery. I have received no physical therapy for my disease because at this point it affects only the oculomotor (eye movement control) portion of my vision.

*—David Hughes*

**David's story is classic for myasthenia gravis. The autoimmune system attacks the postsynaptic muscle membrane receptors, interfering with signaling between neurons and muscle cells. Despite neurons releasing the normal amount of acetylcholine neurotransmitter at the neuromuscular junction, the muscle cells fail to receive most of the signals. As in David's case, often the muscles that move the eyes and elevate the top eyelids are most affected. The drug Tensilon is a short-acting anticholinesterase that rapidly improves muscle strength by increasing muscle response to nerve impulses. The muscle strength increase occurs within a minute of administration of the drug and lasts only a few minutes. Myasthenia gravis is discussed further later in this chapter.**

Neural communication takes place at synapses. Diseases and disorders that interfere with synaptic communication can disrupt any aspect of neural function, from thinking to nerve-muscle signaling to regulation of mood. Most drugs that affect the central nervous system act at the synapse. This chapter discusses how synapses function, including the roles of neurotransmitters and neuromodulators, synaptic receptors, and neurotransmitter agonists and antagonists. This chapter also covers some of the diseases and disorders caused by synaptic failure.

## STRUCTURE OF THE SYNAPSE

At a synapse, a neuron and a postsynaptic cell communicate. The postsynaptic cell can be any cell of an organ, gland, blood vessel, muscle cell, or another neuron. A synapse comprises a presynaptic terminal, a postsynaptic terminal, and the synaptic cleft (Figure 3-1). The *presynaptic terminal,* located at the end

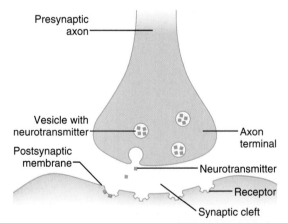

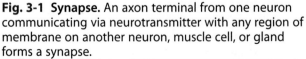

**Fig. 3-1  Synapse.** An axon terminal from one neuron communicating via neurotransmitter with any region of membrane on another neuron, muscle cell, or gland forms a synapse.

of the axon, is a projection specialized for the release of chemicals. The membrane region of the receiving cell is the *postsynaptic terminal*. The space between the two terminals is called the *synaptic cleft*. The presynaptic terminal contains vesicles (small membrane-bound packets) of chemicals called *neurotransmitters*. Neurotransmitters transmit information across the cleft. The postsynaptic membrane contains *receptors,* with specialized molecules designed to bind specific neurotransmitters.

## EVENTS AT THE SYNAPSE

The following steps summarize synaptic communication. This sequence is shown in Figure 3-2.
1. An action potential (a brief pulse of electrical current that travels along the axon) arrives at the presynaptic terminal.
2. The membrane of the presynaptic terminal depolarizes, opening voltage-gated calcium ($Ca^{2+}$) channels.
3. Influx of $Ca^{2+}$ into the neuron terminal, combined with liberation of $Ca^{2+}$ from intracellular stores, triggers the movement of synaptic vesicles, which contain neurotransmitters, toward a release site in the membrane.[1]
4. Synaptic vesicles fuse with the membrane, releasing neurotransmitter into the cleft.
5. Neurotransmitter diffuses across the synaptic cleft.
6. Neurotransmitter that contacts a receptor on the postsynaptic membrane binds to that receptor.
7. The receptor changes shape. The changed configuration of the receptor either:
   • Opens an ion channel associated with the membrane receptor, or
   • Activates intracellular messengers associated with the membrane receptor.

Synaptic communication between neurons can occur on the cell body (axosomatic), the dendrites (axodendritic), or the axon (axoaxonic) of the postsynaptic neuron (Figure 3-3). A single neuron can have multiple synaptic inputs in each region. The total number of action potentials reaching the terminal directly influences the amount of neurotransmitter released. Strong excitatory stimuli to the presynaptic cell lead to a greater number of action potentials reaching the presynaptic terminal. Also, the duration of the stimulus to the presynaptic cell influences the series of subsequent action potentials: when the presynaptic cell is stimulated for a longer time, the series of action potentials is longer.

---

**Clinical Pearl**

An increase in the strength or the duration of an excitatory stimulus to the presynaptic cell results in the release of greater quantities of neurotransmitter.

---

## ELECTRICAL POTENTIALS AT SYNAPSES

Some of the neurotransmitters released into the synaptic cleft bind with receptors on the postsynaptic membrane. The chemical stimulation of these receptors can result in the opening of membrane ion channels. If the synapse is neuromuscular, axosomatic, or axodendritic, the flux of ions in the postsynaptic membrane generates a local postsynaptic potential. Axoaxonic activity produces presynaptic effects, which will be discussed later under presynaptic facilitation and inhibition.

## Postsynaptic Potentials

*Postsynaptic potentials* are local changes in ion concentration across the postsynaptic membrane. When a neurotransmitter binds to a receptor that opens ion channels on the postsynaptic membrane, the effect may be local depolarization or hyperpolarization. A local depolarization is an *excitatory postsynaptic potential* (EPSP). A local hyperpolarization is an *inhibitory postsynaptic potential* (IPSP).

### Excitatory Postsynaptic Potential

An EPSP occurs when neurotransmitters bind to postsynaptic membrane receptors that open ion channels, allowing a local, instantaneous flow of $Na^+$ or $Ca^{2+}$ into the neuron. The flux of positively charged ions into the cell causes the postsynaptic cell membrane to become depolarized (less negative), creating an EPSP (Figure 3-4). Summation of EPSPs can lead to generation of an action potential (see Chapter 2).

EPSPs are common throughout the central and peripheral nervous systems. For example, at the synapse between a neuron and a muscle cell (neuromuscular junction), the neuron releases the neurotransmitter acetylcholine (ACh). Binding of ACh is excitatory, opening ligand-gated channels that allow $Na^+$ influx into the muscle cell, initiating a series of events leading to mechanical contraction of the muscle cell. Every action potential in a motor neuron (a neuron that innervates muscle) elicits a contraction of the muscle cell because motor neurons release sufficient amounts of transmitter to bind to and activate the many receptors on a muscle cell membrane.

### Inhibitory Postsynaptic Potential

An IPSP is a local hyperpolarization of the postsynaptic membrane, which decreases the possibility of an action potential. In contrast to the EPSP, an IPSP involves a local flow of $Cl^-$ and/or $K^+$ in response to a neurotransmitter binding to postsynaptic membrane receptors (Figure 3-5). The postsynaptic ion channels open, allowing $Cl^-$ into the cell or $K^+$ out of the cell. This causes the local postsynaptic cell membrane to become hyperpolarized (more negative). Hyperpolarization can inhibit the generation of an action potential in the postsynaptic cell. If EPSPs coincide with IPSPs, summation determines whether an action potential will be generated. If the preponderance of input to a neuron is inhibitory, an action potential is not generated in the postsynaptic neuron. Only if sufficient depolarization occurs to reach threshold is an action potential generated in the postsynaptic cell.

---

**Clinical Pearl**

At the postsynaptic membrane, changes in membrane potential can be excitatory or inhibitory to the neuron.

---

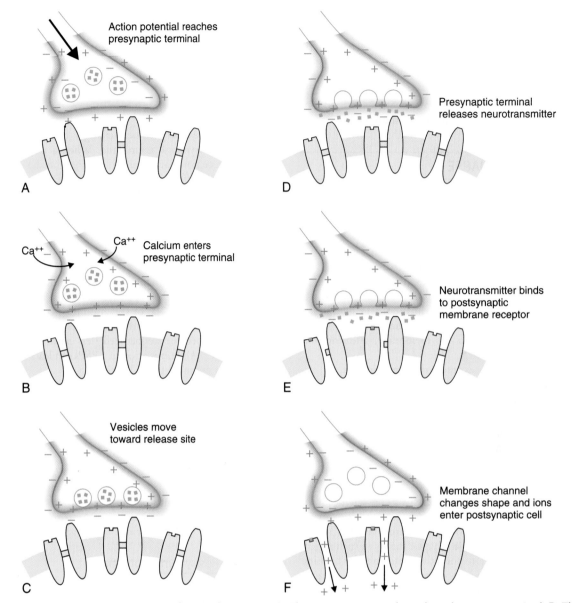

**Fig. 3-2  Series of events at an active chemical synapse. A,** The action potential reaches the axon terminal. **B,** The change in electrical potential causes the opening of voltage-dependent Ca²⁺ channels and the influx of Ca²⁺. **C,** Elevated levels of Ca²⁺ then promote the movement of synaptic vesicles to the membrane. **D,** The synaptic vesicles bind with the membrane, then release neurotransmitter into the synaptic cleft. **E,** Neurotransmitter diffuses across the synaptic cleft and activates a membrane receptor. **F,** In this case, the receptor is associated with an ion channel that opens when the receptor site is bound by neurotransmitter, allowing positively charged ions to enter the postsynaptic cell.

## Presynaptic Facilitation and Inhibition

Activity at a synapse can be influenced by *presynaptic facilitation,* which allows more neurotransmitter to be released, or *presynaptic inhibition,* which allows less (Figure 3-6). For example, presynaptic facilitation intensifies signals that are interpreted as pain. Presynaptic inhibition diminishes the same signals. Clinically, this phenomenon can be seen when a patient concentrates on a painful shoulder. Mentally focusing on the pain can increase the level of activation of brain areas associated

with the pain experience; distraction can lessen the brain activity.

Presynaptic effects occur when the amount of neurotransmitter released by a neuron is influenced by previous activity in an axoaxonic synapse. Neurotransmitter released from the axon terminal of one neuron binding with receptors on the axon terminal of a second neuron alters the membrane potential of the second terminal. For example, activity at axoaxonic synapses between axons descending from the brain and axons of somatosensory neurons can facilitate or inhibit signals

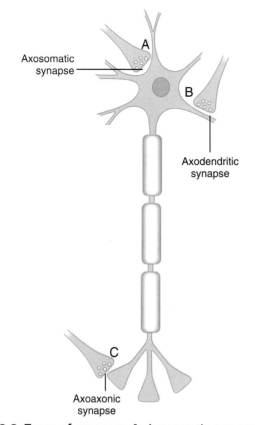

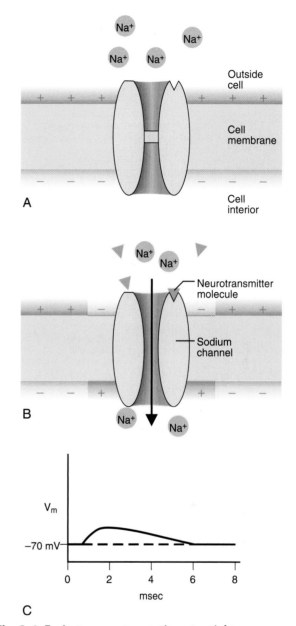

**Fig. 3-3 Types of synapses. A,** Axosomatic synapse between the axon of a presynaptic neuron and the cell body or soma of a postsynaptic neuron. **B,** Axodendritic synapse between the axon of a presynaptic neuron and a dendrite of a postsynaptic neuron. **C,** Axoaxonic synapse between the axon of a presynaptic neuron and the axon of a postsynaptic neuron.

**Fig. 3-4 Excitatory postsynaptic potential. A,** The resting membrane, with Na$^+$ channels closed. **B,** Neurotransmitter released into the synaptic cleft binds with membrane receptors that stimulate the opening of ligand-gated Na$^+$ channels. A resulting influx of Na$^+$ depolarizes the membrane and causes excitation of the neuron. **C,** The resulting postsynaptic membrane potential is more positive than the resting membrane potential.

interpreted as painful. This presynaptic effect intensifies or relieves the perception of pain.

Presynaptic facilitation occurs when a presynaptic axon releases neurotransmitter that slightly depolarizes the axon terminal of a second neuron. This causes a small Ca$^{2+}$ influx into the postsynaptic terminal of the second neuron. Because of this small Ca$^{2+}$ influx, the duration of an action potential in the second neuron increases. The prolonged action potential allows more Ca$^{2+}$ than normal to enter the postsynaptic terminal of the second neuron. The increased Ca$^{2+}$ concentration causes more vesicles of neurotransmitter than usual to move to the cell membrane and release transmitter into the synapse to bind to receptors on the postsynaptic cell (Figure 3-6, *A*).

Presynaptic inhibition occurs when an axon releases neurotransmitter that slightly hyperpolarizes the axonal region of a second neuron. When this happens, the duration of the action potential is decreased in the axon terminal of the second neuron owing to local inhibition of the axon terminal membrane. As a result of the decreased duration of the action potential, Ca$^{2+}$ influx is reduced. Accordingly, the inhibited neuron releases less neurotransmitter onto its target postsynaptic cell (Figure 3-6, *B*). When a therapist asks a patient to

focus on the task at hand and to block out thoughts concerning the pain, the therapist is asking the patient to activate presynaptic inhibition.

> ◎ *Clinical Pearl*
>
> The release of neurotransmitters from an axon terminal can be facilitated or inhibited by the chemical action at an axoaxonic synapse.

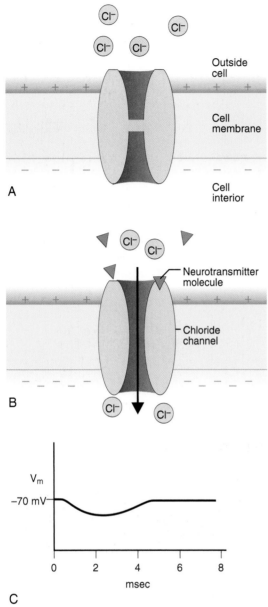

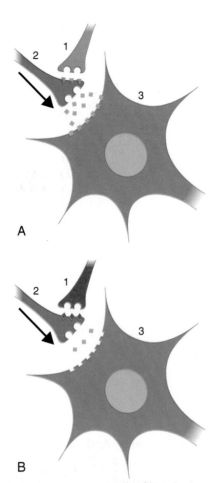

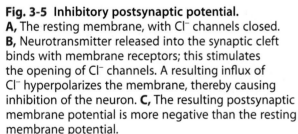

**Fig. 3-5  Inhibitory postsynaptic potential.**
**A,** The resting membrane, with Cl⁻ channels closed.
**B,** Neurotransmitter released into the synaptic cleft
binds with membrane receptors; this stimulates
the opening of Cl⁻ channels. A resulting influx of
Cl⁻ hyperpolarizes the membrane, thereby causing
inhibition of the neuron. **C,** The resulting postsynaptic
membrane potential is more negative than the resting
membrane potential.

**Fig. 3-6  Presynaptic facilitation and presynaptic
inhibition.** In both panels, the interneuron is labeled *1*,
the presynaptic neuron is labeled *2*, and the postsynaptic
neuron is labeled *3*. In **A,** the interneuron *(1)* has just
been fired, releasing neurotransmitter that is bound to
receptors on the axon terminal of the presynaptic neuron
*(2)*. Binding of the neurotransmitter will facilitate the
release of neurotransmitter by the presynaptic neuron *(2)*.
Thus, when an action potential *(indicated by the arrow)*
reaches the axon terminal of the presynaptic neuron,
more $Ca^{2+}$ enters the presynaptic terminal, and more
transmitter than normal is released by the presynaptic
neuron. The result is increased stimulation of the
postsynaptic neuron *(3)* due to increased release of
neurotransmitter. **B,** The opposite effect. The interneuron
*(1)* has released a neurotransmitter that is bound to the
axon terminal of the presynaptic neuron *(2)*. Binding of
this transmitter will inhibit the release of neurotransmitter
by the presynaptic neuron. Thus, when an action
potential reaches the axon terminal of the presynaptic
neuron, less $Ca^{2+}$ than normal enters the terminal and less
neurotransmitter is released by the presynaptic neuron.
The result is decreased stimulation of the postsynaptic
cell membrane *(3)*, owing to decreased release of
neurotransmitter into the synaptic cleft between the
presynaptic neuron and the postsynaptic neuron.

## NEUROTRANSMITTERS AND NEUROMODULATORS

*Neurotransmitters* and *neuromodulators* are chemicals that convey information among neurons. A neurotransmitter is released by a presynaptic neuron and acts directly on postsynaptic ion channels or activates proteins inside the postsynaptic neuron. Neuromodulators are released into extracellular fluid and adjust the activity of many neurons. Most drugs administered to patients with diseases of the nervous system mimic the action of a neurotransmitter or neuromodulator, or block the ability of the neurotransmitter or neuromodulator to interact with its receptor.

Neurotransmitters may excite or inhibit the postsynaptic neuron, depending on the molecule released and the receptors present on the postsynaptic membrane. Neurotransmitters may affect the postsynaptic neuron directly, by activating ion channels (ionotropic), or indirectly, by activating proteins inside the postsynaptic neuron (metabotropic). Neurotransmitters that act directly are classified as fast-acting, because their effects are extremely short-lived—less than $\frac{1}{1000}$ of a second. Neurotransmitters that act indirectly are classified as slow-acting, because their transmission requires $\frac{1}{10}$ of a second to minutes. Slow-acting neurotransmitters regulate fast synaptic transmission by controlling the amount of neurotransmitter released from presynaptic terminals. They can also influence the actions of fast-acting neurotransmitters on the postsynaptic membrane.[2]

Neuromodulators alter neural function by acting at a distance away from the synaptic cleft (Figure 3-7). Their effects manifest more slowly and usually last longer than those of neurotransmitters. In general, neuromodulators require seconds before their cellular effects are observed, and these effects last from minutes to days. Although neuromodulators are not released directly into the synaptic cleft, they often act in conjunction with neurotransmitters. The same molecule can act as a neurotransmitter or a neuromodulator, depending on whether the molecule is released only at specific synapses or is released into the extracellular space. For example, substance P, a short-chain polypeptide discussed later in this chapter, acts as a neurotransmitter between certain neurons in the spinal cord, but as a neuromodulator in the hypothalamus.

Chemical synaptic transmission requires several steps. The neurotransmitter must be synthesized, stored, and released, then must interact with the postsynaptic receptor, and finally must be removed from the synaptic cleft. Neurons often contain more than one neurotransmitter ready for release and may release multiple transmitters simultaneously. Researchers frequently identify new compounds as possible neurotransmitters. These findings greatly complicate the classification of neurons and synapses. The chemicals that most commonly function as neurotransmitters and neuromodulators are listed in Table 3-1. This chapter focuses on the neurotransmitters and neuromodulators that have been characterized extensively.

## SPECIFIC NEUROTRANSMITTERS AND NEUROMODULATORS

### Acetylcholine

Acetylcholine (ACh) is the major conveyor of information in the peripheral nervous system. All neurons that synapse with skeletal muscle fibers (motor neurons) use ACh to elicit

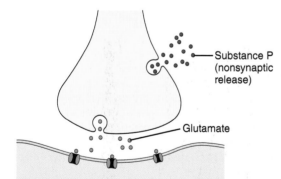

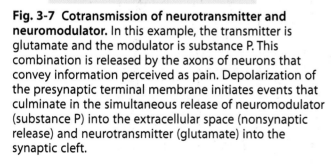

**Fig. 3-7 Cotransmission of neurotransmitter and neuromodulator.** In this example, the transmitter is glutamate and the modulator is substance P. This combination is released by the axons of neurons that convey information perceived as pain. Depolarization of the presynaptic terminal membrane initiates events that culminate in the simultaneous release of neuromodulator (substance P) into the extracellular space (nonsynaptic release) and neurotransmitter (glutamate) into the synaptic cleft.

**TABLE 3-1   COMMON NEUROTRANSMITTERS/ NEUROMODULATORS**

| Category | Transmitter/ Modulator | Action on Postsynaptic Membrane |
|---|---|---|
| Cholinergic | Acetylcholine (ACh) | Excitatory |
| Amino acid | γ-Aminobutyric acid (GABA) | Inhibitory |
|  | Glutamate (Glu) | Excitatory |
|  | Glycine (Gly) | Inhibitory, primarily in spinal cord |
|  | Aspartate | Excitatory |
| Amine | Dopamine (DA) | Inhibitory or excitatory depending upon receptor |
|  | Histamine | Usually inhibitory |
|  | Norepinephrine (NE) | Inhibitory or excitatory depending upon receptor |
|  | Serotonin (5-HT) | Usually inhibitory |
| Peptide | Endorphins | Usually inhibitory |
|  | Enkephalins | Usually inhibitory |
|  | Substance P | Usually excitatory |
|  | Galanin | Usually inhibitory |
| Gas | Nitric oxide | Excitatory |

fast-acting effects on muscle membranes. Myasthenia gravis, the autoimmune disease described by David Hughes at the beginning of this chapter, destroys ACh receptors on the skeletal muscle, leading to muscle weakness or paralysis. ACh also has slow-acting effects in the peripheral nervous system that regulate heart rate and other autonomic functions.

In the brain, ACh is produced by neurons in the basal forebrain (area inferior to the striatum) and in the midbrain. In the central nervous system, slow action and neuromodulation by ACh are involved in control of movement and selection of objects of attention.[3,4]

## Amino Acids

Amino acid transmitters—glutamate, aspartate, glycine, and gamma-aminobutyric acid (GABA)—are typically fast-acting. Glutamate and aspartate have powerful excitatory effects on neurons in virtually every region of the brain.

## Glutamate

*Glutamate,* the principal fast excitatory transmitter of the central nervous system,[5] elicits neural changes that occur with learning and development. However, glutamate may also contribute to neuron death following central nervous system damage.[6] Chapter 4 discusses the destructive role of glutamate.

## Glycine and GABA

Both glycine and GABA are inhibitory transmitters. *Glycine* inhibits postsynaptic membranes, primarily in the brainstem and spinal cord. *GABA* is the major inhibitory neurotransmitter in the central nervous system, particularly at interneurons within the spinal cord. Inhibitory effects produced by GABA and glycine prevent excessive neural activity. Low levels of these transmitters can cause neural overactivity, leading to seizures, unwanted skeletal muscle contractions, and anxiety.

### ◎ *Clinical Pearl*

The most prevalent fast-acting neurotransmitters are glutamate (excitatory) and GABA (inhibitory).

## Amines: Slow-Acting Transmitters

Amines are distributed widely throughout the nervous system. Each amine transmitter has a single amino group ($NH_2$) as part of its chemical structure. Members of this family include dopamine, norepinephrine (NE), serotonin, and histamine. Dopamine, NE, and serotonin are produced by neurons in the brainstem that project throughout the cerebral cortex and other gray matter areas. In the central nervous system, amines act both as slow-acting neurotransmitters and as neuromodulators.[4]

## Dopamine

*Dopamine* affects motor activity, cognition, and behavior. Dopamine action is associated with feelings of pleasure and reward, and thus motivates certain behaviors. These feelings of reward affect behaviors as important as eating, and as destructive as addiction.

Signaling pathways that use dopamine have been implicated in the pathophysiology of schizophrenia (a disorder of thinking) and Parkinson's disease (a disorder of movement). The involvement of dopamine in certain aspects of psychosis is demonstrated by the action of some antipsychotic medications that prevent the binding of dopamine to certain receptor sites. These drugs decrease hallucinations, delusions, and disorganized thinking. However, because these drugs prevent the binding of dopamine in motor areas of the brain, in addition to thinking areas, involuntary muscle contractions are a side effect of many of these medications.[7]

Dopamine is produced by neurons in the substantia nigra and a nearby region of the midbrain (ventral tegmental area).

Cocaine and amphetamines directly affect dopamine signaling by interfering with dopamine *reuptake* into the presynaptic neuron.[8] Impeding dopamine reuptake prolongs dopamine activity, allowing it to continue to bind and activate receptors repeatedly. Cocaine produces euphoria and stereotyped behaviors including pacing and nail biting by interfering with the reuptake protein.[9] Amphetamines energize users by increasing the release of dopamine and blocking dopamine and NE reuptake.

## Norepinephrine

*Norepinephrine* (also called *noradrenaline*) plays a vital role in active surveillance by increasing attention to sensory information. The highest levels of NE are associated with vigilance (e.g., when driving on a crowded freeway), and the lowest levels occur during sleep. NE is essential in producing the "fight-or-flight" reaction to stress. In the periphery, NE is released by neurons in the autonomic nervous system and is secreted by the adrenal gland. In the central nervous system, NE is produced in brainstem nuclei, the hypothalamus and in the thalamus.

Overactivity of the NE system produces fear and, in extreme cases, panic by acting on cortical and limbic regions. Excessive levels of NE can produce *panic disorder,* the abrupt onset of intense terror, a sense of loss of personal identity, and the perception that familiar things are strange or unreal, combined with signs of increased sympathetic nervous system activity.[10] Post-traumatic stress disorder also involves excessive NE.[11] Veterans with post-traumatic stress disorder experience flashbacks to traumatic events, panic, grief, intrusive thoughts about the traumatic event, and loss of emotions when given a drug that stimulates NE activity. Control subjects not diagnosed with post-traumatic stress disorder reported few effects of the same drug.[12]

## Serotonin

*Serotonin* affects mood and perception of pain, adjusts the general arousal level, and can suppress sensory information. The highest levels of serotonin occur with alertness, and low levels are associated with rapid eye movement (REM) sleep. Low levels of serotonin are also associated with depression and suicidal behavior. However, recent data indicate that depression cannot be solely attributed to low serotonin levels, and that other neuromodulatory molecules probably play a more

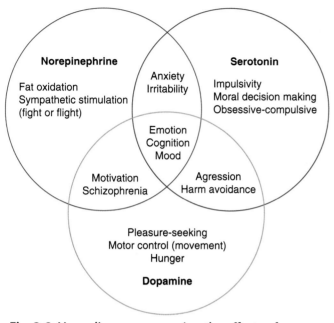

**Fig. 3-8** Venn diagram comparing the effects of serotonin, norepinephrine, and dopamine.

important role.[13] The antidepressant Prozac (fluoxetine) is a selective blocker of serotonin reuptake. By blocking serotonin reuptake, the drug ensures that serotonin will remain in the synapses longer, providing more opportunity for serotonin to bind with receptors. At least 14 different subtypes of serotonin receptors are known. This diversity gives the system several ways of responding to the same neurotransmitter.

### Histamine

Although it is often referred to as an amine modulator, histamine is chemically a distant relative to the other compounds in this category. As a neurotransmitter, histamine is concentrated in the hypothalamus, an area of the brain known for regulating hormonal function, and increases arousal.[14]

### Amine Neurotransmitter Summary

Together the amine neurotransmitters act in the brain to control many behaviors. Figure 3-8 illustrates the interplay between NE, serotonin, and dopamine to control mood, anxiety, appetite, motivation, and a number of other emotions and behaviors. This interplay provides the brain with multiple redundant pathways to alter feelings and behaviors, but at the same time makes it very difficult to design drugs to treat specific psychological disorders. For example, drugs designed to specifically inhibit impulsive behavior are likely to have side effects on emotions, cognition, aggression, and anxiety.

---

**○ Clinical Pearl**

Dopamine, NE, serotonin, and histamine function as slow-acting neurotransmitters and neuromodulators.

---

### Peptides

Neuroactive peptides can affect neuronal signaling by acting as traditional hormones, neurotransmitters, or neuromodulators. Peptides in the central nervous system may act as single neurotransmitters within the synaptic junction, but most researchers believe they work in conjunction with other neurotransmitters and neuromodulators within the same synapse.

### Substance P

One of the most common neuropeptides is *substance P.* When tissue is injured, substance P stimulates nerve endings at the site of injury, and then within the central nervous system, substance P acts as a neurotransmitter, carrying information from the spinal cord to the brain. Substance P has been strongly implicated as a neuromodulator in the pathophysiology of pain syndromes that involve perception of normally innocuous stimuli as painful.[15] In the substantia nigra, amygdala, hypothalamus, and cerebral cortex, substance P acts as a neuromodulator, usually producing long-duration excitation of postsynaptic cells. In addition, it modulates the immune system and neuronal activity in times of high stress.[16]

### Calcitonin Gene-Related Peptide

*Calcitonin gene-related peptide* frequently acts as a neuromodulator. By activating a series of events in the postsynaptic cell, calcitonin gene-related peptide phosphorylates the ACh receptor, resulting in a decreased likelihood that ACh will activate its own receptor when bound. This is a classic example of a neuromodulator affecting synaptic transmission through a neurotransmitter. Neuromodulator effects of calcitonin gene-related peptide also appear to be involved in long-term neural changes in response to painful stimuli, especially in migraine headache.[17]

### Galanin

Galanin tends to play an inhibitory or modulatory role at the synapse. It has an important role in a wide variety of behaviors and disorders, including control of food intake, cognition, emotions and mood, alertness, seizures, and pain perception.[18] Galanin is widely expressed in the brain (hypothalamus, cortex, and brainstem), the spinal cord, and the gut. It plays a critical role in inhibiting insulin release through autonomic neurons that innervate the pancreas.[19]

### Opioid Peptides

Another group of neuroactive peptides are called *endogenous opioid peptides,* because they bind the same receptors that the drug opium binds. This group includes endorphins, enkephalins, and dynorphins. Opioids inhibit neurons in the central nervous system that are involved in the perception of pain. Opioid receptors are predominantly found in the spinal cord, hypothalamus, and specific brainstem gray matter areas (see Chapter 7).

### Diffusible Transmitter: Nitric Oxide

Nitric oxide regulates the vascular system in the periphery and is also active in the brain. Nitric oxide does not require a receptor on the outer cell membrane to bind for activation. Rather, it diffuses through the cell membrane and acts on messenger systems within the postsynaptic cell. It appears to be involved in persistent changes in the postsynaptic response to repeated stimuli and in cell death of neurons. These processes, called *long-term potentiation (LTP)* and *excitotoxicity,* respectively, are explained in Chapter 4. As part of LTP, nitric oxide plays a role in seizure development associated with abnormal mitochrondrial function.[20]

## SYNAPTIC RECEPTORS

Once a neurotransmitter is released into the synaptic cleft, it must bind to a receptor on the postsynaptic membrane to have an effect. Receptors on the postsynaptic neuron are typically named for the neurotransmitter/neuromodulator to which they bind. For example, the receptors that bind GABA are called *GABA receptors.* Most neurotransmitters can bind to several different types of receptors. Thus, the effect of a neurotransmitter is based not on the chemical itself, but on the type of receptor to which it binds.

Receptors may produce direct or indirect actions. Neurotransmitter receptors act directly as ion channels when the receptor and the ion channel constitute a single functional unit. Receptors may act indirectly by using a cascade of intracellular molecules to activate ion channels or may cause other changes within the postsynaptic neuron. Examples of receptors in each of these categories are provided later.

Postsynaptic receptors use three mechanisms to transduce signals. When activated, receptors produce fast or slow responses, by:
1. Directly opening ion channels (fast synaptic transmission)
2. Indirectly opening ion channels (slow synaptic transmission)
3. Activating a cascade of intracellular events, including activation of genes (slow synaptic transmission)

### Direct Activation of Ion Channels: Ligand-Gated Ion Channels

*Ligand-gated ion channels* consist of proteins that function both as receptors for the neurotransmitter and as ion channels (ionotropic receptors). The gates of these channels open in response to a specific chemical ligand binding to the receptor surface (see Figures 3-4 and 3-5). Neurotransmitters and hormones are endogenous ligands because they are produced within the organism. Drugs, because they are produced outside the organism, are exogenous ligands.

In the resting state, ligand-gated channels are closed, blocking the flow of ions through the channels. When a specific neurotransmitter binds to the receptor, the gate opens, and specific ions diffuse down their electrochemical gradient across the membrane of the neuron. For example, when glutamate binds to a ligand-gated channel, $Na^+$ or $Ca^{2+}$ flows into the neuron, producing local depolarization (an EPSP). Even inhibitory neurotransmitters act by opening ion channels. When GABA binds to certain receptors, channels selective for $Cl^-$ open. Chloride ions diffuse down their electrochemical gradient and into the cell, carrying the negative charge. Although the ion channel may be open for only a few milliseconds, enough ions cross the membrane to make substantial changes in the local membrane potential. The additional negative charge entering the cell hyperpolarizes the membrane, making it less likely to reach threshold and fire an action potential. Thus some ligand-gated ion channels inhibit neuronal activation, but others are excitatory.

In general, ion channels will open and close rapidly as long as the neurotransmitter is present in the synaptic cleft. Some ligand-gated channels have shut-off mechanisms that inactivate the channel after a certain period of time, even when the ligand is still present in the extracellular fluid. All other receptors become inactivated when the neurotransmitter is removed from the synaptic cleft by degradation or by reuptake of the neurotransmitter back into the presynaptic axon terminal.

> ## ◎ *Clinical Pearl*
>
> Rapid and brief opening of membrane channels occurs when a neurotransmitter binds to the receptor site of the membrane channel. Ion channel receptors act like a lock and key. The neurotransmitter is analogous to the key; using the key opens the lock.

### Indirect Activation of Ion Channels: G-Proteins

Ion channels can also be opened indirectly using metabotropic receptors, causing reactions slower than those of direct activation. Guanine nucleotide–binding proteins (G-proteins) indirectly open ion channels by acting as cytoplasmic shuttles, moving between the receptor and target effector proteins on the internal surface of the cell membrane.

When a neurotransmitter binds to a G-protein receptor, the following sequence takes place (Figure 3-9)[21]:
1. The receptor protein changes shape.
2. The G-protein becomes activated (via replacement of guanosine diphosphate by guanosine triphosphate).
3. The active subunits of G-proteins, α and βγ, break free from the receptor to act as cytoplasmic signaling shuttles.
4. The subunits bind to a membrane ion channel.
5. The ion channel changes shape and opens.
6. The subunits become deactivated and reassociated with the receptor.

When the membrane receptor is not activated, the αβγ-complex is bound to the receptor.

> ## ◎ *Clinical Pearl*
>
> When a neurotransmitter binds to an extracellular membrane receptor with an associated intracellular G-protein, activation of the G-protein elicits cellular events that develop slowly and last longer than the effects of ligand-gated channels. The G-protein can also cause persistent opening of membrane channels.

### Cascade of Intracellular Events

#### G-Protein Second-Messenger System

The G-protein second-messenger system is responsible for some of the most profound and long-lasting changes in the

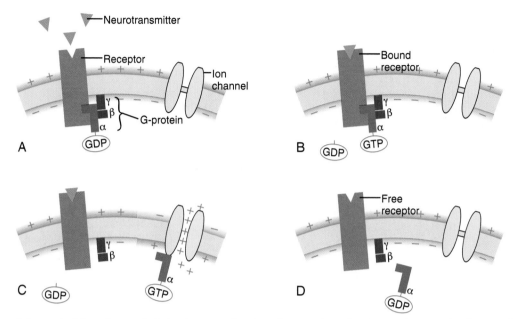

**Fig. 3-9 G-protein–gated ion channel. A,** In the nonstimulated state, the αβγ–G-protein complex is associated with a membrane receptor. **B,** Neurotransmitter binds to the membrane receptor, causing a conformational change and activation of the G-protein. The α-chain detaches from the membrane receptor. **C,** The α–guanosine triphosphate (GTP) complex binds to a membrane-spanning G-protein channel. A conformational change in the protein channel causes the channel to open, and ions flow into the cell. **D,** The α-chain is inactivated and released from the protein channel. The channel closes, and the α-chain returns to its host membrane receptor to bind with the βγ-chain. *GDP,* Guanosine diphosphate.

nervous system. In the entire human genome, genes for G-protein receptors are the most abundant.[22] Via their second-messenger pathways, G-proteins affect long-acting systems that regulate mood, pain perception, movement, motivation, and cognition.[5]

By activating intracellular target proteins, initiating a cascade of intracellular events, G-proteins can:

- Activate genes, causing the cell to manufacture different neurotransmitters or other specific cellular products
- Open membrane ion channels
- Modulate $Ca^{2+}$ concentrations inside the cell. Internal stores of $Ca^{2+}$ liberated in response to second-messenger systems regulate metabolism and other cellular processes. In this case, $Ca^{2+}$ acts as a third messenger.

In second-messenger systems, the neurotransmitter is the first messenger, delivering the signal to the receptor but remaining outside the cell. The second messenger, produced inside the cell, conveys the message and activates responses inside the cell (Figures 3-10 and 3-11). This can alter a variety of cellular functions. All of the amine transmitters and substance P bind to and activate G-protein receptors.

A second-messenger system is similar to a fire department's response to an emergency: the first messenger (neurotransmitter) is analogous to a caller reporting a fire. A receptor conveys relevant information, as an emergency dispatcher does. Second messengers are analogous to firefighters, activating responses within the cell itself. Sometimes only one fire truck is required. Other signals indicate that a variety of different responses are needed, analogous to a fire truck, ambulance, and emergency response vehicle all called by the same signal. In these cases, a single neurotransmitter might turn on a molecular pathway that

ends with a change in gene expression, opening of ion channels, and phosphorylation of a structural protein.

Along with the ability to activate several different downstream molecules with the binding of a single neurotransmitter, the G-protein signaling pathway offers the ability to dramatically amplify a signal. One activated receptor can stimulate a number of G-proteins (Figure 3-12). Each subunit of the G-protein can carry a different signal to the second messengers. Each of the second messengers may activate a number of other downstream molecules. For example, one second-messenger system produces prostaglandins—substances that regulate vasodilation and increase inflammation. Aspirin and other nonsteroidal anti-inflammatory drugs reduce pain and inflammation by inhibiting one of the enzymes in this G-protein–initiated cascade. The difference in effects between activating ligand-gated channels and G-protein–mediated receptors are illustrated in Figure 3-13.

## Receptor Tyrosine Kinase

The receptor tyrosine kinase (RTK) is another class of receptors that act through second messengers. Most frequently, these receptors are involved in cell growth, cellular movement, and cell death.[23] Dysfunction of specific RTKs, or their agonists, has been implicated in multiple sclerosis,[24] schizophrenia,[25] and sensory neuropathies.[26] RTK is named for a site in the intracellular side of the protein that contains at least one tyrosine amino acid. Upon ligand binding on the extracellular side of the receptor protein, the receptor alters its own properties by adding phosphate groups to tyrosine. Then the receptor phosphorylates downstream molecules, thus initiating the signaling cascade.

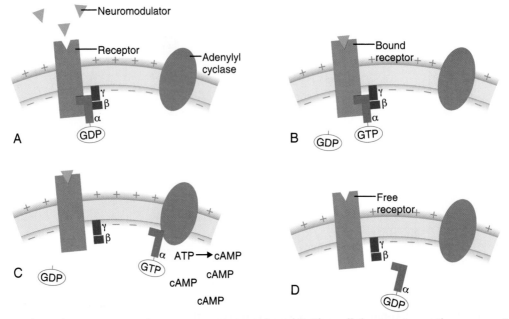

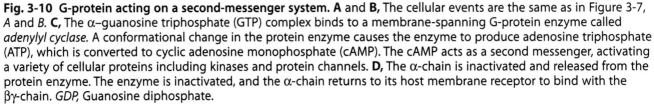

**Fig. 3-10  G-protein acting on a second-messenger system. A** and **B,** The cellular events are the same as in Figure 3-7, *A* and *B.* **C,** The α–guanosine triphosphate (GTP) complex binds to a membrane-spanning G-protein enzyme called *adenylyl cyclase.* A conformational change in the protein enzyme causes the enzyme to produce adenosine triphosphate (ATP), which is converted to cyclic adenosine monophosphate (cAMP). The cAMP acts as a second messenger, activating a variety of cellular proteins including kinases and protein channels. **D,** The α-chain is inactivated and released from the protein enzyme. The enzyme is inactivated, and the α-chain returns to its host membrane receptor to bind with the βγ-chain. *GDP,* Guanosine diphosphate.

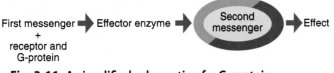

**Fig. 3-11  A simplified schematic of a G-protein–mediated second-messenger system.** These systems involve (1) binding of a neurotransmitter to a G-protein–associated membrane receptor, (2) activation of an effector enzyme, (3) increased levels of a second messenger that elicit a final effect, depending upon the cell type.

Neuropeptides and hormones typically activate RTKs instead of using G-protein receptors. The actions of kinase receptors are important in maintaining healthy neurons in the brain and periphery. When the RTK called musk is missing in developing animals, synaptic terminals do not develop normally.[27]

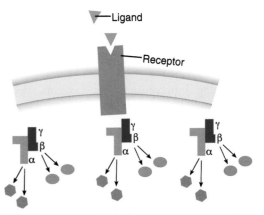

**Fig. 3-12  G-protein action.** A neurotransmitter (a type of ligand) binds to one receptor, activating it. The receptor sequentially binds three G-protein molecules. The G-protein molecules dissociate from the receptor and split into α- and βγ-subunits. The α- and βγ-subunits of the G-protein molecules each transmit the signal to multiple effector molecules. Thus the signal generated by the binding of a neurotransmitter with a receptor is diversified and amplified.

---

### SPECIFIC RECEPTORS

#### Acetylcholine Receptors

Receptors that bind ACh fall into two categories: nicotinic and muscarinic. These receptors are distinguished by their ability to

---

> ◎ **Clinical Pearl**
>
> Second-messenger systems action is similar to the ignition system in a car: using the key (the neurotransmitter) starts the motor. The second messenger initiates many events inside the neuron.

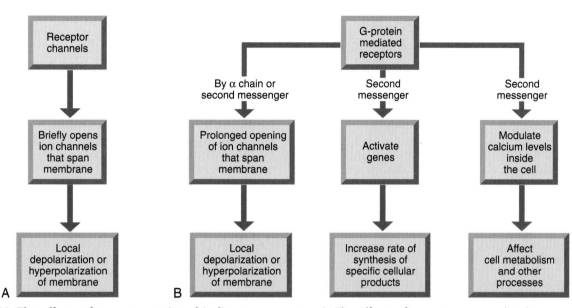

**Fig. 3-13 The effects of neurotransmitter binding to a receptor. A,** The effects of neurotransmitter binding to an ionotropic receptor. **B,** The effects with metabotropic receptors.

bind certain drugs. Nicotine, derived from tobacco, selectively activates the nicotinic receptors. Muscarine, a poison derived from mushrooms, activates only the muscarinic receptors. The nicotinic receptors are ionotropic, directly opening ion channels. These fast-acting receptors allow a rapid increase in intracellular $Na^+$ and $Ca^{2+}$, producing local depolarization. Nicotinic receptors are found at the neuromuscular junction, at autonomic ganglia, and in some areas of the central nervous system. The nicotinic receptors of the brain have been implicated in a number of functions, including neuronal development, memory, and learning.[28] Nonsynaptic nicotinic receptors are prevalent in the hippocampus and the sensory cortex. Loss of nicotinic receptor–expressing neurons in the brain is a hallmark of Alzheimer's disease; three currently licensed drugs used to treat Alzheimer's disease (rivastigmine, galantamine, and donepezil) act by increasing the concentration of ACh in the brain.[29] Nicotine addiction is discussed in Chapter 18.

Muscarinic receptors are G-protein receptors. Their activation produces a slow, prolonged response that may be excitatory or inhibitory. Muscarinic receptors are found mainly on autonomic effector cells in the heart, on other autonomic effectors, and in some regions of the brain. Thus, the actions of ACh on muscarinic receptors mainly contribute to the regulation of cardiac muscle, smooth muscle, and glandular activity (see Chapter 9). Many subtypes of muscarinic receptors are distributed throughout the nervous system. For example, the M1 subtype of muscarinic receptor is essential in normal cortical formation during development.[30]

## Glutamate Receptors

Glutamate receptors may be ionotropic (ligand-gated) or metabotropic (G-protein–coupled). Ligand-gated ion channels that bind glutamate are called AMPA (alpha-amino-3-hydroxy-5-methyl-4-isoxazolepropionic acid), kainate, or NMDA (*N*-methyl-D-aspartate) receptors. Activation of AMPA and kainate receptors causes fast depolarization of the postsynaptic neuron.[31]

The NMDA receptor is unique, because to open the ion channel, glutamate must be bound to the receptor and the membrane must depolarize simultaneously. Thus the NMDA receptor is both voltage- and ligand-gated. Activation of an NMDA receptor causes the associated channel to open and close very slowly. The channel is permeable to $Na^+$, $Ca^{2+}$, and $K^+$. Resulting prolonged ionic changes inside the postsynaptic neuron produce LTP, a prolonged increase in the size of the postsynaptic response to a given stimulus.[32] LTP, important in development and in learning, is described further in Chapter 4.

In contrast to these positive roles for NMDA receptors, abnormal activity of these receptors is associated with numerous disorders. The level of glutamate in the local environment of the NMDA receptors must be finely regulated because exposure of neurons to high concentrations of glutamate for only a few minutes can lead to neuronal cell death (see Chapter 4). Overactivity of NMDA receptors may cause epileptic seizures.[33] Changes in glutamate transmission are associated with chronic pain, depression, Parkinson's disease, schizophrenia, and neuronal injury associated with acute stroke.[33] The illicit drug phencyclidine ("angel dust") binds to the NMDA receptor and blocks the flow of ions, causing users to feel separate from their surroundings, to feel strong and invulnerable, and to experience hallucinations (vivid perceptions of something that is not present) and severe mood disorders. Phencyclidine may cause acute anxiety, paranoia and violent hostility, and occasionally psychoses (loss of contact with reality) indistinguishable from schizophrenia.

## GABA Receptors

As was previously discussed, GABA is the most common fast-acting inhibitory neurotransmitter in the brain. GABA binds to two types of receptors, referred to as $GABA_A$ and $GABA_B$.

$GABA_A$ receptors are found in nearly every neuron. $GABA_A$ receptors are ionotropic $Cl^-$ channels that open when GABA binds to the receptor, producing hyperpolarization of the post-synaptic membrane. Benzodiazepines (antianxiety and anticonvulsant drugs) and barbiturate drugs mimic the action of GABA and bind to the GABA$_A$ receptor subtype. Barbiturates are used pharmacologically for sedation, to decrease anxiety, and as anticonvulsants for treating seizures. In addition, they provide a feeling of euphoria. All of this can be explained by the ability of these drugs to activate GABA$_A$ receptors and inhibit neuronal excitation.

GABA also activates slow-acting responses. GABA$_B$ receptors are linked to ion channels via second-messenger systems. Baclofen, a muscle relaxant used to treat excessive muscle contraction in chronic spinal cord injury, increases the presynaptic release of GABA in the spinal cord, thus activating the GABA$_B$ receptors.

## Dopamine Receptors

Dopamine activates at least five subtypes of receptors. These receptors all use second-messenger systems to suppress the activity of Ca$^{2+}$ channels. Dopamine affects motor activity, motivation, and cognition. Drugs that act on dopamine receptors alter movement, motivation, and thinking. In Parkinson's disease (a movement disorder covered in Chapter 11), dopamine levels are inadequate and can be supplemented by the drug L-dopa. L-Dopa is a precursor to dopamine that crosses the blood-brain barrier (dopamine does not cross the blood-brain barrier) and is converted into dopamine in the brain.

## Norepinephrine Receptors

NE receptors are G-protein–mediated receptors with two major subtypes: α and β. In the brain, activation of NE receptors can produce excitatory or inhibitory responses. Activation of α NE receptors in the gut causes relaxation of intestinal smooth muscle. Activation of β-receptors in the heart increases the force and rate of heart contraction. β-blockers, drugs that bind with β-receptors and prevent activation of the receptors, prevent the sweating, rapid heartbeat, and other signs of sympathetic activation that may otherwise occur in stressful situations. Musicians and actors often take the β-blocker propranolol before a performance.

## Serotonin Receptors

Serotonin receptors come in multiple forms and are coupled to different signaling pathways. Some are G-protein receptors, and others are ligand-gated channels that open Na$^+$ and K$^+$ channels. A multitude of brain functions are regulated by serotonin receptors, including sleep, cognition, perception (including pain), motor activity, and mood. Lysergic acid diethylamide (LSD), a hallucinogenic drug, activates one set of serotonin receptors. Low levels of serotonin are associated with depression and suicidal behavior. The antidepressant Prozac (fluoxetine) is a selective blocker of serotonin reuptake.

## Other Receptors

Other neurotransmitters (glycine, galanin, substance P, and the opioids) have receptors similar to those already described and thus will not be discussed in detail here. Neurotransmitter actions are summarized in Table 3-2.

## RECEPTOR REGULATION

Cells regulate receptor activity in several ways, including limiting the number of receptors that are available for activation on the cell surface. In response to frequent stimulation by a ligand, the cell will decrease receptor activity by:
- Receptor internalization or
- Receptor inactivation

Overstimulation of postsynaptic receptors can cause a decrease in the number of receptors at the surface. Activated receptors are *internalized* when part of the postsynaptic membrane folds into the cell, creating a receptor-containing vesicle that buds off into the cytoplasm. These "used" receptors may be recycled back to the membrane, ready for subsequent activation, or they may be degraded by the cell and replaced with newly formed receptor molecules.

*Inactivation* leaves the total number of receptors at the membrane constant but switches some off, so that the number of functional receptors decreases. An example of this mechanism is the β-adrenergic receptor, which binds NE. Following receptor activation, an intracellular kinase phosphorylates the receptor. Phosphorylation blocks the ability of subsequent NE molecules to activate the receptor. Only when the receptor has been dephosphorylated can it be activated by a ligand.

Neurons can increase the number of active receptors on the surface in response to low levels of a neurotransmitter or infrequent receptor activation. This increases the likelihood that the ligand will bind to a functional receptor.

> ## ◎ Clinical Pearl
>
> Neurotransmitters and neuromodulators are the chemicals released from an axon terminal. Their effects depend on the type of receptor they bind with. Neurotransmitter effects are local, acting on the postsynaptic membrane. Neuromodulators are released into the extracellular fluid and affect the function of many neurons.

## NEUROTRANSMITTER AGONISTS AND ANTAGONISTS

Drugs that affect the nervous system usually bind with receptors or prevent the release of neurotransmitters or neuromodulators. If a drug binds to the receptor and mimics the effects of naturally occurring neurotransmitters, the drug is called an *agonist*. If, on the other hand, a drug prevents the release of neurotransmitters or binds to the receptor and impedes the effects of a naturally occurring transmitter, the drug is called an *antagonist*. Because nicotine binds to certain ACh receptors and elicits the same effects as are elicited by the neurotransmitter, nicotine is an ACh agonist.

Botulinum toxin A (Botox) is a neurotransmitter antagonist used to improve the functional abilities of people with movement abnormalities caused by central nervous system disorders.

**TABLE 3-2**  NEUROTRANSMITTERS AND NEUROMODULATORS

| Neurotransmitter/ Modulator | Sites of Action | Transmitter Binding Causes | Clinical Application |
|---|---|---|---|
| **Acetylcholine (ACh)** Receptors: nicotinic, muscarinic Agonists: nicotine, muscarine Antagonists: curare, atropine, Botulinum toxin | PNS: excitatory at all neuromuscular junctions | Initiation of skeletal muscle contraction | Myasthenia gravis (disease destroys ACh receptors) Botulinum toxin inhibits ACh release Nerve gas and organophosphate insecticides (prolong ACh effect, causing tetanic muscle contractions) Curare blocks nicotinic ACh receptors, causing skeletal muscle paralysis |
| | PNS autonomic: direct action at all preganglionic receptors (nicotinic) | Facilitation of postsynaptic autonomic neurons | |
| | PNS autonomic: second-messenger action at parasympathetic postganglionic muscarinic receptors | Slowing of heart rate; increased digestive secretions and smooth muscle contraction; constriction pupil of eye | Atropine competitively binds with muscarinic ACh receptors, causing increased heart rate and dilation of pupils |
| | CNS: ventral striatum and cerebral cortex | Arousal and feelings of reward | Nicotine binding to nicotinic receptors in ventral striatum may explain pleasurable and addictive effects of smoking In Alzheimer's disease the number of ACh cortical receptors is diminished |
| **Norepinephrine (NE)** Receptors: $\alpha 1$, $\alpha 2$ $\beta 1$, $\beta 2$ Agonists: amphetamines and cocaine Antagonists: propranolol | PNS: sympathetic nervous system and by adrenal gland | Increased heart rate and force of contraction (thus increases blood pressure); dilation of bronchioles, inhibition of peristalsis | Propranolol blocks $\beta$-receptors, preventing heart rate increase, sweating, and other sympathetic nervous system actions that occur during stage fright in actors, public speakers |
| | CNS: limbic system; some areas of cerebral cortex | Control of mood; increased attention to sensory information | Amphetamines and cocaine increase the release of NE and block reuptake of NE Reuptake blocked by tricyclic antidepressants Excessive NE: feeling fearful, panic disorder, post-traumatic stress disorder |
| **Dopamine (DA)** Receptors: $D_1$, $D_2$, $D_3$, $D_4$, $D_5$ Agonists: cocaine, amphetamines, L-dopa Antagonists: antipsychotics | Limbic system: ventral striatum, amygdala, hippocampus | Feelings of pleasure; reinforcement of behaviors, including behaviors associated with drug abuse | Amphetamines increase release of DA Cocaine blocks reuptake |
| | Basal ganglia: caudate head and putamen | Decision making and goal-directed behavior (caudate head); control of movement (putamen) | Parkinson's disease (movement and cognitive disorder): DA levels in caudate and putamen are inadequate L-Dopa, a drug used to treat Parkinson's disease, is converted to DA in the brain Drugs for Parkinson's to increase dopamine can induce involuntary movements |
| | Frontal lobe | Cognitive activity, including planning | May be involved in some aspects of schizophrenia and attention deficit hyperactivity disorder[37] Antipsychotic drugs that decrease hallucinations, delusions, and disorganized thinking (e.g., clozapine) act on $D_2$ receptors |

*Continued*

**TABLE 3-2    NEUROTRANSMITTERS AND NEUROMODULATORS—cont'd**

| Neurotransmitter/ Modulator | Sites of Action | Transmitter Binding Causes | Clinical Application |
|---|---|---|---|
| **Serotonin (5-HT)** Receptors: 5-HT$_1$, 5-HT$_2$, 5-HT$_3$ Agonists: antidepressants (e.g., fluoxetine [Prozac]) Antagonists: none are used clinically | Throughout gray matter in spinal cord and brain | Regulation of sleep, appetite, arousal, mood | Low levels of 5-HT are associated with depression and anxiety Serotonin reuptake inhibitors (including Prozac) treat depression and anxiety High levels of 5-HT associated with obsessive-compulsive disorder and with some symptoms of schizophrenia |
| **GABA** (main inhibitory transmitter in brain) Receptors: GABA$_A$, GABA$_B$ Agonists: benzodiazepines (e.g., Valium), barbiturates, baclofen Antagonists: none are used clinically | Hypothalamus, cerebellum, spinal cord | Sedation, antianxiety, antiseizure, sleep-inducing | Alcohol potentiates effects of GABA (causes impaired motor coordination) Benzodiazepines (including Valium) enhance action of GABA In epilepsy, drugs that increase GABA levels can decrease the excessive neural activity |
| **Glutamate** (main excitatory transmitter in brain) Receptors: NMDA, AMPA, kainate Agonists: none are used clinically Antagonists: phencyclidine | CNS | Learning and memory | Excessive glutamate levels can cause epileptic seizures Excessive release of glutamate by dying neurons causes excitotoxicity, death of neurons due to overstimulation |
| **Glycine** Receptors: glycine Agonists: none are used clinically Antagonists: strychnine (poison) | Spinal cord | Usually inhibition | Strychnine blocks glycine receptors, causing convulsions and respiratory paralysis |
| **Endorphins** (opioid peptides) Receptors: $\mu_1$, $\mu_2$, $\delta$, $\kappa_1$, $\kappa_2$ (opiate) Agonists: opioids: morphine, heroin, oxycodone Antagonists: naloxone | CNS | Inhibition of pain signaling | Opiates activate receptors and decrease pain signals Of people taking oral opiates primarily for low back pain, approximately 23% discontinued owing to adverse effects and 10% discontinued owing to inadequate pain relief[38] Naloxone reverses the effects of opiate overdose |
| **Substance P** Receptors: NK 1 (neurokinin l) Agonists: none are used clinically Antagonists: none are used clinically | PNS: released by nerve endings in skin, muscles, joints CNS: substantia nigra, amygdala, hypothalamus, cerebral cortex | Sensation of pain Respiratory and cardiovascular control; mood regulation; signals interpreted as pain | Levels of substance P are excessive in some pathologic pain conditions |

*AMPA*, Alpha-amino-3-hydroxy-5-methyl-4-isoxazolepropionic acid; *CNS*, central nervous system; *GABA*, gamma-aminobutyric acid; *NMDA*, N-methyl-D-aspartate; *PNS*, peripheral nervous system.

Botulinum toxin A is naturally produced by a family of bacteria and, when ingested, causes widespread paralysis by inhibiting the release of ACh at the neuromuscular junction. When small doses of botulinum toxin A are therapeutically injected directly into an overactive muscle, the local effect is muscle paralysis.[34] This paralysis lasts for up to 12 weeks and can result in improved range of motion, resting limb position, and functional movement for people with cerebral palsy, spinal cord injury, and stroke.[34,35] Botulinum toxin is also used to treat headache, arthritis, GI disorders, and chronic pain disorders.[36]

## DISORDERS OF SYNAPTIC FUNCTION

Diseases that affect the neuromuscular junction and ion channels in the central nervous system interfere with synaptic function.

### Diseases Affecting the Neuromuscular Junction

Signaling between efferent nerve terminals and muscle cells can be disrupted by disease. For example, in Lambert-Eaton syndrome, antibodies destroy voltage-gated $Ca^{2+}$ channels in the presynaptic terminal. Blockage of $Ca^{2+}$ influx into the terminal causes decreased release of neurotransmitter and decreased excitation of the muscle, leading to muscle weakness. Lambert-Eaton syndrome typically occurs in people with small cell cancers of the lung.

Another disease that affects synaptic transmission at the neuromuscular junction is *myasthenia gravis*. In this autoimmune disease, antibodies attack and destroy nicotinic receptors on muscle cells. Normal amounts of ACh are released into the cleft, but few receptors are available for binding. In myasthenia gravis, repetitive use of the muscle leads to increased weakness.

Muscles that contract frequently—eye movement and eyelid muscles, for instance—become weak, causing drooping of the eyelids and misalignment of the eyes. Other commonly affected muscles control facial expression, swallowing, proximal limb movements, and respiration. Proximal limb weakness typically causes difficulty reaching overhead, climbing stairs, and rising from a chair. Onset in women typically occurs between the ages of 20 and 30 years; in men, onset most commonly occurs between the ages of 60 and 70 years.

Drugs that inhibit the breakdown of ACh usually improve function because they increase the amount of time ACh is available to bind with remaining receptors. The autoimmune assault on ACh receptors can be countered with:
- Removal of the thymus gland, an immune organ that functions abnormally in myasthenia gravis, contributing to the damage of ACh receptors
- Immunosuppressive drugs
- Plasmapheresis (the process of removing blood from the body, centrifuging the blood to separate plasma from cells, then returning the blood cells and replacing the plasma with a plasma substitute)

These treatments produce a relatively good prognosis in myasthenia gravis; the survival rate is better than 90%. Occasionally, remissions occur in the course of the disease, but stabilization and progression are more frequent outcomes (Pathology 3-1).[39,40]

> ◎ *Clinical Pearl*
>
> Diseases that affect the neuromuscular junction generally impede the transmission of a signal by decreasing the release of neurotransmitter at the synapse or preventing the transmitter from activating the postsynaptic membrane receptor.

| **PATHOLOGY 3-1** | **MYASTHENIA GRAVIS** |
|---|---|
| Pathology | Decreased number of muscle membrane acetylcholine receptors |
| Etiology | Autoimmune |
| Speed of onset | Chronic |
| Signs and symptoms | Usually affects eye movements or eyelids first |
|    Consciousness | Normal |
|    Cognition, language, and memory | Normal |
|    Sensory | Normal |
|    Autonomic | Normal |
|    Motor | Fluctuating weakness; weakness increases with muscle use |
|    Cranial nerves | Cranial nerves are normal; however, skeletal muscles innervated by cranial nerves show fluctuating weakness (because the disorder affects the muscle membrane receptors) |
| Region affected | Peripheral |
| Demographics | Can occur at any age; women more often affected than men |
|    Incidence | 3 per 100,000 people per year[39] |
|    Lifetime prevalence | 0.4 per 1000[40] |
| Prognosis | Stable or slowly progressive; with medical treatment, >90% survival rate |

## Channelopathy

Channelopathy is a disease that involves dysfunction of ion channels. For example, genetic mutations in both voltage-gated and ligand-gated ion channels are implicated in several inherited neurologic disorders, especially in diseases that disrupt skeletal muscle coordination.[41] Channelopathies cause some cases of epilepsy[42] and migraine. Channelopathies affecting skeletal muscles cause paralysis or slow relaxation following muscle contraction.[43]

## SUMMARY

Scientific understanding of synaptic transmission has changed dramatically over the past 15 years. Researchers have discovered that multiple neurotransmitters may be released simultaneously from a single presynaptic terminal, have found new categories of molecules that act as synaptic neurotransmitters, and have begun to comprehend the role of neuromodulators. The complexity of events at the synaptic cleft leaves researchers much to discover. Because most drugs that act on the central nervous system act at the synapse, both past and future research efforts in this field are critical for understanding health and disease.

## CLINICAL NOTES

### Case 1

M.J., a 54-year-old woman, suffers from small cell cancer of the lung and exhibits generalized, progressive muscle weakness. Medical evaluation determines that M.J.'s weakness is related to a neuromuscular junction disorder consistent with Lambert-Eaton syndrome. In this syndrome, voltage-gated $Ca^{2+}$ channels in the axon terminals at the synapse between the motor neuron and the muscle are disrupted. Plasmapheresis—the process of removing blood from the body, centrifuging the blood to separate the plasma from the cells, then returning the blood cells and replacing the plasma with a plasma substitute—effectively reduces M.J.'s weakness. The benefit derived from plasmapheresis supports the hypothesis that the disease involves circulating antibodies to $Ca^{2+}$ channels in the motor axon terminals, because the circulating antibodies are removed with the plasma.

#### Questions

1. The neurotransmitter released at the synapse between the motor axon and the muscle is ACh. Why would destruction of $Ca^{2+}$ channels in the axon terminal disrupt the release of ACh from the axon terminal?
2. Would therapy be beneficial for increasing M.J.'s strength if antibodies to the $Ca^{2+}$ channel continue to circulate?

### Case 2

S.B., a 12-year-old girl, has significant gait abnormalities resulting from cerebral palsy. She walks on her toes and exhibits a scissor gait, with her legs strongly adducted with each step. S.B. has shown no significant improvements in gait with standard therapy, including exercises, gait training, and training in activities of daily living. Her physicians now want to inject a small amount of botulinum toxin into the gastrocnemius and adductor magnus muscles of both legs in an effort to reduce involuntary muscle activity and improve gait.

#### Questions

1. By what mechanism could injection of botulinum toxin reduce involuntary muscle activity?
2. At the neuromuscular junction, ACh acts via a ligand-gated receptor. Is the action of ACh on the nicotinic, ligand-gated receptor the same as its action on the muscarinic, G-protein–mediated receptor?

## REVIEW QUESTIONS

1. What is the difference between postsynaptic inhibition and presynaptic inhibition? Which one results in a decreased release of neurotransmitter?
2. The release of neurotransmitter from synaptic vesicles is dependent on the influx of what ion into the presynaptic terminal?
3. What is an EPSP?
4. Does direct activation of a membrane ion channel by a neurotransmitter or indirect activation via second-messenger systems result in faster generation of a synaptic potential?
5. How long do the effects of neurotransmitter binding persist? How long do the effects of neuromodulator binding persist?
6. How does binding of a neurotransmitter to the receptor of a ligand-gated ion channel cause the channel to open?
7. How do G-proteins contribute to a cascade of cellular events?
8. Is the effect of a neurotransmitter determined by the transmitter itself or by the type of receptor?
9. When glutamate binds to a ligand-gated receptor, what happens?
10. Which neurotransmitter is involved in feelings of pleasure and reward and in the disorders schizophrenia and Parkinson's disease?
11. What are the actions of substance P?
12. What is the role of endogenous opioid peptides?
13. What transmitter and which type of receptor are essential for long-term potentiation?
14. Is the number of receptors on the cell membrane of a neuron constant throughout the life of the neuron?

## References

1. Trikha S, Lee EC, Jeremic AM: Cell secretion: current structural and biochemical insights. *Sci World J* 10:2054–2069, 2010.
2. Greengard P: The neurobiology of slow synaptic transmission. *Science* 294:1024–1030, 2001.
3. Pepeu G, Giovannini MG: Changes in acetylcholine extracellular levels during cognitive processes. *Learn Mem* 11:21–27, 2004.
4. Aston-Jones G, Cohen JD: An integrative theory of locus coeruleus-norepinephrine function: adaptive gain and optimal performance. *Annu Rev Neurosci* 28:403–450, 2005.
5. Niswender CM, Conn PJ: Metabotropic glutamate receptors: physiology, pharmacology, and disease. *Annu Rev Pharmacol Toxicol* 50:295–322, 2010.
6. Dong XX, Wang Y, Qin ZH: Molecular mechanisms of excitotoxicity and their relevance to pathogenesis of neurodegenerative diseases. *Acta Pharmacol Sin* 30:379–387, 2009.
7. Mailman RB, Murthy V: Third generation antipsychotic drugs: partial agonism or receptor functional selectivity? *Curr Pharm Des* 16:488–501, 2010.
8. Cosgrove KP: Imaging receptor changes in human drug abusers. *Curr Top Behav Neurosci* 3:199–217, 2010.
9. Chen JC, Chen PC, Chiang YC: Molecular mechanisms of psychostimulant addition. *Chang Gung Med J* 32:148–154, 2009.
10. Ravindran LN, Stein MB: The pharmacological treatment of anxiety disorders: a review of progress. *J Clin Psychiatry* 71:839–854, 2010.
11. Krystal JH, Neumeister A: Noradrenergic and serotonergic mechanisms in the neurobiology of posttraumatic stress disorder and resilience. *Brain Res* 1293:13–23, 2009.
12. Bremner JD, Innis RB, Salomon RM, et al: Positron emission tomography measurement of cerebral metabolic correlates of yohimbine administration in combat-related posttraumatic stress disorder. *Arch Gen Psychiatry* 54:246–254, 1997.
13. Aanhet Rot M, Mathew SJ, Charney DS: Neurobiological mechanisms in major depressive disorder. *CMAJ* 180:305–313, 2009.
14. Goutagny R, Verret L, Fort P, et al: Posterior hypothalamus and regulation of vigilance states. *Arch Ital Biol* 142:487–500, 2004.
15. Zamponi GW, Lewis RJ, Todorovic SM, et al: Role of voltage-gated calcium channels in ascending pain pathways. *Brain Res Rev* 60:84–89, 2009.
16. Dragos D, Tranasescu MD: The effect of stress on the defense systems. *J Med Life* 3:10–18, 2010.
17. Recober A, Goadsby PJ: Calcitonin gene-related peptide: a molecular link between obesity and migraine? *Drug News Perspect* 23:112–117, 2010.
18. Mitsukawa K, Lu X, Bartfai T: Galanin, galanin receptors, and drug targets. *Cell Mol Life Sci* 65:1796–1805, 2008.
19. Ahren B, Pacini G, Wynick D, et al: Loss-of-function mutation of the galanin gene is associated with perturbed islet function in mice. *Endocrinology* 124:3190–3196, 2004.
20. Chuang YC: Mitochondrial dysfunction and oxidative stress in seizure-induced neuronal cell death. *Acta Neurol Taiwan* 19:3–15, 2010.
21. Pin JP, Comps-Agrar L, Maurel D, et al: G-protein-coupled receptor oligomers: two or more for what? Lessons from mGlu and GABAB receptors. *J Physiol* 587:5337–5344, 2009.
22. Pin JP, Galvez T, Prezeau L: Evolution, structure, and activation mechanism of family 3/C G-protein-coupled receptors. *Pharmacol Ther* 98:325–354, 2003.
23. Manning G, Whyte DB, Martinez R, et al: The protein kinase complement of the human genome. *Science* 298:1912–1934, 2002.

24. Sobel RA: Ephrin A receptors and ligands in lesions and normal-appearing white matter in multiple sclerosis. *Brain Pathol* 15:35–45, 2005.
25. Kwon OB, Longart M, Vullhorst D, et al: Neuregulin-1 reverses long-term potentiation at CA1 hippocampal synapses. *J Neurosci* 25:9378–9383, 2005.
26. Mutoh T, Tachi M, Yano S, et al: Impairment of the Trk-neurotrophin receptor by the serum of a patient with subacute sensory neuropathy. *Arch Neurol* 62:1612–1615, 2005.
27. Wu H, Xiong WC, Mei L: To build a synapse: signaling pathways in neuromuscular junction assembly. *Development* 137:1017–1033, 2010.
28. Placzek AN, Zhang TA, Dani JA: Nicotinic mechanisms influencing synaptic plasticity in the hippocampus. *Acta Pharmacol Sin* 30:752–760, 2009.
29. Buckingham SD, Jones AK, Brown LA, et al: Nicotinic acetylcholine receptor signaling: roles in Alzheimer's disease and amyloid neuroprotection. *Pharmacol Rev* 61:39–61, 2009.
30. Shideler KK, Yan J: M1 muscarinic receptor for the development of auditory cortical function. *Mol Brain* 3:29, 2010.
31. Traynelis SF, Wollmuth LP, McBain CJ, et al: Glutamate receptor ion channels: structure, regulation, and function. *Pharmacol Rev* 62:405–496, 2010.
32. Yashiro K, Philpot BD: Regulation of NMDA receptor subunit expression and its implications for LTD, LTP, and metaplasticity. *Neuropharmacology* 55:1081–1094, 2008.
33. Monaghan DT, Jane DE: Pharmacology of NMDA receptors. In Van Dongen AM, editor: *Biology of the NMDA receptor*, Boca Raton, Fla, 2009, CRC Press.
34. Olvey EL, Armstrong EP, Grizzle AJ: Contemporary pharmacologic treatments for spasticity of the upper limb after stroke: a systemic review. *Clin Ther* 32:2282–2303, 2010.
35. Balbaloglu O, Basaran A, Ayoglu H: Functional outcomes of multilevel botulinum toxin and comprehensive rehabilitation in cerebral palsy. *J Child Neurol* 26:482–487, 2011.
36. Brashear A: Botulinum toxin type A: exploring new indications. *Drugs Today* 46:671–682, 2010.
37. Beaulieu JM, Gainetdinov RR: The physiology, signaling, and pharmacology of dopamine receptors. *Pharmacol Rev* 63:182–217, 2011.
38. Noble M, Treadwell JR, Tregear SJ, et al: Long-term opioid management for chronic noncancer pain. *Cochrane Database Syst Rev* (1):CD006605, 2010.
39. McGrogan A, Sneddon S, de Vries CS: The incidence of myasthenia gravis: a systematic literature review. *Neuroepidemiology* 34:171–183, 2010.
40. MacDonald BK, Cockerell OC, Sander JW, et al: The incidence and lifetime prevalence of neurological disorders in a prospective community-based study in the UK (see comments). *Brain* 123:665–676, 2000.
41. Lory P, Mezghrani A: Calcium channelopathies in inherited neurological disorders: relevance to drug screening for acquired channel disorders. *IDrugs* 13:467–471, 2010.
42. Mantegazza M, Rusconi R, Scalmani P, et al: Epileptogenic ion channel mutations: from bedside to bench and, hopefully, back again. *Epilepsy Res* 92:1–29, 2010.
43. Ryan DP, Ptácek LJ: Episodic neurological channelopathies. *Neuron* 68:282–292, 2010.

# 4 Neuroplasticity

**Catherine Siengsukon, PT, PhD**

## Chapter Outline

**Habituation**

**Experience-Dependent Plasticity: Learning and Memory**
Long-Term Potentiation and Depression
Transcranial Magnetic Stimulation
Astrocytes Contribute to Experience-Dependent Plasticity

**Cellular Recovery From Injury**
Axonal Injury
*Axonal Injury in the Periphery*
*Axonal Injury in the Central Nervous System*
Synaptic Changes Following Injury
Functional Reorganization of the Cerebral Cortex
Activity-Related Changes in Neurotransmitter Release
Neurogenesis

**Metabolic Effects of Brain Injury**

**Effects of Rehabilitation on Plasticity**

**Summary**

**Clinical Notes**

**Review Questions**

**References**

Previous versions of this chapter were written by Anne Burleigh-Jacobs (1st edition) and Lisa Stehno-Bittel (2nd and 3rd editions).

Our experiences and our states of health or disease continuously create and break neuronal communication sites. *Neuroplasticity* is the ability of neurons to change their function, chemical profile (quantities and types of neurotransmitters produced), or structure.[1] Neuroplasticity is involved in learning and creation of new memories and is essential for recovery from damage to the central nervous system (CNS). By definition, neuroplasticity lasts longer than a few seconds and is not periodic.

Researchers have demonstrated neuroplasticity by studying animals raised in environments with toys and challenging obstacles. These animals develop more dendritic branching and a greater number of synapses per neuron, and they have higher gene expression for certain protein products in the brain, than animals raised without toys and challenging obstacles.[2]

*Neuroplasticity* is a general term used to encompass the following mechanisms:

- Habituation
- Experience-dependent plasticity: learning and memory
- Cellular recovery after injury

## HABITUATION

*Habituation,* one of the simplest forms of neuroplasticity and a type of nonassociative learning, is a decrease in response to a repeated, benign stimulus. In studies of animal posture and locomotion performed in the late 1800s, the pioneering neuroscientist Charles Sherrington observed that certain reflexive behaviors, such as withdrawing a limb from a mildly painful stimulus, ceased after several repetitions of the same stimulus. Sherrington proposed that the decreased responsiveness resulted from a functional decrease in the synaptic effectiveness of stimulated pathways to the motor neuron.[3] Later studies confirmed that habituation of the withdrawal reflex is due to a decrease in synaptic activity between sensory neurons and interneurons. The cellular mechanisms responsible for habituation are not completely understood. However, with habituation there is a decrease in the release of excitatory neurotransmitters, including glutamate, and perhaps a decrease in free intracellular $Ca^{2+}$. After a period of rest in which the stimulus is no longer applied, the effects of habituation are no longer present or are partially resolved, and behavior can be elicited in response to sensory stimuli.

However, with prolonged repetition of stimulation, more permanent structural changes occur: the number of synapses decreases. For example, people with tinnitus (ringing in the ear) can use hearing aids to habituate to the ringing over a prolonged period of time.[4] Habituation is thought to allow other types of learning to occur by letting people pay attention to important stimulation while tuning out stimulation that is less important.[5] For example, it would be very difficult to listen to a lecture while paying attention to the feel of the shirt on your back.

In occupational and physical therapy, the term *habituation* is applied to techniques and exercises intended to decrease the neural response to a stimulus. For example, some children are extremely reactive to stimulation on their skin. Therapists treat this abnormal sensitivity, called *tactile defensiveness,* by gently stimulating the child's skin, then gradually increasing the intensity of stimulation. This is intended to achieve habituation to the tactile stimulation. In people with specific types of vestibular disorders, movements that induce dizziness and nausea are repeatedly performed, again with the purpose of achieving habituation to the movements.

> ### ◎ *Clinical Pearl*
>
> Short-term changes in neurotransmitter release and postsynaptic receptor sensitivity can result in a decreased response to specific, repetitive stimuli.

## EXPERIENCE-DEPENDENT PLASTICITY: LEARNING AND MEMORY

Unlike the short-term, reversible effects of habituation, learning and memory require experience-dependent plasticity (also referred to as *use-dependent* or *activity-dependent plasticity*). This complex process involves persistent, long-lasting changes in the strength of synapses between neurons and within neural networks.[6] Functional magnetic resonance imaging (fMRI) reveals that during the initial phases of motor learning, large and diffuse regions of the brain are active. With repetition of a task, the number of active regions in the brain is reduced. Eventually, when a motor task has been learned, only small, distinct regions of the brain show increased activity during performance of the task.[7] For example, learning to play a musical instrument requires numerous brain regions. As skill increases, fewer areas are activated because less attention is required, motor control is optimized, and only brain areas required to perform the task efficiently are active. Eventually, playing the instrument requires only a few small, specific regions.[8] Specific brain areas involved in playing the instrument show increased but focal activity. Because the fingers of the musician receive more sensory information than is received by fingers in nonmusicians, the finger representation area in the brain enlarges.

Experience-dependent plasticity requires the synthesis of new proteins, the growth of new synapses, and the modification of existing synapses. With repetition of a specific stimulus or the pairing of presynaptic and postsynaptic firing, synthesis and activation of proteins alter the excitability of the neuron and promote or inhibit the growth of new synapses, especially at dendritic spines.[6]

Several mechanisms of experience-dependent plasticity occur, depending on the type of synapse and location involved. These mechanisms include:

- Plasticity of the intrinsic excitability of neurons by functional changes in ion channels
- Plasticity at inhibitory GABAergic synapses
- Homeostatic plasticity to stabilize neural circuits[9]
- Long-term potentiation
- Long-term depression

Long-term potentiation and depression are discussed further in the following section.

### Long-Term Potentiation and Depression

The best-known types of plasticity in learning and memory formation are *long-term potentiation* (LTP) and *long-term*

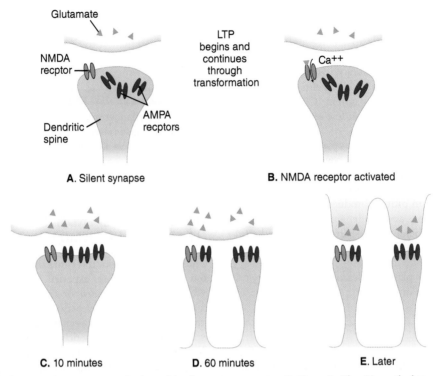

**Fig. 4-1 Structural changes in a synapse induced by long-term potentiation. A,** The *N*-methyl-D-aspartate (NMDA) receptor crosses the membrane, allowing cations to pass through either direction. The receptor binds glutamate *(green)*. The bud-like shape of the postsynaptic membrane represents a dendritic spine. Dendritic spines are protrusions on dendrites that are preferential sites of synapses. This is a silent synapse, with alpha-amino-3-hydroxy-5-methyl-4-isoxazolepropionic acid (AMPA) receptors located in the cytoplasm, not in the cell membrane. **B,** Then, long-term potentiation is initiated by the activity of NMDA receptors. **C,** In response to increased $Ca^{2+}$ from NMDA receptor activity, AMPA receptors are inserted into the cell membrane. **D,** With continued stimulation, the postsynaptic membrane generates a new dendritic spine. **E,** Finally, structural changes occur in the presynaptic cell, producing a new synapse.
*(Modified with permission from Luscher C, Nicoll RA, Malenka RC, Muller D: Synaptic plasticity and dynamic modulation of the postsynaptic membrane. Nat Neurosci 3:547, 2000.)*

*depression* (LTD) of excitatory glutamatergic synapses. LTP and LTD can occur presynaptically through changes in neurotransmitter release, or postsynaptically through changes in receptor density and efficiency. Different forms of LTP and LTD can occur simultaneously, depending on the type and location of the synapse.[1]

The mechanism of LTP is the conversion of *silent synapses* to active synapses (Figure 4-1). Silent synapses lack functional glutamate alpha-amino-3-hydroxy-5-methyl-4-isoxazolepropionic acid (AMPA) receptors. Because these synapses lack functional AMPA receptors, they are inactive under normal conditions. Silent synapses can be converted to active synapses by highly correlated presynaptic and postsynaptic firing. A set of mobile AMPA receptors cycles between the cytoplasm and the synaptic membrane.[10] Silent synapses become active when mobile AMPA receptors are inserted into the synaptic membrane because glutamate in the synaptic cleft can bind to the exposed receptors. LTD is the conversion of an active synapse to a silent synapse by the removal of AMPA receptors from the membrane into the cytoplasm.[10] LTD is illustrated in Figure 4-2.

The morphology, or shape, of the postsynaptic membrane can change with LTP.[11-13] The bud-like shape on the postsynaptic membrane is a dendritic spine, a preferential site for synapse formation. Morphologic remodeling of the synaptic membrane and functional changes in synaptic strength are probably related. First, $Ca^{2+}$ enters the postsynaptic cell through channels associated with *N*-methyl-D-aspartate (NMDA) glutamate receptors, resulting in phosphorylation of AMPA receptors and insertion of AMPA receptors into the membrane.[11] Subsequently, the postsynaptic membrane remodels, generating a new dendritic spine. For a neuron to structurally change, genetic alterations must occur in the cell during the learning process. Calcium is a predominant regulator of gene activity; this is important because the nucleus itself contains $Ca^{2+}$ ion channels,[14] which may regulate transport across the nuclear membrane.[15] This localization of calcium to the nucleus can "turn on" particular genes important in neuronal function.[16] Thus, changes in calcium within the cell are likely to be one of the signals leading to altered gene regulation during the learning process.[17]

LTP and LTD have been intensively studied in the hippocampus and cortex.[6,9] The hippocampus, in the temporal lobe,

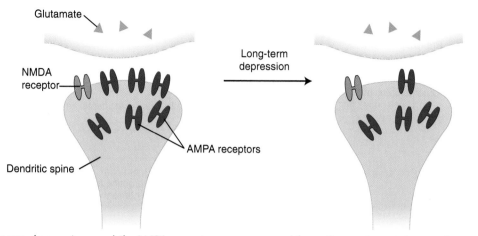

**Fig. 4-2** In long-term depression, mobile AMPA receptors are removed from the postsynaptic membrane, making the postsynaptic membrane less likely to be depolarized when glutamate is released from the presynaptic neuron.

is essential for processing memories that can be easily verbalized. For example, the hippocampus is important in remembering names and events (declarative memory), but not in remembering how to perform motor acts like riding a bicycle (procedural memory). LTP and depression occur in motor, somatosensory, visual, and auditory cortices and in the cerebellum, contributing to motor, somatosensory, visual, and auditory learning.[6,10,18]

Experience-dependent plasticity is essential for neural recovery following an injury or insult. Additionally, plasticity may have harmful consequences; it may contribute to the development of chronic pain syndromes, including low back pain (see Chapter 8).

## Transcranial Magnetic Stimulation

Transcranial magnetic stimulation (TMS) to the motor cortex and other brain areas involved in motor learning can enhance or inhibit motor learning and memory formation, depending on the frequency and the experimental protocol used.[19-21] For example, TMS of the primary motor cortex enhances the duration of motor memory,[22] and stimulation of the dorsal premotor cortex enhances motor memory consolidation.[23] TMS can also be used to induce a transient "virtual lesion" to assess the impact that different brain areas have on motor learning. For example, inhibitory TMS applied to the primary somatosensory cortex impairs motor learning.[24] Magnetic stimulation of the brain is thought to induce synaptic plasticity via LTP- or LTD-type mechanisms.

## Astrocytes Contribute to Experience-Dependent Plasticity

Astrocytes, a type of glia cell discussed in Chapter 2, play a critical role in brain and spinal cord plasticity. Communication between astrocytes and neurons occurs via the release of neurotransmitter by the neuron, which stimulates the release of gliotransmitters by the astrocyte. Gliotransmitters modulate neuronal activity and synaptic transmission, although the mechanisms of modulation appear complex and are not well understood.[25] Astrocytes likely influence synaptic plasticity by modulating neurotransmitter release and receptor expression at the postsynaptic membrane.[26] Astrocytes may also be important for new synapse formation following stroke.[27]

> **◎ Clinical Pearl**
>
> Long-term changes, including synthesis of new proteins and growth of new synapses, result in a maintained response and memory of specific, repetitive stimuli.

## CELLULAR RECOVERY FROM INJURY

Injuries that damage or sever axons cause degeneration but may not result in cell death. Some neurons have the ability to regenerate the axon. In contrast to injury to the axon, injuries that destroy the cell body of a neuron invariably lead to death of the cell. When a neuron dies, the nervous system promotes recovery by altering specific synapses, functionally reorganizing the CNS, and changing neurotransmitter release in response to neural activity. These processes are described in greater detail in the following section.

### Axonal Injury

When an axon in the peripheral or central nervous system is severed, the part connected to the cell body is referred to as the *proximal segment*, and the part isolated from the cell body is called the *distal segment*. Immediately after injury, the cytoplasm leaks out of the cut ends, and the segments retract away from each other. Once isolated from the cell body, the distal segment of the axon undergoes a process called *wallerian degeneration* (Figure 4-3). When the distal segment of an axon degenerates, the myelin sheath pulls away from that

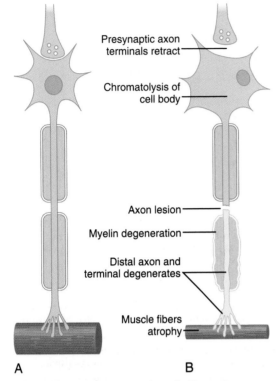

A                              B

**Fig. 4-3 Wallerian degeneration. A,** Normal synapses before an axon is severed. **B,** Degeneration following severance of an axon. Degeneration following axonal injury involves several changes: (1) the axon terminal degenerates, (2) myelin breaks down and forms debris, and (3) the cell body undergoes metabolic changes. Subsequently, (4) presynaptic terminals retract from the dying cell body, and (5) postsynaptic cells degenerate. In this illustration, the postsynaptic cell is a muscle cell.

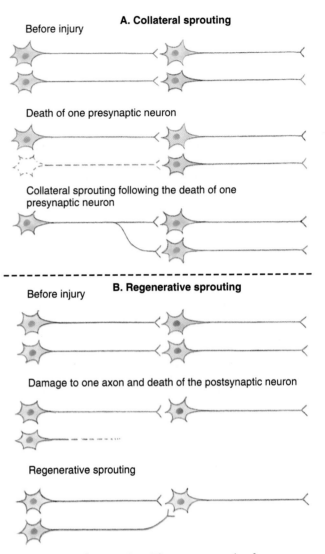

**Fig. 4-4 Axonal sprouting.** The new growth of axons following injury involves two types of sprouting: collateral sprouting **(A),** in which a denervated neuron attracts side sprouts from nearby undamaged axons, and regenerative sprouting **(B),** in which the injured axon issues side sprouts to form new synapses with undamaged neurons.

segment. The axon swells and breaks into shorter segments. The terminals rapidly degenerate, and their loss is followed by death of the entire distal segment. Glial cells scavenge the area, cleaning up debris from the degeneration. In addition to axonal degeneration, the associated cell body undergoes degenerative changes called *central chromatolysis*, which occasionally leads to cell death. If a postsynaptic cell loses most of its synaptic inputs owing to damage to the presynaptic neurons, the postsynaptic cell degenerates and may die.

### Axonal Injury in the Periphery

Axon severance injuries frequently occur in the peripheral nervous system, where the axons extend a long distance and are not protected by the vertebral column or skull. Axons may be severed by injuries from sharp objects (knives, machinery) or by extreme stretch that pulls the axon apart.

The growth of a new branch of an intact axon or the regrowth of damaged axons is called *sprouting*. Sprouting takes two forms: collateral and regenerative (Figure 4-4). Collateral sprouting occurs when a denervated target is reinnervated by branches of intact axons of neighboring neurons. Regenerative sprouting occurs when an axon and its target cell (a neuron, muscle, or gland) have been damaged. The injured axon sends out side sprouts to a new target. Functional regeneration of axons occurs

more frequently in the peripheral system than in the CNS owing to the production of nerve growth factor (NGF) by Schwann cells, the effective clearing of debris, and the formation of bands of Büngner to guide axonal regrowth to the target. Recovery is slow, with approximately 1 mm of growth per day, or about 1 inch of recovery per month. Of clinical importance, exercise begun 5 days after a peripheral nerve lesion increases axonal regeneration and reinnervation of muscle.[28]

Peripheral axon sprouting can cause problems when an inappropriate target is innervated. For example, after peripheral nerve injury, motor axons may innervate different muscles than previously, resulting in unintended movements when the neurons fire.[29] These unintended movements, called *synkinesis,* may be short-lived, as the affected individual relearns muscle control, or may require treatment including botulinum toxin injection, biofeedback, neuromuscular re-education, or surgical correction.[30] Similarly, in the sensory systems, innervation of sensory receptors by axons that previously innervated a different type of sensory receptor can cause confusion of sensory modalities.

---

### ◎ *Clinical Pearl*

Damaged axons of peripheral neurons can recover from injury, and targets deprived of input from damaged axons can attract new inputs to maintain nervous system function.

---

## Axonal Injury in the Central Nervous System

The same processes that follow peripheral axonal injury, including axonal retraction, wallerian degeneration, and central chromatolysis, also occur following damage to the CNS, including spinal cord injury (SCI) and traumatic brain injury (TBI). Although axonal tearing and breakage occur following SCI or TBI, most of the damage evolves hours and days following the initial injury owing to a cascade of cellular events.[31] Damage to the white fiber tracts following SCI or TBI leads to increased permeability of the axons and dysregulation of $Na^+$-$Ca^{2+}$ channels, causing an influx of $Ca^{2+}$. The influx of $Ca^{2+}$ leads to disruption of axonal transport and accumulation of intra-axonal components. This buildup causes the axons to swell until they break at the site of damage. The proximal axon retracts, forming an axonal retraction ball. This eventually leads to central chromatolysis of the cell body and wallerian degeneration of the distal axon.[32,33]

Following SCI, the extent of motor and sensory deficits largely depends on the degree of damage to white fiber tracts in the spinal cord, as well as the vertebral level at which damage occurs. SCI can occur for many reasons and may vary in severity from a contusion to complete severing of the spinal cord.

The inertial forces of a TBI cause widespread tearing and stretching of axons within the brain. The initial damage and the resultant cascade of cellular events lead to *diffuse axonal injury* and widespread disconnection between neurons. Although the initial brain injury is detrimental, the subsequent widespread disconnection can lead to devastating functional consequences.[32]

Functional axon regeneration does not occur in CNS axons. Development of glial scars and limited expression or complete absence of NGF prevents axonal regeneration in the brain and spinal cord. Glial scars, formed by astrocytes and microglia, physically block axonal regeneration and release many different growth-inhibiting factors, including neurite outgrowth inhibitor (Nogo). Nogo is expressed in oligodendrocytes but not in Schwann cells. The exact role of Nogo in halting recovery after injury is unclear, although progress has been made in identifying receptors and components of the signaling pathway.[34] When monkeys with a spinal cord lesion were infused with antibodies to reduce the activity of Nogo, the corticospinal tract underwent sprouting, and the monkeys demonstrated improved functional use of their upper extremity.[35] Furthermore, when rats received a Nogo inhibitor and motor training following stroke, motor recovery was hastened compared with motor training alone.[36] Drugs currently in development block the effects of Nogo and other growth inhibitors—and could become useful in CNS recovery—by targeting inhibitory proteins, blocking receptor-binding sites, or inhibiting the second-messenger signaling cascade.[37] As discussed in Chapter 2, stem cells are another therapeutic agent under investigation to promote regeneration of the CNS. Transplantation of stem cells into the brain of mice resulted in myelination of axons and reduced the activity of glial cells.[38] Stem cells may provide another method of treating white matter injuries such as SCI and demyelinating diseases such as MS.

## Synaptic Changes Following Injury

Following CNS injury, the body uses several mechanisms to overcome damage. Synaptic mechanisms include recovery of synaptic effectiveness, denervation hypersensitivity, synaptic hypereffectiveness, and unmasking of silent synapses (Figure 4-5). After injury, local edema may compress the cell body or axon of a presynaptic neuron, producing focal ischemia and interfering with microvascular function.[39] The reduced blood flow interferes with neural function, including synthesis and transport of neurotransmitters, causing some synapses to become inactive. Once edema has resolved, relief of pressure on the presynaptic neuron restores normal cellular function, allowing the synthesis and transport of neurotransmitters to resume and *synaptic effectiveness* to return. *Denervation hypersensitivity* occurs when presynaptic axon terminals are destroyed and new receptor sites develop on the postsynaptic membrane in response to the reduction in neurotransmitter released. When neurotransmitters are released from other nearby axons, an increased or hypersensitive response occurs owing to the additional receptor sites on the postsynaptic membrane.[40] *Synaptic hypereffectiveness* occurs when only some branches of a presynaptic axon are destroyed. The remaining axon branches receive all of the neurotransmitter that would normally be shared among the terminals, resulting in the release of larger than normal amounts of transmitter onto postsynaptic receptors. Another synaptic change is *unmasking (disinhibition) of silent synapses.* In the normal nervous system, many synapses seem to be unused unless injury to other pathways results in their activation.[41,42]

Researchers are identifying the mechanisms responsible for these synaptic changes. Many of the same mechanisms responsible for brain plasticity during learning are involved in the recovery period following neuronal injury. These include NMDA receptor activity and changes in the levels of $Ca^{2+}$ ions and of the neurotransmitter substance P.[43] Transmission by nitric oxide, the diffusible neuromodulator discussed in Chapter 3, has also been implicated in modulation of synaptic function.[44]

## Functional Reorganization of the Cerebral Cortex

In the adult brain, cortical areas routinely adjust the way they process information. Cortical areas also retain the ability to develop new functions. Changes at individual synapses reorganize the brain, which can have significant functional consequences. Researchers map functional areas of the cerebral cortex by recording neuron activity in response to sensory stimulation or during active muscle contractions. Cortical representation

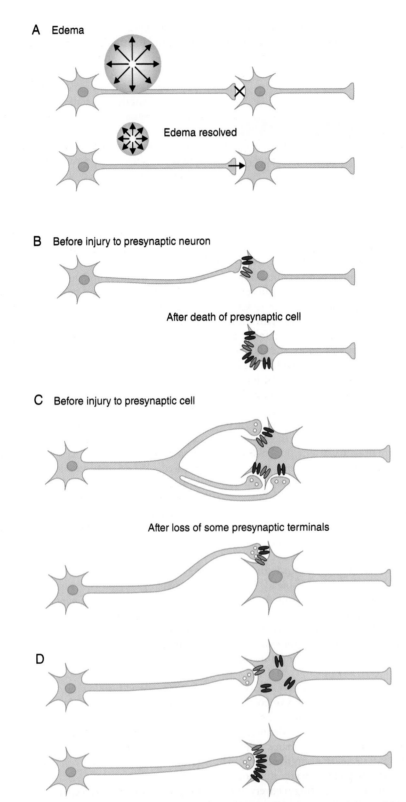

**Fig. 4-5  Synaptic changes following injury. A,** Recovery of synaptic effectiveness occurs with the reduction in local edema that interfered with action potential conduction. **B,** Denervation hypersensitivity occurs after destruction of presynaptic neurons deprives postsynaptic neurons of an adequate supply of neurotransmitter. The postsynaptic neurons develop new receptors at the remaining terminals. **C,** Synaptic hypereffectiveness occurs after some presynaptic terminals are lost. Neurotransmitter accumulates in the undamaged axon terminals, resulting in excessive release of transmitter at the remaining terminals. **D,** Unmasking of a silent synapse. When a synapse is silent, only *N*-methyl-D-aspartate (NMDA) receptors are present on the postsynaptic membrane, and synaptic transmission does not occur. The synapse becomes unmasked when alpha-amino-3-hydroxy-5-methyl-4-isoxazolepropionic acid (AMPA) receptors move into the postsynaptic membrane and the synapse becomes active.

areas, called *cortical maps* or homunculus, can be modified by sensory input, experience, learning, peripheral injury, or brain injury. If a person regularly performs a skilled motor task, the cortical representation of that area will be enlarged. For example, proficient string instrument players have an enlarged area in the somatosensory cortex representing fingers of the left hand caused by years of increased sensory stimulation, while their right hands have only an average finger map.[45]

TMS, positron emission tomography (PET), and fMRI of the cortex indicate reassignment of neuron function in adults following nervous system injury. Using fMRI to map the somatosensory cortex in individuals with complete SCI demonstrates that leg representation is reorganized into hand representation. Furthermore, the intensity of pain that seems to arise below the lesion following SCI is significantly correlated with the amount of reorganization in the somatosensory cortex.[46] Cortical reorganization also occurs following amputation; this is discussed in Chapter 8.

Cortical plasticity and reorganization are likely mechanisms driving functional recovery following stroke.[47] After a cortical stroke, fMRI and PET studies show increased bilateral sensorimotor cortex activity as well as increased bilateral activity in other cortical areas. As time and recovery progress, a shift in brain activity to a more normal lateralized pattern is observed.[48,49] Individuals with stroke experience reorganization of the sensorimotor cortex representation into surrounding motor areas. This reorganization can progress over 2 years.[50]

fMRI shows significant brain reorganization in patients who develop hand paresis following surgery for brain tumor.[51] Figure 4-6 shows changes in the fMRI before and after surgery. Preoperatively, the motor cortex on the right side of the image *(A)* was the major area activated, but after resection of the tumor, the same task was accomplished with activation in multiple areas of the brain, including the ipsilateral side *(B)*.

Brain reorganization has also been demonstrated in people with deafness. Individuals with congenital deafness have enhanced peripheral vision to moving stimuli, compared with hearing subjects.[52] Although cochlear implants placed earlier in life activate cortical areas normally associated with auditory input, cochlear implants placed after 7 years of age activate cortical areas not normally associated with auditory input, indicating cortical reorganization due to lack of auditory sensory input to the auditory cortex.[53] People with blindness also experience brain reorganization. For example, fMRI studies show that individuals with blindness use a visual area of the cortex when reading Braille[54] or performing a memory task.[55]

Functional reorganization after nerve injury is probably also a factor in some chronic pain syndromes, in which pain persists despite apparent healing of the precipitating injury. This type of plasticity is discussed in Chapter 8.

A person's genetic makeup influences the ability of the cortex to reorganize and undergo plasticity. Individuals with a variation of the brain-derived neurotrophic factor (BDNF) gene, which is important for CNS plasticity and repair, displayed decreased motor map reorganization following training.[56] Individuals with a BDNF variation also demonstrated altered patterns of brain activity associated with reduced learning of a motor task.[57] Genes may influence recovery following brain injury or stroke. Individuals with the variant BDNF gene had poorer recovery following subarachnoid hemorrhage.[58] Researchers are beginning to understand how genetics influences recovery following CNS injury and possible therapeutic interventions.

Although nervous system plasticity research is in its infancy, researchers are beginning to explain mechanisms of learning and recovery from injury. Plasticity allows for recovery from nervous system injury; however, active movement is crucial for optimizing motor recovery.

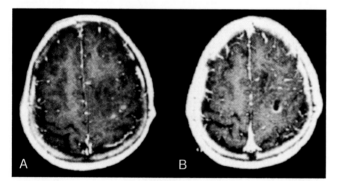

**Fig. 4-6** A functional magnetic resonance image (fMRI) illustrates changes in brain activity during finger and thumb movement before and after surgery to remove a brain tumor. **A,** Before surgery, hand movement was normal, and the primary motor area of the cerebral cortex was most active during movement. **B,** After surgery, the hand was paretic, and activity in the primary motor area of the cerebral cortex decreased. However, activity in other motor areas of the cerebral cortex increased post surgery. *(From Reinges MH, Krings T, Rohde V, et al: Prospective demonstration of short-term motor plasticity following acquired central paresis. Neuroimage 24:1252, 2005.)*

> **◎ Clinical Pearl**
>
> Cortical areas routinely adjust to changes in sensory input and develop new functions dependent on required motor output.

### Activity-Related Changes in Neurotransmitter Release

Neuronal activity regulates neurotransmitter production and release. Repeated stimulation of somatosensory pathways can cause increases in inhibitory neurotransmitters, decreasing the sensory cortex response to overstimulation. Understimulation can have the opposite effect, causing the cortex to be more responsive to weak sensory inputs.[59,60] Improved understanding of cellular mechanisms involved in plasticity may lead to improved clinical rehabilitation of peripheral and CNS disorders in both children and adults.

One potentially beneficial treatment of neurochemical disorders uses genetic manipulation to influence neuroplasticity. Researchers are designing procedures to genetically modify existing neurons, so the neurons can make and secrete chemicals that are deficient in the brain. Laboratory studies have shown that transfer of a gene for NGF into neurons that secrete the neurotransmitter dopamine can protect those neurons from degenerative changes.[61] Furthermore, increased levels of NGF and other neurotropic factors may protect neurons by promoting neuron survival, resistance to injury, and plasticity.[61] Preliminary clinical trials are under way to assess the use of gene therapy to treat various neurologic disorders, including stroke, Alzheimer's disease, Parkinson's disease, Huntington's disease, and amyotrophic lateral sclerosis (ALS).[62]

## Neurogenesis

As discussed in Chapter 2, stem cells in the adult human brain are capable of creating new neurons. Stem cells are suspected to be involved in brain remodeling following neurologic injury, including stroke, TBI, and neurodegenerative disease.[63] Neural precursor cells migrate toward the ischemic area following stroke.[64] Many precursor cells that arrive near the ischemic area do not survive, possibly owing to inflammation present.[63] Researchers are intently examining how and why neurogenesis occurs, what drives neural precursor cells to their target location, how to create a conducive environment for them to survive once they reach their target, and whether neural precursor cells can be used for treatment for neurologic injury and neurodegenerative disease. Neurogenesis is an exciting avenue for the discovery of novel therapies to treat brain injury or disease.

## METABOLIC EFFECTS OF BRAIN INJURY

When the brain suffers a stroke or traumatic injury, neurons deprived of oxygen for a prolonged period die and do not regenerate. This damage is not always limited to directly affected neurons. *Excitotoxicity* (cell death caused by overexcitation of neurons) may add more damage. Oxygen-deprived neurons release large quantities of glutamate, an excitatory neurotransmitter, from their axon terminals.[65] Excessive glutamate kills postsynaptic neurons that receive particularly high concentrations. Glutamate at normal concentrations is crucial for CNS function; however, at excessive concentrations, glutamate is toxic to neurons.

The processes involved in excitotoxicity are diagrammed in Figure 4-7. First, glutamate binds persistently to the NMDA-type glutamate receptor in the cell membrane.[66] Stimulation of this receptor results in an influx of $Ca^{2+}$ into the cell and indirectly facilitates the release of internal $Ca^{2+}$ stores. An influx of $Na^+$ into the cell results in further stimulation of NMDA receptors and additional influx of $Ca^{2+}$ into the cell.[67] Also, channels that are permeable to $Ca^{2+}$ open owing to injury.[68] With the increase in $Ca^{2+}$ inside the cell, more $K^+$ diffuses out of the cell, requiring increased glycolysis to provide energy for the $Na^+$-$K^+$ pump to actively transport $K^+$ into the cell. Together, increased glycolysis and increased $Ca^{2+}$ lead to several destructive consequences for neurons:

- Increased glycolysis liberates excessive amounts of lactic acid, lowering the intracellular pH and resulting in acidosis that can break down the cell membrane.

- High intracellular $Ca^{2+}$ levels activate $Ca^{2+}$-dependent digestive enzymes called *proteases*. These activated proteases break down cellular proteins.
- $Ca^{2+}$ activates protein enzymes that liberate arachidonic acid, producing substances that cause cell inflammation and produce oxygen free radicals. Oxygen free radicals are charged oxygen particles detrimental to mitochondrial functions of the cell. Oxidative stress also results in increased production of nitric oxide (NO), which causes further damage to the neuron.
- An influx of water associated with the ionic influx causes cell edema.

Ultimately, these cellular events lead to cell death and potential propagation of neural damage if the dying cell releases glutamate and overexcites its surrounding cells. Excitotoxicity contributes to neuronal damage in stroke, TBI, and neural degenerative disease. Glutamate receptors and some $Ca^{2+}$ channels have been implicated in the neuronal disruption associated with acquired immunodeficiency syndrome (AIDS). Future pharmaceutical treatment of stroke, brain injury, and neural degenerative disease may be directed toward blocking the NMDA type of glutamate receptor and thus preventing the cascade of cell death related to excitotoxicity. However, blocking these receptors may kill cells on the peripheral region of the ischemia owing to low $Ca^{2+}$ levels.[65] Toxic effects of $Ca^{2+}$ at both low and high concentrations mean that researchers are challenged to find successful pharmacologic interventions. Researchers are attempting to understand how to allow the normal activity of NMDA receptors, which is critical for neuron activity and survival, while blocking the cascade that leads to excitotoxicity.[69,70] One drug that has shown promise is Riluzole, a drug used to treat ALS, which was shown in vitro to be neuroprotective by inhibiting glutamate activity that resulted in excitotoxicity.[71]

In addition to possible pharmaceutical blocking of NMDA-type glutamate receptors for management of an ischemic insult to the brain, other treatments may be directed specifically toward blocking the effects of $Ca^{2+}$ and free radicals. In animals, when oxygen and blood glucose levels are diminished by occlusion of blood flow to the brain, levels of the intracellular messenger inositol triphosphate ($IP_3$) are increased. This increase stimulates the release of $Ca^{2+}$ from intracellular storage sites and promotes a variety of cellular activities. With high cellular activity in the absence of adequate glucose, an increase in lactose, free radicals, and other metabolic end-products poison the cell. Also, when $IP_3$ is broken down by the cell, its by-product, diacylglycerol, breaks down into free fatty acid metabolites that can be poisonous to the cell. Future pharmaceutical treatment of stroke and TBI may be directed toward blocking the $IP_3$ pathway or administering drugs that act as scavengers for oxygen free radicals. These treatments could potentially prevent the cascade of cell death related to the production of fatty acid metabolites.

Despite continued examination of various pharmacologic agents to prevent or reduce the effects of excitotoxicity at different levels of the cascade of events leading to cell death, no pharmacologic agents have yet been identified that provide significant neuroprotection when tested in individuals with stroke, TBI, or neurodegenerative disease.[72,73] Researchers continue to study the complex cascade of cellular events associated with excitotoxicity to seek an effective intervention, but they

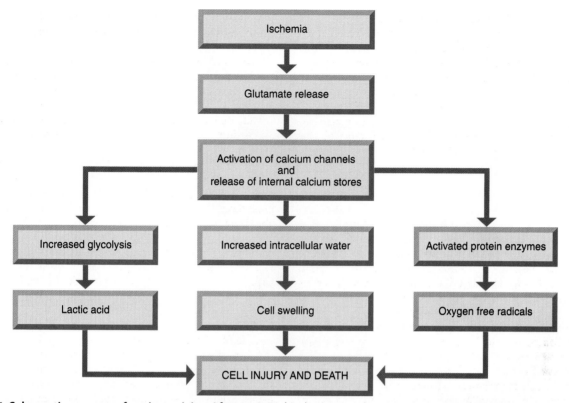

**Fig. 4-7 Schematic process of excitotoxicity.** After an initial ischemic insult, excessive intracellular calcium concentrations result in three pathways of cellular destruction: increased glycolysis, increased intracellular water, and activated protein enzymes.

are also exploring other therapeutic avenues focused on neuro-restoration, including promoting angiogenesis (formation of new blood vessels) and neurogenesis.[72,73]

> ### ◎ *Clinical Pearl*
>
> In response to ischemia, cells can die directly from lack of oxygen or indirectly from the cascade of events resulting from increased stimulation of glutamate receptors.

## EFFECTS OF REHABILITATION ON PLASTICITY

Following brain injury, both the intensity of rehabilitation and the amount of time between injury and initiation of rehabilitation influence the recovery of neuronal function. Prolonged lack of active movement following cortical injury may lead to subsequent loss of function in adjacent, undamaged regions of the brain. However, retraining movements prevent subsequent damage in adjacent areas of cortex.[74] Using monkeys, researchers mimicked a stroke by damaging a small part of the motor cortex associated with hand movement control. When retraining of hand movements was initiated 5 days after the original injury occurred, researchers found no loss of function in undamaged adjacent cortical regions. In some cases, neural reorganization took place, and the hand representation of the cortex extended into regions of the cortex formerly occupied by shoulder and elbow representations.[74] Because functional reorganization coincides with the recovery of fine finger movements, some researchers believe that rehabilitation has a direct effect on the integrity and reorganization of adjacent, undamaged regions of motor cortex.

Conclusive evidence indicates that early rehabilitation is key to improved recovery.[75,76] Investigators produced small lesions in the sensorimotor cortices of rats and then initiated enriched rehabilitation 5 days or 30 days post stroke. The enriched rehabilitation consisted of housing four to six rats in a cage with a variety of objects designed to encourage (not force) coordinated use of the impaired forelimb. After receiving 5 weeks of treatment, rats whose rehabilitation began 5 days post lesion retrieved more than twice as many food pellets using the impaired forelimb as rats who also received 5 weeks of treatment, but whose rehabilitation began 30 days post lesion. Delay reduces the impact of therapy.

Although early initiation of rehabilitation is critical, fMRI and TMS studies show that brain reorganization and plasticity occur in individuals with chronic stroke who undergo training of the upper extremity (subjects more than 1½ years post stroke; subjects more than 6 months post stroke).[77,78] Furthermore, adjunctive therapies such as TMS combined with rehabilitation may induce plastic changes to enhance upper extremity function in individuals with chronic stroke.[79]

The type of therapy offered is also important to the ultimate success of treatment. Task-specific practice is essential for motor learning.[80] TMS and fMRI show that task-specific training, as opposed to traditional stroke rehabilitation, produces long-lasting cortical reorganization in the brain areas activated.[81] Task-specific training induces a more normal pattern of brain activation compared with general use training of the upper extremity in individuals with stroke.[78]

Constraint-induced movement therapy (CIMT) is one type of task-specific training used in people with chronic dysfunction resulting from a stroke. With this technique, use of the

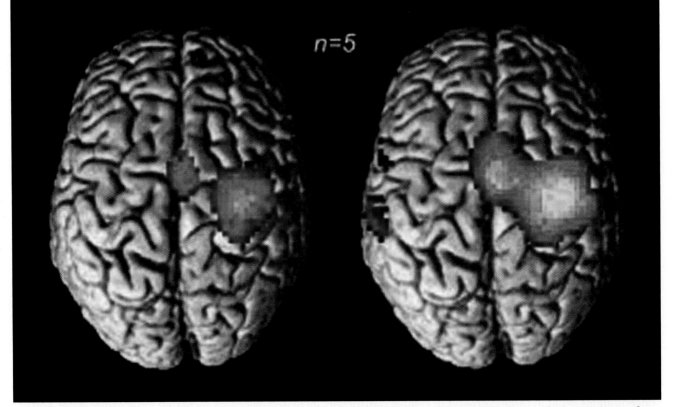

**Fig. 4-8 Functional magnetic resonance imaging during active movement of the paretic hand.** These results are for a group of five people, all of whom had a stroke near their time of birth and participated in constraint-induced movement therapy for 2 weeks when they were between 10 and 20 years old. The image on the left shows cortical activity before movement therapy, and the image on the right shows cortical activity afterward. Affected sensory and motor cortices show increased activation after therapy. *(From Walther M, Juenger H, Kuhnke N, et al: Motor cortex plasticity in ischemic perinatal stroke: a transcranial magnetic stimulation and functional MRI study. Pediatr Neurol 41:171–178, 2009.)*

unaffected upper limb is constrained by a sling. The patient then undergoes intense practice of functional movements with the affected upper extremity. Selected patients (only 20% to 25% of patients have enough hand movement to qualify for the therapy)[82] in a multisite trial experienced greater improvement in upper limb function compared with those individuals who received customary care,[83] and these improvements persisted for at least 2 years.[84] CIMT induces functional reorganization of the cortex in individuals with stroke. CIMT increases sensory and motor cortex activity during hand movement (Figure 4-8) and the size of the cortical area devoted to hand movement.[85,86]

However, excessively vigorous rehabilitation of motor function too soon after injury can be counterproductive. Constraint-induced movement of an impaired limb immediately after an experimental lesion of the sensorimotor cortex in adult rats has been shown to dramatically increase neuronal injury and result in long-lasting deficits in limb placement, decreased response to sensory stimulation, and defective use of the limb for postural support.[87] Furthermore, the cortices of these animals showed large increases in the volume of the lesions, and absence of dendritic growth or sprouting. These results suggest that immediate, intense, constraint-induced movement of an impaired limb may expand brain injury. Preliminary data indicate that excitotoxicity, caused by use-dependent increases in cortical activity, is a possible explanation for the increase in lesion size (Figure 4-9).[87] In people, intense CIMT initiated around 10 days following stroke produced less functional

improvement of the impaired upper extremity compared with customary therapy or standard CIMT.[88] Intense CIMT did not increase the size of the stroke lesion[88] as immediate intense rehabilitation had in adult rats.

These harmful effects of CIMT occur only with extreme overuse of the impaired extremity immediately after the lesion. If rats have lesions induced in the sensorimotor cortex and are able to freely use both forelimbs after surgery, dendritic complexity increases in the part of the cortex that controls the impaired extremity, and no increase in cortical damage occurs.[89] In rats, rehabilitation training initiated 3 to 5 days after a lesion does not increase lesion size or worsen behavioral outcomes.[76]

## SUMMARY

Researchers have made remarkable progress in understanding the ability of the nervous system to heal and adapt following injury. Neuroplasticity, which enables people to recover from neural injury, is an essential concept for those designing therapeutic interventions. An understanding of this key concept is essential for physical and occupational therapists, as well as for those designing pharmacologic treatments. Therapists can optimize recovery by initiating therapy early, avoiding vigorous use or overuse of impaired extremities during the first few days post CNS injury, and practicing specific tasks to elicit beneficial adaptive neuroplasticity.

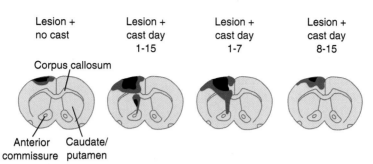

Lesion +
no cast

Lesion +
cast day
1-15

Lesion +
cast day
1-7

Lesion +
cast day
8-15

Corpus callosum

Anterior
commissure

Caudate/
putamen

**Fig. 4-9 Effects of forced movement on brain lesion size in rats.** Unilateral brain damage was induced in some of the rats; some had the ipsilateral forelimb casted during recovery, and others were not casted. Experimental groups were as follows: no lesion, with or without cast; lesion without cast; lesion with cast on days 1 to 15; lesion with cast on days 1 to 7; and lesion with cast on days 8 to 15. In the group with no lesion, no effect of casting was found in the brain. Drawings of coronal sections indicate average lesions in each lesioned group. The black areas indicate minimum damage, and the red regions show the maximum extent of brain damage. Brain lesion size increased with constraint-induced movement that occurred on days 1 to 7 or days 1 to 15; constraint-induced movement on days 8 to 15 did not increase lesion size. *(Modified from Humm JL, Kozlowski DA, James DC, et al: Use-dependent exacerbation of brain damage occurs during an early post-lesion vulnerable period. Brain Res 783:286–292, 1998.)*

## CLINICAL NOTES

### Case 1

B.G., a 37-year-old woman, suffered a compound fracture of her right distal radius and ulna following a fall while ice skating. Internal fixation of the fracture was required, and B.G. was restricted to very limited use of her dominant right arm and hand. Postoperatively, B.G. reported decreased sensation in the fourth and fifth fingers of her right hand. Owing to the severity of the fracture, some of the ulnar nerve fibers had been damaged. Six weeks after injury, B.G. was referred to therapy for range-of-motion exercises of the right wrist and hand and low-resistance exercise. Grip strength in the right hand was two thirds that in the left hand. During therapy, B.G. reported "burning sensations" and "pins and needles" in the digits of her right hand.

#### Questions

1. Is it possible for damaged or severed ulnar nerve axons to recover after injury?
2. Should the therapist anticipate the abnormal sensory sensations to diminish over the course of a few months?

### Case 2

K.S., a 52-year-old man, experienced some right-sided weakness and then collapsed while working on his farm. Several hours passed before K.S. was found. He was transported to the local hospital, where doctors determined he had suffered a stroke. The stroke resulted from sudden blockage of an artery, preventing blood flow to a region of the brain. K.S. experienced a right facial droop, inability to move his right arm and leg, and decreased sensation on the right side of the body. K.S. required maximal assistance for all mobility and was referred to occupational and physical therapy.

#### Questions

1. Was the brain damage associated with the stroke most likely confined only to the cells that were deprived of oxygen owing to decreased blood flow?
2. If excitotoxicity was in part responsible for the severity of the stroke, which principal excitatory neurotransmitter would be involved?

## REVIEW QUESTIONS

1. Define *neuroplasticity.*
2. When therapists repeatedly provoke unwanted reactions in people with tactile defensiveness, what is the intent?
3. What is the mechanism of long-term potentiation?
4. Define *wallerian degeneration.*
5. What are some consequences of axonal sprouts innervating inappropriate targets?
6. Can cortical motor and sensory maps of adult mammals change?
7. Define the term *excitotoxicity.*

8. Name one end-product of glycolysis that contributes to cell death.

9. Identify two mechanisms by which excessive levels of intracellular calcium promote cell death.

10. Can some of the brain damage associated with stroke, traumatic injury, and degenerative disease potentially be reduced with the administration of pharmaceutical agents?

11. What are the effects of constraint-induced movement following a stroke?

## References

1. Kim SJ, Linden DJ: Ubiquitous plasticity and memory storage. *Neuron* 56:582–592, 2007.

2. Johansson BB: Brain plasticity and stroke rehabilitation. *Stroke* 31:223–230, 2000.

3. French RD: Some concepts of nerve structure and function in Britain, 1875–1885: background to Sir Charles Sherrington and the synapse concept. *Med Hist* 14:154–165, 1970.

4. Sweetow RW, Sabes JH: Effects of acoustical stimuli delivered through hearing aids on tinnitus. *J Am Acad Audiol* 21:461–473, 2010.

5. Rankin CH, Abrams T, Barry RJ, et al: Habituation revisited: an updated and revised description of the behavioral characteristics of habituation. *Neurobiol Learn Mem* 92:135–138, 2009.

6. Feldman D: Synaptic mechanisms for plasticity in neocortex. *Annu Rev Neurosci* 32:33–55, 2009.

7. Steele CJ, Penhune VB: Specific increases within global decreases: a functional magnetic resonance imaging investigation of five days of motor sequence learning. *J Neurosci* 30:8332–8341, 2010.

8. Meister I, Krings T, Foltys H, et al: Effects of long-term practice and task complexity in musicians and nonmusicians performing simple and complex motor tasks: implications for cortical motor organization. *Hum Brain Mapp* 25:345–352, 2005.

9. Nelson SB, Turrigiano GG: Strength through diversity. *Neuron* 60:477–482, 2008.

10. Citri A, Malenka R: Synaptic plasticity: multiple forms, functions, and mechanisms. *Neuropsychopharmacology* 33:18–41, 2008.

11. Luscher C, Nicoll RA, Malenka RC, Muller D: Synaptic plasticity and dynamic modulation of the postsynaptic membrane. *Nat Neurosci* 3:545–550, 2000.

12. Matsuzaki M, Honkura N, Ellis-Davies GC, Kasai H: Structural basis of long-term potentiation in single dendritic spines. *Nature* 429:761–766, 2004.

13. Fortin DA, Davare MA, Srivastava T, et al: Long-term potentiation-dependent spine enlargement requires synaptic Ca2+-permeable AMPA receptors recruited by CaM-kinase I. *J Neurosci* 30:11565–11575, 2010.

14. Stehno-Bittel L, Lückhoff A, Clapham DE: Calcium release from the nucleus by InsP3 receptor channels. *Neuron* 14:163–167, 1995.

15. Stehno-Bittel L: Calcium signalling in normal and abnormal brain function. *Neurol Rep* 19:12–17, 1995.

16. Bading H, Ginty DD, Greenberg ME: Regulation of gene expression in hippocampal neurons by distinct calcium pathways. *Science* 260:181–186, 1993.

17. Bading H: Nuclear calcium-activated gene expression: possible roles in neuronal plasticity and epileptogenesis. *Epilepsy Res* 36:225–231, 1999.

18. Llansola M, Sanchez-Perez A, Cauli O, Felipo V: Modulation of NMDA receptors in the cerebellum. 1. Properties of the NMDA receptor that modulate its function. *Cerebellum* 4:154–161, 2005.

19. Fitzgerald PB, Fountain S, Daskalakis ZJ: A comprehensive review of the effects of rTMS on motor cortical excitability and inhibition. *Clin Neurophysiol* 117:2584–2596, 2006.

20. Censor N, Cohen LG: Using repetitive transcranial magnetic stimulation to study the underlying neural mechanisms of human motor learning and memory. *J Physiol* 589:21–28, 2011.

21. Chouinard PA, Paus T: What have we learned from "perturbing" the human cortical motor system with transcranial magnetic stimulation? *Front Hum Neurosci* 19:2–14, 2010.

22. Butefisch CM, Khurana V, Kopylev L, Cohen LG: Enhancing encoding of a motor memory in the primary motor cortex by cortical stimulation. *J Neurophysiol* 91:2110–2116, 2004.

23. Boyd LA, Lindell MA: Excitatory repetitive transcranial magnetic stimulation to left dorsal premotor cortex enhances motor consolidation of new skills. *BMC Neurosci* 10:72, 2009.

24. Vidoni ED, Acerra NE, Dao E, et al: Role of the primary somatosensory cortex in motor learning: an rTMS study. *Neurobiol Learn Mem* 93:532–539, 2010.

25. Perea G, Araque A: GLIA modulates synaptic transmission. *Brain Res Rev* 63:93–102, 2010.

26. Barker AJ, Ullian EM: Astrocytes and synaptic plasticity. *Neuroscientist* 16:40–50, 2010.

27. Liauw J, Hoang S, Choi M, et al: Thrombospondins 1 and 2 are necessary for synaptic plasticity and functional recovery after stroke. *J Cereb Blood Flow Metab* 28:1722–1732, 2008.

28. Udina E, Puigdemasa A, Navarro X: Passive and active exercise improve regeneration and muscle reinnervation after peripheral nerve injury in the rat. *Muscle Nerve* 43:500–509, 2011.

29. Freidenberg SM, Hermann RC: The breathing hand: obstetric brachial plexopathy reinnervation from thoracic roots? *J Neurol Neurosurg Psychiatry* 75:158–160, 2004.

30. Husseman J, Mehta RP: Management of synkinesis. *Facial Plast Surg* 24:242–249, 2008.

31. Kilinc D, Gallo G, Barbee KA: Mechanical membrane injury induces axonal beading through localized activation of calpain. *Exp Neurol* 219:553–561, 2009.

32. Büki A, Povlishock JT: All roads lead to disconnection? Traumatic axonal injury revisited. *Acta Neurochir* 148:181–193, 2006.

33. Beirowski B, Nógrádi A, Babetto E, et al: Mechanisms of axonal spheroid formation in central nervous system Wallerian degeneration. *J Neuropathol Exp Neurol* 69:455–472, 2010.

34. Llorens F, Gil V, Del Río JA: Emerging functions of myelin-associated proteins during development, neuronal plasticity, and neurodegeneration. *FASEB J* 25:463–475, 2011.

35. Freund P, Schmidlin E, Wannier T, et al: Nogo-A-specific antibody treatment enhances sprouting and functional recovery after cervical lesion in adult primates. *Nat Med* 12:790–792, 2006.

36. Fang PC, Barbay S, Plautz EJ, et al: Combination of NEP 1-40 treatment and motor training enhances behavioral recovery after a focal cortical infarct in rats. *Stroke* 41:544–549, 2010.

37. Cao Z, Gao Y, Deng K, et al: Receptors for myelin inhibitors: structures and therapeutic opportunities. *Mol Cell Neurosci* 43:1–14, 2010.

38. Cristofanilli M, Harris VK, Zigelbaum A, et al: Mesenchymal stem cells enhance the engraftment and myelinating ability of allogeneic oligodendrocyte progenitors in dysmyelinated mice. *Stem Cells Dev* 2011 March 12. [Epub ahead of print]

39. del Zoppo GJ: Inflammation and the neurovascular unit in the setting of focal cerebral ischemia. *Neuroscience* 158:972–982, 2009.

40. Obata K, Noguchi K: BDNF in sensory neurons and chronic pain. *Neurosci Res* 55:1–10, 2006.

41. Poncer JC: Hippocampal long term potentiation: silent synapses and beyond. *J Physiol Paris* 97:415–422, 2003.

42. Kerchner GA, Nicoll RA: Silent synapses and the emergence of a postsynaptic mechanism for LTP. *Nat Rev Neurosci* 9:813–825, 2008.

43. Zipfel GJ, Babcock DJ, Lee JM, Choi DW: Neuronal apoptosis after CNS injury: the roles of glutamate and calcium. *J Neurotrauma* 17:857–869, 2000.

44. Kara P, Friedlander MJ: Dynamic modulation of cerebral cortex synaptic function by nitric oxide. *Prog Brain Res* 118:183–198, 1998.

45. Elbert T, Pantev C, Wienbruch C, et al: Increased cortical representation of the fingers of the left hand in string players. *Science* 270:305–307, 1995.

46. Wrigley PJ, Press SR, Gustin SM, et al: Neuropathic pain and primary somatosensory cortex reorganization following spinal cord injury. *Pain* 141:52–59, 2009.

47. Rossini PM, Altamura C, Ferreri F, et al.: Neuroimaging experimental studies on brain plasticity in recovery from stroke. *Eura Medicophys* 43:241–254, 2007.

48. Carey LM, Abbott DF, Egan GF, et al: Evolution of brain activation with good and poor motor recovery after stroke. *Neurorehabil Neural Repair* 20:24–41, 2006.

49. Askim T, Indredavik B, Vangberg T, Håberg A: Motor network changes associated with successful motor skill relearning after acute ischemic stroke: a longitudinal functional magnetic resonance imaging study. *Neurorehabil Neural Repair* 23:295–304, 2009.

50. Jaillard A, Martin CD, Garambois K, et al: Vicarious function within the human primary motor cortex? A longitudinal fMRI stroke study. *Brain* 128:1122–1138, 2005.

51. Reinges MH, Krings T, Rohde V, et al: Prospective demonstration of short-term motor plasticity following acquired central paresis. *Neuroimage* 24:1248–1255, 2005.

52. Tharpe AM, Ashmead D, Sladen DP, et al: Visual attention and hearing loss: past and current perspectives. *J Am Acad Audiol* 19:741–747, 2008.

53. Gilley PM, Sharma A, Dorman MF: Cortical reorganization in children with cochlear implants. *Brain Res* 1239:56–65, 2008.

54. Fujii T, Tanabe HC, Kochiyama T, Sadato N: An investigation of cross-modal plasticity of effective connectivity in the blind by dynamic causal modeling of functional MRI data. *Neurosci Res* 65:175–186, 2009.

55. Park HJ, Chun JW, Park B, et al: Activation of the occipital cortex and deactivation of the default mode network during working memory in the early blind. *J Int Neuropsychol Soc* 22:1–16, 2011.

56. Kleim JA, Chan S, Pringle E, et al: BDNF val66met polymorphism is associated with modified experience-dependent plasticity in human motor cortex. *Nat Neurosci* 9:735–737, 2006.

57. McHughen SA, Rodriguez PF, Kleim JA, et al: BDNF val66met polymorphism influences motor system function in the human brain. *Cereb Cortex* 20:1254–1262, 2010.

58. Siironen J, Juvela S, Kanarek K, et al: The Met allele of the BDNF Val66Met polymorphism predicts poor outcome among survivors of aneurysmal subarachnoid hemorrhage. *Stroke* 38:2858–2860, 2007.

59. Rosselet C, Zennou-Azogui Y, Xerri C: Nursing-induced somatosensory cortex plasticity: temporally decoupled changes in neuronal receptive field properties are accompanied by modifications in activity-dependent protein expression. *J Neurosci* 26:10667–10676, 2006.

60. Benali A, Weiler E, Benali Y, et al: Excitation and inhibition jointly regulate cortical reorganization in adult rats. *J Neurosci* 28:12284–12293, 2008.

61. Sun M, Kong L, Wang X, et al: Comparison of the capability of GDNF, BDNF, or both, to protect nigrostriatal neurons in a rat model of Parkinson's disease. *Brain Res* 1052:119–129, 2005.

62. Lim ST, Airavaara M, Harvey BK: Viral vectors for neurotrophic factor delivery: a gene therapy approach for neurodegenerative diseases of the CNS. *Pharmacol Res* 61:14–26, 2010.

63. Kernie SG, Parent JM: Forebrain neurogenesis after focal ischemic and traumatic brain injury. *Neurobiol Dis* 37:267–274, 2010.

64. Ohab JJ, Fleming S, Blesch A, Carmichael ST: A neurovascular niche for neurogenesis after stroke. *J Neurosci* 26:13007–13016, 2006.

65. Zipfel GJ, Lee JM, Choi DW: Reducing calcium overload in the ischemic brain. *N Engl J Med* 341:1543–1544, 1999.

66. Waxman EA, Lynch DR: N-methyl-D-aspartate receptor subtypes: multiple roles in excitotoxicity and neurological disease. *Neuroscientist* 11:37–49, 2005.

67. Yu XM, Groveman BR, Fang XQ, Lin SX: The role of intracellular sodium (Na) in the regulation of calcium (Ca)-mediated signaling and toxicity. *Health* 2:8–15, 2010.

68. Deshpande LS, Limbrick DD, Jr, Sombati S, DeLorenzo RJ: Activation of a novel injury-induced calcium-permeable channel that plays a key role in causing extended neuronal depolarization and initiating neuronal death in excitotoxic neuronal injury. *J Pharmacol Exp Ther* 322:443–452, 2007.

69. Aarts M, Liu Y, Liu L, et al: Treatment of ischemic brain damage by perturbing NMDA receptor-PSD-95 protein interactions. *Science* 298:846–850, 2002.

70. Fan J, Vasuta OC, Zhang LY, et al: N-methyl-D-aspartate receptor subunit- and neuronal-type dependence of excitotoxic signaling through post-synaptic density 95. *J Neurochem* 115:1045–1056, 2010.

71. Cifra A, Nani F, Nistri A: Riluzole is a potent drug to protect neonatal rat hypoglossal motoneurons in vitro from excitotoxicity due to glutamate uptake block. *Eur J Neurosci* 33:899–913, 2011.

72. Xiong Y, Mahmood A, Chopp M: Emerging treatments for traumatic brain injury. *Exp Opin Emerg Drugs* 14:67–84, 2009.

73. Lau A, Tymianski M: Glutamate receptors, neurotoxicity and neurodegeneration. *Pflugers Arch* 460:525–542, 2010.

74. Nudo RJ, Wise BM, SiFuentes S, Milliken GW: Neural substrates for the effects of rehabilitative training on motor recovery after ischemic infarct. *Science* 272:1791–1794, 1996.

75. Teasell R, Bitensky J, Salter K, Bayona NA: The role of timing and intensity of rehabilitation therapies. *Top Stroke Rehabil* 12:228–237, 2005.

76. Biernaskie J, Chernenko G, Corbett D: Efficacy of rehabilitative experience declines with time after focal ischemic brain injury. *J Neurosci* 24:1245–1254, 2004.

77. Hamzei F, Liepert J, Dettmers C, et al: Two different reorganization patterns after rehabilitative therapy: an exploratory study with fMRI and TMS. *Neuroimage* 31:710–720, 2006.

78. Boyd LA, Vidoni ED, Wessel BD: Motor learning after stroke: is skill acquisition a prerequisite for contralesional neuroplastic change? *Neurosci Lett* 482:21–25, 2010.

79. Koganemaru S, Mima T, Thabit MN, et al: Recovery of upper-limb function due to enhanced use-dependent plasticity in chronic stroke patients. *Brain* 133:3373–3384, 2010.

80. Bayona NA, Bitensky J, Salter K, Teasell R: The role of task-specific training in rehabilitation therapies. *Top Stroke Rehabil* 12:58–65, 2005.

81. Classen J, Liepert J, Wise SP, et al: Rapid plasticity of human cortical movement representation induced by practice. *J Neurophysiol* 79:1117–1123, 1998.

82. Wolf SL, Thompson PA, Morris DM, et al: The EXCITE trial: attributes of the Wolf Motor Function Test in patients with subacute stroke. *Neurorehabil Neural Repair* 19:194–205, 2005.

83. Wolf SL, Winstein CJ, Miller JP, et al: Effect of constraint-induced movement therapy on upper extremity function 3 to 9 months after stroke: the EXCITE randomized clinical trial. *JAMA* 296:2095–2104, 2006.

84. Wolf SL, Winstein CJ, Miller JP, et al: Retention of upper limb function in stroke survivors who have received constraint-induced movement therapy: the EXCITE randomised trial. *Lancet Neurol* 7:33–40, 2008.

85. Sawaki L, Butler AJ, Leng X, et al: Constraint-induced movement therapy results in increased motor map area in subjects 3 to 9 months after stroke. *Neurorehabil Neural Repair* 22:505–513, 2008.

86. Gauthier LV, Taub E, Perkins C, et al: Remodeling the brain: plastic structural brain changes produced by different motor therapies after stroke. *Stroke* 39:1520–1525, 2008.

87. Kozlowski DA, James DC, Schallert T: Use-dependent exaggeration of neuronal injury after unilateral sensorimotor cortex lesions. *J Neurosci* 16:4776–4786, 1996.

88. Dromerick AW, Lang CE, Birkenmeier RL, et al: Very early constraint-induced movement during stroke rehabilitation (VECTORS): a single-center RCT. *Neurology* 73:195–201, 2009.

89. Schallert T, Fleming SM, Woodlee MT: Should the injured and intact hemispheres be treated differently during the early phases of physical restorative therapy in experimental stroke or parkinsonism? *Phys Med Rehabil Clin N Am* 14(1 Suppl):S27–S46, 2003.

# 5 Development of the Nervous System

Laurie Lundy-Ekman

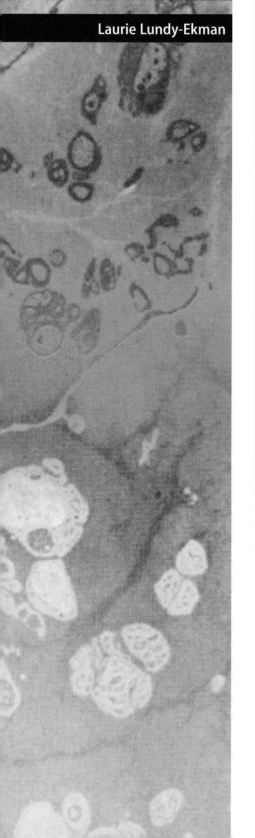

I am a 22-year-old student. Next year I will complete my master's degree in physical therapy, and I plan to specialize in pediatrics. Helping children with neurologic deficits is very important to me, as I was diagnosed with cerebral palsy at 2 years of age. At that time, a friend asked my parents if they would let me be seen by a pediatric specialist because the friend noticed that I was still crawling while all the children I was playing with were walking. I had no other signs of delayed development, verbally, cognitively, or socially, but motorically, I was far behind my peers. Unlike the pediatricians that I had seen previously, who said that I would outgrow my motoric delay, this specialist confirmed what my parents had suspected. A diagnosis of mild spastic diplegic cerebral palsy* was made, and my parents searched for things they could do to encourage my development.

I have yet to understand why my doctors did not tell my parents about physical therapy. Fortunately, I started school 3 years later, and my physical education teacher took an interest. To the best of his abilities, he used his skills as an educator and read extensively over the next 6 years to provide opportunities for me to develop motor skills. My first formal therapy session came in eighth grade, when I was referred by the school to an occupational therapist for an evaluation and to develop a physical education program that I could do independently. That visit sparked my interest in rehabilitation, shaping my choice of career.

As I mentioned, my cerebral palsy is mild. My cognitive skills are not affected, and my upper limb coordination is near normal. One physician's record states that there was some involvement of my left upper limb, but I do not notice any problems except when my reflexes are tested. I am inclined to think that any decrease in upper limb coordination is due to lack of challenges at a younger age, but I cannot confirm this suspicion. The most significant physical impact cerebral palsy has had on my life is on my gait pattern and recreational activities. As a child, motor dysfunction was more a daily problem than it is now because I could not keep up with my friends. I still struggle at times. Most recently, I struggled with learning to perform dependent-patient transfers in physical therapy school. Personally, I think that the greatest impact cerebral palsy has had on my life is a psychological one. There are still some things I would like to learn to do, but failing with motor activities as a child has influenced what I am willing to try now. On the other hand, that is why I am becoming a physical therapist: I want children and adults to know that physical limitations do not have to prevent them from enjoying life as much as anyone else.

—*Heidi Boring*

*Bilateral excessive muscle stiffness with weakness, usually affecting the lower limbs.*

From a single fertilized cell, an entire human being can develop. How is the exquisitely complex nervous system generated during development? Genetic and environmental influences act on cells throughout the developmental process, stimulating cell growth, migration, differentiation, and even cell death and axonal retraction to create the mature nervous system. Some of these processes are completed in utero; others continue during the first several years after birth. Understanding the beginnings of the nervous system is vital for comprehending developmental disorders and helpful for understanding the anatomy of the adult nervous system.

## DEVELOPMENTAL STAGES IN UTERO

Humans in utero undergo three developmental stages:
- Pre-embryonic
- Embryonic
- Fetal

### Pre-embryonic Stage

The pre-embryonic stage lasts from conception to about day 14. Fertilization of the ovum usually occurs in the uterine tube. The fertilized ovum, a single cell, begins cell division as it moves down the uterine tube and into the cavity of the uterus (Figure 5-1). Through repeated cell division, a solid sphere of cells is formed. Next, a cavity opens in the sphere of cells. At this stage of development, the sphere is called a *blastocyst*. The outer layer of the blastocyst will become the fetal contribution to the placenta, and the inner cell mass will become the embryo. The blastocyst implants into the endometrium of the uterus. During

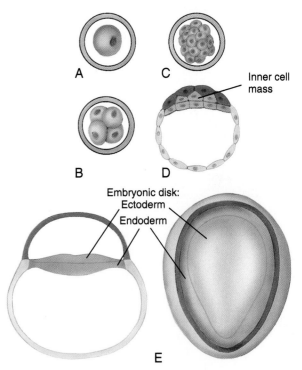

**Fig. 5-1 A,** Fertilized ovum, a single cell. **B,** Four-cell stage. **C,** Solid sphere of cells. **D,** Hollow sphere of cells. The inner cell mass will become the embryonic disk. **E,** The two-layered embryonic disk, shown in cross-section *(left)* and from above *(right)*. The upper layer of the disk is the ectoderm, and the lower layer is the endoderm.

implantation, the inner cell mass develops into the embryonic disk, consisting of two cell layers: ectoderm and endoderm. Soon, a third cell layer, mesoderm, is formed between the other two layers.

## Embryonic Stage

During the embryonic stage, from day 15 to the end of the eighth week, the organs are formed (Figure 5-2). The ectoderm develops into sensory organs, epidermis, and the nervous system. The mesoderm develops into dermis, muscles, skeleton, and the excretory and circulatory systems. The endoderm differentiates to become the gut, liver, pancreas, and respiratory system.

## Fetal Stage

The fetal stage lasts from the end of the eighth week until birth. The nervous system develops more fully, and myelination (insulation of axons by fatty tissue) begins.

> **◎ Clinical Pearl**
>
> The nervous system develops from ectoderm, the outer cell layer of the embryo.

## FORMATION OF THE NERVOUS SYSTEM

Formation of the nervous system occurs during the embryonic stage and consists of two phases. First, tissue that will become the nervous system coalesces to form a tube running along the back of the embryo. When the ends of the tube close, the second phase, brain formation, commences.

### Neural Tube Formation (Days 18 to 26)

The nervous system begins as a longitudinal thickening of the ectoderm, called the *neural plate* (Figure 5-2, *A*). The plate forms on the surface of the embryo, extending from the head to the tail region, in contact with amniotic fluid. The edges of

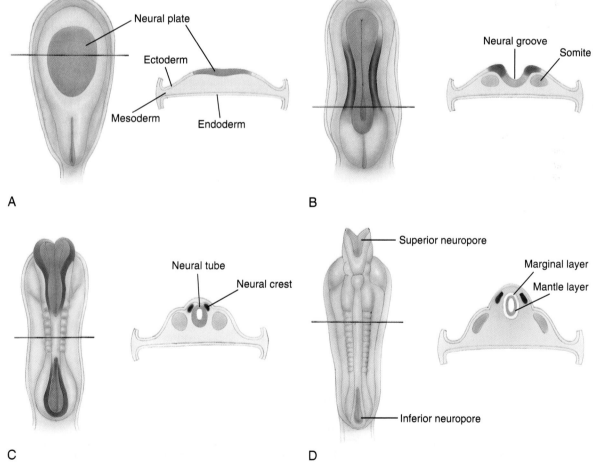

**Fig. 5-2** On the left in each panel, the view is from above the embryo. On the right in each panel, cross-sections through the embryo are shown. **A,** Day 16. Compare with Figure 5-1, *E.* **B,** The midline section of the neural plate moves toward the interior of the embryo, creating the neural groove (day 18). **C,** The folds of the neural plate meet, forming the neural tube. The neural crest separates from the tube and from the remaining ectoderm (day 21). **D,** The open ends of the neural tube are neuropores. The neural tube differentiates into an inner mantle layer and an outer marginal layer.

the plate fold to create the *neural groove,* and the folds grow toward each other (Figure 5-2, *B*). When the folds touch (day 21), the neural tube is formed (Figure 5-2, *C*). The neural tube closes first in the future cervical region. Next, the groove rapidly zips closed rostrally and caudally, leaving open ends called *neuropores* (Figure 5-2, *D*). Cells adjacent to the neural tube separate from the tube and the remaining ectoderm to form the *neural crest.* When the crest has developed, the neural tube and the neural crest move inside the embryo. The overlying ectoderm (destined to become the epidermal layer of skin) closes over the tube and the neural crest. The superior neuropore closes by day 27, and the inferior neuropore closes about 3 days later.

By day 26, the tube differentiates into two concentric rings (see Figure 5-2, *D*). The *mantle layer* (inner wall) contains cell bodies and will become gray matter. The *marginal layer* (outer wall) contains processes of cells whose bodies are located in the mantle layer. The marginal layer develops into white matter, consisting of axons and glial cells.

---

◎ **Clinical Pearl**

The brain and spinal cord develop entirely from the neural tube.

---

## Relationship of Neural Tube to Other Developing Structures

As the neural tube closes, the adjacent mesoderm divides into spherical cell clusters called *somites* (see Figure 5-2, *B*). Developing somites cause bulges to appear on the surface of the embryo (Figure 5-3). The somites first appear in the future occipital region, and new somites are added caudally. The anteromedial part of a somite, the *sclerotome,* becomes the vertebrae and the skull. The posteromedial part of the somite, the *myotome,*

becomes skeletal muscle. The lateral part of the somite, the *dermatome,* becomes dermis (Figure 5-4).

As the cells of the mantle layer proliferate in the neural tube, grooves form on each side of the tube, separating the tube into ventral and dorsal sections (see Figure 5-4). The ventral section is the *motor plate* (also called *basal plate*). Axons from cell bodies located in the motor plate grow out from the tube to innervate the myotome region of the somite. As development continues, this association leads to the formation of a *myotome:* a group of muscles derived from one somite and innervated by a single spinal nerve. Thus, myotome has two meanings: (1) an embryologic section of the somite, and (2) after the embryonic stage, a group of muscles innervated by a segmental spinal nerve. Neurons whose cell bodies are in the basal plate become motor neurons, which innervate skeletal muscle, and interneurons. In the mature spinal cord, the gray matter derived from the basal plate is called the *ventral horn.*

The dorsal section of the neural tube is the *association plate* (also called *alar plate*). In the spinal cord, these neurons proliferate and form interneurons and projection neurons. In the mature spinal cord, the gray matter derived from the association plate is called the *dorsal horn* (see Figure 5-4).

---

◎ **Clinical Pearl**

Neurons in the dorsal region of the neural tube process sensory information. Neurons with cell bodies in the ventral region innervate skeletal muscle.

---

The *neural crest* separates into two columns, one on each side of the neural tube. The columns break up into segments that correspond to the dermal areas of the somites. Neural crest cells form peripheral sensory neurons, myelin cells, autonomic neurons, and endocrine organs (adrenal medulla and pancreatic islets). The cells that become peripheral sensory neurons grow two processes: one connects to the spinal cord, and the other

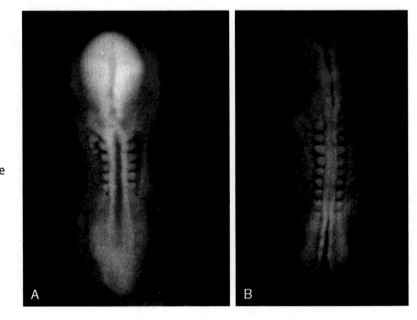

**Fig. 5-3 Photographs of embryos early in the fourth week.** In **A,** the embryo is essentially straight, whereas the embryo in **B** is slightly curved. In **A,** the neural groove is deep and is open throughout its entire extent. In **B,** the neural tube has formed between the two rows of somites but is widely open at the rostral and caudal neuropores. The neural tube is the primordium of the central nervous system (brain and spinal cord). *(From Moore KL, Persaud TVN: The developing human, clinically oriented embryology, ed 8, Philadelphia, 2008, Saunders.)*

A                                        B

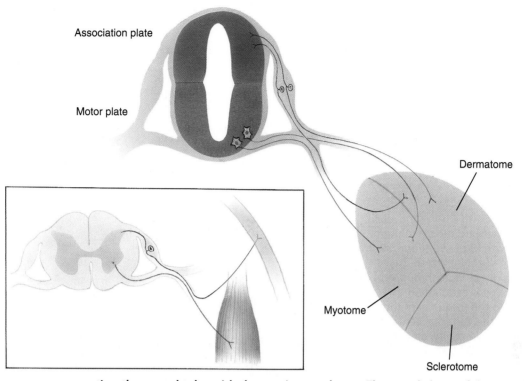

**Fig. 5-4 The neurons connecting the neural tube with the somite are shown.** The mantle layer of the neural tube has differentiated into a motor plate (ventral) and an association plate (dorsal). The inset illustrates the same structures in maturity. The following changes have occurred: part of the neural plate→spinal cord, motor plate→ventral horn, association plate→dorsal horn, myotome→skeletal muscle, and dermatome→dermis.

innervates the region of the somite that will become dermis. Similar to the term *myotome, dermatome* has two meanings: (1) the area of the somite that will become dermis, and (2) after the embryonic stage, the dermis innervated by a single spinal nerve. The peripheral sensory neurons, also known as *primary sensory neurons,* convey information from sensory receptors to the association plate. The cell bodies of the peripheral sensory neurons are outside the spinal cord, in the dorsal root ganglion.

### ◎ Clinical Pearl

The peripheral nervous system, with the exception of motor neuron axons, develops from the neural crest.

Until the third fetal month, spinal cord segments are adjacent to corresponding vertebrae, and the roots of spinal nerves project laterally from the cord. As the fetus matures, the spinal column grows faster than the cord. As a result, the adult spinal cord ends at the L1-L2 vertebral level. The end of the spinal cord is the *conus medullaris.*

Caudal to the thoracic levels, roots of the spinal nerves travel inferiorly to reach the intervertebral foramina (Figure 5-5). The collection of lumbosacral nerve roots that extend inferior to the end of the spinal cord is the *cauda equina* (named for resemblance to a horse's tail; Figure 5-6). Disorders of the cauda equina are discussed in Chapter 13. The filum terminale is a

continuation of the dura, pia, and glia connecting the end of the spinal cord with the coccyx.

### Brain Formation (Begins Day 28)

When the superior neuropore closes, the future brain region of the neural tube expands to form three enlargements (Figure 5-7): *hindbrain, midbrain,* and *forebrain.* The enlargements, like their precursor neural tube, are hollow. In the mature nervous system, the fluid-filled cavities are called *ventricles.*

The hindbrain divides into two sections: the lower section becomes the *myelencephalon,* and the upper section becomes the *metencephalon.* These later differentiate to become the medulla, pons, and cerebellum. In the upper hindbrain, the central canal expands to form the fourth ventricle. The pons and the upper medulla are anterior to the fourth ventricle, and the cerebellum is posterior. In the cerebellum, the mantle layer gives rise to both deep nuclei and the cortex. To become the cortex, the mantle layer cell bodies migrate through the white matter to the outside.

The *midbrain* enlargement retains its name, midbrain, throughout development. The central canal becomes the cerebral aqueduct in the midbrain, connecting the third and fourth ventricles.

The posterior region of the forebrain stays in the midline to become the *diencephalon.* Major structures are the *thalamus* and the *hypothalamus.* The midline cavity forms the third ventricle.

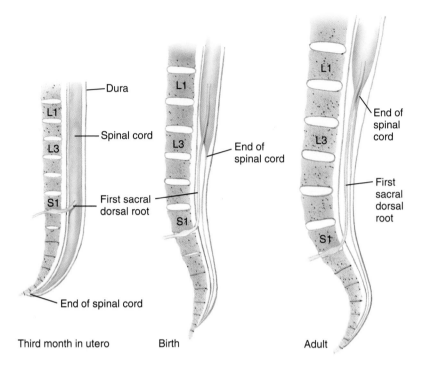

**Fig. 5-5** After the third month in utero, the rate of growth of the vertebral column exceeds that of the spinal cord. The passage of the nerve roots through specific vertebral foramina is established early in development, so the lower nerve roots elongate within the vertebral canal to reach their passage. For simplicity, only the first sacral nerve root is illustrated.

| TABLE 5-1 | | SUMMARY OF NORMAL BRAIN DEVELOPMENT | | |
|-----------|---|---|---|---|
| Hindbrain | → | Metencephalon | → | Pons, upper medulla, cerebellum, fourth ventricle |
| | | Myelencephalon | → | Lower medulla |
| Midbrain | → | Midbrain | → | Midbrain, cerebral aqueduct |
| Forebrain | → | Diencephalon | → | Thalamus, hypothalamus, third ventricle |
| | | Telencephalon | → | Cerebral hemispheres, including basal ganglia, cerebral cortex, lateral ventricles |

The anterior part of the forebrain becomes the *telencephalon.* The central cavity enlarges to form the two lateral ventricles (Figure 5-8). The telencephalon becomes the *cerebral hemispheres;* the hemispheres expand so extensively that they envelop the diencephalon. The cerebral hemispheres consist of deep nuclei, including the basal ganglia (groups of cell bodies); white matter (containing axons); and the cortex (layers of cell bodies on the surface of the hemispheres). As the hemispheres expand ventrolaterally to form the temporal lobe, they attain a C shape. As a result of this growth pattern, certain internal structures, including the caudate nucleus (part of the basal ganglia) and the lateral ventricles, also become C-shaped (Figure 5-9).

### Continued Development During Fetal Stage

Lateral areas of the hemispheres do not grow as much as other areas, with the result that a section of cortex becomes covered by other regions. The covered region is the *insula* (see Atlas A-4), and the edges of the folds that cover the insula meet to form the lateral sulcus. In the mature brain, if the lateral sulcus is pulled open, the insula is revealed. The surfaces of the cerebral and cerebellar hemispheres begin to fold, creating sulci, grooves into the surface, and gyri, which are elevations of the surface. Table 5-1 summarizes normal brain development.

### CELLULAR-LEVEL DEVELOPMENT

The progressive developmental processes of cell proliferation, migration, and growth; extension of axons to target cells; formation of synapses; and myelination of axons are balanced by the regressive processes that extensively remodel the nervous system during development.

Epithelial cells that line the neural tube divide to produce neurons and glia. The neurons migrate to their final location by one of two mechanisms:
1. Sending a slender process to the brain surface and then hoisting themselves along the process
   or
2. Climbing along radial glia (long cells that stretch from the center of the brain to the surface).[1]

The neurons differentiate appropriately after migrating to their final location. The function of each neuron—visual, auditory, motor, and so on—is not genetically determined. Instead,

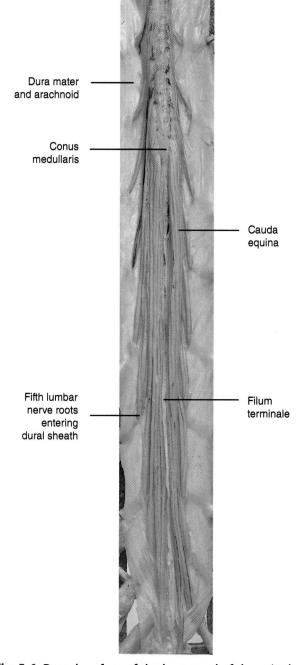

Dura mater
and arachnoid

Conus
medullaris

Cauda
equina

Fifth lumbar
nerve roots
entering
dural sheath

Filum
terminale

**Fig. 5-6 Dorsal surface of the lower end of the spinal cord and the cauda equina.** Because the spinal cord does not grow as long as the vertebral column, the lumbosacral nerve roots extend below the end of the spinal cord, forming the cauda equina. *(With permission from Abrahams PH, Marks SC, Hutchings R: McMinn's color atlas of human anatomy, ed 5, Philadelphia, 2003, Mosby.)*

function depends on the area of the brain to which the neuron migrates.[2] Daughter cells of a specific mother cell may assume totally different functions, depending on the location of migration.[3]

How do neurons in one region of the nervous system find the correct target cells in another region? For example, how do neurons in the cortex direct their axons down through the brain to synapse with specific neurons in the spinal cord? A process emerges from the neuron cell body. The forward end of the process expands to form a *growth cone* that samples the environment, contacting other cells and chemical cues. The growth cone recoils from some chemicals it encounters and advances into other regions where the chemical attractors are specifically compatible with the growth cone characteristics.

When the growth cone contacts its target cell, synaptic vesicles soon form, and microtubules that formerly ended at the apex of the growth cone project to the presynaptic membrane. With repeated release of neurotransmitter, the adjacent postsynaptic membrane develops a concentration of receptor sites. In early development, many neurons develop that do not survive. *Neuronal death* claims as many as half of the neurons formed during the development of some brain regions. The neurons that die are probably those that failed to establish optimal connections with their target cells, or that were too inactive to maintain their connection. Thus, development is partially dependent on activity. Some neurons that survive retract their axons from certain target cells while leaving other connections intact. For example, in the mature nervous system, a muscle fiber is innervated by only one axon. During development, several axons may innervate a single muscle cell. This polyneuronal innervation is eliminated during development.[4] These two regressive processes—neuronal death and *axon retraction*—sculpt the developing nervous system.

Neuronal connections also sculpt the developing musculature. Experiments that change motor neuron connections to a muscle fiber demonstrate that muscle fiber type (fast or slow twitch) is dependent on innervation. *Fast twitch muscle* is converted to slow twitch if innervated by a slow motor neuron, and *slow twitch muscle* can be converted to fast twitch if innervated by a fast motor neuron.[5]

Before neurons with long axons become fully functional, their axons must be insulated by a *myelin sheath,* composed of lipid and protein. The process of acquiring a myelin sheath is called *myelination.* This process begins in the fourth fetal month; most sheaths are completed by the end of the third year of life. The process occurs at different rates in each system. For instance, the motor roots of the spinal cord are myelinated at about 1 month of age, but tracts sending information from the cortex to activate motor neurons are not completely myelinated, and therefore are not fully functional, until a child is approximately 2 years old. Thus, if neurons that project from the cerebral cortex to motor neurons were damaged perinatally, motor deficits might not be observed until the child is older. For example, if some of the cortical neurons that control lower limb movements were damaged at birth, the deficit might not be recognized until the child is older than 1 year and has difficulty standing and walking. This is an example of *growing into deficit:* nervous system damage that occurred earlier is not evident until the damaged system would normally have become functional.

## DEVELOPMENTAL DISORDERS: IN UTERO AND PERINATAL DAMAGE TO THE NERVOUS SYSTEM

The central nervous system is most susceptible to major malformations between day 14 and week 20, as the fundamental structures of the central nervous system are forming. After this

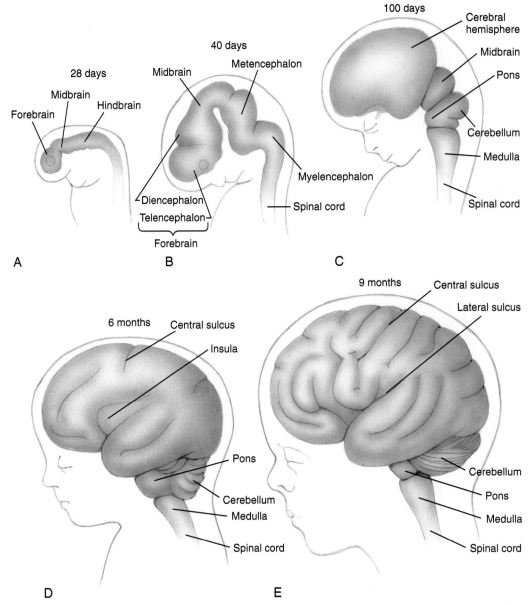

**Fig. 5-7  Brain formation. A,** Three-enlargement stage. **B,** Five-enlargement stage. **C,** The telencephalon has grown so extensively that the diencephalon is completely covered in a lateral view. **D,** The insula is being covered by continued growth of adjacent areas of the cerebral hemisphere. **E,** Folding of the surface of the cerebral and cerebellar hemispheres continues.

period, growth and remodeling continue; however, insults cause functional disturbances and/or minor malformations.

## Neural Tube Defects

*Anencephaly,* formation of a rudimentary brainstem without cerebral and cerebellar hemispheres, occurs when the cranial end of the tube remains open and the forebrain does not develop. The skull does not form over the incomplete brain, leaving the malformed brainstem and meninges exposed. Anencephaly can be detected by maternal blood tests, amniotic fluid tests, and ultrasound imaging. Causes include chromosomal

abnormalities, maternal nutritional deficiencies, and maternal hyperthermia. Most fetuses with this condition die before birth, and almost none survive longer than a week after birth.

*Arnold-Chiari malformation* is a developmental deformity of the hindbrain. There are two types of Arnold-Chiari malformation. Arnold-Chiari type I is not associated with defects of the lower neural tube and consists of herniation of the cerebellar tonsils through the foramen magnum into the vertebral canal. Both the medulla and the pons are small and deformed. Often, people with Arnold-Chiari I malformation have no symptoms. If symptoms do occur, they begin during adolescence or early adulthood. The most frequent complaints are severe head and

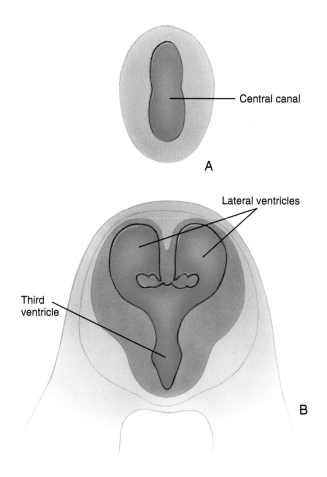

**Fig. 5-8  Formation of ventricles. A,** Central canal in neural tube. **B,** Coronal section of developing telencephalon.

neck pain, usually suboccipital. Headache may be induced by coughing, sneezing, or straining. The deformity may be associated with restriction of cerebrospinal fluid (CSF) flow, producing hydrocephalus (see Chapter 19). Hydrocephalus is an excessive volume of CSF. Pressure exerted by the CSF may interfere with the function of adjacent structures, causing sensory and motor disorders. Malformation of lower cranial nerves and of the cerebellum may result in problems with tongue and facial weakness, decreased hearing, dizziness, weakness of lateral eye movements, and problems with coordination of movement. Visual disturbances include flashing lights, loss of vision from part of the visual field, and discomfort in response to light.[6] The visual disturbances are a result of CSF in the third ventricle pressing on the optic chiasm.[7] If the deficits are stable, no medical treatment is indicated. If the deficits are progressing, surgical removal of the bone immediately surrounding the malformation may be indicated. Abnormalities of the upper cervical cord may cause loss of pain and temperature sensation on the shoulders and lateral upper limbs (see Chapter 13). (See Milhorat et al [1999][8] for clinical and magnetic resonance imaging [MRI] findings in a large group of people with symptomatic Arnold-Chiari type I.)

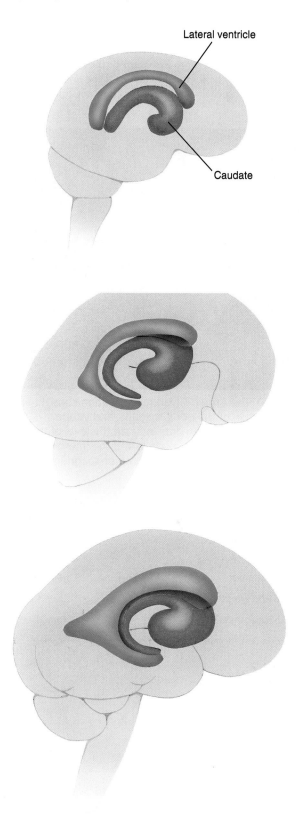

**Fig. 5-9** The growth pattern of the cerebral hemispheres results in a C shape of some of the internal structures. The changing shapes of the caudate nucleus and the lateral ventricle are shown.

In Arnold-Chiari type II (Figure 5-10), the signs are present in infancy. Type II consists of malformation of the brainstem and cerebellum, leading to extension of the medulla and cerebellum through the foramen magnum. Type II often produces progressive hydrocephalus (blockage of flow of CSF; see Chapter

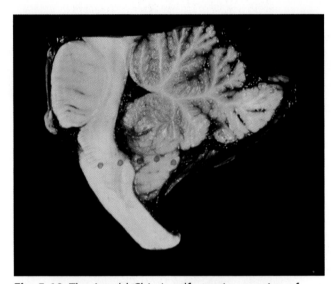

**Fig. 5-10** The Arnold-Chiari malformation consists of malformation of the pons, medulla, and inferior cerebellum. The green dots indicate the level of the foramen magnum. The medulla and the inferior cerebellum protrude into the foramen magnum.

19), paralysis of the sternocleidomastoid muscles, deafness, bilateral weakness of lateral eye movements, and facial weakness (Pathology 5-1).[9,10] Arnold-Chiari type II is almost always associated with another disorder—incomplete closure of the neural tube, called *meningomyelocele* (see later).

*Spina bifida* is the neural tube defect that results when the inferior neuropore does not close (Figure 5-11). Developing vertebrae do not close around an incomplete neural tube, resulting in a bony defect at the distal end of the tube. Maternal nutritional deficits (e.g., eating less than 400 mg of folic acid per day during early pregnancy) are associated with a higher incidence of the disorder. The severity of the defect varies; if neural tissue does not protrude through the bony defect (spina bifida occulta), spinal cord function is usually normal.

In spina bifida cystica, the meninges and in some cases the spinal cord protrude through the posterior opening in the vertebrae. The three types of spina bifida cystica, in order of increasing severity, are meningocele, meningomyelocele, and myeloschisis. *Meningocele* is protrusion of the meninges through the bony defect. In some cases, meningocele may be asymptomatic. In other cases, spinal cord function may be impaired. In *meningomyelocele*, neural tissue with the meninges protrudes outside the body (Figure 5-12). Meningomyelocele always results in abnormal growth of the spinal cord and some degree of lower extremity dysfunction; often, bowel and bladder control is impaired. Associated cognitive deficits include problems with abstract reasoning, visual perception, and visual-motor integration.[11] No consensus exists on proper medical management of meningomyelocele. *Myeloschisis* is the most severe defect, consisting of a malformed spinal cord open to the

| PATHOLOGY 5-1 | ARNOLD-CHIARI MALFORMATION |
| --- | --- |
| Pathology | Developmental abnormality |
| Etiology | Unknown |
| Speed of onset | Unknown |
| Signs and symptoms | |
| Consciousness | Normal |
| Cognition, language, and memory | Normal |
| Sensory | Headache, usually suboccipital, initiated by or exacerbated by coughing, straining, and sneezing; may have loss of pain and temperature sensation on shoulders and lateral upper limbs if upper central spinal cord is abnormal |
| Autonomic | Vomiting secondary to hydrocephalus |
| Motor | Uncoordinated movements, paresis, impaired fine motor coordination of hands |
| Cranial nerves | Vertigo (sensation of spinning); deafness; tongue, facial muscle, and lateral eye movement weakness; difficulty swallowing |
| Vision | Temporary visual disturbances |
| Region affected | Upper spinal cord, brainstem, and cerebellum |
| Demographics | |
| Prevalence | Affects only developing nervous system. 1 per 1000[9] |
| Incidence | Type II: 7.9 per 100,000 live births (based on incidence of meningomyelocele) |
| Prognosis | Defect is stable; symptoms are stable or progressive; symptoms may be precipitated by trauma[9,10] |

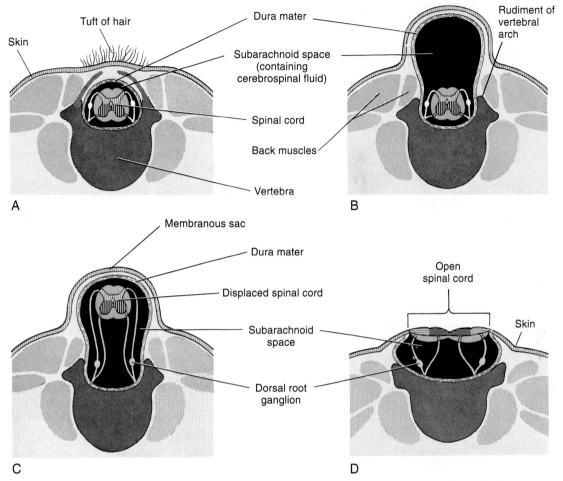

**Fig. 5-11 Various types of spina bifida and commonly associated malformations of the nervous system. A,** Spina bifida occulta. About 10% of people have this vertebral defect in L5, S1, or both. Neural function is usually normal. **B,** Spina bifida with meningocele. **C,** Spina bifida with meningomyelocele. **D,** Spina bifida with myeloschisis. The types illustrated in **B** to **D** are often referred to collectively as *spina bifida cystica* because of the cyst-like sac that is associated with them. *(From Moore KL, Persaud TVN: The developing human: clinically oriented embryology, ed 8, Philadelphia, 2008, Saunders.)*

surface of the body, which occurs when the neural folds fail to close (Pathology 5-2).[12-15]

## Tethered Spinal Cord

During normal development, spinal cord length increases less than vertebral length, resulting in the conus medullaris ending at L4 at birth and between L1-L2 in adults. Rarely, the end of the spinal cord adheres to one of the lower vertebra, thus tethering the spinal cord to the bone (Figure 5-13). As the person grows, resulting traction on the inferior spinal cord causes dermatomal and myotomal deficits in the lower limbs, pain in the saddle region (part of the body that would contact a horse saddle) and lower limbs, and bowel and bladder dysfunction. Less often, a tethered cord syndrome interferes with movement control signals descending from the brain. If traction on the spinal cord is mild, signs may occur only when mechanical stress increases and/or the onset of signs may not occur until adolescence or later. Clinical signs include progressive lower limb weakness, deterioration of walking, back pain, leg pain,

excessive muscle resistance to stretch, increasing scoliosis, increasing foot deformity, and deterioration in bladder and bowel function.

## Spinal Muscular Atrophy

In this autosomal recessive disorder, motor neurons with cell bodies in the spinal cord that innervate skeletal muscles degenerate. The most common genetic defect is deletion of the survival motor neuron-1 gene. The resulting muscle weakness and atrophy typically lead to premature death. The incidence is 1 in 6000 live births. Severity is variable; type I (also known as Werdnig-Hoffmann disease) is the most severe form. Type II is intermediate in severity, and type III is less severe.[16]

## Forebrain Malformation

The forebrain normally divides into two cerebral hemispheres. Rarely, this division does not occur, resulting in a single cerebral hemisphere, often associated with facial abnormalities

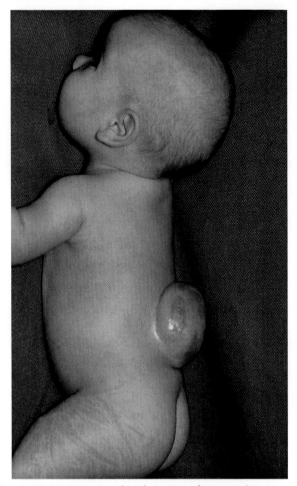

**Fig. 5-12** Meningomyelocele in an infant, resulting in paralysis of the lower limbs. *(From Moore KL, Persaud TVN: The developing human: clinically oriented embryology, ed 8, Philadelphia, 2008, Saunders.)*

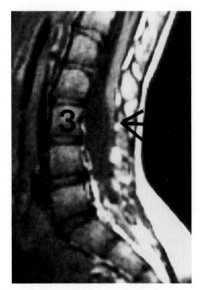

**Fig. 5-13** Magnetic resonance image showing a tethered spinal cord at L3. *(From Freeman BL: Scoliosis and kyphosis. In Canale ST, Beaty JH, editors: Campbell's operative orthopaedics, ed 11, Philadelphia, 2008, Mosby.)*

including a single eye (or no eye), a deformed nose, or cleft lip and palate. The defect is called *holoprosencephaly.* Genetic factors have been implicated in the disorder. This disorder can be identified in utero by genetic testing and by ultrasound.

## Exposure to Alcohol or Cocaine in Utero

What are the consequences of maternal substance abuse? Fetal alcohol syndrome (consisting of impairment of the central nervous system, growth deficiencies before and/or after birth, and facial anomalies) and the milder syndrome of alcohol-related birth defects are examples of substance abuse interfering with development during gestation. Both syndromes are due to maternal alcohol intake. Physical characteristics include an abnormally small head, an indistinct philtrum (groove above upper lip), a thin upper lip, and a short vertical space between the open eyelids. Malformation of the cerebellum, cerebral nuclei, corpus callosum, neuroglia, and neural tube leads to cognitive, movement, and behavioral problems. Intelligence, memory, language, attention, reaction time, visuospatial abilities, decision making, goal-oriented behavior, fine and gross motor skills, and social and adaptive functioning are impaired.[17] Prevalence is 0.2 to 2 per 1000 live births.[18]

The effects of in utero exposure to cocaine depend on the stage of development. Disturbance of neuronal proliferation is the most frequent consequence of cocaine exposure during neural development, but interference with other neurodevelopmental processes also occurs. Cocaine exposure in utero causes difficulties with attention and impulse control.[19]

## Abnormal Locations of Cells

What happens when the process of cell migration goes awry? Cells fail to reach their normal destination. In the cerebral cortex, this results in abnormal gyri, due to abnormal numbers of cells in the cortex, and heterotopia, the displacement of gray matter, commonly into the deep cerebral white matter. Seizures are often associated with heterotopia.

## Intellectual Disability

Abnormalities of dendritic spines are found in many cases of intellectual disability.[20,21] Dendritic spines are projections from the dendrites, common in cerebral and cerebellar cortex projection neurons, which are the preferential sites of synapses. Figure 5-14 shows normal dendritic spines.

## Cerebral Palsy

*Cerebral palsy* (CP) is a movement and postural disorder caused by permanent, nonprogressive damage to a developing brain. In premature infants, the brain damage usually occurs postnatally. CP is classified according to the type of motor dysfunction. The most common types are as follows:
- Spastic (Figure 5-15)
- Dyskinetic
- Ataxic
- Hypotonic
- Mixed

*Spasticity* is neuromuscular overactivity, resulting in excessive involuntary skeletal muscle contraction. Spasticity makes

| PATHOLOGY 5-2 | SPINA BIFIDA CYSTICA |
| --- | --- |
| Pathology | Developmental abnormality |
| Etiology | Some cases due to maternal nutritional deficits |
| Speed of onset | Unknown |
| Signs and symptoms | Signs and symptoms vary, depending on location and severity of the malformation |
| Consciousness | Normal |
| Cognition, language, and memory | Usually normal in meningocele; intellectual disability frequently accompanies meningomyelocele and myeloschisis |
| Somatosensation in lower limbs | Meningocele: may be impaired<br>Meningomyelocele: impaired or absent<br>Myeloschisis: absent |
| Autonomic | Meningomyelocele/myeloschisis: lack of bladder and bowel control |
| Motor | Meningocele and meningomyelocele: paresis of lower limbs<br>Myeloschisis: paralysis of the lower limbs |
| Cranial nerves | Meningomyelocele and myeloschisis are almost always associated with Chiari type II malformation, so eye movement abnormalities, headache, problems with swallowing, and impaired hearing occur[12] |
| Region affected | Inferior spinal cord |
| Demographics | |
| Prevalence | Affects only developing nervous system; 7.9 per 100,000 live births[13] |
| Prognosis | Defect is stable. In utero surgery to close meningomyelocele decreases incidence and severity of associated brainstem abnormalities[14]; 85% survive to adulthood[15] |

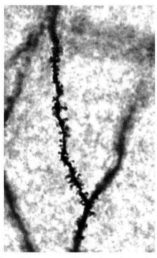

**Fig. 5-14** A silver-impregnated dendrite (Golgi stain). The dendritic spines, small lateral projections from the dendrite, are specialized to receive synaptic input from other neurons. *(Courtesy Dr. Bryan Luikart.)*

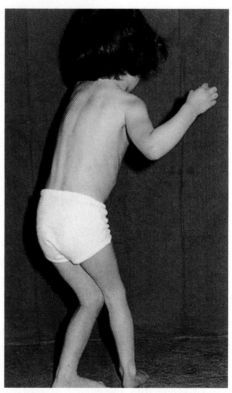

**Fig. 5-15** Child with spastic cerebral palsy. Note the flexion contractures of the right arm and both knees, and the internal rotation of the left lower limb. *(From Forbes CD, Jackson WF (1997). Color atlas and text of clinical medicine, 2nd edition. London: Mosby.)*

muscles more stiff than normal. In spastic CP, muscle stiffness and shortening often result in toe walking and a scissor gait. In scissor gait, one leg swings in front of the other instead of straight forward, producing a crisscross motion of the legs during walking. Spastic CP is caused by damage to axons adjacent to the lateral ventricles.

In dyskinetic CP, muscle tone (muscle resistance to stretch) fluctuates, ranging from hypertonia to hypotonia. Hypertonia is excessive resistance to stretch, producing unwanted stiffness. Hypotonia is inadequate muscle contraction for movements and to maintain normal head and trunk posture. The most common form of dyskinetic CP is choreoathetoid, characterized by involuntary choreiform (jerky, abrupt, irregular) and athetoid (slow, writhing) movements. The less common dystonic form of dyskinetic CP comprises involuntary sustained skeletal muscle contractions. In dyskinetic cerebral palsy, the neuronal damage is in the basal ganglia.

Ataxic CP consists of incoordination, weakness, and shaking during voluntary movement. In ataxic CP, the damage is in the cerebellum. Hypotonic cerebral palsy is characterized by very low muscle tone, often described as floppy. The person with hypotonic CP has little or no ability to move. The site of damage in hypotonic CP is unknown. If more than one type of abnormal movement coexists in a person, the disorder is classified as mixed type. Cerebral palsy is also classified according to the area of the body affected: hemiplegia affects both limbs on one side of the body, quadriplegia affects all four limbs equally, and diplegia indicates that the upper limbs are less severely affected than both lower limbs.

Traditionally, CP was believed to result from difficulties during the birth process. However, epidemiologic studies indicate that 80% of cases result from events that occur before the onset of labor, including genetic, metabolic, immune, endocrine, and coagulation disorders, and maternal infection.[22,23] Hypoxia during birth is rarely a cause of cerebral palsy.[22,24] Further, only 20% of cases of spastic quadriplegic CP are associated with difficulties during labor or delivery, and dyskinetic CP is infrequently associated with difficult labor or delivery. Hemiplegic CP, spastic diplegia, and ataxic CP are not associated with difficult labor or delivery.[25] Neuroimaging (Figure 5-16) reveals the variety of pathologies that cause CP.[26]

Cognitive, somatosensory, visual, auditory, and speech deficits are frequently associated with CP. *Growing into deficit* is common in CP. Although the nervous system damage is not progressive, new problems appear as the child reaches each age for normal developmental milestones, for example, when the child reaches the age when most children walk, the inability of

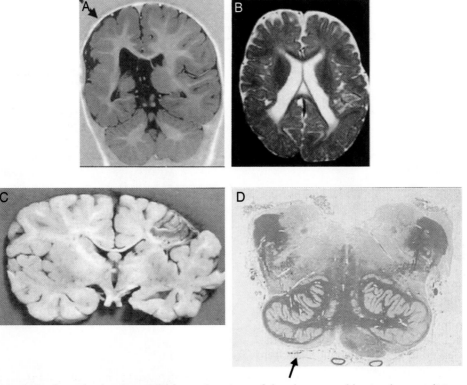

**Fig. 5-16 Neuroimaging of cerebral palsy pathology.** A variety of developmental brain abnormalities can cause cerebral palsy. **A,** Patient has hemiplegic cerebral palsy and began walking at the typical age for hemiplegia (18 to 22 months). The arrow indicates abnormal right hemisphere development, with many small folds of the cerebral cortex. **B,** Horizontal section showing enlarged ventricles secondary to the death of adjacent white matter. The corpus callosum is extremely thin. The clinical presentation is spastic diplegia. **C,** Coronal section through the hemispheres of an 8-month-old infant shows a cortical-subcortical infarct and a small internal capsule. **D,** Transverse section of the medulla from the same infant as in **C.** The arrow points to the absence of the medullary pyramid caused by loss of corticospinal tract axons. *(From Lin JP: The cerebral palsies: a physiological approach. J Neurol Neurosurg Psychiatry 74[Suppl 1]:i27, 2003. Reproduced with permission from the BMJ Publishing Group.)*

**PATHOLOGY 5-3**  CEREBRAL PALSY

| | |
|---|---|
| Pathology | Developmental abnormality |
| Etiology | Abnormal development in utero, metabolic abnormalities, disorders of the immune system, coagulation disorders, infection, trauma, or, rarely, hypoxia; central nervous system damage occurs before the second birthday |
| Speed of onset | Unknown |
| Signs and symptoms | |
| Consciousness | Normal |
| Cognition, language, and memory | Frequently associated with intellectual disability and language deficits, although some people with cerebral palsy have above normal intelligence and memory |
| Sensory | Usually impaired |
| Autonomic | Voiding dysfunction in ≈50%[27] |
| Motor | Spastic type: paresis, muscle shortening, increased muscle resistance to movement; dyskinetic type: slow, writhing movements; and jerky movements, or sustained involuntary postures; ataxic type: incoordination, weakness, shaking during voluntary movements; hypotonic type: very low muscle tone, impaired ability to move. |
| Cranial nerves | Not directly affected; however, owing to abnormal neural input, the output of motor cranial nerves is impaired |
| Vision | Eye movements and vision are frequently impaired[27] |
| Associated disorders | Seizures affect ≈50%[23] |
| Region affected | Brain; some abnormalities in spinal cord |
| Demographics | Only developing nervous system affected |
| Prevalence | 230 per 100,000 live births per year[28] |
| Prognosis | The abnormality is stable, but functional limitations may become obvious as the person grows |

the child with CP to walk independently at the usual age becomes apparent (Pathology 5-3).[27,28]

Even at birth, the infant brain is far from its adult form. Thus, damage during development has different consequences than injury of a fully developed brain.

## Developmental Coordination Disorder

Children with normal intellect without traumatic brain injury or CP or other neurologic problems who lack the motor coordination to perform tasks that most children their age are able to perform are considered to have *developmental coordination disorder (DCD)*. The condition is usually permanent, continuing into adulthood.[29] These children lag behind their peers in dressing, using utensils, handwriting, and/or athletics. Currently, a variety of standards and tests are used to diagnose DCD. Slowed movement time and longer movement planning times differentiate children with DCD from those without the disorder.[30] Mood, anxiety disorders, behavioral problems, and social difficulties are frequently associated with DCD.[31]

## Attention Deficit Hyperactivity Disorder

*Attention deficit hyperactivity disorder (ADHD)* is characterized by developmentally inappropriate inattention, impulsivity, and motor restlessness. Approximately half of people with ADHD have impaired handwriting or clumsiness, and are delayed in achieving motor milestones. Three percent to 7% of

school-aged children are affected by ADHD. Estimates of heritability range from 60% to 90%. Additional factors associated with increased incidence include maternal alcohol use and smoking, low birth weight, and early social deprivation.[32] A meta-analysis of studies indicates that food coloring increases hyperactive behavior in some children with ADHD.[33] Depending on the criteria used, childhood ADHD persists into adulthood in 15% to 65% of people.[34]

Individuals with ADHD have reduced volume of the prefrontal cortex, caudate and putamen, dorsal cingulate cortex, and cerebellum. Inadequate myelination of axons connecting these areas further decreases function. Stimulant drugs (including methylphenidate hydrochloride) increase the availability of dopamine and norepinephrine in synapses, improving function in some people with ADHD.[32]

## Autism Spectrum Disorders

*Autism* indicates a range of abnormal behaviors including impaired social skills (Pathology 5-4). Three disorders comprise the autism spectrum: autistic disorder, Asperger's disorder, and pervasive developmental disorder not otherwise specified. Individuals with autistic disorder engage in repetitive behaviors, have limited interests, appear to lack imagination, and are uninterested in interacting with other people. Some of those with autistic disorder are mute; others can speak but do not initiate conversation. People with Asperger's disorder speak and have normal or better intelligence. However, their limited social

**PATHOLOGY 5-4**    AUTISM SPECTRUM DISORDERS

| | |
|---|---|
| Pathology | Developmental disorder |
| Etiology | Epigenetic disorder (activation and deactivation of genes without modifying the DNA[41]). Factors that increase risk: Older parents (due to increased mutations of sperm and increased complications during pregnancy in older mothers), maternal infection, low birth weight, multiple births[42] |
| Speed of onset | Unknown |
| Signs and symptoms | |
| Consciousness | Normal |
| Cognition, language, and memory | 75% have cognitive impairment; social use of language is often impaired; working memory is impaired |
| Sensory | Variable; some are under-responsive to stimuli (example: walk into things), some are over-responsive (distressed by loud sounds), and others seek repetitive sensory stimuli[43] |
| Autonomic | Less skin conduction response to emotional faces in people with autism than in controls[44] |
| Motor | Variable; dyspraxia (impaired ability to perform gestures on request, imitate movements, and use tools), clumsy gait, balance problems[36] |
| Cranial nerves | Usually normal |
| Region affected | Cerebrum; decreased connections among cerebral cortical areas, and larger amygdala in children but not adults with autism[35]; abnormal shape of caudate and putamen[36] |
| Demographics | |
| Prevalence | 0.6%; 4:1 male-to-female ratio[41] |
| Prognosis | Variable; those with least impairment improve most |

skills, their narrow range of interests, and their repetitive and frequently obsessive behaviors interfere with school, work, and/or social life. Pervasive developmental disorder not otherwise specified indicates atypical behaviors similar to autism or Asperger's, yet not meeting all of the criteria for a diagnosis of autism or Asperger's.

Infants who later develop signs of autism show the following traits at 12 months of age: poor eye contact and decreased shared attention, communication, and social interaction.[35] Shared attention is responding to other people's nonverbal cues, including pointing or eye movements toward an object. Brain differences in autism include reduced communication among cerebral areas and during childhood larger than normal amygdala, although the amygdala size difference does not persist into adulthood.[35] Abnormal shape of the caudate and putamen correlates with motor, social, and communication impairment.[36]

The physician who reported an association between the development of autism and the measles, mumps, rubella (MMR) vaccine had his medical license revoked for dishonesty because only 12 children were included in the study, several children had been referred to the physician by a lawyer advocating for vaccine damages in the courts, he had an undisclosed patent on an alternative vaccine, and invasive tests were performed on the children without ethics approval.[37,38] The journal that published the falsified original article fully retracted the article.[39] Subsequent high-quality research involving 555,815 children in Canada, the United Kingdom, and Denmark found no relationship between the MMR vaccine and autism.[40] In Canada during the time studied, the rate of MMR vaccination declined while the incidence of autism increased.[40]

## Summary of Developmental Disorders

Major deformities of the nervous system occur before week 20 because the gross structure is developing during this time. After 20 weeks of normal development, damage to the immature nervous system causes minor malformations and/or disorders of function. Table 5-2 summarizes the processes of development and the consequences of damage during the peak time of each process. Table 5-3 lists the timing of developmental disorders.

## NERVOUS SYSTEM CHANGES DURING INFANCY

Many animal experiments have investigated the consequences of sensory deprivation for the infant nervous system. These experiments indicate that *critical periods* during development are crucial for normal outcomes. Critical periods are the times when neuronal projections compete for synaptic sites; thus, the nervous system optimizes neural connections during the critical periods.

One example of changing the functional properties of the nervous system was demonstrated in infant monkeys. Monkeys raised with one eyelid sutured shut from birth to 6 months were permanently unable to use vision from that eye, even after the sutures were removed. Recordings indicate that the retinal cells responded normally to light and the information was relayed correctly to the visual cortex, but the visual cortex did not respond to the information.[45] Occluding vision in one eye in an adult monkey for an equivalent period of time had relatively little effect on vision once visual input was restored. Thus the

**TABLE 5-2   SUMMARY OF DEVELOPMENTAL PROCESSES AND THE CONSEQUENCES OF INTERFERENCE WITH SPECIFIC DEVELOPMENTAL PROCESSES**

| Developmental Process | Peak Time of Occurrence | Disorders Secondary to Interference With Developmental Process |
|---|---|---|
| Neural tube formation | In utero weeks 3–4 | Anencephaly, Arnold-Chiari malformation, spina bifida occulta, meningocele, meningomyelocele, myeloschisis |
| Formation of brain enlargements | In utero months 2–3 | Holoprosencephaly |
| Cellular proliferation | In utero months 3–4 | Fetal alcohol syndrome, cocaine-affected nervous system |
| Neuronal migration | In utero months 3–5 | Heterotopia, seizures |
| Organization (differentiation, growth of axons and dendrites, synapse formation, selective neuron death, retraction of axons) | In utero month 5–early childhood | Intellectual disability, trisomy 21, cerebral palsy |
| Myelination | Birth–3 years after birth | Unknown |

**TABLE 5-3   TIMING OF EVENTS THAT MAY CAUSE NEURODEVELOPMENTAL DISORDERS**

| Time | Disorder |
|---|---|
| 0–6+ weeks | Neural tube disorders, chromosomal disorders, drugs, chemicals, and TORCH infections (toxoplasmosis, other [syphilis, varicella-zoster, parvovirus B19], rubella, cytomegalovirus [CMV], and herpes infections are infections during pregnancy that are associated with congenital abnormalities) |
| 1 month–birth | Neurocutaneous syndromes (autosomal dominant disorders with skin abnormalities and increased risk of nervous system tumors) and maternal problems including diabetes, toxemia, multiple pregnancies, and placental dysfunction |
| Perinatal | Prematurity, trauma, aspiration |
| Postnatal | Progressive encephalopathies, infections, trauma, childhood nervous system tumors, complications of spina bifida cystica |

critical period for tuning the visual cortex is during the first 6 months of development in monkeys.

> ### ◎ *Clinical Pearl*
>
> Critical periods are times when axons are competing for synaptic sites. Normal function of neural systems is dependent on appropriate experience during the critical periods.

Changes analogous to functional disuse in the monkeys explain the decrease in ability to learn a new language after early childhood. At birth, the cerebral cortex hearing areas are sensitive to all speech sounds. By 6 months, non-native speech sound distinctions (for example, Japanese-only speakers cannot distinguish between the sounds of the English letters "r" and "l" ) have been eliminated from the auditory-perceptual map.[46] Therefore older children and adults have great difficulty hearing, as well as pronouncing, non-native speech sounds. However, in normal 9-month-old American infants, 5 hours of exposure to Chinese speakers during a 1-month period preserves the ability to distinguish among Mandarin speech sounds.[45] This indicates that critical periods do not end abruptly; however, neuroplasticity is optimal for learning a specific task during a particular critical period. Learning a new language is possible during adulthood, but the adult probably will never sound like a native speaker. During critical periods, experience regulates the competition between inputs, affecting the electrical activity, molecular mechanisms, and inhibitory actions that produce permanent structural changes in the nervous system.[47]

Interruption of development during a critical period may explain some of the differences in outcome between perinatal and adult brain injury. In individuals with CP, damage to fibers descending from the cerebrum to the spinal cord during fetal development or at birth may eliminate some competition for synaptic sites during a critical period, causing persistence of inappropriate connections and abnormal development of spinal motor centers.[48] These inappropriate connections and developmental deficits in spinal motor centers, in addition to the deficiency of descending control, result in abnormal movement. The adult with brain damage loses descending control, but because development is complete, inappropriate connections or abnormal spinal motor circuits do not compound the dysfunction.

## SUMMARY

During the pre-embryonic stage, three layers of cells are formed: ectoderm, mesoderm, and endoderm. During the embryonic stage, the nervous system develops from ectoderm. During the fetal stage, the nervous system continues to develop, and myelination of axons begins.

Somites appear during the embryonic stage. Parts of the somite include the myotome, destined to become skeletal muscle, and the dermatome, destined to become dermis. The association of a single spinal nerve with a specific spinal nerve leads to the formation of a myotome—a group of skeletal muscles innervated by a spinal nerve. Similarly, the skin innervated by a single spinal nerve is a dermatome.

The inferior part of the neural tube becomes the spinal cord. The superior part of the neural tube differentiates to become the medulla, pons, midbrain, cerebellum, diencephalons, and cerebral hemispheres. During development, neural cells multiply, migrate, and grow. Neurons extend their axons to target cells, synapses form, and axons are myelinated. Neuronal death, claiming up to half of the neurons that develop in some brain regions, and axon retraction prune the developing nervous system. Damage to the developing nervous system may cause deficits that are not recognized until later in development, when the system that was damaged would become functional. This delayed loss of function is called *growing into deficit*.

Malformations of the central nervous system include anencephaly, Arnold-Chiari malformation, spina bifida, and forebrain malformation. Other disorders that occur during development include tethered spinal cord, intellectual disability, cerebral palsy, developmental coordination disorder, and autism.

## CLINICAL NOTES

### Case 1

A 2-year-old boy has no reaction to any stimulation below the level of the umbilicus. He does not voluntarily move his lower limbs, his lower limb muscles are atrophied, and he has no voluntary control of his bladder or bowels. His mother reports that he had surgery on his back 2 days after birth. Above the level of the umbilicus, sensation and movement are within normal limits.

#### Questions

1. Nervous system deficits affect which of these systems: sensory, autonomic, or motor?
2. The lesion is in what region of the nervous system: the peripheral, spinal, brainstem, or cerebral region?

### Case 2

Mary, a 2-year-old girl, is not yet attempting to stand. She has been slower than her peers in developing motor skills. The mother reports that Mary's lower body always felt "stiff as a board" when she was lifted and held. The mother also reports difficulty dressing and changing Mary when Mary is agitated, because the girl's legs strongly adduct. Mary is not yet toilet trained. Even when Mary is calm, her muscles are stiffer than normal. The therapist finds that Mary's somatosensation is intact throughout the body, her upper body has normal strength for her age, and the muscles of her lower limbs are weak.

#### Questions

1. Nervous system deficits affect which of these systems: sensory, autonomic, or motor?
2. The lesion is in what region of the nervous system?
3. What is the most likely diagnosis?

## REVIEW QUESTIONS

1. When do the organs form during development?
2. List the steps in formation of the neural tube.
3. What is a myotome?
4. Describe the changes in the neural tube that lead to formation of the brain.
5. List the progressive processes of cellular-level development.
6. Describe the regressive processes of cellular-level development.
7. Explain the concept of *growing into deficit*.
8. Describe the anatomic deficit in each of the following: anencephaly, Arnold-Chiari malformation, and the four types of spina bifida.
9. What are the differences between Arnold-Chiari type I and type II?
10. About half of cases of severe intellectual disability are associated with what developmental defect?
11. What is cerebral palsy? List the major types of cerebral palsy. What causes cerebral palsy?
12. What is autism? Does the measles/mumps/rubella vaccine cause autism? What is the most common cause of autism?
13. What are critical periods? Give an example of a critical period.

# References

1. Chotard C, Salecker I: Neurons and glia: team players in axon guidance. *Trends Neurosci* 27:655–661, 2004.
2. Gaspard N, Vanderhaeghen P: Mechanisms of neural specification from embryonic stem cells. *Curr Opin Neurobiol* 20:37–43, 2010.
3. Gotz M: Glial cells generate neurons—master control within CNS regions: developmental perspectives on neural stem cells. *Neuroscientist* 9:379–397, 2003.
4. Martin JH: The corticospinal system: from development to motor control. *Neuroscientist* 11:161–173, 2005.
5. Chakkalakal JV, Nishimune H, Ruas J, et al: Retrograde influence of muscle fibers on their innervation revealed by a novel marker for slow motoneurons. *Development* 137:3489–3499, 2010.
6. Erdogan E, Cansever T, Secer HI, et al: The evaluation of surgical treatment options in the Chiari malformation type I. *Turk Neurosurg* 20:303–313, 2010.
7. Holsgrove D, Leach P, Herwadkar A, et al: Visual field deficit due to downward displacement of optic chiasm. *Acta Neurochir (Wien)* 151:995–997, 2009.
8. Milhorat TH, Chou MW, Trinidad EM, et al: Chiari I malformation redefined: clinical and radiographic findings for 364 symptomatic patients. *Neurosurgery* 44:1005–1017, 1999.
9. Vannemreddy P, Nourbakhsh A, Willis B, et al: Congenital Chiari malformations. *Neurol India* 58:6–14, 2010.
10. Yarbrough CK, Powers AK, Park TS, et al: Patients with Chiari malformation Type I presenting with acute neurological deficits: case series. *J Neurosurg Pediatr* 7:244–247, 2011.
11. Sandler AD: Children with spina bifida: key clinical issues. *Pediatr Clin North Am* 57:879–892, 2010.
12. Juranek J, Salman MS: Anomalous development of brain structure and function in spina bifida myelomeningocele. *Dev Disabil Res Rev* 16:23–30, 2010.
13. Centers for Disease Control and Prevention: Racial/ethnic differences in the birth prevalence of spina bifida—United States, 1995–2005. *MMWR Morb Mortal Wkly Rep* 57:1409–1413, 2009.
14. Danzer E, Finkel RS, Rintoul NE, et al: Reversal of hindbrain herniation after maternal-fetal surgery for myelomeningocele subsequently impacts on brain stem function. *Neuropediatrics* 39:359–362, 2008.
15. Davis BE, Daley CM, Shurtleff DB, et al: Long-term survival of individuals with myelomeningocele. *Pediatr Neurosurg* 41:186–191, 2005.
16. Lorson CL, Rindt H, Shababi M: Spinal muscular atrophy: mechanisms and therapeutic strategies. *Hum Mol Genet* 19:R111–118, 2010.
17. Riley EP, Infante MA, Warren KR: Fetal alcohol spectrum disorders: an overview. *Neuropsychol Rev* 21:73–80, 2011.
18. Frost EA, Gist RS, Adriano E: Drugs, alcohol, pregnancy, and the fetal alcohol syndrome. *Int Anesthesiol Clin* 49:119–133, 2011.
19. Ackerman JP, Riggins T, Black MM: A review of the effects of prenatal cocaine exposure among school-aged children. *Pediatrics* 125:554–565, 2010.
20. Halpain S, Spencer K, Graber S: Dynamics and pathology of dendritic spines. *Prog Brain Res* 147:29–37, 2005.
21. Carlisle HJ, Kennedy MB: Spine architecture and synaptic plasticity. *Trends Neurosci* 28:182–187, 2005.
22. Johnston MV: Encephalopathies. In Kliegman RM, editor: *Nelson textbook of pediatrics*, ed 18, Philadelphia, 2007, Saunders.
23. Green LB, Hurvitz EA: Cerebral palsy. *Phys Med Rehabil Clin N Am* 18:859–882, vii, 2007.
24. Longo M, Hankins GD: Defining cerebral palsy: pathogenesis, pathophysiology and new intervention. *Minerva Ginecol* 61:421–429, 2009.
25. Task Force on Neonatal Encephalopathy and Cerebral Palsy: Neonatal encephalopathy and cerebral palsy: defining the pathogenesis and pathophysiology. Presented at American College of Obstetricians and Gynecologists (in collaboration with the American Academy of Pediatrics), Washington, DC, May 9, 2003.
26. Kin JP: The cerebral palsies: a physiological approach. *J Neurol Neurosurg Psychiatry* 74(Suppl 1):i23–i29, 2003.
27. Pakula AT, Van Naarden Braun K, Yeargin-Allsopp M: Cerebral palsy: classification and epidemiology. *Phys Med Rehabil Clin N Am* 20:425–452, 2009.
28. Jan MM: Cerebral palsy: comprehensive review and update. *Ann Saudi Med* 26:123–132, 2006.
29. Kirby A, Sugden D, Beveridge S, Edwards L: Developmental co-ordination disorder (DCD) in adults and adolescents. *JORSEN* 8:120–131, 2008.
30. Elders V, Sheehan S, Wilson AD, et al: Head-torso-hand coordination in children with and without developmental coordination disorder. *Dev Med Child Neurol* 52(3):238–243, 2010.
31. Kirby A, Sugden DA: Developmental coordination disorder. *Br J Hosp Med (Lond)* 71:571–575, 2010.
32. Curatolo P, D'Agati E, Moavero R: The neurobiological basis of ADHD. *Ital J Pediatr* 36:79, 2010.
33. Artificial food colouring and hyperactivity symptoms in children. *Prescrire Int* 18:215, 2009.
34. Steinhausen H-C: The heterogeneity of causes and courses of attention-deficit/hyperactivity disorder. *Acta Psychiatr Scand* 120:392–399, 2009.
35. Dawson G, Murias M: Autism. In Squire L, editor: *Encyclopedia of neuroscience*, St Louis, Mo, 2009, Elsevier, pp 799–884.
36. Qiu A, Adler M, Crocetti D, et al: Basal ganglia shapes predict social, communication, and motor dysfunctions in boys with autism spectrum disorder. *J Am Acad Child Adolesc Psychiatry* 49:539–551, 551.e1–551.e4, 2010.
37. Greenhalgh T: Why did *The Lancet* take so long? *BMJ* 340:c644, 2010.
38. Kmietowicz Z: Wakefield is struck off for the "serious and wide-ranging findings against him." *BMJ* 340:c2803, 2010.
39. Editors of the Lancet: Retraction—ileal-lymphoid-nodular hyperplasia, non-specific colitis, and pervasive developmental disorder in children. *Lancet* 375:445, 2010.
40. Kemp ML, Hart MB: MMR vaccine and autism: is there a link? *JAAPA* 23:48, 50, 2010.
41. Grafodatskaya D, Chung B, Szatmari P, et al: Autism spectrum disorders and epigenetics. *J Am Acad Child Adolesc Psychiatry* 49:794–809, 2010.
42. Hallmayer J, Cleveland S, Torres A, et al: Genetic heritability and shared environmental factors among twin pairs with autism. *Arch Gen Psychiatry.* Published online July 4, 2011.
43. Ben-Sasson A, Hen L, Fluss R, et al: A meta-analysis of sensory modulation symptoms in individuals with autism spectrum disorders. *J Autism Dev Disord* 39:1–11, 2009.
44. Hubert BE, Wicker B, Monfardini E, et al: Electrodermal reactivity to emotion processing in adults with autistic spectrum disorders. *Autism* 13:9–19, 2009.
45. Hubel DH, Wiesel TN: Ferrier lecture: Functional architecture of macaque monkey visual cortex. *Proc R Soc Lond B Biol Sci* 198:1–59, 1977.
46. Kuhl P: Brain mechanisms in early language acquisition. *Neuron* 67:713–727, 2010.
47. Tropea D, Majewska AK, Garcia R, et al: Structural dynamics of synapses in vivo correlate with functional changes during experience-dependent plasticity in visual cortex. *J Neurosci* 30:11086–11095, 2010.
48. Eyre JA, Taylor JP, Villagra F, et al: Evidence of activity-dependent withdrawal of corticospinal projections during human development. *Neurology* 57:1543–1554, 2001.

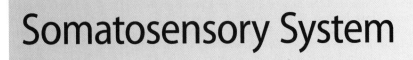

# 6

# Somatosensory System

Laurie Lundy-Ekman, PhD, PT

Sensation allows us to investigate the world, move accurately, and avoid or minimize injuries. This chapter discusses somatosensation—sensory information from the skin and musculoskeletal systems. The special senses of smell, vision, hearing, and equilibrium and sensations from the viscera are discussed in subsequent chapters.

Sensory information from the skin is called *superficial* or *cutaneous.* Superficial sensory information includes touch, pain, and temperature. Touch sensation includes superficial pressure and vibration. In contrast, sensory information from the musculoskeletal system includes proprioception and pain. Proprioception provides information regarding stretch of muscles, tension on tendons, positions of joints, and deep vibration. Proprioception includes both static joint position sense and kinesthetic sense—sensory information about movement.

All pathways that convey somatosensory information share similar anatomic arrangements. Receptors in the periphery encode the mechanical, chemical, or thermal stimulation received into receptor potentials (see Chapter 2). If the receptor potentials exceed the threshold of the trigger zone, an action potential is generated in a peripheral axon. The action potential is conducted along a peripheral axon, to a soma in a dorsal root ganglion, then along the proximal axon into the spinal cord. Within the spinal cord, information ascends via axons in the white matter to various regions of the brain. Information is transmitted through a series of neurons and synapses.

### ◎ Clinical Pearl

Information in the somatosensory system proceeds from the receptor through a series of neurons to the brain.

The diameter of the axons, the degree of axonal myelination, and the number of synapses in the pathway determine how quickly information is processed. Much somatosensory information is not consciously perceived but is processed at the spinal level in local neural circuits or by the cerebellum to adjust movements and posture. The distinction between sensory information (nerve impulses generated from the original stimuli) and sensation (awareness of stimuli from the senses) should be noted throughout this chapter. Perception, the interpretation of sensation into meaningful forms, occurs in the cerebrum. Perception is an active process of interaction between the brain and the environment. To perceive involves acting on the environment—moving the eyes, moving the head, or touching objects—and interpreting sensation.

## PERIPHERAL SOMATOSENSORY NEURONS

### Sensory Receptors

Sensory receptors are located at the distal ends of peripheral neurons. Each type of receptor is specialized, responding only to a specific type of stimulus, the adequate stimulus, under normal conditions. Based on the characteristics of the adequate stimulus, somatosensory receptors are classified as follows:

- Mechanoreceptors, responding to mechanical deformation of the receptor by touch, pressure, stretch, or vibration
- Chemoreceptors, responding to substances released by cells, including damaged cells following injury or infection
- Thermoreceptors, responding to heating or cooling

A subset of each type of somatosensory receptors is classified as nociceptors. Nociceptors are preferentially sensitive to stimuli that damage or threaten to damage tissue. Stimulation of nociceptors results in a sensation of pain. For example, when pressure mechanoreceptors are stimulated by stubbing a toe, the sensation experienced is pain rather than pressure. The receptors that encode the pain message are nociceptors, not the lower-threshold pressure receptors that convey information experienced as nonpainful pressure. Information from each of these types of receptors may reach awareness, but much of the information is used to make automatic adjustments and is selectively prevented from reaching consciousness by descending and local inhibitory connections.

Receptors that respond as long as a stimulus is maintained are called *tonic receptors.* For example, some stretch receptors in muscles, the tonic stretch receptors, fire the entire time a muscle is stretched. Receptors that adapt to a constant stimulus and stop responding are called *phasic receptors.* Muscles also contain phasic stretch receptors, which respond only briefly to a quick stretch. Another example of skin phasic receptors is the brief response of pressure receptors after putting on a wrist watch.

### Somatosensory Peripheral Neurons

The cell bodies of most peripheral sensory neurons are located outside the spinal cord in dorsal root ganglia or outside the brain in cranial nerve ganglia. Peripheral sensory neurons have two axons:

- Distal axons conduct messages from receptor to the cell body.
- Proximal axons project from the cell body into the spinal cord or brainstem.

Some proximal axons that enter the spinal cord extend as far as the medulla before synapsing.

Peripheral axons, also called *afferents,* are classified according to axon diameter. The most commonly used system for classifying peripheral sensory axons designates the axons in order of declining diameter: Ia, Ib, II, or Aβ, Aδ, C. The diameter of an axon is functionally important: larger-diameter axons transmit information faster than smaller-diameter axons C (Figure 6-1). The faster conduction occurs because resistance to current flow is lower in large-diameter axons, and because large-diameter axons are myelinated, allowing saltatory conduction of the action potential (see Chapter 2).

### Cutaneous Innervation—Peripheral Versus Dermatomal Intervention

The area of skin innervated by a single afferent neuron is called the *receptive field* for that neuron (Figure 6-2). Receptive fields tend to be smaller distally and larger proximally. Distal regions of the body also have a greater density of receptors than proximal areas. The combination of smaller receptive fields and greater density of receptors distally enables us to distinguish

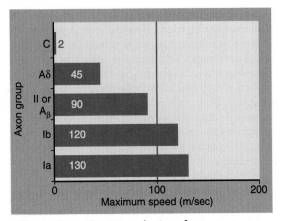

**Fig. 6-1** Conduction velocity of sensory axons.

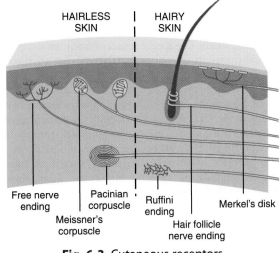

**Fig. 6-3** Cutaneous receptors.

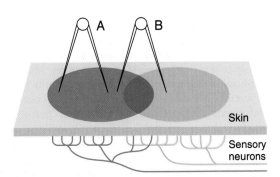

**Fig. 6-2 Receptive fields.** Areas of skin innervated by each neuron are indicated on the surface of the skin. **A,** The caliper points touching the skin would be perceived as one point, because both points are within the receptive field of a single neuron. **B,** The caliper points would be perceived as two points, because the points are contacting the receptive fields of two neurons.

between two closely applied stimuli on a fingertip, while the same stimuli cannot be perceived as separate stimuli when applied to the back.

Sensations from skin include the following:
- Touch
- Pain
- Temperature

Touch information is categorized as fine touch or coarse touch. *Fine touch* includes a variety of receptors (Figure 6-3) and subsensations. Superficial fine touch receptors have small receptive fields, allowing resolution of closely spaced stimuli. Superficial fine touch receptors include Meissner's corpuscles, sensitive to light touch and vibration, and Merkel's disks, sensitive to pressure. Hair follicle receptors, sensitive to displacement of a hair, also have small receptive fields. Subcutaneous fine touch receptors have large receptive fields, providing less localization and discrimination of stimuli. Subcutaneous fine touch receptors include pacinian corpuscles, responsive to touch and vibration, and Ruffini's corpuscles, sensitive to stretch of the skin. All of the fine touch receptors transmit information on

Aβ afferents. *Coarse touch* is mediated by free endings throughout the skin (see Figure 6-3). These free nerve endings provide information perceived as pleasant touch or pressure and the sensations of tickle and itch.

Nociceptors are free nerve endings, responsive to stimuli that damage or threaten tissue. Nociceptors provide information perceived as pain. *Thermal receptors,* also free nerve endings, respond to warmth or cold within the temperature range that does not damage tissue. Information from all of the free nerve endings is conveyed by Aδ and C afferents. Although the various tactile receptors respond to different types of stimuli, natural stimuli typically activate several types of tactile receptors.[1]

As noted in Chapter 5, the area of skin innervated by axons from cell bodies in a single dorsal root is a dermatome. In the brachial and lumbosacral plexus, sensory axons innervating specific parts of the limbs are separated from other axons arising in the same dorsal root and regrouped to form peripheral nerves. Thus peripheral nerves, such as the median nerve, have a different pattern of innervation than the dermatomes. Dermatomes and the cutaneous distribution of peripheral nerves in the posteromedial upper limb are illustrated in Figure 6-4. Dermatomes and the cutaneous distribution of peripheral nerves throughout the body are illustrated in Figures 6-5 and 6-6.

Although cutaneous receptors are not proprioceptors, the information from cutaneous receptors contributes to our sense of joint position and movement. The contribution of cutaneous receptors is primarily kinesthetic, responding to stretching of or increasing pressure on the skin. However, Ruffini's corpuscles discharge in response to static joint angles.

---

**◎ Clinical Pearl**

Cutaneous receptors respond to touch, pressure, vibration, stretch, noxious stimuli, and temperature.

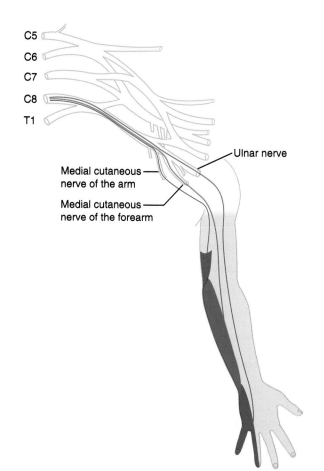

**Fig. 6-4 Cutaneous innervation of the posteromedial upper limb.** All afferent axons enter the spinal cord through the C8 dorsal root, so the dermatome innervating the posteromedial upper limb is C8. However, three peripheral nerves distribute the axons of sensory neurons to the periphery. Thus, afferents from the posteromedial hand travel in the ulnar nerve, afferents from the posteromedial forearm travel in the medial cutaneous nerve of the forearm, and afferents from the upper posteromedial arm travel in the medial cutaneous nerve of the arm. Therefore, a complete lesion of the ulnar nerve superior to the wrist would deprive the area colored blue of sensation, yet the green and red regions would still be innervated. A C8 dorsal root lesion would deprive the entire posteromedial upper limb of sensation.

## Musculoskeletal Innervation

### Muscle Spindle

The sensory organ in muscle is the *muscle spindle*, consisting of muscle fibers, sensory endings, and motor endings (Figure 6-7). The sensory endings of the spindle respond to stretch, that is, changes in muscle length and the velocity of length change. Quick and tonic stretch of the spindle is registered by type Ia afferents. Tonic stretch of a muscle is monitored by type II afferents. Small efferent fibers to the ends of muscle spindle

fibers adjust spindle fiber stretch so that the spindle is responsive through the physiologic range of muscle lengths.

### Intrafusal and Extrafusal Fibers

Muscle spindles are embedded in skeletal muscle. Because the spindle is fusiform (tapered at the ends), specialized muscle fibers inside the spindle are designated *intrafusal fibers;* ordinary skeletal muscle fibers outside the spindle are *extrafusal.* The ends of the intrafusal fibers connect to the extrafusal fibers, so stretching the muscle stretches the intrafusal fibers. To serve the dual purposes of providing information about the length and rate of change in length of the muscle, the spindle has two types of muscle fibers, two types of sensory afferents, and two types of efferents.

Intrafusal fibers are contractile only at their ends; the central region cannot contract. The arrangement of nuclei in the central region characterizes the two types of intrafusal fibers:
- *Nuclear bag fibers* have a clump of nuclei in the central region.
- *Nuclear chain fibers* have nuclei arranged single file.

For spindles to monitor muscle length and rate of change in length, two different sensory endings are required:
- *Primary endings* of type Ia neurons wrap around the central region of each intrafusal fiber.
- *Secondary endings* of type II afferents end mainly on nuclear chain fibers adjacent to the primary endings.

Because of their appearance, primary endings are also known as *annulospiral endings,* and secondary endings are called *flower-spray endings.* The discharge of primary endings is both phasic and tonic. Phasic discharge is maximal during quick stretch and fades quickly, as when a tendon is tapped with a reflex hammer. Tonic discharge is sustained during constant stretch; the rate of firing is proportional to the stretch of spindle fibers. Secondary endings respond only tonically.

If a muscle is passively stretched, the muscle spindles respond to the stretch (Figure 6-8, *A*). If the ends of intrafusal fibers were not contractile, the sensory endings would register change only when the muscle was fully elongated; if the muscle were contracted even slightly, the spindle would be slack, rendering the sensory endings insensitive to stretch (Figure 6-8, *B*). To maintain the sensitivity of the spindle throughout the normal range of muscle lengths, *gamma motor neurons* fire, causing the ends of intrafusal fibers to contract. Contracting the ends of the intrafusal fibers stretches the central region, thus maintaining sensory activity from the spindle (Figure 6-8, *C*). Gamma efferent control is dual, with *gamma dynamic axons* ending on nuclear bag fibers to adjust the sensitivity of primary afferents, and *gamma static axons* innervating both types of intrafusal fibers to tune the sensitivity of both primary and secondary afferents.[2]

> **◯ Clinical Pearl**
>
> Muscle length is signaled by type Ia and II afferents, reflecting stretch of the central region of both types of intrafusal fibers. Spindle sensitivity to changes in length is adjusted by gamma static efferents. Velocity of change in muscle length is signaled only by type Ia afferents, with information mainly from nuclear bag fibers, whose sensitivity is adjusted by gamma dynamic efferents.

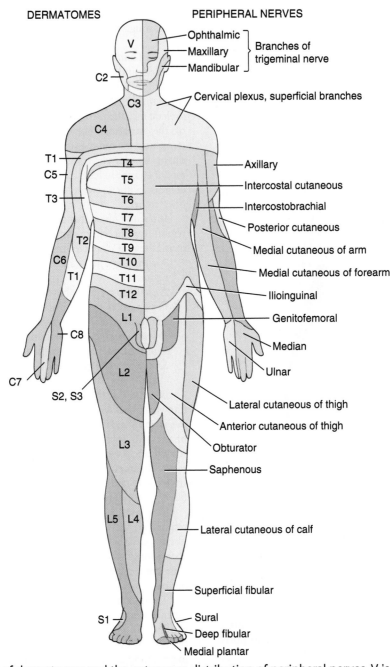

**Fig. 6-5** Anterior view of dermatomes and the cutaneous distribution of peripheral nerves. V is Roman Numeral V, indicating the fifth cranial nerve (trigeminal nerve). *(Dermatome distributions are based on information from Lee MW, McPhee RW, Stringer MD: An evidence-based approach to human dermatomes. Clin Anat 21:363–373, 2008.)*

## Golgi Tendon Organs

Tension in tendons is relayed from Golgi tendon organs, encapsulated nerve endings woven among the collagen strands of the tendon near the musculotendinous junction (Figure 6-9, *A*). Golgi tendon organs are sensitive to very slight changes (<1 g) in tension on a tendon and respond to tension exerted both by active contraction and by passive stretch of muscle.[3] Information is transmitted from Golgi tendon organs into the spinal cord by type Ib afferents.

## Joint Receptors

Joint receptors respond to mechanical deformation of the capsule and ligaments (Figure 6-9, *B*). Ruffini's endings in the joint capsule signal the extremes of joint range and respond more to passive than to active movement. Paciniform corpuscles respond to movement, but not when joint position is constant. Ligament receptors are similar to Golgi tendon organs and signal tension. Free nerve endings are most often stimulated by inflammation. The afferents associated with the joint receptors are as follows:

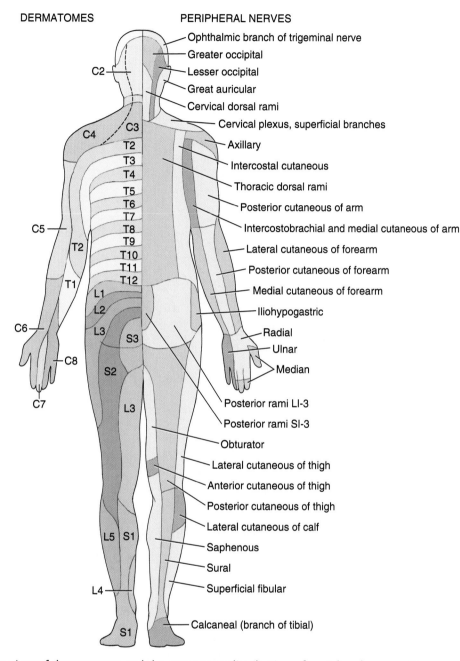

DERMATOMES        PERIPHERAL NERVES

- Ophthalmic branch of trigeminal nerve
- Greater occipital
- Lesser occipital
- Great auricular
- Cervical dorsal rami
- Cervical plexus, superficial branches
- Axillary
- Intercostal cutaneous
- Thoracic dorsal rami
- Posterior cutaneous of arm
- Intercostobrachial and medial cutaneous of arm
- Lateral cutaneous of forearm
- Posterior cutaneous of forearm
- Medial cutaneous of forearm
- Iliohypogastric
- Radial
- Ulnar
- Median
- Posterior rami LI-3
- Posterior rami SI-3
- Obturator
- Lateral cutaneous of thigh
- Anterior cutaneous of thigh
- Posterior cutaneous of thigh
- Lateral cutaneous of calf
- Saphenous
- Sural
- Superficial fibular
- Calcaneal (branch of tibial)

**Fig. 6-6** Posterior view of dermatomes and the cutaneous distribution of peripheral nerves. *(Dermatome distributions are based on information from Lee MW, McPhee RW, Stringer MD: An evidence-based approach to human dermatomes. Clin Anat 21:363–373, 2008.)*

- Ligament receptors—type Ib
- Ruffini's and paciniform endings—type II
- Free nerve endings

Fully normal proprioception requires muscle spindles, joint receptors, and cutaneous mechanoreceptors. This redundancy probably reflects the importance of proprioception to the control of movement. People with total hip joint replacements retain good hip proprioception, despite the loss of joint proprioceptors.[4]

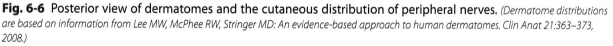

### ◎ *Clinical Pearl*

Muscle spindles respond to quick and to prolonged stretch of the muscle. Tendon organs signal the force generated by muscle contraction or by passive stretch of the tendon. Joint receptors respond to mechanical deformation of joint capsules and ligaments.

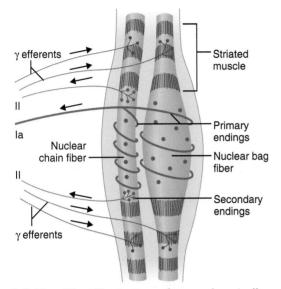

**Fig. 6-7  Simplified illustration of a muscle spindle.**
Intrafusal muscle fibers include nuclear chain and nuclear bag fibers. Stretch of the central region of intrafusal fibers is sensed by primary and secondary endings. Sensory information is conveyed to the central nervous system by type Ia and type II afferents. Efferent control of intrafusal fibers is provided by gamma motor neurons.

## Summary: Function of Different-Diameter Axons

Large-diameter afferents transmit information from specialized receptors in muscles, tendons, and joints. Medium-sized afferents transmit information from joint capsules, muscle spindles, and cutaneous touch, stretch, and pressure receptors. The smallest-diameter afferents convey crude touch, nociceptive, and temperature information from both the musculoskeletal system and the skin. Table 6-1 summarizes axon types, associated receptors, and adequate stimuli for the somatosensory system. Two systems are used to classify somatosensory axons: Roman numerals for proprioceptive axons, and letters for all others.

## PATHWAYS TO THE BRAIN

Three types of pathways bring sensory information to the brain (Table 6-2):
- Conscious relay pathways
- Divergent pathways
- Unconscious relay pathways

An important distinction among types of pathways is the fidelity of information conveyed. Pathways that transmit signals with high fidelity provide accurate details regarding the location of the stimulation. For example, high-fidelity signals from the fingertips allow people to recognize two points separated by as little as 1.6 mm as being distinct points, and to identify precisely where on the fingertip the stimulation occurred. The ability to identify the location of stimulation is achieved by the anatomic arrangement of axons in the pathways. In high-fidelity pathways, a somatotopic arrangement of information is created. *Somatotopic* refers to information arranged similarly to the anatomic organization of the body. To create somatotopic

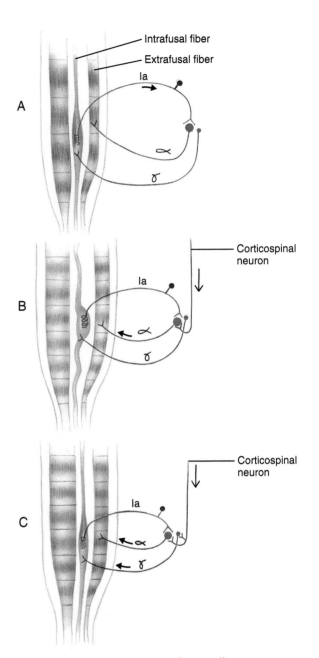

**Fig. 6-8  A,** During passive stretch, spindles are elongated as the muscle is stretched. This stretch activates the spindle sensory receptors. The arrow indicates action potentials transmitted by the type Ia afferent. **B,** Excitation of the α-motor neuron via the corticospinal neuron results in contraction of extrafusal muscle fibers. If γ-motor neurons do not fire when α-motor neurons to the extrafusal muscles fire, the intrafusal central region will be relaxed and the afferent neurons inactive. This does not occur in a normal neuromuscular system. **C,** Normally, during active muscle contraction, α- and γ-motor neurons are simultaneously active. The firing of gamma motor neurons causes the ends of intrafusal fibers to contract, thus maintaining the stretch on the intrafusal central region and preserving the ability of sensory endings to indicate stretch.

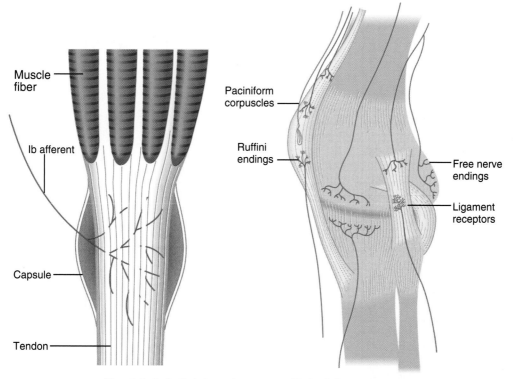

**Fig. 6-9** *Left,* Golgi tendon organ. *Right,* Joint receptors.

arrangement, axons from one part of the body are close to axons carrying signals from adjacent parts of the body and are segregated from axons carrying information from distant parts of the body. For example, axons carrying information from the thumb are near axons carrying information from the index finger and relatively distant from axons carrying information from the toes.

In describing pathways in the nervous system, only neurons with long axons that connect distant regions of the nervous system are counted. These neurons with long axons are called *projection neurons.* The convention for numbering or naming only the projection neurons omits the small, integrative interneurons interposed between the projection neurons. Thus, a three-neuron pathway means three projection neurons, but a number of interneurons may also be linked in the pathway.

Within the central nervous system, a bundle of axons with the same origin and a common termination is called a *tract.* Somatosensory pathways are often named for the origin and termination of the tract that contains the second neuron in the series. The second neuron in the spinothalamic pathway originates in the spinal cord and terminates in the thalamus. Thus, the second neuron in the pathway travels in the *spinothalamic tract,* and the tract lends its name to the entire pathway. The pathway includes the neuron that brings the information into the central nervous system, the neuron in the spinothalamic tract, and the neuron from the thalamus to the cerebral cortex.

The first type of pathway, *the conscious relay pathway,* brings information about location and type of stimulation to the cerebral cortex. The information in conscious relay pathways is transmitted with high fidelity, thus providing accurate details regarding the stimulus and its location. Because the information in these pathways allows us to make fine distinctions about stimuli, the term *discriminative* is used to describe the

sensations conveyed in conscious relay pathways. Information about discriminative touch and proprioception ascends ipsilaterally in the posterior spinal cord. Information about discriminative pain and temperature crosses the midline soon after entering the cord and then ascends contralaterally.

The second type of pathway, *the divergent pathway,* transmits information to many locations in the brainstem and cerebrum and uses pathways with varying numbers of neurons. The sensory information is used at both conscious and unconscious levels. Aching pain is a form of sensation that is transmitted via divergent pathways in the central nervous system.

The third type of pathway, *the unconscious relay pathway,* brings unconscious proprioceptive and other movement-related information to the cerebellum. This information plays an essential role in automatic adjustments of our movements and posture.

---

### ◎ *Clinical Pearl*

Conscious relay pathways convey high-fidelity, somatotopically arranged information to the cerebral cortex. Divergent pathways convey information that is not somatotopically organized to many areas of the brain. Unconscious relay pathways convey movement-related information to the cerebellum.

---

### Conscious Relay Pathways to Cerebral Cortex

All four types of somatosensation reach conscious awareness:
- Touch
- Proprioception

**TABLE 6-1   AXON CLASSIFICATIONS, ASSOCIATED RECEPTORS, AND ADEQUATE STIMULI FOR THE SOMATOSENSORY SYSTEM**

| Axon Type* | PROPRIOCEPTION | | | CUTANEOUS AND SUBCUTANEOUS TOUCH AND PRESSURE | | | PAIN AND TEMPERATURE | | |
|---|---|---|---|---|---|---|---|---|---|
| | Roman Numeral Classification | Receptors | Stimulus | Letter Classification | Receptors | Stimulus | Letter Classification | Receptors | Stimulus |
| Large myelinated | Ia | Muscle spindles | Muscle stretch | — | | | — | | |
| | Ib | Golgi tendon organs Ligament receptors | Tendon tension Ligament tension | — | | | — | | |
| Medium myelinated | II | Muscle spindles Paciniform and Ruffini-type receptors in joint capsules | Muscle stretch Joint movement | Aβ | Meissner's Pacinian Ruffini's Merkel's Hair follicle | Touch, vibration Touch, vibration Skin stretch Pressure Pressure | — | | |
| Small myelinated | | | | | | | Aδ | Free nerve ending | Tissue damage, temperature, coarse touch |
| Small unmyelinated | | | | | | | C | Free nerve ending | Tissue damage, temperature, itch, tickle |

*The axon diameter correlates with speed of conduction; thus, the large, myelinated fibers conduct fastest, and the unmyelinated fibers have the slowest conduction speeds.

**TABLE 6-2**   SOMATOSENSORY PATHWAYS

| Type | Information Conveyed | Anatomic Name | Termination |
|------|---------------------|---------------|-------------|
| Conscious relay | Discriminative touch and conscious proprioception | Dorsal column/medial lemniscus | Primary sensory area cerebral cortex |
| | Discriminative pain and temperature | Spinothalamic | Primary sensory area cerebral cortex |
| Divergent | Slow, aching pain | Spinomesencephalic | Midbrain |
| | | Spinoreticular | Reticular formation |
| | | Spinolimbic | Amygdala, basal ganglia, many areas of cerebral cortex |
| Unconscious relay | Movement-related information | Spinocerebellar | Cerebellum |

- Pain
- Temperature

The pathways involve three projection neurons. The pathways to consciousness travel upward in the spinal cord via two routes:

- Dorsal columns
- Anterolateral tracts

The routes in the spinal cord are composed of white matter, because myelin promotes rapid conduction along the axons. The dorsal columns carry sensory information about discriminative touch and conscious proprioception; discriminative pain and temperature information travels in the anterolateral tracts. To be aware of sensory information, the information must reach the thalamus, where crude awareness is possible.[5] For discriminative perception of stimuli localized with fine resolution, information must be processed by the cerebral cortex.

If peripheral afferent information is absent, awareness of body parts can be lost. Oliver Sacks, a neurologist, recounts his strange experience of believing that he had lost his leg following severe damage to several nerves in a climbing accident. The complete loss of sensation from his leg led to lack of awareness of the limb. Although he was not paralyzed, he was unable to voluntarily take a step until his physical therapist moved his leg passively, giving him the concept of how to move the injured leg.[6]

## Discriminative Touch and Conscious Proprioception

*Discriminative touch* includes localization of touch and vibration and the ability to discriminate between two closely spaced points touching the skin. *Conscious proprioception* is the awareness of movements and of the relative position of body parts. Integration of touch and proprioceptive information in the cerebral cortex allows identification of an object by touch and pressure information. *Stereognosis* is the ability to use touch and proprioceptive information to identify an object, for example, a key in the hand can be identified without vision. Information conveyed in this pathway is important for recognizing objects by touch, controlling fine movements, and making movements smooth.

The pathway for discriminative touch and conscious proprioception uses a three-neuron relay (see Figures 6-9 and 6-10):

- The primary, or first-order, neuron conveys information from the receptors to the medulla.
- The secondary, or second-order, neuron conveys information from the medulla to the thalamus.
- The tertiary, or third-order, neuron conveys information from the thalamus to the cerebral cortex.

The anatomic name for the pathway that conveys discriminative touch and conscious proprioception is the dorsal column/medial lemniscus system.

### Dorsal Column/Medial Lemniscus System

Stimulation of receptors at the distal end of the primary neuron is conveyed to the cell body in the dorsal root ganglion. The proximal axon of the primary neuron enters the spinal cord via the dorsal root, then ascends in the ipsilateral dorsal column. Axons from the lower limb occupy the more medial section of the dorsal column, called the *fasciculus gracilis*. Axons from the upper limb occupy the lateral section of the dorsal column, called the *fasciculus cuneatus*. This pattern occurs because nerve fibers entering the dorsal column from higher segments are added laterally to fibers already in the dorsal column from lower segments.

Axons that ascend in the fasciculus gracilis synapse with second-order neurons in the *nucleus gracilis* of the medulla. Axons in the fasciculus cuneatus synapse with second-order neurons in the *nucleus cuneatus* of the medulla. Thus, in a tall person, a primary neuron could be 6 feet long, extending from a toe to the medulla.

Throughout the spinal cord, primary neurons of the discriminative touch/conscious proprioception pathway have many collateral branches entering the gray matter. Some collaterals contribute to motor control, some influence activity in neurons in other sensory systems, and others influence autonomic regulation.

Cell bodies of the second-order neurons are located in the nucleus gracilis or cuneatus. Axons from the second-order neurons cross the midline as internal arcuate fibers, then ascend to the thalamus as the *medial lemniscus*. The second-order neurons end in an area of the thalamus named for its location, the *ventral posterolateral (VPL) nucleus*.

Third-order neurons connect the thalamus to the sensory cortex. Axons form part of the thalamocortical radiations—fibers connecting the thalamus to the cerebral cortex. Thalamocortical axons travel through the internal capsule.

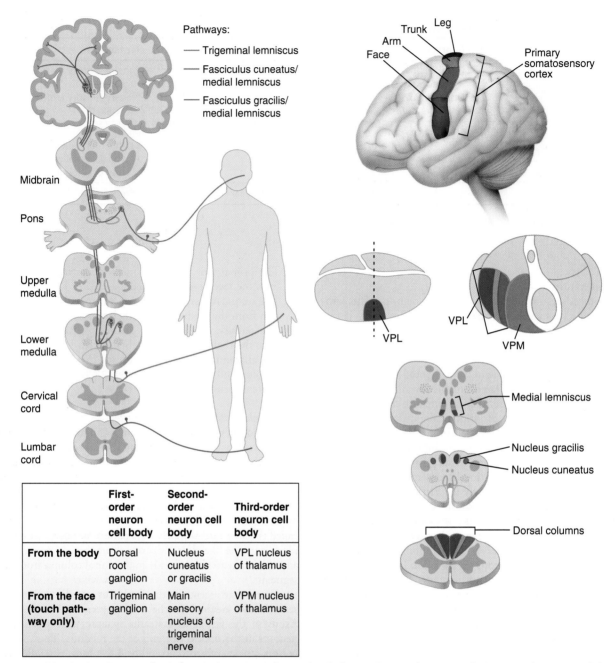

| | First-order neuron cell body | Second-order neuron cell body | Third-order neuron cell body |
|---|---|---|---|
| **From the body** | Dorsal root ganglion | Nucleus cuneatus or gracilis | VPL nucleus of thalamus |
| **From the face (touch pathway only)** | Trigeminal ganglion | Main sensory nucleus of trigeminal nerve | VPM nucleus of thalamus |

**Fig. 6-10  Discriminative touch and conscious proprioceptive information pathways.** *Left,* A coronal section of the cerebrum, shown above horizontal sections of the brainstem and spinal cord. *Right,* The distribution of information from the face, arm, trunk, and leg. *Middle right,* A lateral view of the cerebrum is shown. Below the cerebrum are lateral and coronal views of the thalamus. The lateral view of the thalamus shows the location of the ventroposterolateral nucleus (VPL). The dotted line indicates the plane of the coronal section of the thalamus. The coronal section of the thalamus reveals the ventroposteromedial nucleus (VPM). The medulla and the spinal cord are shown in horizontal section on the right. Color coding is indicated at top right.

**Discriminative Touch Information From the Face.** Sensory innervation for the face is supplied by the three divisions of the *trigeminal nerve* (see Figures 6-10 and 6-11) (see Chapter 14 for additional details on the trigeminal nerve). Some of the neurons in the trigeminal nerve are first-order neurons for discriminative touch information from the face. Their cell bodies are in the trigeminal ganglion, and the proximal axons

end in the *trigeminal main sensory nucleus.* Second-order neuron cell bodies are located in the trigeminal main sensory nucleus. Second-order axons cross the midline in the pons to travel in the *trigeminal lemniscus* and end in the *ventral posteromedial (VPM) nucleus* of the thalamus. Third-order axons continue to the cerebral cortex. Details regarding sensation from the face are presented in Chapter 14. The effects of lesions in the

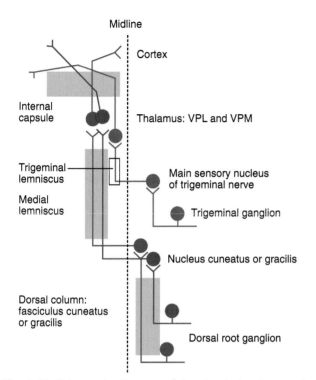

**Fig. 6-11** Schematic diagram of the discriminative touch and conscious proprioceptive pathways. Blocks of color indicate groups of axons, as labeled on the left side. Compare with Figure 6-10.

cortical representation corresponds to the relatively high density of receptors in these regions and the associated degree of fine motor control.

**Somatosensory Areas of the Cerebral Cortex.** The primary sensory cortex discriminates the size, texture, or shape of objects. Another area of the cerebral cortex, the *somatosensory association area,* analyzes information from the primary sensory area and the thalamus and provides stereognosis and memory of the tactile and spatial environment.

> **◎ Clinical Pearl**
>
> Sensory information essential for identifying objects by palpation, distinguishing between closely spaced stimuli, and controlling fine movement and smoothness of movement travels in dorsal columns, then in the medial lemniscus, to the primary sensory cortex. Tactile information from the face travels in the trigeminal nerve, then to the thalamus, then to the sensory cortex.

## Discriminative Pain and Temperature, Coarse Touch

### Anterolateral Columns: Pain and Temperature

The anterolateral white matter in the spinal cord contains axons that transmit discriminative information about coarse touch, pain, and temperature. Coarse touch conveys less localized information than is conveyed by the dorsal column/medial lemniscus system. Coarse touch, transmitted by C-fiber unmyelinated axons from low-threshold mechanoreceptors, is vital for perceiving pleasant touch and pleasurable skin-to-skin contacts. The coarse touch information projects to the left insula, an area associated with positive emotional feelings.[7,8] Anterolateral column lesions interfere with the emotional aspects of touch but not with discriminative touch.[8]

Several parallel tracts ascend in the anterolateral spinal cord. One of the tracts, the *spinothalamic tract,* is part of a three-neuron conscious relay pathway called the *spinothalamic pathway.* Phylogenetically older, slower-conducting divergent pathways include the spinolimbic, spinoreticular, and spinomesencephalic.

**Temperature Sensation.** Warmth and cold are detected by specialized free nerve endings of small myelinated and unmyelinated neurons. Aδ fibers carry impulses produced by cooling, and C fibers carry information regarding heat. In the spinothalamic pathway, the proximal axon of the first-order neuron branches to spread vertically to adjacent segments of the spinal cord, then synapses with second-order neurons in the dorsal horn. Second-order axons cross the midline and then ascend contralaterally to project to the VPL nucleus of the thalamus. The axons of third-order neurons project from the thalamus to the sensory cortex.

**Pain.** Pain is an extremely complex phenomenon. Persistent pain affects emotional, autonomic, and social function. Pain is composed of both protective sensation and the emotional response to this sensation. The term *nociceptive* describes receptors or neurons that receive or transmit information about stimuli that damage or threaten to damage tissue. Nociceptive information travels in several different pathways.

discriminative touch/conscious proprioception pathways are illustrated in Figure 6-12.

**Somatotopic Arrangement of Information.** Although the axons in the dorsal column are arranged segmentally as they enter the dorsal columns, these axons are rearranged into a somatotopic organization as they ascend. The somatotopic arrangement is maintained throughout the second- and third-order neurons, so that the area of cerebral cortex devoted to discriminative somatosensation, the *primary sensory (primary somatosensory) cortex,* receives somatotopically organized information. The primary sensory cortex is located in the gyrus posterior to the central sulcus, that is, the postcentral gyrus.

The size of the area of primary sensory cortex devoted to a specific part of the body is represented by the *homunculus* surrounding the cortex in Figure 6-13. The homunculus is a map, developed by recording the responses of awake individuals during surgery. Small areas of the cerebral cortex are electrically stimulated, and individuals report what they feel. When the sensory cortex is stimulated, they report feeling sensations that seem to originate from the surface of the body. For example, stimulation of the medial postcentral gyrus elicits sensations that seem to originate in the contralateral lower limb. Another method of testing is to stimulate areas on the body and record from the cerebral cortex. For example, touching a fingertip activates neurons in the superolateral postcentral gyrus. The homunculus illustrates the proportions and arrangement of cortical areas that contain representations of the surface of the body. The fingers and lips of the homunculus are much larger than their proportion of the body would indicate. The large

LESION IN:

EFFECT ON DISCRIMINATIVE
TOUCH AND CONSCIOUS
PROPRIOCEPTIVE INFORMATION:

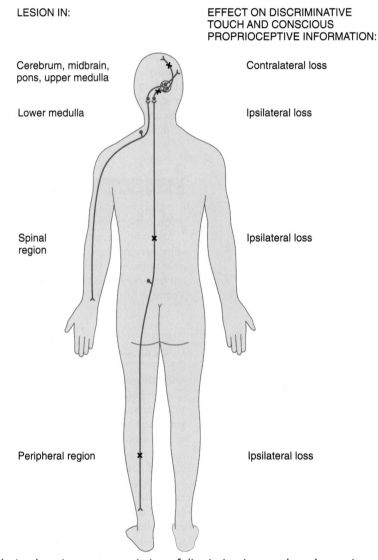

Cerebrum, midbrain,
pons, upper medulla

Contralateral loss

Lower medulla

Ipsilateral loss

Spinal
region

Ipsilateral loss

Peripheral region

Ipsilateral loss

**Fig. 6-12** The effect of lesion location on transmission of discriminative touch and conscious proprioceptive information.

A common patient report of back pain secondary to lifting a heavy object consists of an initial immediate sharp sensation that indicates the location of the injury; this is called fast or *spinothalamic pain.* Fast pain is often followed by a dull, throbbing ache that is not well localized. The latter pain is called slow or *spinolimbic pain.* Both types of pain occur in acute pain. Impulses that convey both fast and slow pain travel together in the anterolateral section of the spinal cord, and then their paths become separate in the brain (Figure 6-14). Fast pain uses a conscious relay pathway and therefore is discussed in this section; slow pain is discussed in a subsequent section on divergent pathways.

### Fast, Localized Pain: Lateral Pain System
Fast pain uses a three-neuron system (Figures 6-14, *A* and *C,* and 6-15A):

- The first-order neuron brings information into the dorsal horn of the spinal cord.
- The axon of the second-order neuron crosses the midline and projects from the spinal cord to the thalamus.
- The third-order neuron projects from the thalamus to the cerebral cortex.

The primary neuron in the fast pain pathway is a small myelinated Aδ fiber. Aδ fibers transmit information from free nerve endings in the periphery to the spinal cord. The endings respond to noxious mechanical stimulation (high-threshold mechanoreceptor afferents) or to mechanical or thermal stimulation (mechanothermal afferents). The peripheral axon brings an impulse to the cell body in the dorsal root ganglion. The central axon enters the cord, then branches to several levels in the *dorsolateral tract* (Lissauer's marginal zone) before entering into and terminating in lamina I, II, or V of the dorsal horn

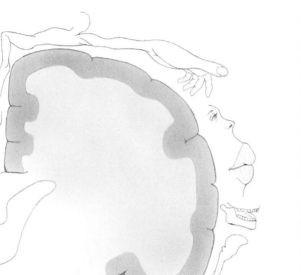

**Fig. 6-13 Primary sensory cortex.** Areas of the cortex responding to somatosensory stimulation are indicated by the homunculus.

(Figure 6-16). *Laminae* are histologic divisions of the spinal cord gray matter. The primary neuron releases the neurotransmitter glutamate.

The cell body of the second-order neuron is in lamina I, II, or V of the dorsal horn. The axon of the second-order neuron crosses the midline in the anterior white commissure, then ascends to the thalamus via the *spinothalamic tract*. Most spinothalamic tract neurons end in the VPL nucleus of the thalamus. The name *lateral pain system* derives from this termination of the tract in the lateral thalamus. The third-order neurons arise in the VPL nucleus and project to the primary and secondary sensory cortex. Although localizing noxious stimuli requires information in the fast pain pathway, the posterior parietal cortex must provide additional processing for spatial localization.[9] A lesion in the VPL nucleus interrupts the pathway to the cortex, causing inability to localize painful stimuli despite feeling the affective (emotional) aspects of pain.

---

© *Clinical Pearl*

Information that enables individuals to localize noxious sensations and consciously distinguish between warmth and cold travels to the cerebral cortex via spinothalamic pathways.

---

*Comparison of Dorsal Column/Medial Lemniscus and Spinothalamic Systems*

The spinothalamic and dorsal column systems are anatomically similar, consisting of three neuron relay pathways. Unlike the

dorsal columns, which contain axons of primary neurons and ascend ipsilaterally, ascending axons in the anterolateral columns are second-order neurons, and most ascend contralaterally. In both the dorsal column paths and the spinothalamic tract, the second-order axon crosses the midline. However, in the dorsal column path, the crossing occurs in the medulla, but in the spinothalamic pathway, the crossing occurs in the spinal cord before the axon ascends. The second neuron in both dorsal column and spinothalamic paths ends in the VPL nucleus of the thalamus. In both pathways, third-order neurons project from the thalamus to the primary sensory cortex, where the information can be localized.

In contrast to the discriminative touch and conscious proprioceptive information traveling in the dorsal columns, the anterolateral white matter contains axons that transmit information about pain, temperature, and coarse touch. However, functions of the dorsal and anterolateral columns are not rigidly segregated; information about nondiscriminative (coarse) touch travels in the anterolateral system, and some pain and temperature information ascends in the dorsal columns.[10]

*Fast Pain Information From the Face*

Afferent information interpreted as fast pain from the face travels in the *trigeminal nerve*. Fibers in this pathway enter the pons, then travel down into the medulla and upper cervical cord in the descending tract of the trigeminal nerve before synapsing in the spinal nucleus of the trigeminal nerve (see Figure 6-14, *A*). Second-order fibers cross the midline and ascend in the trigeminal lemniscus to the VPM nucleus of the thalamus. Touch and temperature information also travels in the trigeminal lemniscus. Third-order neurons project to the cerebral cortex. Figure 6-17 summarizes the effects of various lesions on transmission of fast pain and discriminative temperature information. Lesions that interrupt the pathways conveying nociceptive information produce analgesia. *Analgesia* is the absence of pain in response to stimuli that normally would be painful. The term *crossed analgesia* indicates that a single lesion can cause pain sensation to be lost on the side of the face ipsilateral to the lesion and on the opposite side of the body (contralateral to the lesion).

*Fast versus Slow Pain*

When fast pain information reaches the somatosensory cortex, a person is consciously aware of sharp pain in a specific location. If tissue damage has occurred, the fast pain is followed by slow, aching pain. The onset of slow pain occurs later than fast pain because the impulses travel on smaller, unmyelinated axons. The difference in conduction velocities cause C fibers to require about 0.5 second to transmit information to the spinal cord, while Aδ fibers require as little as 0.03 second.

## Divergent Pathways

### Medial Pain System: Slow Pain

Many responses to nociception depend on a divergent ascending network of neurons called the *medial pain system*. Activity of the medial pain system elicits affective, motivational, withdrawal, arousal, and autonomic responses. Most of the medial pain system projection neurons synapse in medial locations in

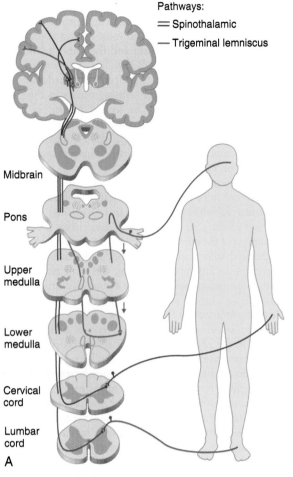

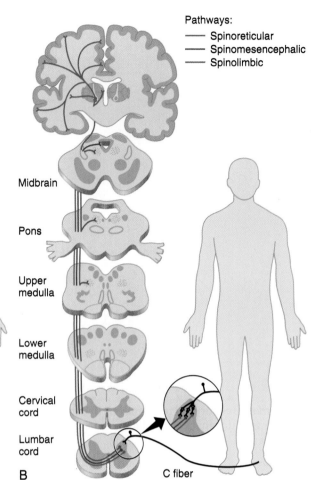

| | First-order neuron cell body | Second-order neuron cell body | Third-order neuron cell body |
|---|---|---|---|
| **From the body** | Dorsal root ganglion | Dorsal horn of spinal cord | VPL nucleus of thalamus |
| **From the face** | Trigeminal ganglion | Spinal nucleus of trigeminal nerve | VPM nucleus of thalamus |

**Fig. 6-14 Pathways for nociceptive information. A,** Sharp, localized pain travels in a three-neuron pathway. All sections are horizontal except the coronal section of the cerebrum at the top. The box below **A** lists the location of the cell bodies in this pathway. **B,** Slowly conducted nociceptive information from the body travels in the spinoreticular, spinomesencephalic, and spinolimbic tracts. Efferents from the thalamic nuclei project to widespread areas of the cerebral cortex and to the striatum.

the central nervous system.[11,12] The medial pain system uses several pathways with variable numbers of projection neurons, not a three-neuron pathway, as is used by fast pain. Information from the medial pain system is not somatotopically organized, so slow pain cannot be precisely localized.

### First Neuron
The first neuron is a small, unmyelinated C fiber. The receptors are free nerve endings that are sensitive to noxious heat,

chemical, or mechanical stimulation (polymodal afferents). High-threshold C fiber endings become *sensitized* with repeated stimulation. Thus, after injury, these neurons can be fired with less stimulation than is usually required. Tissue damage also results in release of chemicals—histamine, prostaglandins, and others—that sensitize pain receptors. For example, a gentle touch on sunburned skin can be painful.

Information from free nerve endings in the periphery travels in peripheral axons to the cell body in the dorsal root

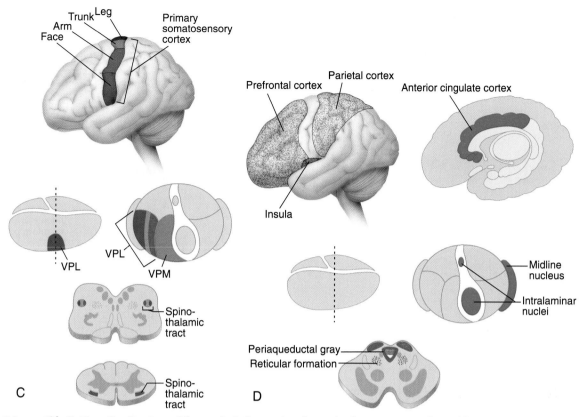

**Fig. 6-14, cont'd  C,** The distribution of fast pain information from the face, arm, trunk, and leg. *Top,* Lateral view of the cerebrum. Below the cerebrum is a lateral view of the thalamus, showing the location of the ventroposterolateral nucleus (VPL). The dotted line indicates the plane of the coronal section of the thalamus. The coronal section of the thalamus reveals the ventroposteromedial nucleus (VPM). The upper medulla and the cervical spinal cord are shown in horizontal sections. **D,** Sites of synapse and termination for slowly conducted nociceptive information. Lateral and midsagittal views of the cerebrum, lateral and coronal views of the thalamus, and a horizontal view of the midbrain are illustrated. Stippled blue in the cerebral cortex and blue in the anterior cingulate cortex indicate the termination of the spinolimbic pathway. The blue areas in the midline and intralaminar nuclei of the thalamus indicate sites of synapse of the spinolimbic tract. Red indicates the termination of the spinomesencephalic tract in the superior colliculus and the periaqueductal gray. Green indicates the termination of the spinoreticular tract in the midbrain reticular formation.

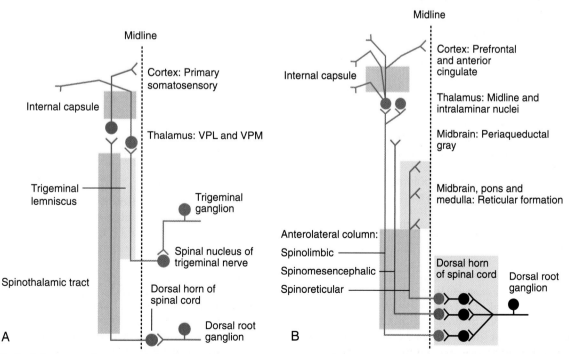

**Fig. 6-15  A,** Schematic diagram of the fast nociceptive pathways: spinothalamic and trigeminothalamic systems. (Compare with Figure 6-14, *A.*) **B,** Schematic diagram of the slow nociceptive pathways. (Compare with Figure 6-14, *B.*)

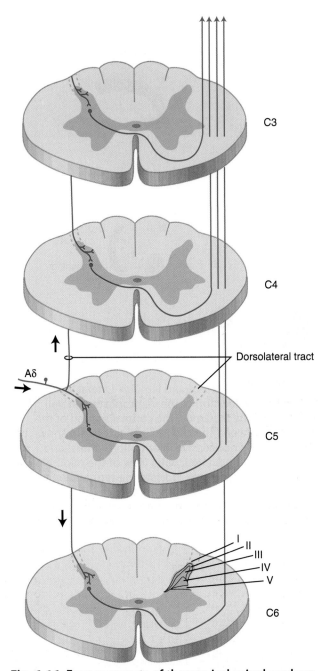

C3

C4

Dorsolateral tract

Aδ

C5

I
II
III
IV
V

C6

**Fig. 6-16 Four segments of the cervical spinal cord are illustrated.** The numbered areas are the laminae in the dorsal horn. The dorsolateral tract conveys nociceptive information from one dermatome to adjacent levels of the spinal cord. Thus nociceptive information that enters the C5 cervical segment is conveyed to the C3, C4, and C6 segments via the dorsolateral tract. After synapse in the dorsal horn, information crosses the midline in the tract neurons and ascends to the brain.

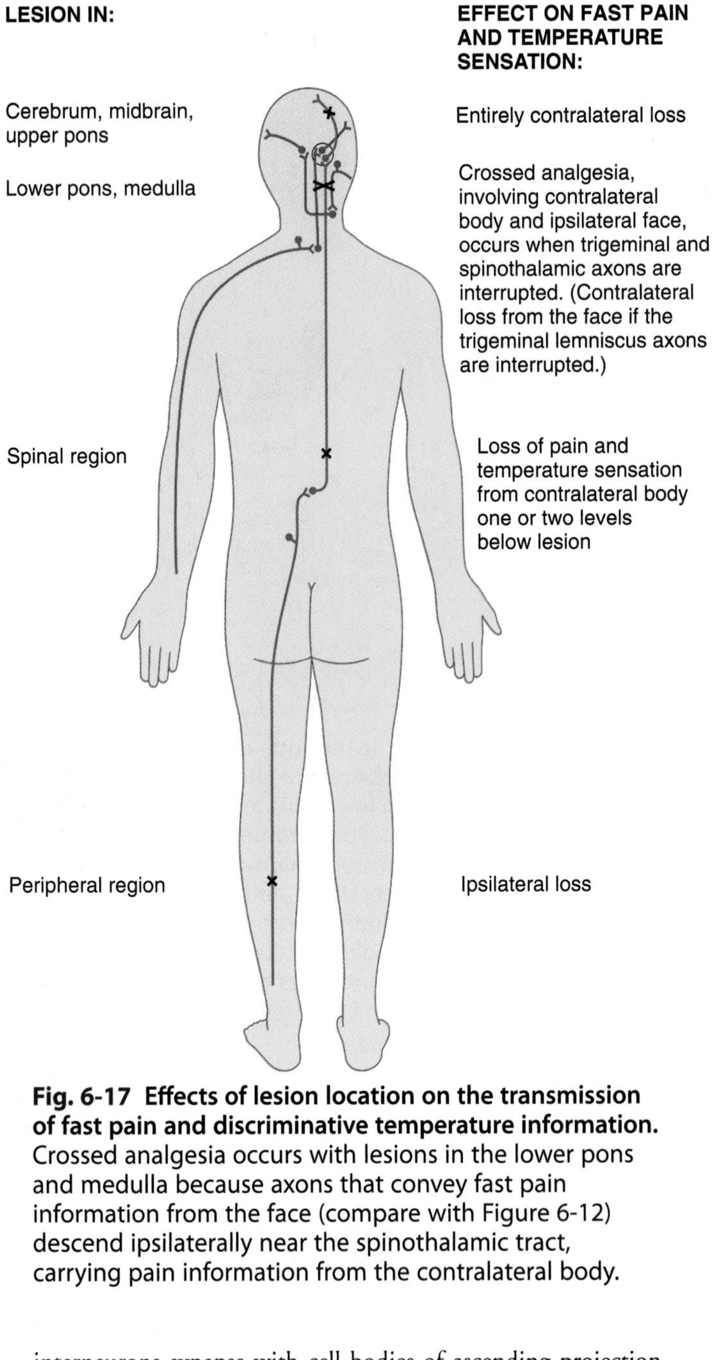

**LESION IN:**

Cerebrum, midbrain, upper pons

Lower pons, medulla

Spinal region

Peripheral region

**EFFECT ON FAST PAIN AND TEMPERATURE SENSATION:**

Entirely contralateral loss

Crossed analgesia, involving contralateral body and ipsilateral face, occurs when trigeminal and spinothalamic axons are interrupted. (Contralateral loss from the face if the trigeminal lemniscus axons are interrupted.)

Loss of pain and temperature sensation from contralateral body one or two levels below lesion

Ipsilateral loss

**Fig. 6-17 Effects of lesion location on the transmission of fast pain and discriminative temperature information.** Crossed analgesia occurs with lesions in the lower pons and medulla because axons that convey fast pain information from the face (compare with Figure 6-12) descend ipsilaterally near the spinothalamic tract, carrying pain information from the contralateral body.

ganglion. The central axon enters the cord, branches in the dorsolateral tract, and then synapses with interneurons in lamina I, II, or V of the dorsal horn. Lamina I is called the *marginal layer,* and lamina II is called the *substantia gelatinosa.* The neurotransmitter is *substance P.* Axons from the interneurons synapse with cell bodies of ascending projection neurons in laminae V to VIII.

*Ascending Projection Neurons*
The axons of ascending projection neurons reach the midbrain, reticular formation, and limbic areas via three tracts in the anterolateral spinal cord (see Figure 6-14, *B* and *D*):
• Spinomesencephalic
• Spinoreticular
• Spinolimbic
    These three tracts are parallel ascending tracts. Among these tracts, only information in the spinolimbic tract is perceived as pain. Information in the other tracts serves arousal, motivational, and reflexive functions and/or activates descending projections that control the flow of sensory information.[11]

### Spinomesencephalic Tract

This tract carries nociceptive information to two areas in the midbrain: to the superior colliculus, and to an area surrounding the cerebral aqueduct, the periaqueductal gray.[12] The spinomesencephalic tract is involved in turning the eyes and head toward the source of noxious input and in activating descending tracts that control pain. The periaqueductal gray is part of the descending pain control system (discussed in Chapter 7).

### Spinoreticular Tract

These ascending neurons synapse in the brainstem reticular formation. The *reticular formation* is a neural network in the brainstem that includes the reticular nuclei and their connections. Arousal, attention, and sleep/waking cycles are modulated by the reticular formation. Thus severe pain commands attention and interferes with sleep. From the reticular formation, axons project to the midline and to intralaminar nuclei of the thalamus.

### Spinolimbic Tract

Axons of the spinolimbic tract transmit slow pain information to the medial and intralaminar nuclei in the thalamus. Neurons located in these thalamic nuclei have large receptive fields, sometimes from the entire body. Their axons project to the anterior cingulate cortex, insula, amygdala, and dorsolateral prefrontal cortex.[13] Direct electrical stimulation of the posterior insula evokes pain in humans.[14] When the anterior cingulate gyrus is removed as a treatment for chronic pain, the pain intensity is unchanged, but the pain interferes less with thinking, behavior, and social activities.[15] The ability to localize painful stimuli remains intact, but the affective dimension is eliminated.

Eventually, spinolimbic information projects to areas of the cerebral cortex involved with emotions, sensory integration, personality, and movement, as well as to the basal ganglia, the amygdala, and the hypothalamus. Activity in the spinoreticular and spinolimbic tracts results in arousal, withdrawal, and autonomic and affective responses to pain.[12,16]

If someone breaks a bone in the hand, divergent pain pathways provide information that contributes to automatically directing the eyes and head toward the injury, automatically moving the hand away from the cause of injury, becoming pale, and feeling faint, nauseous, and emotionally distressed. The information provided by the divergent pathways is not well localized, so the entire hand seems to hurt.

---

> **◎ Clinical Pearl**
>
> Slow pain pathways provide information that produces automatic movements and autonomic and emotional responses to noxious stimuli.

---

### Trigeminoreticulolimbic Pathway

Slow pain information from the face proceeds in the *trigeminoreticulolimbic pathway*.[17] The first neurons are C fibers in the trigeminal nerve that synapse in the reticular formation with ascending projection neurons. These neurons project to the intralaminar nuclei in the thalamus. Projections from the intralaminar nuclei are similar to the spinolimbic pathway, with projections to many areas of the cerebral cortex.

Although intact sensory and parietal cortex is required for localization of pain, crude awareness of slow pain can be achieved in many cortical areas, and possibly in the thalamus and basal ganglia.

## Temperature Information

Temperature information is transmitted in phylogenetically older pathways to the reticular formation, to the nonspecific nuclei of the thalamus, to subcortical nuclei, and to the hypothalamus. Temperature information that does not reach conscious awareness contributes to arousal, provides gross localization, and contributes to autonomic regulation.

## Unconscious Relay Tracts to the Cerebellum

Information from proprioceptors and information about activity in spinal interneurons are transmitted to the cerebellum via the *spinocerebellar tracts*. Information relayed by these tracts is critical for adjusting movements. For example, one of the complications of diabetes is dysfunction of proprioceptive neurons. If, as often occurs in diabetes, proprioceptive information from the ankle is decreased, sway during stance increases. Inadequate proprioceptive input can also cause ataxia (uncoordinated movement) because loss of sensory feedback disrupts movement control (see Chapter 11 regarding types of ataxia).

Two of the spinocerebellar pathways deliver information from receptors in muscles, tendons, and joints from peripheral neurons to the cerebellum. These two neuron pathways relay high-fidelity, somatotopically arranged information to the cerebellar cortex. In contrast, two other spinocerebellar tracts are specialized to provide feedback to the cerebellum about the activity in spinal interneurons and in the descending motor tracts. These one-neuron internal feedback tracts do not directly convey information from any peripheral receptors.

### High-Fidelity Pathways

Two pathways relay high-fidelity, somatotopically arranged information to the cerebellar cortex (Figure 6-18):
- Posterior spinocerebellar pathway
- Cuneocerebellar pathway

### Posterior Spinocerebellar Pathway

The *posterior* (dorsal) *spinocerebellar pathway* transmits information from the legs and the lower half of the body. The proximal axon of the first-order neuron travels in the dorsal column to the thoracic or upper lumbar spinal cord, then synapses in the area of the dorsal gray matter called the *nucleus dorsalis* (Clarke's nucleus). The nucleus dorsalis extends vertically from spinal segment T1 to L2. Second-order axons form the posterior spinocerebellar tract. The tract remains ipsilateral and projects to the cerebellar cortex via the inferior cerebellar peduncle.

### Cuneocerebellar Pathway

The *cuneocerebellar pathway* begins with primary afferents from the arm and upper half of the body; central axons travel via the posterior columns to the lower medulla. The synapse between the first- and second-order neurons occurs in the *lateral cuneate*

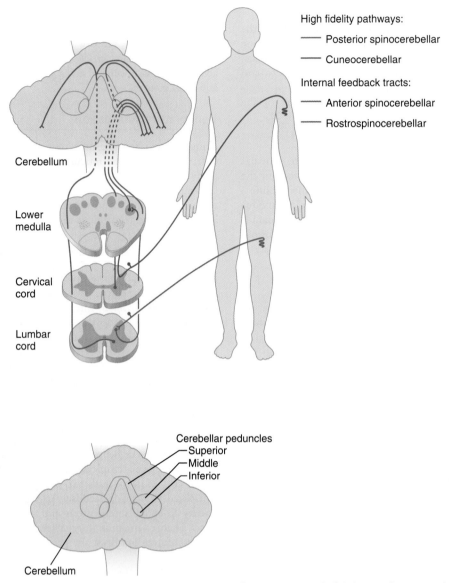

**Fig. 6-18  Tracts transmitting unconscious proprioceptive information.** High-fidelity pathways include the posterior spinocerebellar, from the lower body, and the cuneocerebellar, from the upper body. Internal feedback tracts include the anterior spinocerebellar, from the lower spinal cord, and the rostrospinocerebellar, from the cervical cord. *Inset,* Location of the three cerebellar peduncles.

*nucleus,* a nucleus in the medulla analogous to the nucleus dorsalis in the spinal cord. Second-order neurons form the cuneocerebellar tract, enter the ipsilateral inferior cerebellar peduncle, and end in the cerebellar cortex. Target neurons for the posterior spinocerebellar and cuneocerebellar tracts are arranged somatotopically in the cerebellar cortex.

### Internal Feedback Tracts

The two internal feedback tracts monitor the activity of spinal interneurons and of descending motor signals from the cerebral cortex and brainstem (see Figure 6-18):
* Anterior spinocerebellar tract
* Rostrospinocerebellar tract

### Anterior Spinocerebellar Tract

The *anterior spinocerebellar tract* transmits information from the thoracolumbar spinal cord. The tract begins with cell bodies in the lateral and ventral horns, in the area of the spinal cord that contains the greatest number of interneurons. The axons cross to the opposite side and ascend in the contralateral anterior spinocerebellar tract to the midbrain. Leaving the midbrain, the axons enter the cerebellum via the superior cerebellar peduncle. Most fibers recross the midline before entering the cerebellum, so each side of the cerebellum gets information from both sides of the lower body. The bilateral projection may reflect the normally automatic coordination of lower limb activities, as opposed to the typically more voluntary control of the upper limbs.

### Rostrospinocerebellar Tract

The *rostrospinocerebellar tract* transmits information from the cervical spinal cord to the ipsilateral cerebellum and enters the cerebellum via the inferior and superior cerebellar peduncles.

The anterior and rostrospinocerebellar tracts apprise the cerebellum of descending commands delivered to the neurons that control muscle activity via interneurons located between descending motor tracts and motor neurons that innervate muscles. Internal feedback tracts also convey information about the activity of spinal reflex circuits.

### Function of Spinocerebellar Tracts

Information that travels in the spinocerebellar tracts is not consciously perceived. Information in the spinocerebellar tracts is used for unconscious adjustments to movements and posture. Because the internal feedback tracts convey descending motor information to the cerebellum before the information reaches the motor neurons, and the high-fidelity pathways convey information from muscle spindles, tendon organs, and cutaneous mechanoreceptors, the cerebellum obtains information about movement commands and about the movements or postural adjustments that followed the commands. Thus the cerebellum can compare the intended motor output versus the actual movement output. The cerebellum uses this information to make corrections to neural commands through its connections with other brain areas (see Chapter 10).

> **◎ Clinical Pearl**
>
> Information in the spinocerebellar tracts is received from proprioceptors, spinal interneurons, and descending motor pathways. This information, which does not reach conscious awareness, contributes to automatic movements and postural adjustments.

### Differentiating Spinocerebellar Tract From Cerebellar Lesions

Damage to the spinocerebellar tracts can be differentiated from lesions of the cerebellum by comparing the coordination of movement with vision versus that of movements without vision. In spinocerebellar tract lesions, movements are more coordinated when vision is present and are clumsier when the eyes are closed. Imaging studies can distinguish between spinocerebellar and cerebellar lesions.

## SUMMARY

Somatosensory pathways provide information about the external world—information used in movement control and to prevent or minimize injury. Conscious information about external objects can be provided by all four types of discriminative sensation: touch, proprioception, pain, and temperature. Discriminative sensation requires analysis of sensory signals by the somatosensory area of the cerebral cortex. The dorsal column/medial lemniscus and spinothalamic pathways deliver high-fidelity, somatotopically arranged information to the cerebral cortex. This conscious information contributes to our understanding of the physical world and to control of fine movements.

Unconscious information that contributes to control of posture and movement is delivered to the cerebellum by the spinocerebellar tracts. Unconscious nociceptive information provides information about stimuli that threaten to damage or have damaged tissue. Spinolimbic, spinoreticular, and spinomesencephalic tracts deliver information to the thalamus and cortex, reticular formation, and midbrain that elicit emotional and automatic responses to nociceptive stimuli.

## REVIEW QUESTIONS

1. What are the three types of somatosensory receptors?
2. What are nociceptors?
3. To what do primary and secondary sensory endings in muscle spindles respond?
4. How is the sensitivity of sensory endings in a muscle spindle maintained when the muscle is shortened?
5. What type of information is transmitted by large-diameter type Ia and Ib axons?
6. What classes of axons convey nociceptive and temperature information?
7. What are the three types of pathways that convey information to the brain?
8. High-fidelity, somatotopically arranged somatosensory information is conveyed to what area of the cerebral cortex?
9. Neural signals that are interpreted as dull, aching pain travel in what pathway?
10. What are the functions of the spinoreticular, spinomesencephalic, and spinolimbic pathways?
11. All of the unconscious relay tracts end in what part of the brain?
12. Where do synapses occur between neurons conveying discriminative touch information from the left lower limb?
13. Where do synapses occur between neurons conveying discriminative pain information from the left lower limb?
14. Name the tracts that relay unconscious proprioceptive information to the cerebellum. Name the tracts that provide unconscious information about activity in spinal interneurons and descending motor commands.

## References

1. Vallbo AB: Single-afferent neurons and somatic sensation in humans. In Gazzaniga MS, editor: *The cognitive neurosciences*, Cambridge, Mass, 1995, M.I.T. Press, pp 237–252.

2. Taylor A, Durbaba R, Ellaway PH: Direct and indirect assessment of gamma-motor firing patterns. *Can J Physiol Pharmacol* 82:793–802, 2004.

3. Chalmers G: Re-examination of the possible role of Golgi tendon organ and muscle spindle reflexes in proprioceptive neuromuscular facilitation muscle stretching. *Sports Biomech* 3:159–183, 2004.

4. Nallegowda M, Singh U, Bhan S, et al: Balance and gait in total hip replacement: a pilot study. *Am J Phys Med Rehabil* 82:669–677, 2003.

5. Min BK: A thalamic reticular networking model of consciousness. *Theor Biol Med Model* 7:10, 2010.

6. Sacks O: *A leg to stand on*, New York, 1984, Harper & Row.

7. Löken LS, Wessberg J, Morrison I, et al: Coding of pleasant touch by unmyelinated afferents in humans. *Nat Neurosci* 12:547–548, 2009.

8. Olausson H, Lamarre Y, Backlund Y, et al: Unmyelinated tactile afferents signal touch and project to insular cortex. *Nat Neurosci* 5:900–904, 2002.

9. Oshiro Y, Quevedo AS, McHaffie JG, et al: Brain mechanisms supporting spatial discrimination of pain. *J Neurosci* 27:3388–3394, 2007.

10. Palecek J, Paleckova V, Willis WD: Fos expression in spinothalamic and postsynaptic dorsal column neurons following noxious visceral and cutaneous stimuli. *Pain* 104:249–257, 2003.

11. Brooks J, Tracey I: From nociception to pain perception: imaging the spinal and supraspinal pathways. *J Anat* 207:19–33, 2005.

12. Almeida TF, Roizenblatt S, Tufik S: Afferent pain pathways: a neuroanatomical review. *Brain Res* 1000:40–56, 2004.

13. Wasan AD, Sullivan MD, Clark MR: Psychiatric illness, depression, anxiety, and somatoform pain disorders. In Ballantyne JC, Fishman SM, Rathmell JP, editors: *Bonica's management of pain*, ed 4, Baltimore, 2010, Lippincott Williams & Wilkins.

14. Ostrowsky K, Magnin M, Ryvlin P, et al: Representation of pain and somatic sensation in the human insula: a study of responses to direct electrical cortical stimulation. *Cereb Cortex* 12:376–385, 2010.

15. Lorenz J, Hauck M: Supraspinal mechanisms of pain and nociception. In Ballantyne JC, Fishman SM, Rathmell JP, editors: *Bonica's management of pain*, ed 4, Baltimore, 2010, Lippincott Williams & Wilkins.

16. Chapman RC: The psychophysiology of pain. In Ballantyne JC, Fishman SM, Rathmell JP, editors: *Bonica's management of pain*, ed 4, Baltimore, 2010, Lippincott Williams & Wilkins.

17. van Bijsterveld OP, Kruize AA, Bleys RL: Central nervous system mechanisms in Sjogren's syndrome. *Br J Ophthalmol* 87:128–130, 2003.

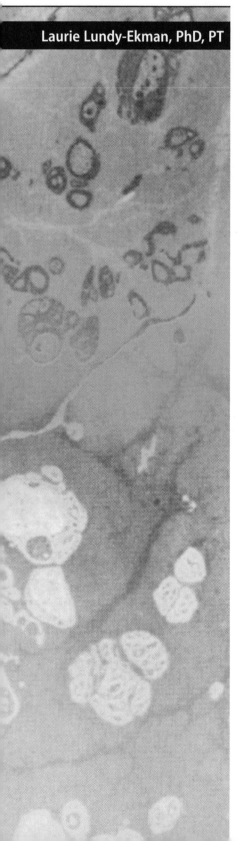

# 7 Somatosensation: Clinical Application

Laurie Lundy-Ekman, PhD, PT

## FUNCTIONS OF SENSATION

Somatosensation contributes to smooth, accurate movements, to the prevention or minimization of injury, and to our understanding of the external world. The first two of these topics are considered in this chapter. Perception, the ability to interpret somatosensation as meaningful information, is discussed in Chapters 17 and 18.

### Contribution of Somatosensory Information to Movement

The role of sensation in movement is complex. In the early 1900s, Sherrington[1] performed an experiment on a monkey to determine the effect of loss of information conveyed by the dorsal roots. He cut the dorsal roots entering the spinal cord from one arm, severing the sensory axons. Sherrington found that even after recovery from surgery, the monkey avoided using that limb. This experimental outcome reinforced the assumption that sensation is essential for movement. Similarly, people who lack sensation in one upper limb tend to avoid using the limb, substituting with the unimpaired limb whenever possible.

However, Taub and associates[2] tested the effects of bilateral deafferentation. His group deafferented both forelimbs in newborn monkeys and sewed their eyelids closed to eliminate vision. These monkeys were able to ambulate, climb, and pick up some objects, although their performance was very clumsy and motor development was delayed. The monkeys were permanently unable to use their fingers individually, and thus could not pick up small objects.

The functional problems of a person with a severe peripheral sensory loss were reported by Rothwell and colleagues.[3] Motor power was nearly normal, and the subject could move individual fingers separately. Without vision, he could move his thumb accurately at different speeds and with different levels of force. Yet he could not write, hold a cup, or button his shirt. These difficulties were due to lack of somatosensation, depriving him of normal, automatic corrections to movement. When he tried to hold a pen to write, his grip did not automatically adjust because he lacked unconscious somatosensory information about appropriate changes in pressure.

### Somatosensory Information Protects Against Injury

Individuals with somatosensory deficits are prone to pressure-induced skin lesions, burns, and joint damage because they are unaware of excessive pressure, temperature, or stretch. People with congenital insensitivity to pain tend to self-inflict injuries, have bone fractures, joint deformities, and amputations, and to die young.[4]

---

**◉ *Clinical Pearl***

Somatosensation is necessary for accurate control of movements and protects against injury.

---

## TESTS FOR SOMATOSENSATION

Clinically, the sensory examination covers conscious relay pathways:
- Discriminative touch
- Conscious proprioception
- Fast pain
- Discriminative temperature

These pathways are tested because the findings give information that can be used to localize a lesion.

The purpose of the sensory examination is to establish whether there is sensory impairment and, if so, its location, type of sensation affected, and severity of the deficit. The following guidelines serve to improve the reliability of sensory testing.
1. Administer tests in a quiet, distraction-free setting.
2. Position the subject seated or lying supported by a firm, stable surface to avoid challenging balance during testing.
3. Explain the purpose of the testing.
4. Demonstrate each test before administering the test. During the demonstration, allow the subject to see the stimulus.
5. During testing, block the subject's vision by having the subject close the eyes or wear a blindfold, or by placing a barrier between the part being tested and the subject's eyes.
6. Apply stimuli near the center of the dermatomes being tested. Record the results after each test. The time interval between stimuli should be irregular to prevent the subject from predicting stimulation. Comparing the subject's responses on the left and right sides is often informative, especially if one side of the body or face is neurologically intact.

An important limitation of sensory testing is the reliance on conscious awareness of sensory stimulation. Most somatosensory information is used at subconscious levels. For example, massive amounts of somatosensory information are processed by the cerebellum; however, there is no conscious awareness of this processing. Thus, testing proprioception by having the patient report whether he or she can sense the position of a limb tests conscious awareness of proprioception, but not the ability to use proprioceptive information to adjust movements.

### Quick Screening

Quick screening for sensory impairment consists of testing proprioception and vibration in the fingers and toes and testing fast pain sensation in the limbs, trunk, and face with pinprick. This quick screening evaluates the function of some large-diameter and some small-diameter axons. Because of the possibility of spreading blood-borne diseases, care should be taken during pinprick testing to prevent puncturing the skin, and each pin should be discarded after use on a single person. A paper clip or plastic toothpick may serve as an alternative to the pin and is less likely to puncture the skin. If loss or impairment of sensation is found, additional testing is performed to determine the precise pattern of sensory loss.

Indications for more thorough testing include the following:
- Any complaints of sensory abnormality or loss
- Nonpainful skin lesions
- Localized weakness or atrophy

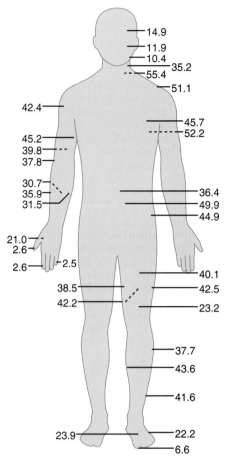

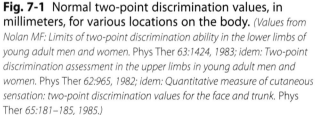

**Fig. 7-1** Normal two-point discrimination values, in millimeters, for various locations on the body. *(Values from Nolan MF: Limits of two-point discrimination ability in the lower limbs of young adult men and women. Phys Ther 63:1424, 1983; idem: Two-point discrimination assessment in the upper limbs in young adult men and women. Phys Ther 62:965, 1982; idem: Quantitative measure of cutaneous sensation: two-point discrimination values for the face and trunk. Phys Ther 65:181–185, 1985.)*

## Complete Somatosensory Evaluation

A complete sensory evaluation includes measuring *sensitivity* and *thresholds* for stimulation of each conscious sensation (except proprioceptive thresholds are not measured). For example, a measure of conscious touch sensitivity is the ability to distinguish between two closely applied points on the skin; threshold is the lowest intensity of a stimulus that can be perceived, as when the person barely perceives being touched. Table 7-1 explains the testing procedures. Figure 7-1 shows normal values for touch sensitivity (two-point discrimination) on various parts of the body. A sensory assessment form is shown in Figure 7-2.

## Interpreting Test Results

The results derived from these testing procedures can be used to map a person's pattern of sensory loss. The resulting map can be compared with standardized maps of *peripheral nerve distribution* and of dermatome distributions to determine whether the person's pattern of sensory loss is consistent with a peripheral nerve or a spinal region pattern (see Figures 6-5 and 6-6). Because every individual is unique and adjacent dermatomes overlap one another, the maps presented represent common but not definitive nerve distributions. The overlap of adjacent dermatomes also ensures that if only one sensory root is severed, complete loss of sensation does not occur in any area.

The primary somatosensory cortex is essential for two-point discrimination, graphesthesia, stereognosis, and simultaneous awareness of stimulation on both sides of the body. For predicting hand function from sensory tests, only two-point discrimination scores correlate well with hand function. Individuals on ventilators or with communication disorders may present unusual challenges to sensory testing. The therapist may be able to establish a communication system using eye blinks (one for yes, two for no) or finger movements with cooperative people.

> **◎ Clinical Pearl**
>
> Caveat: All somatosensory testing requires that the client has conscious awareness and cognition. These tests do not test the ability to use somatosensation to prepare for and during movements.

## ELECTRODIAGNOSTIC STUDIES

Recording electrical activity from nerves reveals the location of pathology and is often diagnostic. Two methods of examining sensory nerve function are as follows:
- Nerve conduction studies (NCSs)
- Somatosensory evoked potentials (SEPs)

Nerve conduction studies evaluate only the function of peripheral nerves. Somatosensory evoked potentials test transmission of sensory information in both peripheral nerves and central nervous system pathways. In both NCS and SEP testing, electrical stimulation is applied to the peripheral nerve so that all axons are depolarized simultaneously. In electrodiagnostic studies, measurements of latencies, amplitudes, and conduction velocities obtained can be compared with those of unaffected nerves in the same patient or with published normal values. Some physical therapists specialize in performing NCSs, but therapists typically do not perform SEPs.

### Sensory Nerve Conduction Studies

To test nerve conduction, surface recording electrodes are placed along the course of a peripheral nerve, and then the nerve is electrically stimulated. Nerve conduction studies quantify the function of only the fastest-conducting axons. Because large-diameter axons normally conduct fastest, NCS testing in intact nerves measures only the performance of large-diameter fibers. Because the velocity of nerve conduction depends on an intact myelin sheath, conduction velocity is slowed throughout a nerve that has been demyelinated. If myelin has been damaged by a focal injury, conduction is slowed only at the injured segment.

## TABLE 7-1 TESTING THE SOMATOSENSORY SYSTEM

### DISCRIMINATIVE TOUCH: PRIMARY SENSATION

#### Location of Touch

**Test:** Before testing touch, ask subject to "Say yes when you feel the touch and then point to or tell me where you feel it." Lightly touch the pad of the subject's fingertips or toes with your fingertip or a wisp of cotton. If answers are accurate, assume that proximal location of touch is normal. If distal touch location is impaired, test dermatomes.* Once the extent of the impairment has been mapped, test peripheral nerve distributions (see Figures 6-5 and 6-6) to determine whether the loss is in a dermatomal or peripheral nerve distribution.

**Interpretation:** If subject's responses are accurate, this indicates that the pathway for discriminative touch (dorsal column/medial lemniscus system) is intact from the periphery to the cerebral cortex. Failure to localize fine touch despite accurate reporting when touched indicates a lesion superior to the thalamus.

#### Tactile Thresholds

**Test:** Ask subject to "Say yes if you feel the touch." Touch a monofilament (nylon filaments available in sets of 5 to 10; bending pressure ranges from 0.02 to 40.0 g) to the subject's skin. The monofilament must be applied perpendicular to the skin. Press so that the filament bends. If answers are accurate, assume that proximal location of touch is normal. If distal touch location is impaired, test dermatomes.* Once the extent of the impairment has been mapped, test peripheral nerve distributions (Figure 6-5) to determine whether the loss is in a dermatomal or peripheral nerve distribution. If testing for diabetic neuropathy, test six sites on plantar surface of each foot: pulp of hallux, first, second, third, fourth, and fifth metatarsal phalangeal joints[5]

**Interpretation:** Normal response: able to feel the 6 g filament anywhere on the foot. The filaments that apply greater force are used to quantify decreased tactile sensitivity. Inability to sense the 10 g filament indicates loss of protective sensation.[5] This test is not sufficiently accurate to be used as the only test of protective sensation.[6]

### DISCRIMINATIVE TOUCH: CORTICAL SENSATION

(Because these tests depend on touch sense, they cannot be performed when primary touch sensation is abnormal.)

#### Two-Point Discrimination

**Test:** Ask subject to "Tell me whether you feel one point or two points." Using calipers, apply light, equal pressure to two points. Begin with the points of the calipers farther apart than the mean value for the body part being tested. With each trial, move the points closer together until the subject cannot distinguish two points as separate. Measure the distance between the points with a ruler. Alternatively, use a two-point discriminator to apply pressure. To prevent anticipation, randomly stimulate with a single point. Typically, only test the subject's hands and feet.

**Interpretation:** Ability to accurately discriminate in normal ranges (see Figure 7-1) indicates that the pathway for discriminative touch (dorsal column/medial lemniscus system) is intact from the periphery to the cerebral cortex. Normal value about 8 mm in plantar areas. People with diabetic foot ulcers had discriminations of about 14 mm.[7]

#### Bilateral Simultaneous Touch

**Test:** Ask subject to say "left" if the left side is touched, "right" if the right side is touched, and "both" if both sides are touched. Lightly touch one limb, the opposite limb, or both sides of the body simultaneously. Typically, test the forearms and the shins.

**Interpretation:** Tests for sensory extinction. Used to determine whether a person can attend to stimuli on both sides of the body simultaneously. If a person can accurately report stimuli presented on each side of the body separately but not when presented simultaneously, this indicates a lesion in the parietal lobe contralateral to the side of the body where sensory extinction occurs.

#### Graphesthesia

**Test:** Ask subject to "Tell me what letter I draw in the palm of your hand." The subject's palm should be positioned facing the examiner, with the fingers pointed upward as if signaling "stop." Using a key or similar object, draw a letter in the palm of the subject's hand.

**Interpretation:** Tests the dorsal column/medial lemniscus system and parietal lobe. Normal response: able to identify numbers or letters. If touch sensation is intact yet the person cannot perform this task, this indicates a lesion in the contralateral parietal cortex or adjacent white matter.

**TABLE 7-1  TESTING THE SOMATOSENSORY SYSTEM—cont'd**

**CONSCIOUS PROPRIOCEPTION**

*Joint Movement*

| | |
|---|---|
| **Test:** Ask subject to "Tell me whether I am bending or straightening your joint." Firmly hold the sides of the phalanx (usually big toe or a finger), and passively flex or extend the joint approximately 10 degrees. Randomize the order of flexions/extensions. | **Interpretation:** Normal response: no errors. Errors indicate dysfunction in the peripheral nerves, spinal cord, brainstem, or cerebrum. |

*Joint Position*

| | |
|---|---|
| **Test:** Tell subject you are going to move a joint. After the movement has stopped, ask the subject to match the final joint position with the opposite limb, or to report the position of the joint. Passively flex or extend the joint (usually elbow or ankle). Maintain a static position before asking subject to respond. | **Interpretation:** Normal response: no errors. Errors indicate dysfunction in the peripheral nerves, spinal cord, brainstem, or cerebrum. |

*Vibration*

| | |
|---|---|
| **Test:** Use a tuning fork with a frequency of 128 Hz. (1) Ask subject to "Tell me when the vibration stops," then touch a vibrating tuning fork to a bony prominence, *or* (2) Ask subject to "Tell me if the tuning fork is vibrating or not," then randomly apply a vibrating or nonvibrating tuning fork to a bony prominence. Test distal interphalangeal joints of the index fingers and big toes; if finger vibration sense is impaired, test wrists, elbows, clavicles. If toe vibration sense is impaired, test medial malleoli, patellae, and anterior superior iliac spines. | **Interpretation:** Primarily tests the large, Aβ peripheral nerve fibers and the dorsal column/medial lemniscus neurons. Typically, lesions superior to the thalamus do not impair vibration sensation. |

**DISCRIMINATIVE TOUCH AND CONSCIOUS PROPRIOCEPTION**

*Stereognosis*

| | |
|---|---|
| **Test:** Ask subject to "Tell me what this is. You can move the object around in your hand." Place an object (key, paper clip) in subject's hand. | **Interpretation:** Normal response: able to identify object. If touch sensation is intact yet person cannot identify the object, this indicates a lesion in the contralateral parietal cortex or adjacent white matter. |

**FAST PAIN (LATERAL PAIN SYSTEM)**

*Sharp, Prickling Pain*

| | |
|---|---|
| **Test:** Ask subject to report "sharp" or "dull." If subject reports feeling the stimulus, ask where the stimulus was felt. Gently poke subject with a pin or touch with blunt end of a pin (or use a toothpick). To map an area of decreased or lost sensation, drag a pinwheel lightly along the skin to determine regions of normal and abnormal sensitivity. To use the pinwheel on a limb, circle the circumference of the limb. | **Interpretation:** Normal response: able to differentiate accurately between sharp and dull stimuli. Complete peripheral nerve lesions produce loss of all sensations in the region supplied by the nerve. Lesions of the anterolateral tracts or thalamocortical radiations produce inability to distinguish sharp from dull. Lesions of the primary sensory cortex interfere with ability to localize the stimulus, although the subject may be able to distinguish sharp versus dull. |

**DISCRIMINATIVE TEMPERATURE**

*Heat or Cold*

| | |
|---|---|
| **Test:** Ask subject to report temperature as hot or cold. Touch subject with test tubes filled with warm (40° C) and cool (10° C) water. Maintain contact with subject's skin for about 3 seconds before asking for a response. | **Interpretation:** Normal response: accurate identification of warm or cold. Usually used to map areas of deficiency to determine whether the sensory loss fits a peripheral or dermatomal pattern |

*To test upper limb dermatomes (see Figure 6-5), begin distally and test lateral, then posterior, then medial. For the hand, touch the thumb (C6), middle finger (C7), and little finger (C8). For the forearm, touch lateral (C6), posterior (C7), and medial (C8). For the upper arm, touch anterolateral (C5), lateral (C6), posterior (C7), posteromedial (C8), and anteromedial (T1). For the lower limb, begin distally. On the sole of the foot, touch the big toe (L4), middle toe (L5), little toe (S1), and medial heel (S2). Midcalf: posteromedial (L3), anteromedial (L4), anterolateral (L5), posterolateral (S1), and posterior calf (S2). Anterior knee: L4. Thigh: medial proximal (L2), medial distal (L3), anterior distal (L4), lateral (L5), posterior (S1), and posteromedial (S2). Mnemonic for landmarks in lower limb: Stand on L4-S2; L3 medial knee.

Diagnosis _____

Limb _____

Sketch the distribution of signs and symptoms.

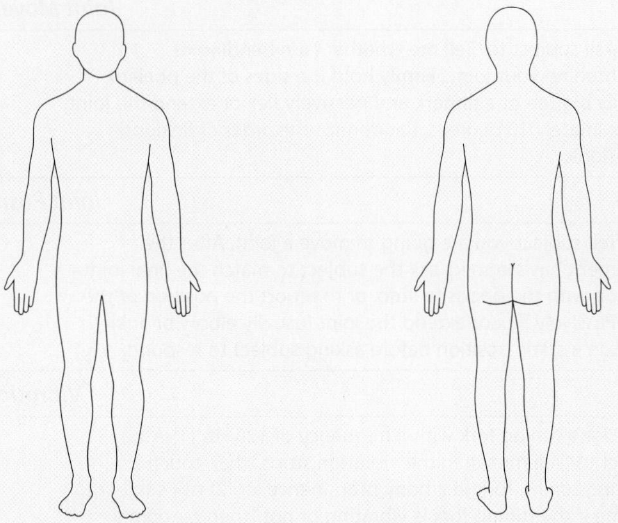

| SYMPTOMS | Right | Left |
|---|---|---|
| Numbness | | |
| Abnormal sensations (paresthesia or dysesthesia) | | |
| SIGNS | | |
| Light Touch | | |
| Two-point discrimination | | |
| Static proprioception | | |
| Kinesthesia | | |
| Vibration | | |
| Pinprick | | |
| Warmth | | |
| Cold | | |
| For symptoms, record the person's report. For signs, record as WNL (within normal limits), I (impaired), or A (absent). | | |

**Fig. 7-2** Sensory examination form.

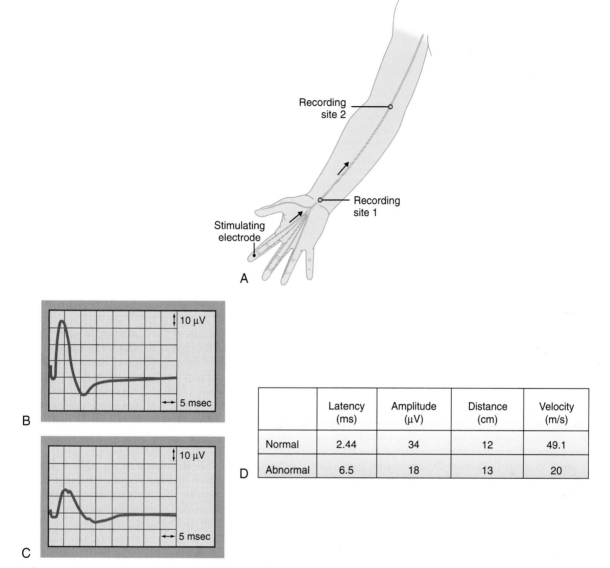

| | Latency (ms) | Amplitude (µV) | Distance (cm) | Velocity (m/s) |
|---|---|---|---|---|
| Normal | 2.44 | 34 | 12 | 49.1 |
| Abnormal | 6.5 | 18 | 13 | 20 |

**Fig. 7-3** Sensory nerve conduction study (NCS): median nerve. **A,** Sites of electrodes for stimulation of index finger and for recording from skin over the median nerve at the wrist and elbow. **B,** Graphic results from a normal median NCS recording at the wrist. **C,** Graph of recording at the wrist from a demyelinated nerve. **D,** Numeric results of the NCS.

The function of the sensory fibers in the median nerve can be tested by electrically stimulating the skin of the middle finger and recording the electrical activity evoked in the median nerve at the wrist and elbow (Figure 7-3). The conduction velocity equals the distance between electrodes divided by the amount of time from the stimulus to the first depolarization at the recording electrode. The amplitude of the depolarization is also measured. Amplitude serves as an indicator of the number of axons conducting. Often the results from two recording sites are compared, for example, the amplitude and latency recorded at the wrist are compared with measurements at the elbow.

To determine whether an NCS is normal, three numeric values are compared:
• Distal latency
• Amplitude of the evoked potential
• Conduction velocity

Distal latency is the time required for the depolarization evoked by the stimulus to reach the distal recording site. The results of an NCS in a normal nerve and in an abnormally functioning nerve are illustrated in Figure 7-3. Sensory nerve conduction may also be studied by stimulating proximal to the recording site. With this method, the recording electrode is picking up impulses that were propagated in the direction opposite the normal physiologic direction of sensory nerve impulse propagation.

## Somatosensory Evoked Potentials

SEPs evaluate the function of the pathway from the periphery to the upper spinal cord or to the cerebral cortex. The skin over a peripheral nerve is electrically stimulated, and the resulting electrical activity is recorded from the skin over the upper cervical spinal cord or from the scalp over the primary somatosensory cortex. Again, the velocity is determined by dividing the distance between the stimulating and recording electrodes by the time required for the action potential to be transmitted. SEPs are used to verify subtle signs and to locate lesions of the dorsal roots, posterior columns, and brainstem. For example, SEPs may be used in people with multiple sclerosis to determine the location of a lesion.

## SENSORY ABNORMALITIES

### Proprioceptive Pathway Lesions: Sensory Ataxia

*Ataxia* is incoordination that is not due to weakness. There are three types of ataxia: sensory, vestibular, and cerebellar. Lesions that produce sensory ataxia are located in peripheral sensory nerves, dorsal roots, dorsal columns of the spinal cord, or medial lemnisci. The Romberg test is used to distinguish between cerebellar ataxia (see Chapter 11) and sensory ataxia. The person is asked to stand with the feet together, first with eyes open, then with eyes closed. Those with cerebellar ataxia have difficulty maintaining their balance regardless of whether their eyes are open or closed. People with sensory ataxia have better balance when their eyes are open but become unsteady when their eyes are closed (Romberg sign). Thus, individuals with sensory ataxia are able to use vision to compensate for decreased or lost somatosensory information. People with sensory ataxia often report that their balance is better when they watch their feet while walking, and that their balance is worse in the dark. Another method to differentiate between sensory ataxia and cerebellar ataxia is to test conscious proprioception and vibratory sense. These sensations are impaired in sensory ataxia yet intact in cerebellar ataxia. Differentiating vestibular ataxia from cerebellar or sensory ataxia is discussed in Chapter 16.

### Peripheral Nerve Lesions

The general term for dysfunction or pathology of one or more peripheral nerves is *neuropathy*. Peripheral nerves are subject to trauma and disease. Complete severance of a peripheral nerve results in lack of sensation in the distribution of the nerve; pain may occur, and sensory changes are accompanied by motor and reflex loss. Compression of a nerve affects large myelinated fibers preferentially, with initial relative sparing of the smaller pain, thermal, and autonomic fibers. For example, when one stands up after prolonged sitting with the legs crossed, occasionally one finds that part of a limb has "fallen asleep." Sensory loss proceeds in the following order:
1. Conscious proprioception and discriminative touch
2. Cold
3. Fast pain
4. Heat
5. Slow pain

When compression is relieved, tingling or prickling sensations occur as the blood supply increases. After compression is removed, sensations return in the reverse order that they were lost. Thus, aching pain occurs first, then a sensation of warmth, then sharp, stinging sensations, then cold, and finally a return of discriminative touch and conscious proprioception.

Because large axons are the most heavily myelinated, demyelination of axons in a peripheral nerve often affects proprioception and vibratory sense most severely, resulting in diminished or lost proprioception. Neuropathy is discussed further in Chapter 12.

> **Clinical Pearl**
> Neuropathy is dysfunction or pathology of one or more peripheral nerves.

### Spinal Region Lesions

Common causes of dysfunction of the spinal region include the following:
- Trauma to the spinal cord, completely or partially severing the cord
- Disorders that compromise the function of specific areas within the spinal cord (These disorders are discussed in Chapter 13.)
- A virus infecting the dorsal root ganglion

### Complete Transection of the Spinal Cord

Complete transection of the cord prevents all sensation one or two levels below the level of the lesion from ascending to higher levels in the cord. Clinically, observed complete loss of sensation begins in dermatomes one or two levels below the level of the lesion owing to the overlap of nerve endings in adjacent dermatomes. Voluntary motor control below the lesion is also lost.

### Hemisection of the Spinal Cord

A hemisection, that is, damage to the right or left half of the cord, interrupts pain and temperature sensation from the contralateral body because the axons transmitting nociceptive and temperature information cross to the opposite side of the cord soon after entering the cord. As a result of collateral branching of nociceptive axons in the dorsolateral tract (Lissauer's marginal zone; see Figure 6-15), complete loss of pain sensation occurs two to three dermatomes below the level of the lesion. Because discriminative touch and conscious proprioception information ascends on the same side of the cord as it entered, these sensations are lost ipsilateral to the lesion. Paralysis also occurs ipsilaterally. The pattern of loss is called *Brown-Séquard syndrome*.

### Posterior Column Lesions

In posterior column lesions, conscious proprioception, two-point discrimination, and vibration sense are lost below the level of the lesion. Immediately after the lesion, movements are uncoordinated, that is, ataxic. If the lesion is above C6, the person may be unable to recognize objects by palpation because ascending sensory information from the hand has been lost.

### Infection

Infection of a dorsal root ganglion or a cranial nerve ganglion with varicella-zoster virus causes *varicella zoster*, also called *shingles* or *herpes zoster*. The varicella-zoster virus causes chickenpox. After a chickenpox infection, the sensory ganglia hold latent components of the varicella-zoster virus. Occasionally, some of the virus reverts to infectiousness. If the level of circulating antibodies is inadequate, the virus begins to multiply and is transported antidromically down sensory peripheral axons. The virus irritates and inflames the nerve, causing pain. The virus is released into the skin around the sensory nerve endings, causing painful eruptions on the skin. The infection, which destroys neurons and supporting cells in the dorsal root ganglion and accompanying dermatome, is usually limited to a single dermatome or trigeminal nerve branch (Figure 7-4; Pathology 7-1). However, in severe or inadequately treated cases, *postherpetic neuralgia* develops. Postherpetic neuralgia is severe pain that persists longer than 120 days after the rash onset.

If varicella zoster is treated with antiviral drugs within 72 hours of rash onset, these drugs reduce viral replication, duration of rash, neural damage, severity and duration of pain, and duration and incidence of postherpetic neuralgia.[8] Analgesic medications are also required. These include acetaminophen alone or in combination with tramadol, nonsteroidal anti-inflammatory drugs (NSAIDs), or opioids. If these are inadequate, drugs used to treat neuropathic pain can be used (see Table 8-6). The zoster vaccine, for people older than 60, prevents varicella zoster or diminishes its severity and duration.

## Brainstem Region Lesions

Because the axons that carry sensory information from the body and face cross the midline at various levels, lesions in the brainstem usually cause a mix of ipsilateral and contralateral signs.

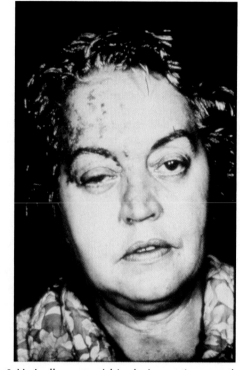

**Fig. 7-4** Varicella-zoster (shingles) eruptions on the skin. One branch of the trigeminal nerve is affected. *(Courtesy of Dr. Melvin J. Ball.)*

| PATHOLOGY 7-1 | VARICELLA ZOSTER |
|---|---|
| Pathology | Infection of sensory root cell bodies, causing inflammation of sensory neurons |
| Etiology | Varicella-zoster virus |
| Speed of onset | Acute or subacute; often preceded for 3–7 days by fatigue, headache, fever, neck stiffness, malaise, and nausea. May have pain and abnormal sensations in a single dermatomal pain prior to the rash |
| Signs and symptoms | |
| Consciousness | Normal |
| Communication and memory | Normal |
| Sensory | Itching, burning, or tingling may precede eruption of vesicles by up to days; pain is often severe. |
| Autonomic | Normal |
| Motor | Normal |
| Region affected | Peripheral plus spinal region or brainstem. Usually limited to one dermatome (often thoracic) or one branch of trigeminal nerve |
| Demographics | Both genders equally affected; incidence increases with aging |
| Incidence: Varicella zoster | Incidence 1.2 to 4.8/1000 people per year. Lifetime prevalence reaches approximately 50% in individuals living to 85 years of age.[8] |
| Incidence: Postherpetic neuralgia | 3.9 per 100,000 people per year[9] |
| Prognosis | Pain usually lasts 1–4 weeks but may persist longer and may progress to postherpetic neuralgia; ultimately, the pain resolves. Early treatment with medications shortens the course of varicella zoster and decreases the duration and pain of postherpetic neuralgia.[8] |

Only in the upper midbrain, after all discriminative sensation tracts have crossed the midline, will sensory loss be entirely contralateral. Throughout the brainstem, a lesion of trigeminal nerve proximal axons or of the trigeminal nerve nuclei causes an ipsilateral loss of sensation from the face.

A lesion in the posterolateral medulla or lower pons can cause a mixed sensory loss consisting of ipsilateral loss of pain and temperature sensation from the face combined with contralateral loss of pain and temperature information from the body (Figure 7-5). This occurs because the trigeminal nerve pain information is ipsilateral in the medulla and lower pons, while ascending pain information from the body crosses in the spinal cord. Discriminative touch and proprioceptive

information from the body is not affected because the tracts conveying this information travel in the medial medulla and pons. Discriminative touch and proprioceptive information from the face is not affected because these tracts and nuclei are superior to the medulla.

A lesion in the medial medulla or lower pons may cause impairment of pain sensation from the contralateral face owing to interruption of some second-order axons conveying information from the trigeminal nerve, combined with loss of discriminative touch and conscious proprioceptive information from the contralateral body. The contralateral loss occurs because the medial lemniscus axons have crossed the midline in the lower medulla.

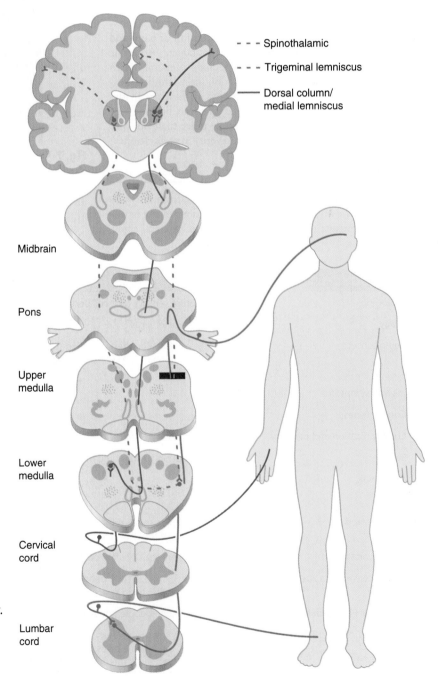

**Fig. 7-5 Mixed sensory loss due to a lesion in the posterolateral medulla.** Black bar indicates the lesion site. Dotted lines indicate pathways that no longer transmit information. Pain and temperature information is lost from the ipsilateral face and the contralateral body. The lesion does not affect discriminative touch and conscious proprioception because the medial lemniscus is medial to the site of the lesion.

Legend (right of figure):
- - - Spinothalamic
- - - Trigeminal lemniscus
— Dorsal column/ medial lemniscus

Labels: Midbrain, Pons, Upper medulla, Lower medulla, Cervical cord, Lumbar cord

A lesion in the posterolateral upper pons or midbrain, after the trigeminothalamic tracts (except proprioceptive) and all of the tracts from the body have crossed the midline, causes contralateral sensory loss from the face (except proprioceptive) and entirely contralateral loss from the body, because all tracts (except proprioceptive) have crossed the midline below the lesion.

> ### ◎ Clinical Pearl
> Lesions in the brainstem often cause mixed sensory impairments, affecting the contralateral body and ipsilateral face.

## Cerebral Region Lesions

### Thalamic Lesions

Lesions in the ventral posterolateral (VPL) or ventral posteromedial (VPM) nucleus of the thalamus result in decreased or lost sensation from the contralateral body or face. Rarely, individuals who have strokes that affect the VPL or VPM nucleus have severe pain in the contralateral body or face.

### Somatosensory Cortex Lesions

The sensory effects of a cortical lesion are contralateral and include decrease or loss of discriminative sensation:
- Conscious proprioception
- Two-point discrimination
- Stereognosis
- Localization of touch and pinprick (nociceptive) stimuli

Cortical processing is essential for discriminative sensation, although crude awareness of sensation is possible at the thalamic level.

In cases of *sensory extinction* (also called *sensory inattention*), loss of sensation is evident only when symmetric body parts are tested bilaterally. For example, if both hands are touched or pricked simultaneously, the person may be aware of stimulation only on the same side of the body as the cortical lesion. If stimuli are not simultaneous, people with sensory extinction are aware of stimulation on either side of the body. Sensory extinction is a form of unilateral neglect because the person neglects stimuli on one side of the body if the other side of the body is stimulated simultaneously. Unilateral neglect is discussed in Chapter 18.

## CLINICAL PERSPECTIVES ON PAIN

Pain is an unpleasant sensory and emotional experience.[10] Pain is frequently associated with tissue damage or potential tissue damage, although pain can be experienced independently of tissue damage. Nociceptors signal injury, yet nociceptor activity is insufficient to cause pain. Pain is a perception.

## Pain From Muscles and Joints

Both A$\delta$ and C fibers are found in skeletal muscle and joints, so signals interpreted as both fast and slow pain can occur with musculoskeletal injury. Under normal circumstances, many nociceptors are "sleeping," that is, not responsive to stimulation.[11] When tissue is injured or ischemic, biochemicals are released that awaken the sleeping nociceptors. The awakened nociceptors are excessively reactive to stimuli; this is called *peripheral sensitization*. The sensitized neurons fire in response to normally innocuous stimuli, even with slight movements, and may fire spontaneously. For example, after an ankle sprain, partial weight bearing may be painful, and the ankle may ache while at rest.

Unlike superficial pain, which encourages withdrawal (movement to escape the source of pain), deep pain usually occurs after tissue has been damaged. The function of deep pain may be to encourage rest of the damaged tissue. After a lower limb injury, pain on weight bearing often produces a modified gait. The modified gait is called *antalgic* and is characterized by a shortened stance phase on the affected side.

## Referred Pain

Referred pain is perceived as coming from a site distinct from the actual site of origin. Usually pain is referred from visceral tissues to skin. For example, during a heart attack, the brain may misinterpret the nociceptive information as arising from the skin or the medial left arm. Similarly, gallbladder pain is often referred to the right subscapular region.

Referred pain is explained by convergence and facilitation of nociceptive information from different sources. Referred pain occurs when branches of nociceptive fibers from an internal organ and branches from nociceptive fibers from the skin converge on the same second-order neurons in the spinal cord or in the thalamus, and the central neurons become sensitized.[12]

Common patterns of referred pain are illustrated in Figure 7-6.

> ### ◎ Clinical Pearl
> Identifying referred pain is important in preventing misdiagnoses and malpractice, so that individuals with disorders not amenable to occupational or physical therapy can be referred to the appropriate practitioner.

## The Pain Matrix

The pain matrix consists of brain structures that process and regulate pain information and are capable of creating pain perception in the absence of nociceptive input. The pain matrix includes parts of the brainstem, amygdala, hypothalamus, and thalamus, and areas of the cerebral cortex.[13] When peripheral nociceptors are stimulated, the signals travel up the pain matrix (Figure 7-7). The person perceives the location and intensity of tissue damage or potential tissue damage (lateral pain system) and has affective and cognitive responses to the signals (medial pain system). Brain scans show differential activation of the medial and lateral systems of the pain matrix (Figure 7-8). Table 7-2 lists the structures of the lateral and medial pain systems.

The experience of pain is strongly linked to emotional, behavioral, and cognitive phenomena.[14] Thus understanding

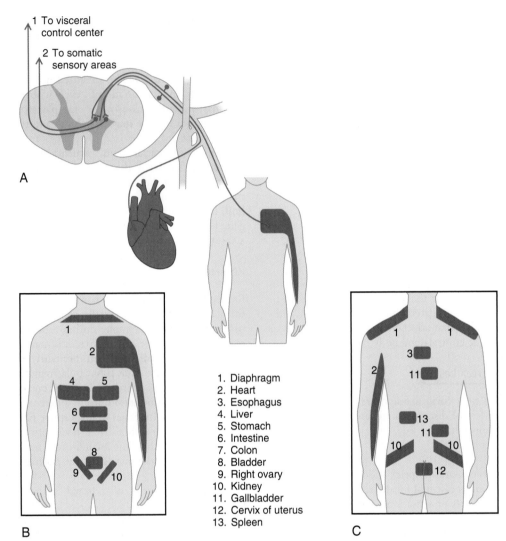

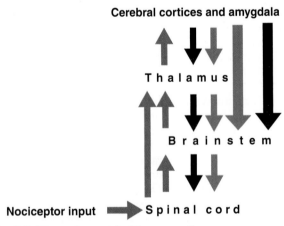

1. Diaphragm
2. Heart
3. Esophagus
4. Liver
5. Stomach
6. Intestine
7. Colon
8. Bladder
9. Right ovary
10. Kidney
11. Gallbladder
12. Cervix of uterus
13. Spleen

**Fig. 7-6  A,** Theoretical mechanism of referred pain. Some visceral afferents synapse with the same second-order neurons as somatosensory afferents. **B** and **C,** Common patterns of referred pain.

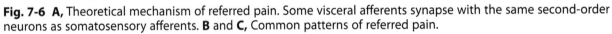

**Fig. 7-7  The pain matrix.** The ascending arrows represent the medial and lateral nociceptive pathways. The descending arrows represent the top-down control of nociceptive signals by the pain matrix. The black arrows indicate antinociception, and the green arrows indicate pronociception.

| TABLE 7-2 | STRUCTURES IN THE LATERAL AND MEDIAL PAIN SYSTEMS | |
|---|---|---|
| | **Lateral System** | **Medial System** |
| Cerebral cortex | Somatosensory cortex Insula | Insula Cingulate cortex Prefrontal cortex |
| Deep cerebrum | — | Amygdala Hypothalamus |
| Thalamus | Ventroposterolateral and ventroposteromedial nuclei | Midline and intralaminar nuclei |
| Brainstem | — | Periaqueductal gray, reticular formation, ventral medulla |

pain requires consideration of multiple aspects of the pain experience: discriminative, motivational-affective, and cognitive-evaluative components.[14] The discriminative aspect refers to the ability to localize the site, timing, and intensity of tissue damage or potential tissue damage. This information travels in the spinothalamic tract and is processed in the somatosensory and insular cortex (lateral pain system). The motivational-affective aspect refers to the effects of the pain experience on emotions and behavior, including increased arousal and avoidance behavior. Nociceptive information that impacts emotions and motivation travels in the spinolimbic and spinoreticular tracts, to the medial and intralaminar nuclei of the thalamus, then to the limbic system. The cognitive-evaluative aspect refers to the meaning that the person ascribes to the pain. Is the pain conceived as a punishment, an unfair burden, a signal of a life-threatening disorder? Cognitive factors, including focusing exclusively on the pain and worry regarding the pain, can increase distress.[15] The separation of the discriminative system from the other systems is verified by the fact that cingulotomy (electrical destruction of the anterior cingulate gyrus) reduces the emotional and cognitive aspects of chronic pain but does not modify the sensory-discriminative aspects.[16] The regions of the brain that respond to pain signals are illustrated in Figure 7-9.

In reaction to nociceptive signals, the pain matrix generates a top-down response that regulates ascending pain signals (see Figure 7-7). The top-down response depends on psychological, physiologic, social, and genetic factors and may suppress or amplify nociceptive signals. Thus the pain matrix determines whether ascending nociceptive processing will be normal, suppressed, sensitized, or reorganized. *Antinociception* is the top-down inhibition of pain signals. *Pronociception* is the biological amplification of pain signals.

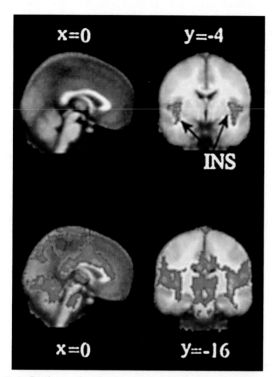

**Fig. 7-8  Brain activation in neurologically normal subjects during pressure on the skin with a stiff nylon filament (Frey hair).** *Left scans,* Midsagittal. *Right scans,* Coronal. *Top scans,* Stimulation of normal skin. Only the insula was activated. *Bottom scans,* Stimulation in the area of secondary hyperalgesia. The area of skin stimulated was adjacent to an area that had received previous application of heat and a topical irritant, capsaicin. *(With permission from Zambreanu L, Wise RG, Brooks JC, et al: A role for the brainstem in central sensitisation in humans: evidence from functional magnetic resonance imaging. Pain 114:397–407, 2005.)*

## How Is Pain Controlled?

What is a typical response to hitting one's thumb with a hammer? A common sequence is to withdraw the thumb, yell (via limbic connections), and then apply pressure to the injured thumb. The first scientific explanation of how pressure and other external stimuli inhibit pain transmission was the *gate theory of pain,* proposed by Melzack and Wall in 1965.[17] They hypothesized that information from first-order low-threshold mechanical afferents and from first-order nociceptive afferents normally converges onto the same second-order neurons. They proposed that the preponderance of activity in the primary afferents determines the pattern of signals transmitted by the second-order neuron. Thus, if low-threshold mechanical afferents are more active than nociceptive afferents, mechanoreceptive information is transmitted and nociceptive information is

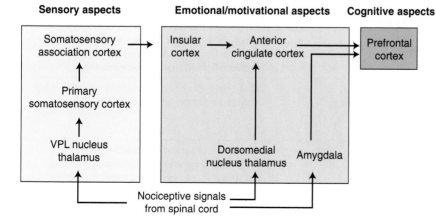

**Fig. 7-9** Contributions to the experience of pain from brain regions that respond to pain signals.

inhibited. According to the theory as initially presented, transmission of pain information is blocked in the dorsal horn, closing the gate to pain.

Although later investigations demonstrated that some details of the original gate theory proposal are incorrect, the original gate theory is important because it inspired inquiry into the mechanics and control of pain. One result of these investigations was the clinical application of transcutaneous electrical nerve stimulation (TENS). TENS uses electrical current applied to the skin to interfere with the transmission of pain information.

### Counterirritant Theory

A theory that has incorporated findings from research stimulated by the gate theory is the *counterirritant theory*. According to the counterirritant theory, inhibition of nociceptive signals by stimulation of non-nociceptive receptors occurs in the dorsal horn of the spinal cord (Figure 7-10). For example, pressure stimulates mechanoreceptive afferents. Theoretically, proximal branches of the mechanoreceptive afferents activate interneurons that release the neurotransmitter *enkephalin*. Enkephalin binds with receptor sites on both the primary afferents and the interneurons of the pain system. Enkephalin binding depresses the release of substance P and hyperpolarizes the interneurons, thus inhibiting the transmission of nociceptive signals.

### Dorsal Horn Processing of Nociceptive Information

Processing of somatosensory information in the dorsal horn can be altered by abnormal neural activity or by tissue injury. Four states of dorsal horn processing occur: normal, suppressed, sensitized, and reorganized[18] (Table 7-3). In the normal state, signals resulting from stimuli are accurate. For example, touch sensation is interpreted as touch, and nociceptive information is interpreted as painful. In the suppressed state, touch, pressure, and vibration information is transmitted normally but nociceptive impulses are inhibited. Medications, TENS,

counterirritants, excitement, distraction, and placebo effects can produce the inhibition. In the sensitized state, changes in the quantities and types of neurotransmitters and receptors produce painful responses to both Aβ and Aδ/C activity. In the reorganized state, the structure of the dorsal horn has changed owing to cell death, degeneration of nociceptive axon terminals, and the sprouting of new Aβ axon terminals that synapse with neurons in the nociceptive pathways. Sensitized and reorganized states are neuropathic states, that is, the pain experienced in these states is due to abnormal neural processing.

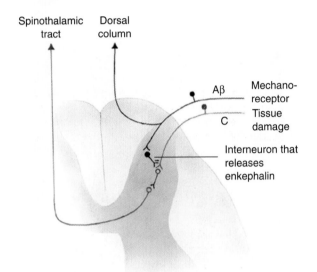

**Fig. 7-10 Counterirritant mechanism.** Circuits in the dorsal horn that may produce inhibition of nociceptive signals. Collaterals of mechanoreceptive afferents stimulate interneurons that release enkephalins. Enkephalin binding inhibits the transmission of nociceptive messages by primary afferents and interneurons in the nociceptive pathway.

| TABLE 7-3 | STATES OF SENSORY PROCESSING IN THE DORSAL HORN OF THE SPINAL CORD | |
|---|---|---|
| **State of Dorsal Horn** | **Response to Activation of Primary Afferent Fibers** | **Mechanism** |
| Normal | Aβ: sensation of touch, pressure, vibration<br>Aδ/C: nociceptive pain | Normal physiologic activity |
| Suppressed nociception | Aβ: normal<br>Aδ/C: reduced response | Activity of segmental and descending inhibition on dorsal horn; includes counterirritation, medications, and psychological factors |
| Sensitized (temporary) | Aβ: allodynia (pain evoked by stimuli that would not normally cause pain)<br>Aδ/C: excessive response | Additional types of neurotransmitters active, plus increased numbers and types of receptors |
| Reorganized (persistent increased pain sensibility) | Aβ: allodynia<br>Aδ/C: excessive response | Structural reorganization, including death of neurons, degeneration of C fiber axon terminals, and sprouting of new Aβ axon terminals to form abnormal synapses with neurons in the nociceptive pathways |

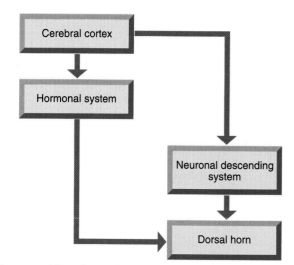

**Fig. 7-11 Flowchart of supraspinal analgesic systems.** Cerebral cortical output activates the hormonal and neuronal descending systems that inhibit the transmission of nociceptive information in the dorsal horn.

---

**◎ Clinical Pearl**

Neuropathic pain results from changes in neuronal activity. Thus, neuropathic pain is produced by neuroplasticity, not by stimulation of nociceptors.

---

## Antinociceptive Systems

Antinociception is suppression of pain in response to stimulation that normally would be painful. The endogenous, or naturally occurring, substances that activate antinociceptive mechanisms are called *endorphins*. Endorphins include enkephalins, dynorphin, and β-endorphin. Opiates, drugs that block nociceptive signals without affecting other sensations, bind to the same receptor sites as endorphins. Because opiates bind to the receptor sites, the receptors are sometimes called *opiate receptors*.

The transmission of nociceptive information can be inhibited by pain matrix activity (Figure 7-11). Brainstem areas that provide intrinsic antinociception form a neuronal descending system, arising in the following:

- Rostral ventromedial medulla
- Periaqueductal gray (PAG) in the midbrain
- Locus coeruleus in the pons

When the rostral ventromedial medulla is electrically stimulated, the raphespinal tracts (axons projecting to the spinal cord) release the neurotransmitter serotonin in the dorsal horn, inhibiting the tract neurons via enkephalin interneurons, and thus interfering with transmission of nociceptive messages. Stimulation of PAG produces antinociception via activation of the rostral ventromedial medulla.[19] The third descending tract, the ceruleospinal (from locus coeruleus) tract, inhibits spinothalamic activity in the dorsal horn but is non–opiate-mediated; instead, binding of the transmitter norepinephrine on the primary afferent neuron directly suppresses the release of nociceptive transmitters.[20]

Narcotics, drugs derived from opium or opium-like compounds, bind to opiate receptor sites in the PAG, rostral ventromedial medulla, and dorsal horn of the spinal cord. By activating the receptor sites, narcotics induce antinociception and stupor (a state of reduced consciousness). If the descending tracts from the rostral ventromedial medulla are severed, administration of morphine or other opiates results in only slight antinociception, because the lesion of the raphespinal tract blocks descending inhibition. The slight antinociception that occurs is the result of morphine binding to opiate receptors in the dorsal horn.

Pain-inhibiting centers do not lie dormant waiting for an electrode or a drug to stimulate them. How are they normally activated? Individuals injured in accidents, disasters, or athletic contests sometimes do not feel pain until after the emergency or game is over. Stress during an emergency or competition may trigger the antinociception systems. *Stress-induced antinociception* requires activation of the raphespinal tracts plus release of hormonal endorphins from the pituitary gland (β-endorphins) and the adrenal medulla (both enkephalins and epinephrine inhibit nociceptive signals in the dorsal horn). The hormonal endorphins bind to opiate receptors in the pain matrix and spinal cord. β-Endorphins are the most potent endorphins, and their effects last for hours. Stress-induced antinociception may be triggered by cortical input to the descending antinociception systems.

## Sites of Antinociception

The transmission of nociceptive information can be altered at several locations in the nervous system. The phenomenon of *antinociception* is summarized by a five-level model (Figure 7-12):

- **Level 1** occurs in the *periphery*. Non-narcotic analgesics (e.g., aspirin) decrease the synthesis of prostaglandins, preventing prostaglandins from sensitizing nociceptors.[21] Both topical menthol and capsaicin desensitize nociceptive C fibers.[22] Membrane-stabilizing medications (anticonvulsants and tricyclic antidepressants) can prevent abnormal axon-generated action potentials, thus decreasing pain.
- **Level II** occurs in the *dorsal horn,* via local inhibitory neurons releasing enkephalin or dynorphin. This is the level of counterirritant effects; examples include superficial heat and high-frequency, low-intensity TENS. Activity in collateral branches of non-nociceptive afferents decreases or prevents the transmission of nociceptive information to the second-order neuron in the spinal cord.
- **Level III** is the fast-acting *neuronal descending system,* involving the PAG, the rostral ventromedial medulla, and the locus coeruleus.
- **Level IV** is the *hormonal system,* involving the periventricular gray (PVG) in the hypothalamus, the pituitary gland (releases β-endorphin), and the adrenal medulla. Direct electrical stimulation of the PVG results in antinociception with 10-minute latency; the effect lasts for hours after stimulation has stopped. Low-frequency TENS may act on this level because its pattern of action has a similar latency and lasting effect.
- **Level V** is the *cortical level.* Here, expectations, excitement, distraction, and placebo all play a role in adjusting the transmission of nociceptive signals. Placebo antinociception activates the same higher-order cognitive and brainstem areas that are activated by opiate drugs.[23]

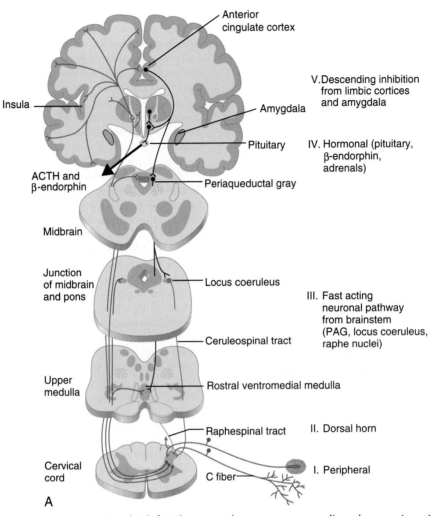

**Fig. 7-12 Antinociceptive systems. A,** On the left side, tracts that convey ascending slow nociceptive information are shown: spinolimbic *(blue)*, spinomesencephalic *(red)*, and spinoreticular *(green)* tracts. Structures indicated in the coronal section are not in the same plane (anterior cingulate and amygdala are anterior to the section of thalamus illustrated). On the right, the five levels of the nervous system involved in pain inhibition are shown. All tracts are bilateral. Signals in the spinoreticular tract facilitate the locus coeruleus neurons.

> ### ◎ Clinical Pearl
>
> Transmission of nociceptive information can be inhibited by binding of endorphins or of analgesic drugs to receptor sites in the dorsal horn, PAG, PVG, and rostral ventromedial medulla. Norepinephrine binding to primary afferents in the dorsal horn inhibits transmission of nociceptive information. In the periphery, signals from nociceptors can be inhibited by non-narcotic analgesics.

Distraction using virtual reality has been shown to decrease ratings of worst pain, pain unpleasantness, and time thinking about pain in people undergoing painful removal of dead, injured, and infected tissue as a treatment for burns. The effect of virtual reality was compared with the same treatment without virtual reality. Participants played a game called Snow World, wearing a virtual reality helmet and using a joystick to glide down an icy canyon and throw snowballs at snowmen, igloos, robots, and penguins.[24]

### Pronociception: Biological Amplification of Nociception

Pain transmission can be intensified at several levels. Edema and endogenous chemicals can sensitize free nerve endings in the periphery. For example, following a minor burn injury, stimuli that normally would be innocuous can cause exquisite pain. Pronociception may occur when a person is anxious or depressed.[25] Pronociceptive pain matrix activity can also produce pain perception in the absence of any nociceptive input.[25] An example of pain perception without nociceptive input is the study of social exclusion conducted by Eisenberger and coworkers.[26] Subjects played a virtual ball game and eventually were excluded. Scans during the experience indicated that brain activity changes in the prefrontal and anterior cingulate cortex that occur during physical pain are the same during social distress. Brain areas involved in antinociception and pronociception are illustrated in Figure 7-13.

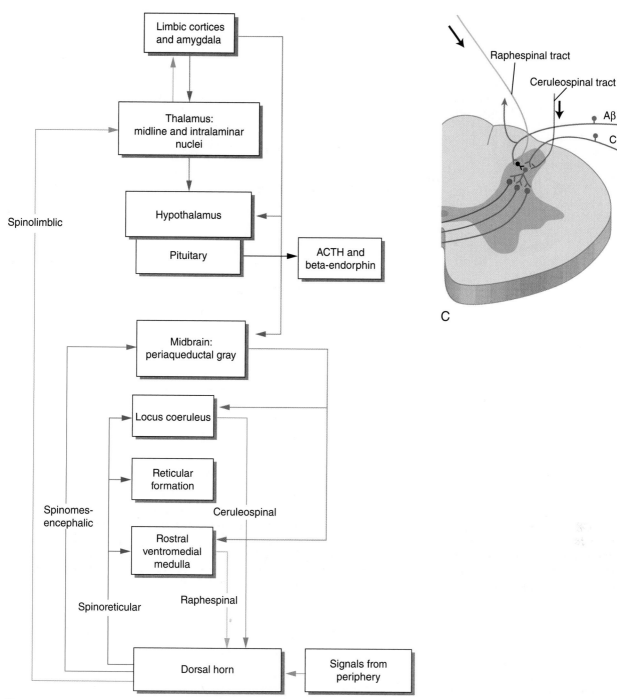

**B**

**Fig. 7-12, cont'd  B,** Flowchart illustrating the same pathways as in **A**. The flow of slow pain information upward is shown on the left, and the descending antinociceptive pathways are shown on the right. The limbic cortices include the medial prefrontal cortex, the anterior cingulate cortex, and the lateral orbitofrontal cortex. **C,** A segment of the spinal cord. The raphespinal tract synapses with an interneuron *(black)* that inhibits the transmission of nociceptive information in the dorsal horn of the spinal cord. The ceruleospinal tract directly inhibits the primary nociceptive afferent.

## CHRONIC PAIN

Therapists must distinguish between acute pain and chronic pain and between pain and activity limitations, so appropriate treatment can be administered. Pain is an unpleasant subjective experience; activity limitation is the lack of ability to perform normal tasks. Characteristics of acute and chronic pain are compared in Table 7-4.

### Nociceptive Chronic Pain

Nociceptive chronic pain is due to continuing stimulation of nociceptive receptors. Examples include chronic pain resulting

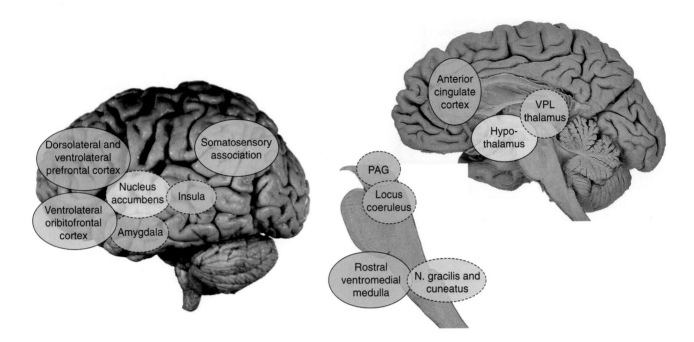

| Brain: | Specific area | Action |
|---|---|---|
| **Cortex** | Dorsal and ventral prefrontal cortex | Both pro- and antinociceptive |
| | Anterior cingulate cortex | Both pro- and antinociceptive (Diederich & Goetz 2008) |
| | Insular cortex | Pronociceptive |
| | Ventrolateral orbitofrontal cortex | Role in development of depressive symptoms in long-standing pain including neuropathic pain |
| **Subcortical** | Amygdala | Emotional aspects of neuropathic pain; contributes to hypersensitivity (Jaggi et al 2011) |
| | Nucleus accumbens | Inhibits pronociceptive cells in rostroventromedial medulla (Hagelberg et al 2004; Scott et al 2007) |
| | Thalamus: VPL nucleus | Pronociceptive role in pain processing |
| | Hypothalamus | Antinociceptive (release of beta-endorphins and ACTH via pituitary) |
| **Brainstem** | Periaqueductal gray (midbrain) | Pronociceptive (Fundytus 2001); antinociceptive (Piché et al 2009) |
| | Locus coeruleus (in pons) | Both pro- and antinociceptive |
| | Nucleus gracilis & cuneatus (in medulla) | Pronociceptive |
| | Rostroventromedial medulla | Both pro- and antinociceptive |

**Fig. 7-13** Orange indicates pro-nociceptive brain areas; purple indicates areas that are both pro- and anti-nociceptive; yellow indicates areas that are anti-nociceptive. *(Citations: Diederich NJ, Goetz CG: The placebo treatments in neurosciences: New insights from clinical and neuroimaging studies. Neurol 71(9):677–684, 2008. Hagelberg N, Jääskeläinen SK, Martikainen I, et al: Striatal dopamine D2 receptors in modulation of pain in humans: a review. Eur J Pharmacol 500:187–192, 2004. Jaggi AS, Singh N: Role of different brain areas in peripheral nerve injury-induced neuropathic pain. Brain Research 2011, in press. Fundytus ME: Glutamate receptors and nociception: implications for the drug treatment of pain. CNS Drugs 15(1):29–58, 2001. Piché M, Arsenault M, Rainville P: Cerebral and cerebrospinal processes underlying counterirritation analgesia. J Neurosci 29(45):14236–14246, 2009. Scott DJ, Stohler CS, Egnatuk CM, et al: Neuron. Individual differences in reward responding explain placebo-induced expectations and effects. 55(2):325–336, 2007. Photographs courtesy of Nolte, John. The Human Brain: An Introduction to Its Functional Anatomy, 6th Edition. Mosby, 082008.)*

**TABLE 7-4**   CHARACTERISTICS OF ACUTE AND CHRONIC PAIN

|  | Acute Pain | Chronic Pain |
|---|---|---|
| Causes | Threat of or actual tissue damage | Continuing tissue damage<br>Environmental factors (operant conditioning)<br>Sensitization of nociceptive pathway neurons<br>Dysfunction of endogenous pain control systems |
| Client report | Clear description of location, pattern, quality, frequency, and duration | Vague description |
| Function | Warning of tissue damage, enforce rest of healing tissue | If tissue damage is not continuing, no biological benefit; may have social or psychological benefit |
| Consequences | Excessive autonomic activity<br>Excessive neuroendocrine activation<br>If not adequately treated, can be as harmful as disease[27] and may progress to chronic pain | Severe financial, emotional, physical, and/or social stresses on the person and family<br>Physiologic consequences of inactivity |

from tissue damage caused by cancer or by a vertebral tumor pressing on nociceptors in the meninges surrounding the spinal cord. The neurons are functioning normally by sending appropriate signals regarding tissue damage. The chemical changes in damaged tissue awaken sleeping peripheral nociceptors. The activity of the awakened nociceptors results in *primary hyperalgesia,* excessive sensitivity to stimuli in the injured tissue. An example is the pain caused by mild heat on burned skin. If a fingertip is burned, picking up a hot plate is more painful than if the skin were uninjured. Nociceptive chronic pain serves a useful biological function as a warning to protect injured tissue.

## SUMMARY

Somatosensation is essential for smooth, accurate movements and to prevent injury. Testing of somatosensation includes testing discriminative touch, conscious proprioception, pin-prick sensation (fast pain), and discriminative temperature sensations. Sensory nerve function can also be evaluated using nerve conduction studies and somatosensory evoked potentials.

Lesions of the proprioceptive pathway produce sensory ataxia. Peripheral nerve lesions may interrupt all somatosensation in the distribution of the nerve. Compression of a nerve primarily affects the function of large-diameter axons. Spinal region lesions affecting somatosensation include complete transection or hemisection of the cord, posterior column lesions, and infection. Varicella zoster selectively infects the cell bodies of somatosensory neurons, causing pain in a specific dermatome or trigeminal nerve branch.

Pain is a complex experience. The lateral pain system discriminates the location of actual or potential tissue damage. The medial pain system processes the motivational-affective and cognitive-evaluative aspects of pain.

Musculoskeletal injury or ischemia sensitizes peripheral nociceptors and thus causes pain in response to stimuli that are not normally painful. Pain can also occur without stimulation of nociceptors, when lesions of the somatosensory system, pain matrix dysfunction, and pain syndromes occur. These causes of pain are discussed in Chapter 8.

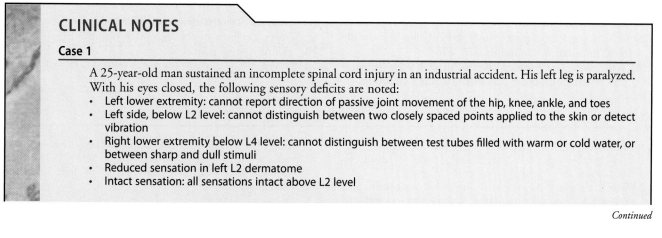

## CLINICAL NOTES

### Case 1

A 25-year-old man sustained an incomplete spinal cord injury in an industrial accident. His left leg is paralyzed. With his eyes closed, the following sensory deficits are noted:
- Left lower extremity: cannot report direction of passive joint movement of the hip, knee, ankle, and toes
- Left side, below L2 level: cannot distinguish between two closely spaced points applied to the skin or detect vibration
- Right lower extremity below L4 level: cannot distinguish between test tubes filled with warm or cold water, or between sharp and dull stimuli
- Reduced sensation in left L2 dermatome
- Intact sensation: all sensations intact above L2 level

*Continued*

## CLINICAL NOTES—cont'd

- Left lower extremity: can distinguish between test tubes filled with warm or cold water and can distinguish between sharp and dull stimuli
- Right lower extremity: can distinguish between two closely spaced points applied to the skin, can accurately report the direction of passive movements of the joints, and can detect vibration

### Question

Explain the pattern of sensory loss seen in this person.

### Case 2

A 42-year-old chef is unable to work because of weakness and altered sensation in her dominant right hand. She reports difficulty lifting heavy skillets that began 2 months ago. Tingling in the thumb, index, and middle fingers and half of the ring finger began 6 weeks ago. Currently, she is unable to stir anything for longer than 5 minutes using her right hand. The thenar muscles are visibly atrophied. Results of motor and sensory testing of the right upper limb are as follows:

- Pinch grip on the right of 30 g (vs. 120 g with left hand)
- Diminished sensation in the lateral three and a half digits
- Strength, reflexes, and sensation within normal limits throughout the remainder of the right upper extremity

### Question

What is the location and probable cause of the lesion?

### Case 3

A 73-year-old man was found unconscious on the floor at home 1 week ago. He is now lucid and cooperative. Sensation and movement are within normal limits on the right side of the body and face. He has sensory extinction on the left side. The lower half of the left side of his face appears to droop, and he cannot actively move the left limbs. When assisted to sitting, he collapses as soon as support is removed.

### Question

What is the location and probable cause of the lesion?

## REVIEW QUESTIONS

1. How is a quick screening for somatosensory impairments performed?
2. What are the important limitations of sensory testing?
3. What signs and/or symptoms indicate that a thorough somatosensory evaluation should be performed?
4. What precautions are essential to ensure valid results of somatosensory testing?
5. How is a sensory nerve conduction study performed?
6. A patient describes spontaneous tingling and prickling in both feet. What clinical term corresponds to this description?
7. How can a clinician distinguish between sensory ataxia and cerebellar ataxia?
8. Which types of somatosensory information are usually most impaired by demyelination? Why?
9. What sensory and motor losses occur with a left hemisection of the spinal cord? Name the resulting syndrome.

10. What is varicella zoster?
11. Describe the sensory loss associated with a lesion in the left posterolateral lower pons.
12. What is sensory extinction?
13. How does the counterirritant theory explain the inhibition of pain messages caused by application of pressure to an injured finger?
14. An inability to sleep due to nociception is an example of what aspect of the pain experience: discriminative, motivational-affective, or cognitive-evaluative?
15. List the origins of the three supraspinal analgesic systems.
16. How do narcotics induce their effects?
17. Name the levels of the antinociception model.
18. Define *referred pain*.

## References

1. Sherrington CS: The muscular sense. In Schafer EA, editor: *Text-book of physiology*, vol 2, Edinburgh, 1900, Pentland, pp 1002–1025.
2. Taub E, Perrella P, Barro G, et al: Behavioral development after forelimb deafferentation on day of birth in monkeys with and without blinding. *Science* 181:959–960, 1973.
3. Rothwell JC, Traub MM, Day BL, et al: Manual motor performance in a deafferented man. *Brain* 105:515–542, 1982.
4. Woolf CJ: What is this thing called pain? *J Clin Invest* 120:3742–3744, 2010.
5. Thomson MP, Potter J, Finch PM, et al: Threshold for detection of diabetic peripheral sensory neuropathy using a range of research

grade monofilaments in persons with type 2 diabetes mellitus. *J Foot Ankle Res* 1:9, 2008.

6. Dros J, Wewerinke A, Bindels PJ, et al: Accuracy of monofilament testing to diagnose peripheral neuropathy: a systematic review. *Ann Fam Med* 7:555–558, 2009.

7. Ferreira MC, Rodrigues L, Fels K: New method for evaluation of cutaneous sensibility in diabetic feet: preliminary report. *Rev Hosp Clin Fac Med Sao Paulo* 59:286–290, 2004.

8. Thakur R, Kent JL, Dworkin RH: Herpes zoster and postherpetic neuralgia. In Ballantyne JC, Fishman SM, Rathmell JP, editors: *Bonica's management of pain*, ed 4, Baltimore, 2010, Lippincott Williams & Wilkins.

9. Koopman JS, Dieleman JP, Huygen FJ, et al: Incidence of facial pain in the general population. *Pain* 147:122–127, 2009.

10. IASP, Task Force on Taxonomy: Classification of chronic pain. In Merskey H, Bogduk N, editors: Seattle, Wash, 1994, IASP Press, pp 209–214.

11. Gold MS, Gebhart GF: Peripheral mechanical and nociceptor sensitization. In Ballantyne JC, Fishman SM, Rathmell JP, editors: *Bonica's management of pain*, ed 4, Baltimore, 2010, Lippincott Williams & Wilkins, p 32.

12. McGuirk BE, Bogduk N: Chronic low back pain. In Ballantyne JC, Fishman SM, Rathmell JP, editors: *Bonica's management of pain*, ed 4, Baltimore, 2010, Lippincott Williams & Wilkins, pp 1105–1122.

13. Zambreanu L, Wise RG, Brooks JC, et al: A role for the brainstem in central sensitisation in humans: evidence from functional magnetic resonance imaging. *Pain* 114:397–407, 2005.

14. Lorenz J, Hauck M: Supraspinal mechanisms of pain and nociception. In Ballantyne JC, Fishman SM, Rathmell JP, editors: *Bonica's management of pain*, ed 4, Baltimore, 2010, Lippincott Williams & Wilkins.

15. Fabian LA, McGuire L, Goodin BR, et al: Ethnicity, catastrophizing, and qualities of the pain experience. *Pain Med* 12:314–321, 2011.

16. Medford N, Critchley HD: Conjoint activity of anterior insular and anterior cingulate cortex: awareness and response. *Brain Struct Funct* 214:535–549, 2010.

17. Melzack R, Wall PD: Pain mechanisms: a new theory. *Science* 150:971–979, 1965.

18. Doubell TP: The dorsal horn: state-dependent sensory processing, plasticity, and the generation of pain. In Wall PD, Melzack R, editors: *Textbook of pain*, Edinburgh, 1999, Churchill Livingstone, pp 165–182.

19. Griffin R, Fink E, Brenner JG: Functional neuroanatomy of the nociceptive system. In Ballantyne JC, Fishman SM, Rathmell JP, editors: *Bonica's management of pain*, ed 4, Baltimore, 2010, Lippincott Williams & Wilkins.

20. Griffin RS, Woolfe CJ: Pharmacology of analgesia. In Golan DE, Tashjian AH, Armstrong EJ, Armstrong AW, editors: *Principles of pharmacology: the pathophysiologic basis of drug therapy*, ed 2, Baltimore, 2008, Lippincott Williams & Wilkins, pp 263–278.

21. Stix G: Better ways to target pain. *Sci Am* 296:84–86, 88, 2007.

22. Patel T, Ishiuji Y, Yosipovitch G: Menthol: a refreshing look at this ancient compound. *J Am Acad Dermatol* 57:873–878, 2007.

23. Ossipov MH, Dussor GO, Porreca F: Central modulation of pain. *J Clin Invest* 120:3779–3787, 2010.

24. Malloy KM, Milling LS: The effectiveness of virtual reality distraction for pain reduction: a systematic review. *Clin Psychol Rev* 30:1011–1018, 2010.

25. Brooks J, Tracey I: From nociception to pain perception: imaging the spinal and supraspinal pathways. *J Anat* 207:19–33, 2005.

26. Eisenberger NI, Lieberman MD, Wiliams KD: Does rejection hurt? An FMRI study of social exclusion. *Science* 302:290–292, 2003.

27. Liebeskind JC: Pain can kill. *Pain* 44:3–4, 1991.

# 8 Neuropathic Pain, Pain Matrix Dysfunction, and Pain Syndromes

Laurie Lundy-Ekman

## Chapter Outline

I am 69 years old, retired from working for the county, and the mother of three children. Nine years ago I awoke with sciatica, a severe pain extending from the left buttock, down the back of my leg, and into my big toe. I could not bend over to put on shoes or socks. A myelogram, an x-ray study of the spinal region in which dye is injected into the spinal region, showed a herniated intervertebral disk. I developed an excruciating headache secondary to the myelogram, and the scheduled surgery to remove part of the disk was cancelled. After two months of bed rest, I recovered.

One year later I again developed sciatic pain in my left leg that rapidly intensified. I couldn't walk at all because of the pain. I had to crawl. The pain was unbelievable. This time, magnetic resonance imaging revealed that two intervertebral disks had herniated. One month later, surgery was performed and when I awoke the sciatic pain was completely gone. Two years later, I was vacuuming and abruptly developed agonizing pain in my left leg. Surgery again repaired the disk. Since then I have had several deep cortisone shots that effectively relieved the pain.

Throughout this time, I didn't have any lack of sensation, weakness, or other problems. My ability to move was curtailed during the periods when I had sciatica. I could only move in ways that didn't hurt, so I couldn't drive or use stairs. The only time I wasn't in pain was when I was lying down, perfectly still. The pain completely dominated my life.

In physical therapy following the second surgery, I learned two exercises that I do daily. The first exercise is back extension. I lie on the floor on my stomach, my palms on the floor under my shoulders, then slowly push with my arms to raise my head and upper trunk off the floor. I hold this position for 20 seconds, then lie flat again. The other exercise is done lying on my side. If I am lying on my left side, I clasp my hands in front of me, then slowly raise both arms in an arc toward the ceiling and then to the floor on my right. When I began this exercise I could only move through half of the arc with my arms, but now I can reach across to the opposite side. This rotation of my spine works very well. I am much more limber now than when I began these exercises. I am free of pain now, except for a dull ache upon awakening that is relieved by the exercises. Also, I am careful not to lift more than ten pounds and I've learned to take breaks when I'm gardening.

—*Pauline Schweizer*

**The sciatic pain described is neuropathic pain, because the pain is caused by compression of the sciatic nerve. Although it may feel as though the big toe, back of the leg, and buttock are the sources of the pain, there is no tissue damage and thus no activation of nociceptors in those regions. Instead the pain is caused by compression of the sciatic nerve by the intervertebral disks, and pain signals arise from the section of nerve irritated by the pressure. Because signals from the sciatic nerve typically arise from stimulation of receptors at the ends of axons, the brain misinterprets the signals from the compressed sciatic nerve as arising from the healthy lower limb and buttock.**

## CHRONIC PAIN AS A DISEASE

Pain is more than a simple sensation arising from tissue injury. Pain involves inhibitory and excitatory circuits in the central nervous system (CNS) that can diminish or amplify pain messages. In neuropathic pain, pain matrix dysfunction, and pain syndromes, the neural mechanisms for regulating pain amplify signals, creating pain in the absence of noxious stimuli. This pathologic pain is similar to a malfunctioning burglar alarm system: there is no burglar, yet the alarm siren blasts a warning. Pathologic pain has no beneficial biological function. For example, chronic low back pain may be caused by abnormal pain processing rather than by current musculoskeletal injury. The neurons are pathologically active.

> ◎ **Clinical Pearl**
>
> In neuropathic pain, pain matrix dysfunction, and pain syndromes, the pain is a disease, not a warning of tissue injury. The pain is produced by pathologic neural activity. Nociception can alter the structure and function of the nervous system.

## NEUROPATHIC PAIN

The International Association for the Study of Pain defines neuropathic pain as "pain arising as a direct consequence of a lesion or disease affecting the somatosensory system."[1]

Individuals whose genetic code results in less production of an enzyme that regulates the levels of catecholamines and enkephalins are twice as likely to develop neuropathic pain as those who produce more of the enzyme.[2]

### Symptoms of Neuropathic Pain

Symptoms of neuropathic pain include paresthesia, dysesthesia, allodynia, and secondary hyperalgesia.

*Paresthesia* is a painless abnormal sensation in the absence of nociceptor stimulation. Paresthesias arise from dysfunction of neurons. Typically, paresthesias are experienced as tingling or prickling sensations. Lesions anywhere along the nociceptive pathways, from peripheral nerves to somatosensory cortex, can produce paresthesia.

*Dysesthesia* is an unpleasant abnormal sensation, whether evoked or spontaneous. Often spontaneous dysesthesia is described as a sensation of burning pain, or shooting or electrical sensations. A similar shooting pain is elicited by striking the ulnar nerve at the elbow. Allodynia and hyperalgesia are specific types of dysesthesia evoked by stimuli.

*Allodynia* is pain evoked by a stimulus that normally would not cause pain. For example, the normally nonpainful stimulus of touch produces pain if skin is sunburned.

*Secondary hyperalgesia* is excessive sensitivity to stimuli that normally are mildly painful in uninjured tissue.

Table 8-1 lists the tests for neuropathic pain. Figure 8-1 lists self-administered questions for determining whether a person has neuropathic pain. A total score greater than 11 indicates

**TABLE 8-1    DETECTING NEUROPATHIC PAIN: SOMATOSENSORY TESTING**

| | Test | Response |
|---|---|---|
| Cold allodynia | Ask patient, "How does this feel?" Place a cold object, for example, the metal handle of a reflex hammer, on the skin. | Normal response: perception of cold<br>Neuropathic response: perception of pain |
| Brush allodynia | Ask patient, "How does this feel?" Lightly stroke the skin with a 1 inch wide foam brush. The stroke should be 3–5 cm (1.5–2 inches) long and should require about 1 second.[3] | Normal response: perception of light touch<br>Neuropathic response: perception of pain |
| Abnormal temporal summation | Tell patient that you are going to tap on the skin with a nylon filament; ask, "How does this feel?" For 5–10 seconds, repeatedly stimulate the same location on the skin with a stiff nylon filament, using the same amount of force each time. | Normal response: perception of the intensity of the stimulus remains constant<br>Neuropathic response: increasing perception of pain |
| Secondary hyperalgesia | Ask patient, "Does this feel the same on both sides?" Prick the skin with a sharp object on a normal area of the skin (contralateral to the affected area), and then prick the skin with the same object near the painful area on the affected side. | Normal response: perception is the same on both sides of the body<br>Neuropathic response: pain is more intense near the painful area |

neuropathic pain. Box 8-1 summarizes the biological factors and consequences of neuropathic pain.

## Four Mechanisms Produce Neuropathic Pain

Neuropathic pain is produced by four mechanisms:
* Ectopic foci
* Ephaptic transmission
* Central sensitization
* Structural reorganization

## Ectopic Foci

When myelin is damaged, signals from the exposed axon alter the gene activity in the cell body, stimulating excessive production of mechanosensitive and chemosensitive ion channels. These channels are inserted into the demyelinated membrane, producing abnormal sensitivity to mechanical and chemical stimuli. The demyelinated region takes on a new, pathologic role: the generation of action potentials, in addition to the normal role of conducting action potentials. The sensitivity of ectopic foci to circulating catecholamines may contribute to the development of pain syndromes.[4]

## Ephaptic Transmission

Also called *cross-talk,* ephaptic transmission occurs in demyelinated regions as a result of lack of insulation between neurons. An action potential in one neuron may induce an action potential in another neuron.

## Central Sensitization

Excessive responsiveness of central neurons, called *central sensitization,* develops in response to ongoing nociceptive input, yet

**BOX 8-1    NEUROPATHIC PAIN: BIOLOGICAL FACTORS AND CONSEQUENCES**

| Biological Factors | Consequences |
|---|---|
| Abnormal sensory processing<br>Psychiatric disorders (primarily depression and anxiety disorders) | Distress, fear of becoming someone they do not want to be<br>Poor memory<br>Psychological reactions, including depression, anxiety, guilt<br>Limitations of social roles (parenting, friendship, partner)<br>Mobility problems<br>Difficulties with activities of daily living |

Developed from Hensing GK, Sverker AM, Leijon GS: Experienced dilemmas of everyday life in chronic neuropathic pain patients—results from a critical incident study. Scand J Caring Sci 21:147-54, 2007; Kindermans HP, Huijnen IP, Goossens ME, et al: "Being" in pain: the role of self-discrepancies in the emotional experience and activity patterns of patients with chronic low back pain. Pain 152:403-9, 2011; Mailis-Gagnon A, Yegneswaran B, Lakha SF, et al: Pain characteristics and demographics of patients attending a university-affiliated pain clinic in Toronto, Ontario. Pain Res Manag 12:93-9, 2007.

the alterations in central neural activity outlast the tissue injury (Pathology 8-1). Normally, when a brief, mild nociceptive message is conveyed into the CNS, a small amount of activity is generated in the central neurons, producing the usual level of output from the central neurons. However, peripheral injury can induce an abnormal increase in CNS responsiveness that

## APPENDIX
## THE S-LANSS PAIN SCORE

Leeds Assessment of Neuropathic Symptoms and Signs (self-complete)

NAME _____    DATE _____

- This questionnaire can tell us about the type of pain that you may be experiencing. This can help in deciding how best to treat it.

- Please draw on the diagram below where you feel your pain. If you have pain in more than one area, **only shade in the one main area where your worst pain is.**

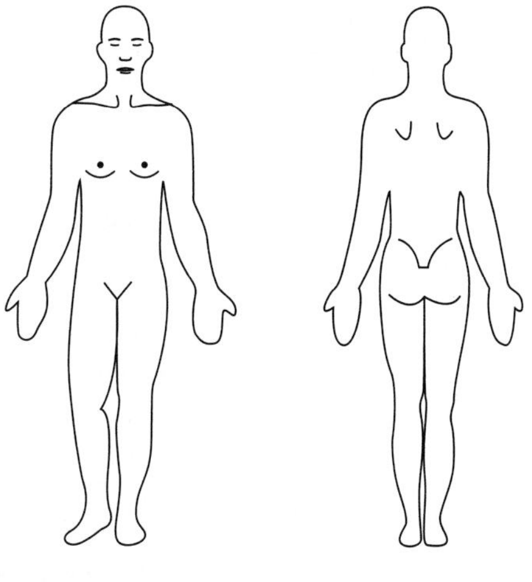

- On the scale below, please indicate how bad your pain (that you have shown on the above diagram) has been in the last week where:
  '0' means no pain and '10' means pain as severe as it could be.

**NONE**   0   1   2   3   4   5   6   7   8   9   10   **SEVERE PAIN**

- On the other side of the page are 7 questions about your pain (the one in the diagram).

- Think about how your pain that you showed in the diagram has felt **over the last week**. Please circle the descriptions that best match your pain. These descriptions may, or may not, match your pain no matter how severe it feels.

- Only circle the responses that describe your pain. **Please turn over.**

**Fig. 8-1  Leeds Assessment of Neuropathic Symptoms and Sign (S-LANSS).** *(With permission from Bennett MI, Smith BH, Torrance N, Potter J: The S-LANSS score for identifying pain of predominantly neuropathic origin: validation for use in clinical and postal research. J Pain. 2005 Mar;6(3):149–58.)*

*Continued*

## S-LANSS

1.   **In the area where you have pain, do you also have 'pins and needles', tingling or prickling sensations?**

     a)     NO – I don't get these sensations                                                                          (0)
     b)     YES – I get these sensations often                                                                        (5)

2.   **Does the painful area change colour (perhaps looks mottled or more red) when the pain is particularly bad?**

     a)     NO – The pain does not affect the colour of my skin                                              (0)
     b)     YES – I have noticed that the pain does make my skin look different from normal      (5)

3.   **Does your pain make the affected skin abnormally sensitive to touch? Getting unpleasant sensations or pain when lightly stroking the skin might describe this.**

     a)     NO – The pain does not make my skin in that area abnormally sensitive to touch     (0)
     b)     YES – My skin in that area is particularly sensitive to touch                                    (3)

4.   **Does your pain come on suddenly and in bursts for no apparent reason when you are completely still? Words like 'electric shocks', jumping and bursting might describe this.**

     a)     NO – My pain doesn't really feel like this                                                             (0)
     b)     YES – I get these sensations often                                                                        (2)

5.   **In the area where you have pain, does your skin feel unusually hot like a burning pain?**
     a)     NO – I don't have burning pain                                                                            (0)
     b)     YES – I get burning pain often                                                                             (1)

6.   **Gently <u>rub</u> the painful area with your index finger and then rub a non-painful area (for example, an area of skin further away or on the opposite side from the painful area). How does this rubbing feel in the painful area?**

     a)     The painful area feels no different from the non-painful area                               (0)
     b)     I feel discomfort, like pins and needles, tingling or burning in the painful
            area that is different from the non-painful area                                                     (5)

7.   **Gently <u>press</u> on the painful area with your finger tip then gently press in the same way onto a non-painful area (the same non-painful area that you chose in the last question). How does this feel in the painful area?**

     a)     The painful area does not feel different from the non-painful area                         (0)
     b)     I feel numbness or tenderness in the painful area that is different from the non-painful
            area                                                                                                                  (3)

**Scoring: a score of 12 or more suggests pain of predominantly neuropathic origin**

**Fig. 8-1, cont'd**

persists after the peripheral injury has healed. The sensitization is created by increased availability of excitatory transmitters and an increased number of excitatory receptors. Central sensitization affects neurons throughout the nociceptive pathways, including cells in the dorsal horn, brainstem, thalamus, and cerebral cortex.

Intense signals from an injury in the periphery may cause central sensitization. In central sensitization, the central neurons produce neural output that is disproportionate to incoming nociceptive signals. Arnstein[5] reported that if severe pain persists longer than 24 hours, neuroplastic changes occur that are associated with intractable chronic pain. Figure 8-2 illustrates the process.

Cellular changes that reflect central sensitization include the following:
- Increased spontaneous activity
- Increased responsiveness to afferent inputs
- Prolonged afterdischarge (the part of the response to a stimulus that persists following termination of the stimulus) in response to repeated stimuli
- Expansion of receptive fields (central neurons receive information from larger areas of tissue than normally)

| PATHOLOGY 8-1 | NEUROPATHIC PAIN |
|---|---|
| Pathology | Ectopic foci, ephaptic transmission, abnormal connections of large afferents (Aβ) with nociceptive projection neurons in the dorsal horn, increased number of excitatory receptors and availability of transmitters in the nociceptive pathways, expansion of receptive fields, and cortical reorganization |
| Etiology | Pathologic neural response following trauma, inflammation, metabolic disorders, infection, tumor, toxin, or autoimmune disorders (e.g., multiple sclerosis) |
| Speed of onset | Chronic |
| Signs and symptoms | |
| Consciousness, communication, and memory | Normal |
| Sensory | Pain, paresthesia, dysesthesia, allodynia, and secondary hyperalgesia |
| Autonomic | May be impaired |
| Motor | May be impaired |
| Region affected | Peripheral, spinal, brainstem, and/or cerebral |
| Demographics | Incidence: 8.2/1000 person-years[7]<br>Prevalence in the general population = 7%; pain moderate to severe in 5%[8] |
| Prognosis | Variable, depending on genetic and environmental factors, type of neuropathic pain, and treatment |

The chemicals that produce these profound changes in physiology include glutamate and neuropeptides (Figure 8-3). Glutamate acts on both ligand-gated ion channels (alpha-amino-3-hydroxy-5-methyl-4-isoxazolepropionic acid [AMPA] and *N*-methyl-D-aspartate [NMDA] receptors) and G-protein–mediated receptors (metabotropic receptors) to increase cellular $Ca^{2+}$. The peptides act via second-messenger systems to increase the activity of protein kinases. These changes lead to activation of genes, triggering increased cellular activity. For example, sensitized neurons in the spinothalamic tract are more easily excited, produce increased spontaneous activity, and undergo structural changes in neural connections.[6] Thus, nociceptive information is not simply delivered to the brain. Instead, nociception can change the structure and function of the CNS.

The central sensitization process described is remarkably similar to long-term potentiation, the process vital for memory formation and learning. Therefore, although currently available NMDA antagonists have demonstrated efficacy in treating neuropathic pain, side effects—primarily cognitive deficits—preclude the use of these agents to treat neuropathic pain. When both peripheral inputs and central sensitization contribute to the maintenance of neuropathic pain, therapies must target both peripheral and central abnormalities.

### Clinical Pearl

Central sensitization is a state of excessive excitability of central neurons in the nociceptive pathways. The critical events are NMDA receptor depolarization, an increase in intracellular $Ca^{2+}$, and reduced inhibition. Nociception can alter the structure and function of the nervous system.

### Structural Reorganization

Prolonged central sensitization leads to rewiring of connections in the CNS. In the dorsal horn, structural changes include withdrawal of C-fiber axon terminals from the dorsal horn and growth of Aβ-fiber axons into regions of the spinal cord that normally receive only C-fiber endings, with the formation of novel synapses between Aβ fibers and central nociceptive neurons. Once the novel synapses have formed, stimulation of Aβ fibers will produce impulses perceived as pain. Reorganization also occurs in the cerebral cortex.[9] The mechanisms of nociceptive pain, neuropathic pain, and pain matrix dysfunction are summarized in Figure 8-4.

### Sites That Generate Neuropathic Pain

Neuropathic pain can arise from abnormal neural activity in:
- The periphery (e.g., nerve compression in carpal tunnel syndrome)
- The CNS in response to deafferentation
- The dorsal horn

### Peripheral Generation of Neuropathic Pain

Injury or disease of peripheral nerves often results in sensory abnormalities. A complete nerve section results in lack of sensation from that nerve's receptive field, but sometimes paresthesia and pain also occur in the denervated region. Partial damage to a nerve can result in allodynia and sensations such as electric shock.

These unusual sensations are the result of aberrant activity in the peripheral nervous system, evoking abnormal responses in the CNS. Peripheral abnormalities causing neuropathic pain include the development of ephaptic transmission and ectopic

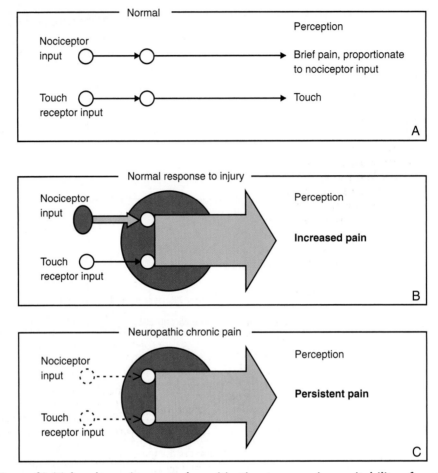

**Fig. 8-2 Contributions of initial and ongoing central sensitization to excessive excitability of central nociceptive neurons.** Open circles indicate the normal amount of activity in a neuron. Red circles indicate excessive neural activity due to sensitization. **A,** In the normal processing of brief, mild nociceptive inputs, there is a close correlation between the amount of input from peripheral nociceptors and the perception of pain. Neural output after central processing, indicated by the black arrow, is proportional to the input. Stimulation of touch receptors generates neural activity perceived as touch. **B,** Following injury, intensified, prolonged nociceptive input occurs owing to peripheral sensitization. In turn, this abnormal input in response to injury produces sensitization of central neurons in the nociceptive pathway. The enlarged red oval for nociceptor input indicates sensitization of nociceptive endings. The enlarged arrow from the peripheral nociceptor indicates increased input into the central nervous system. The large output arrow indicates the amplified output associated with central sensitization. Note that touch receptor information traveling on Aβ fibers now activates increased pain. Before injury, stimulation of the touch receptors produced only signals perceived as touch. **C,** In neuropathic chronic pain, the perception of pain may arise spontaneously, that is, without peripheral input. The central sensitization persists despite the lack of continuing signals from nociceptors. Alternatively, when a brief, small signal is sent from nociceptors or touch receptors, abnormal responses of sensitized neurons produce an amplified perception of pain. In neuropathic chronic pain, no correlation exists between the amount of receptor stimulation and the perception of pain.

foci in an injured nerve. Ephaptic transmission occurs in demyelinated regions. Ectopic foci can occur at the nerve stump, in areas of myelin damage, or in the dorsal root ganglion somas. These foci can become so sensitive to mechanical stimulation that tapping on an injured nerve can elicit pain or tingling *(Tinel's sign)*. Examples of neuropathy that affects a single nerve (mononeuropathy) include median nerve entrapment in carpal tunnel syndrome and ulnar nerve compression at the elbow (see Chapter 12).

## Central Response to Deafferentation

Deafferentation can be complete or partial. When peripheral sensory information is completely absent, as occurs in people with deafferentation or amputation, neurons in the CNS that formerly received information from the body part may become abnormally active.

**Avulsion of dorsal roots** from the spinal cord produces deafferentation and causes people to feel burning pain in the

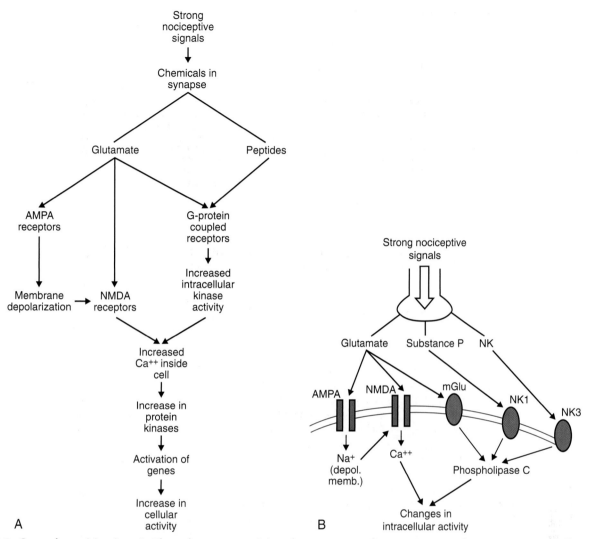

**Fig. 8-3 Central sensitization. A,** Flow chart summarizing the sequence of events in central sensitization. **B,** Effects of intense activation of receptors involved in central sensitization. Strong nociceptive signals elicit the release of glutamate and the peptides substance P and neurokinin (NK). Binding of glutamate to the alpha-amino-3-hydroxy-5-methyl-4-isoxazolepropionic acid (AMPA) receptor depolarizes the membrane of the postsynaptic neuron; then the combination of voltage change and binding of glutamate to the *N*-methyl-D-aspartate (NMDA) receptor opens the NMDA channel. $Ca^{2+}$ flows into the neuron through the NMDA channel. The remaining receptors involved in central sensitization act via second-messenger systems involving phospholipase C. Glutamate activates the metabotropic glutamate receptor (mGlu). Substance P and neurokinin activate neurokinin receptors (NKRs). Activity in these second-messenger systems increases protein kinase activity, which, in turn, activates genes. The outcome is an increase in the activity of ion channels and intracellular enzymes, generating central sensitization.

area of sensory loss. Avulsion of dorsal roots of the brachial plexus sometimes occurs in motorcycle accidents. The extreme neck flexion that occurs when the head impacts the pavement pulls the dorsal roots out of the spinal cord.

### Phantom Pain

Almost all people with amputations report sensation that seems to originate from the missing limb, called *phantom limb sensation.* Less frequently, people with amputations report that their phantom sensation is painful. This condition is called *phantom pain.* Phantom pain must be differentiated

from residual limb pain (pain in the part of the limb that still exists) because some causes of residual limb pain can be successfully treated. Residual limb pain is caused peripherally by neuropathy, neuroma (a tumor of nerve tissue), a poorly fitting prosthesis, or nerve compression. In phantom pain, the absence of sensory information causes neurons in the central nociceptive pathways to become overactive. Maladaptive structural reorganization is found in the spinal cord, thalamus, and cerebral cortex. The cortex shows extensive overlap of cortical representations that are normally separate. For example, the lip and hand representations overlap. Massive

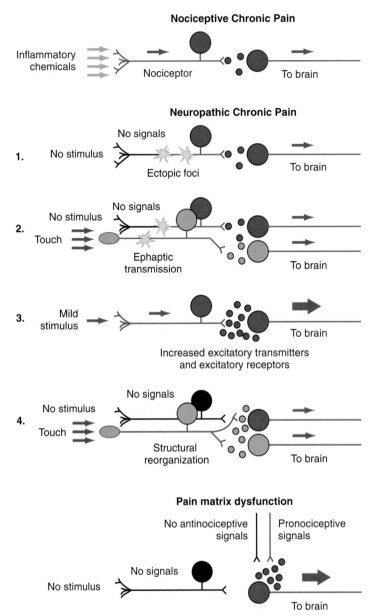

**Fig. 8-4 Mechanisms of nociceptive and neuropathic pain and pain matrix dysfunction.** The top panel illustrates normal physiologic function of the pain system: inflammatory chemicals at the site of injury have sensitized peripheral nociceptors, and signals indicating tissue damage travel to the brain. The numbered panels correspond to the sections in the text on neuropathic mechanisms: *1,* Ectopic foci. *2,* Ephaptic transmission from an Aβ tactile neuron to nociceptive fibers. *3,* Central sensitization, created by increased excitatory transmitter availability and an increased number of excitatory receptors. *4,* Structural reorganization, in this case, the retraction of C-fiber proximal endings from nociceptive tract neurons and growth of Aβ tactile endings to synapse with nociceptive tract neurons. The bottom panel illustrates changes in pain matrix top-down regulation, with silence of antinociceptive signals and excessive pronociceptive signals.

cortical reorganization correlates with the severity of phantom pain.[10]

This cortical reorganization can be reversed with mental practice. Before intervention, functional magnetic resonance imaging (fMRI) showed that when people with hand amputations moved their lips, the hand area of the primary somatosensory and primary motor cortex was activated. The mental practice consisted of relaxation training followed by imagining the phantom limb resting on the couch and the position of each finger, then imagining comfortably moving the phantom limb,

and finally allowing the phantom limb to rest comfortably. After therapy, the hand area of the cortex did not activate when the lips were moved, and most participants had a greater than 50% reduction in pain.[10]

Movement therapy for phantom pain reduces pain significantly more than medical care and physical therapy.[11] Movement therapy is administered in three stages: recognition of whether a photograph shows a right or left hand, imagining moving the phantom hand, followed by mirror therapy. In mirror therapy, a mirror is positioned with the residual limb on

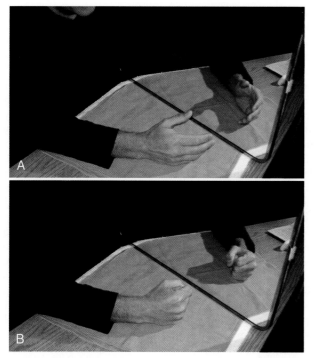

**Fig. 8-5   Mirror therapy.** A mirror is set vertically between the affected limb and the unaffected limb so that the reflection of the unaffected limb appears to replace the affected limb. The patient moves the unaffected hand while imagining moving both hands. This practice is helpful for patients with amputated limbs as well as those recovering from stroke. Repeated practice of the illusion causes central nervous system reorganization and reduces pain. *(From Skirven TM, Osterman AL, Fedorczyk J, et al. Rehabilitation of the Hand and Upper Extremity, ed 6. St. Louis, Mosby, 2012.)*

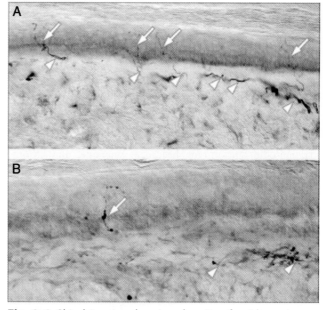

**Fig. 8-6** Skin biopsies showing density of epidermal nociceptive fibers *(arrows)* and dermal nerve bundles *(arrowheads)*. **A,** Biopsy from a healthy control. **B,** Severe loss of epidermal nociceptive fibers in a biopsy from a patient with diabetic neuropathy. Swelling of the epidermal fiber in **B** *(arrow)* indicates axonal degeneration. *(From Sommer C, Lauria G: Skin biopsy in the management of peripheral neuropathy. Lancet Neurol 6:632–42, 2007.)*

the nonreflective side and the intact hand on the reflective side, and is positioned so that the reflection of the intact hand appears to replace the phantom. The person imagines moving both hands, and the visual illusion makes it appear that both hands are moving (Figure 8-5). Only three people need to be treated with movement therapy to have one person achieve significant relief of pain.[11] Similar results have been reported for the foot when only mirror therapy was used without the first two stages. Individuals were divided into three groups: one group viewed a mirror image of the intact foot and attempted to move both the intact foot and the phantom foot, another group viewed a covered mirror and attempted to move both the intact foot and the phantom foot, and another group closed their eyes and imagined moving both the intact foot and the phantom foot. After 4 weeks of 15 minute daily sessions, the mirror group reported significant decreases in pain, the covered mirror group had little change in pain, and the visualization group had significantly increased pain. For the next 4 weeks, all groups used mirror therapy, and all showed a significant reduction in pain.[12]

### Central Pain: Spinal Cord Injury, Stroke, and Multiple Sclerosis

Central pain is caused by a lesion of the CNS and usually is localized to the area of the body deafferented by the lesion.

Neuropathic central pain is often described as a burning, shooting, aching, freezing, and/or tingling pain. In spinal cord injury (SCI) central pain, the thalamus may be the site of pain generation because after SCI, neurons in the ventral posterolateral (VPL) thalamic nucleus are spontaneously active without input from the spinal cord.[13] This type of pain occurs in approximately two thirds of all people with SCI.[13] Central poststroke pain follows lesions of the somatosensory pathways in the brain, most often after lateral medulla infarction or lesions of the ventroposterior thalamus.[14] Lateral medulla lesion pain often involves the ipsilateral face and the contralateral body; thalamic poststroke pain typically involves the contralateral body. The incidence of central poststroke pain has been reported as 1% to 12%.[14] In multiple sclerosis, the location of the pain depends on the location of the lesion. Central pain occurs in 30% of people who have multiple sclerosis.[15]

### Small Fiber Neuropathy: Postherpetic Neuralgia, Diabetic Neuropathy, and Guillain-Barré Syndrome

*Small fiber neuropathy* produces partial deafferentation and central sensitization. Loss of nociceptors is associated with neuropathic pain.[16,17] Postherpetic neuralgia, diabetic neuropathy, and Guillain-Barré syndrome cause deafferentation pain. Postherpetic neuralgia follows varicella virus infection, producing severe axonal loss of somatosensory neurons plus multisegmental dorsal horn atrophy.[18] Diabetic neuropathy (see Chapter 12) and Guillain-Barré syndrome (see Chapter 2) are polyneuropathies (neuropathies that affect more than one nerve) that cause small fiber neuropathy. Figure 8-6 compares the density of nociceptive fibers innervating normal epidermis with the epidermal density of nociceptive fibers in diabetic neuropathy.

## PAIN MATRIX DYSFUNCTION

When the pain matrix malfunctions, top-down regulation of pain is disturbed. Antinociception is reduced and/or pronociception is intensified. The result is increased pain. Fibromyalgia, episodic tension-type headache, migraine, and chronic whiplash-associated disorder involve disturbance of top-down regulation of pain. Because these disorders are not caused by structural lesions of the somatosensory system, they are not included in the neuropathic pain designation.[19]

### Fibromyalgia

People with fibromyalgia (fibro = fibrous tissue + myo = muscle + algos = pain) have tenderness of muscles and adjacent soft tissues, stiffness of muscles, and aching pain (Pathology 8-2). The painful area shows a regional rather than a dermatomal or peripheral nerve distribution. The fundamental problem is abnormal processing of pain information, resulting in the perception of pain without any painful stimulus external to the nervous system. The criteria for a fibromyalgia diagnosis are listed in Figure 8-7.

People with fibromyalgia have structural differences and abnormal pain processing compared with control subjects. The brain in fibromyalgia has significantly less gray matter density than controls in the pain-inhibiting brain areas (medial frontal cortex, mid/posterior cingulate gyrus, and insular cortex) and in stress response areas.[20] In fibromyalgia, pain inhibition areas are significantly less active than in healthy controls. When people with fibromyalgia report identical pain levels to healthy controls in response to pressure on the thumbnail (approximately half as much pressure required for people with fibromyalgia to report identical pain to healthy controls), there is no difference between the groups in brain regions processing somatosensory stimuli, or attention, or in emotional areas. However, the primary region that initiates pain inhibition is activated in healthy controls and is not activated in people with fibromyalgia.[21] Thus pain inhibition is impaired in fibromyalgia (Figure 8-8).

Neural responses to afferent signals are amplified in fibromyalgia. Gracely and associates[22] compared brain activation of people with and without fibromyalgia in response to 10 minutes of blunt, pulsing pressure to the base of the left thumbnail. When the same pressure intensity was used in both groups ($\approx 2.5$ kg/cm$^2$), people with fibromyalgia reported slightly intense pain, and most of the pain matrix was activated. People without fibromyalgia reported that stimulation was not painful, and only part of the contralateral somatosensory cortex was activated. For control subjects to report slightly intense pain and to activate similar areas of the pain matrix required nearly twice as much pressure on the thumbnail. Thus subjects with fibromyalgia demonstrated biological amplification of pain signals.

| PATHOLOGY 8-2 | FIBROMYALGIA |
|---|---|
| Pathology | Abnormal central processing of pain signals: both pain amplification and impaired descending inhibition. Level of substance P (pain neurotransmitter) in cerebrospinal fluid 3× normal,[23] glutamate (excitatory transmitter) in spinal cord 2× normal[23]; decreased pain inhibition from brainstem to dorsal horn[21] |
| Etiology | Genetics affecting transport or metabolism of dopamine, epinephrine, norepinephrine, and/or serotonin accounts for about 50% of risk[24,25]; occurs in psychologically normal people, most do not have depression[23] |
| Speed of onset | Usually chronic |
| Signs and symptoms | Nonrestorative sleep, fatigue |
| Consciousness | Difficulty concentrating |
| Communication and memory | Impaired: working memory (difficulty manipulating recalled information; can be tested by asking person to state the months in reverse order), ability to recall specific events, ability to think quickly and choose appropriate words[26] |
| Sensory | Widespread pain, stiffness |
| Autonomic | Inconsistent reports |
| Motor | Normal |
| Region affected | Central nervous system |
| Incidence and prevalence | Incidence: 6.88 cases per 1000 person-years for males, and 11.28 cases per 1000 person-years for females; women 1.64 times more likely to have fibromyalgia than men[27]<br>Prevalence: 1.5%[28] |
| Prognosis | In the general population, prognosis is good; poor prognosis in tertiary care (patients referred by primary and secondary health professionals to a specialty pain center)[23] |

**Criteria**

A patient satisfies modified ACR 2010 fibromyalgia diagnostic criteria if the following 3 conditions are met:

- Widespread Pain Index ≥ 7 and Symptom Severity Score ≥ 5 –or– Widespread Pain Index between 3–6 and Symptom Severity Score ≥ 9.
- Symptoms have been present at a similar level for at least 3 months.
- The patient does not have a disorder that would otherwise sufficiently explain the pain.

**Widespread Pain Index (WPI)**

Note the number of areas in which the patient has had pain over the last week. In how many areas has the patient had pain? Score will be between 0 and 19.

| Shoulder girdle, L | Hip (buttock, trochanter), L | Jaw, L | Upper Back |
| --- | --- | --- | --- |
| Shoulder girdle, R | Hip (buttock, trochanter), R | Jaw, R | Lower Back |
| Upper Arm, L | Upper Leg, L | Chest | Neck |
| Upper Arm, R | Upper Leg, R | Abdomen | |
| Lower Arm, L | Lower Leg, L | | |
| Lower Arm, R | Lower Leg, R | | |

**Symptom Severity Score**

For the each of these 3 symptoms, indicate the level of severity over the past week using the following scale:

- 0 = No problem;
- 1 = Slight or mild problems; generally mild or intermittent;
- 2 = Moderate; considerable problems; often present and/or at a moderate level;
- 3 = Severe: pervasive, continuous, life-disturbing problems.

| Symptom | Rating |
| --- | --- |
| Fatigue | |
| Waking unrefreshed | |
| Cognitive symptoms | |
| Total | |

The Symptom Severity Score is the sum of the severity of the 3 symptoms (fatigue, waking unrefreshed, and cognitive symptoms) plus the sum of the number of the following symptoms occurring during the previous 6 months: headaches, pain or cramps in lower abdomen, and depression (0–3). The final score is between 0 and 12.

**Fig. 8-7 Fibromyalgia criteria modified from American College of Rheumatology (ACR) diagnostic criteria.** *(From Wolfe F, Clauw DJ, Fitzcharles MA, et al. Fibromyalgia Criteria and Severity Scales for Clinical and Epidemiological Studies: A Modification of the ACR Preliminary Diagnostic Criteria for Fibromyalgia. J Rheumatol 38(6): 1121, 2011.)*

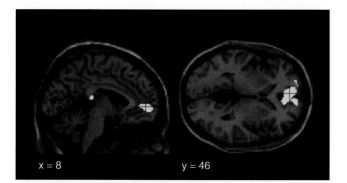

x = 8    y = 46

**Fig. 8-8 People with fibromyalgia have impaired descending pain inhibition.** Regions of the brain where healthy control subjects have significantly more activation than people with fibromyalgia when both groups subjectively report equal pain (functional magnetic resonance imaging [fMRI]). The rostral anterior cingulate cortex is significantly more active in healthy controls. *(Reproduced with permission from Jensen KB, Kosek E, Petzke F, et al: Evidence of dysfunctional pain inhibition in fibromyalgia reflected in rACC during provoked pain. Pain 144:95–100, 2009.)*

Chronic widespread pain, the primary symptom of fibromyalgia, is only moderately correlated with psychological distress, and a weak correlation exists between distress and the development of chronic widespread pain. A large majority of people with fibromyalgia are psychologically normal; most people with fibromyalgia do not have antecedent or subsequent depression.[23,29] Abnormalities of the hypothalamic-pituitary-adrenal (HPA) axis (sympathetic nervous system activity) are most likely due to the pain and do not cause fibromyalgia.[23] Culpepper states that a major obstacle to appropriate care is the attitude of many health care professionals who do not consider fibromyalgia a valid diagnosis or avoid patients with it.[30]

**◎ Clinical Pearl**

People with fibromyalgia have objectively real structural and functional brain abnormalities. A large majority of people with fibromyalgia are psychologically normal.

For fibromyalgia, heated pool therapy, with or without exercise, is effective. For some patients with fibromyalgia syndrome, individually designed aerobic exercise and strength

**TABLE 8-2**  EVIDENCE-BASED PHARMACOTHERAPY FOR NEUROPATHIC PAIN, FIBROMYALGIA, AND LOW BACK PAIN SYNDROME

| Disorder | Tricyclic Antidepressants (Nortriptyline and Desipramine) | SNRI Antidepressants (Duloxetine, Venlafaxine, Milnacipran) | α2δ Ca$^{2+}$ Channel Antagonists (Anticonvulsants: Gabapentin and Pregabalin) | Tramadol | Opioids | Other Medications |
|---|---|---|---|---|---|---|
| Neuropathic pain | Effective[72] | Effective | Effective; in spinal cord injury, pregabalin decreases pain and anxiety and improves sleep[73] | Effective[72] | Used when other drugs fail | Topical lidocaine may be effective; cannabinoids improve sleep and mood, somewhat reduce pain[74] |
| Fibromyalgia | Effective | Milnacipran improves pain, fatigue, and functioning[75]; on fMRI, inhibition of pain-sensitive regions and facilitation of pain suppression areas[76] | Gabapentin and pregabalin both effective[77,78] | Somewhat effective[79] | No evidence of effectiveness[32] | NSAIDs not effective[80]; synthetic cannabinoid reduces pain, improves quality of life and anxiety[81] |
| Low back pain syndrome | Slightly more effective than placebo[82] | Uncertain; reports are inconsistent | Not effective[79] | Somewhat effective[79] | Inconclusive | |

*fMRI,* Functional magnetic resonance imaging.

training and/or cognitive-behavioral therapy may be effective.[31] A combination of occupational, physical, and cognitive therapy has been shown to be effective in people with fibromyalgia.[32] Treatment included physical reconditioning, biofeedback, relaxation training, stress management, activity moderation, chemical health education, and reduction of pain behaviors. Participants reported significantly less pain and improvements in life control, social activity and general activity, and physical and emotional health. The same program significantly reduced the number of participants taking opioids, antianxiety drugs, nonsteroidal anti-inflammatory drugs (NSAIDs), and muscle relaxants, all of which are not effective in treating fibromyalgia.[32] Medications that are effective for treating fibromyalgia are listed in Table 8-2.

## Episodic Tension-Type Headache

The criteria for episodic tension-type headache (ETTH) include mild to moderate pain, usually bilateral, lasting 30 minutes to 7 days, not aggravated by physical activity and not associated with nausea or vomiting. Fear and avoidance of light or sound but not both may accompany the headache. The mechanism of ETTH appears to be supersensitivity to nitric oxide, a molecule used in the transmission of nerve impulses. Nitric oxide sensitizes nociceptive pathways in the CNS.[33] The 1-year prevalence is 87%.[34] Environmental factors appear to be much more important than genetic factors in ETTH.[35] Environmental factors include volatile organic compounds (e.g., fumes from paint, lacquers, plastics), molds, lighting, noise, excessive heating, air conditioning, and psychosocial pressure.[36]

## Migraine

Migraine is a neurogenic disorder. In migraine, a disorder of sensory processing produces pain matrix malfunction that amplifies nociceptive signals in the trigemino-thalamo-cortical pathway.[37]

Migraine headaches are characterized by at least two of the following: unilateral location, pulsating quality, severity that interferes with daily activities, and aggravation by routine physical activity. During the headache, nausea, vomiting, photophobia (fear and avoidance of light), and/or phonophobia (fear and avoidance of sound) are present.[38] Untreated migraines last from 4 to 72 hours in adults and from 2 to 15 hours in children younger than 15 years of age. Eighteen percent of females and 6% of males have one or more migraines per year.[38] The cumulative lifetime migraine incidence is 43% in women and 18% in men.[38]

Some migraines are preceded, accompanied, or followed by an aura. An *aura* is a transient neurologic disorder that involves sensory, motor, or cognitive symptoms. Typically, an aura develops over 5 to 20 minutes and lasts less than an hour. During visual aura, visual cortex neurons rapidly depolarize with a massive redistribution of ions across cell membranes. K$^+$ and organic anions exit and Na$^+$, Ca$^{2+}$, and Cl$^-$ enter the neurons.[39] This depolarization produces visual illusions. Subsequently, the neurons are temporarily unresponsive. The metabolic load during depolarization elicits dilation of the blood vessels in the meninges and activation of the nociceptive fibers that innervate the vessels.

A once prevalent theory of migraine origin—that initial vasoconstriction subsequently produced vasodilation and headache—has not been supported by blood flow studies. In people susceptible

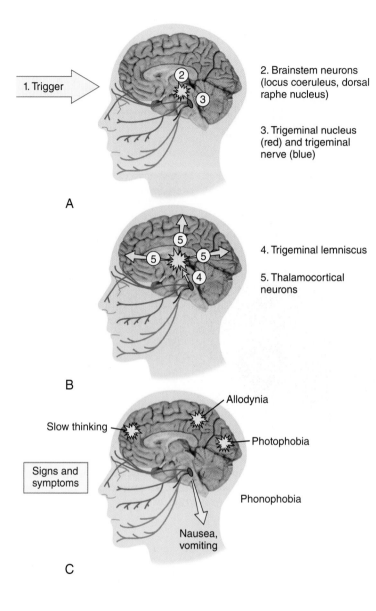

A

B

C

**Fig. 8-9 Sequence of events in migraine.**
**A,** Migraine begins when a trigger (1) activates hyperexcitable brainstem neurons (2) that activate the trigeminal nucleus and sensitize the trigeminal nerve (3). **B,** Signals from the trigeminal nucleus sensitize the trigeminal lemniscus and thalamocortical neurons (4, 5), causing these neurons to fire excessively. **C,** Signs and symptoms of migraine imposed on a midsagittal section. Phonophobia is not indicated by a yellow flash because the auditory area is located in the lateral cerebral cortex. *(Modified from copyright 1994, University of Washington. From Digital Anatomist Interactive Brain Atlas and the Structural Informatics Group.)*

to migraine, cortical and brainstem neurons are hyperexcitable owing to channelopathy (dysfunction of ion channels), mitochondrial dysfunction, or possibly excessive nitric oxide.[40,41] The tendency to have migraines is strongly influenced by genetic factors.[38] The cascade of events in migraine[40,42] proceeds as follows:

1. Migraine trigger (bright light, loud noise, prostaglandins, emotional stress, hormonal changes, specific foods or drinks, or meteorologic changes)
2. Excitation of hyperexcitable brainstem neurons
3. Only in people who experience aura: a wave of intense neural activity spreads through the cerebral cortex, particularly the visual cortex. This is followed by widespread and prolonged neural inhibition.
4. Activation of trigeminal afferents that synapse with trigeminal lemniscus neurons. Trigeminal lemniscus and

thalamocortical neurons become sensitized during a migraine owing to pain matrix malfunction.

Figure 8-9 illustrates the sequence of events in migraine. The pain matrix malfunction disrupts antinociception and promotes pronociception, affecting the trigemino-thalamo-cortical pathway.[37] If taken at migraine onset, aspirin or a combination of aspirin, caffeine, and acetaminophen may stop the headache. Serotonin agonists, including sumatriptan, rizatriptan, and other triptan drugs, reduce neuronal activity in the trigeminal lemniscus and thalamus.[42]

## Red Flags for Headache

The following lists are compiled from the findings of Joubert[43] and Dowson.[44]

Signs that headache may be caused by excessive pressure, including hydrocephalus or tumor:
- Headache present at wakening
- Pain triggered by coughing, sneezing, or straining
- Vomiting (may also indicate migraine)
- Worse when lying down

Signs that headache is caused by serious intracranial disease, including tumor, encephalitis, or meningitis:
- Progressive worsening over days or weeks
- Neck stiffness and vomiting (irritation of meninges)
- Rash and fever (bacterial meningitis or Lyme disease)
- History of cancer, human immunodeficiency virus (HIV) infection

Signs that headache may be caused by hemorrhage:
- Headache following head injury
- Abrupt onset

Headache associated with onset of paralysis or reduced level of consciousness (confusion, drowsiness, memory loss, loss of consciousness) is a strong indication for neuroimaging.[45]

## Chronic Whiplash-Associated Disorder

Whiplash is an injury to the neck that results from rapid acceleration or deceleration. In one study, 34% of people with whiplash had a predominantly neuropathic pain component as assessed by the Leeds Assessment of Neuropathic Symptoms and Signs.[46] The group with neuropathic signs had greater pain/disability, cold hyperalgesia, and cervical mechanical hyperalgesia, and less elbow extension with the brachial plexus provocation test when compared with the group with non-neuropathic pain. There were no differences between the two groups in terms of pressure pain thresholds at distant sites and psychological distress.[46] Because no damage to the somatosensory system has been identified in chronic whiplash-associated disorder,[47] it is considered a pain matrix disorder.

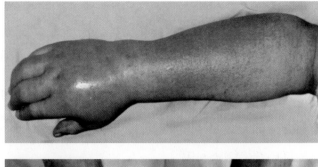

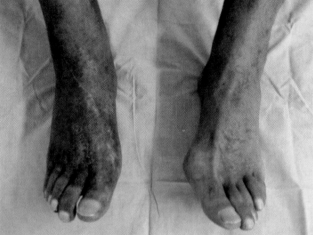

**Fig. 8-10** Complex regional pain syndrome (CRPS) causes intense pain in a limb, swelling, changes in skin color and temperature, and sweating. *(Reproduced with permission from Albrecht PJ, Hines S, Eisenberg E, et al: Pathologic alterations of cutaneous innervation and vasculature in affected limbs from patients with Complex Regional Pain Syndrome. Pain 120:246, 2006.)*

## PAIN SYNDROMES

These two syndromes involve other systems in addition to the pain system. Complex regional pain syndrome affects the somatosensory, autonomic, and motor systems. Chronic low back pain syndrome includes muscle guarding, disuse, and abnormal movements.

### Complex Regional Pain Syndrome

Complex regional pain syndrome (CRPS) is a syndrome of pain, vascular changes, and atrophy (Figure 8-10). The term *regional* indicates that the signs and symptoms present in a regional distribution (upper limb or lower limb) rather than in a peripheral nerve or nerve root distribution. Typically, signs and symptoms are worst in the distal extremity, affecting the entire hand or foot. An aberrant response to trauma, even minor trauma, produces the syndrome. Most frequently, CRPS follows surgery, fracture, crush injury, or sprain.[48] In 5% to 10% of cases, CRPS occurs spontaneously.[49] The time between the trauma and the onset of CRPS is highly variable—from hours to weeks.

The primary complaint is severe, spontaneous pain, out of proportion to the original injury. The pain is aggravated by psychological and physical stimuli (sensitivity to cold, pressure, and touch). Early signs of CRPS include red or pale skin color, excessive sweating, edema, and skin atrophy. Later, the skin becomes dry and cold, and the joints become stiff and swollen. If the condition progresses to its late stage, irreversible muscle atrophy, osteoporosis, and arthritic changes occur. Motor signs that may be associated include paresis, spasms, and tremor.[49] Criteria for diagnosis are listed in Box 8-2. Formerly, reduction of signs and symptoms following injection of an anesthetic into sympathetic ganglia was considered diagnostic for CRPS. However, the response to sympathetic nerve block is not diagnostic, because later in the course of the disorder, the pathology migrates into the CNS.[50]

Disuse of the limb is a primary precipitating factor in the development of CRPS. Classic theories postulate excessive activity of sympathetic efferents, but findings of low serum levels of norepinephrine in the affected limb indicate that sympathetic efferents are not overactive. Pathologic processes in CRPS include increased levels of neurochemicals that produce neurogenic inflammation in the periphery, loss of nociceptor fibers in the skin (Figure 8-11), impairment of sympathetic regulation of blood flow and sweating, sensitization (Figure 8-12), and cortical reorganization (shrinkage of the hand or foot representation

### BOX 8-2 DIAGNOSTIC CRITERIA FOR COMPLEX REGIONAL PAIN SYNDROME

- Continuous pain, disproportionate to the inciting event
- At least one symptom in each of the following categories and one sign in two or more categories.
  - Sensory (allodynia, hyperalgesia, hypoesthesia)
  - Vasomotor (temperature or skin color abnormalities)
  - Sudomotor (edema or sweating abnormalities)
  - Motor/trophic (muscle weakness; tremor; hair, nail, skin abnormalities)

Modified from Harden NR, Bruehl SP: Complex regional pain syndrome. In Ballantyne JC, Fishman SM, Rathmell JP, editors: Bonica's management of pain, ed 4, Baltimore, 2010, Lippincott Williams & Wilkins.

in the cortex).[48] The disorder affects children as well as adults: the youngest CRPS case documented in the literature is a 2½-year-old girl whose upper limb was affected.[51] The tendency to develop CRPS in response to trauma appears to be genetic.[48] Traditionally, CRPS was considered by some to be a psychological disorder or a stress response. However, results from a prospective study indicate that of 88 patients post acute distal radius fracture, 14 patients who had significantly elevated life stresses did not develop CRPS, and the 1 patient who developed CRPS had no major life stresses and average emotional distress levels. People with CRPS are no more likely to have preexisting psychiatric disorders than other people with chronic pain.[52] Pathology 8-3 summarizes CRPS.

Therapy is essential for CRPS.[49] Occupational therapy (specifically, splinting, tactile stimulation, and functional activities) has a positive effect on functional limitations and is likely to have a positive effect on activity levels.[55] Physical therapy (specifically, discussions to optimize coping, relaxation exercises, connective tissue massage, exercises to decrease pain, and activities of daily living training) produces quicker improvement in pain, abnormal skin temperature, mobility, and edema than control treatment.[55] Another effective strategy is movement therapy in three stages: recognition of whether a photograph shows a right or left hand, imagining moving the CRPS hand, followed by mirror therapy (making movements with both hands, but with the CRPS hand concealed and the mirror positioned so that the mirror image of the uninvolved hand appears to be the CRPS hand). Only two people need to be treated with movement therapy to have one person achieve greater than 50% reduction in pain.[56] Overly aggressive therapy may aggravate CRPS, increasing pain, edema, and distress, and worsening inflammation and vascular symptoms.[52]

Drug treatment for CRPS includes the free radical scavengers dimethyl sulfoxide (DMSO) cream and N-acetylcysteine, and glucocorticoids to inhibit proinflammatory cytokines.[49] Vitamin C, a free radical scavenger, reduces the incidence of CRPS following wrist fracture from 10% to 2%.[57] In persistent, severe CRPS, surgery may be indicated. Stimulating electrodes are implanted next to the spinal cord to provide continuous electrical stimulation, or a drug pump delivers opioids or local anesthetics directly into the spinal fluid. Administering drugs via pump allows lower drug doses and increases drug effectiveness.

The terms *causalgia, Sudeck's atrophy, sympathetically maintained pain,* and *reflex sympathetic dystrophy* are often used

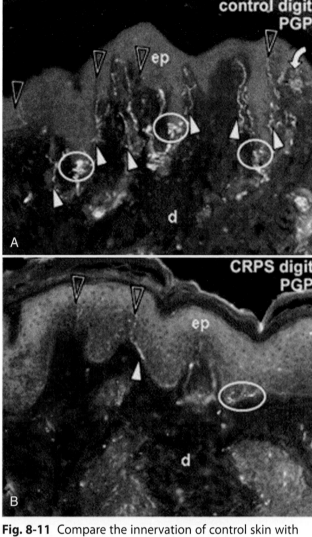

**Fig. 8-11** Compare the innervation of control skin with the partial denervation in complex regional pain syndrome (CRPS). **A,** Control skin has numerous free nerve endings in the epidermis *(open arrowheads)* and small nerves in the upper dermis *(white arrowheads)*. A Meissner corpuscle *(curved arrow, top right)* and three Merkel endings (inside ovals) are also visible. **B,** CRPS skin sample shows a dramatic loss of free nerve endings in the epidermis and small nerves in the upper dermis compared with control skin. Only one Merkel ending (inside oval) and no Meissner corpuscles are visible in the CRPS sample. *d,* Dermis; *ep,* epidermis. *(Reproduced with permission from Albrecht PJ, Hines S, Eisenberg E, et al: Pathologic alterations of cutaneous innervation and vasculature in affected limbs from patients with Complex Regional Pain Syndrome. Pain 12:252, 2006.)*

synonymously with *complex regional pain syndrome,* despite the attempts of some authors to distinguish among these terms. CRPS following stroke is often termed *shoulder-hand syndrome.* A prospective study demonstrated that a prevention program reduced poststroke CRPS from 27% to 8%. The program consisted of daily physical therapy and instruction to all hospital staff and family members on methods to avoid trauma to the paretic upper limb.[58]

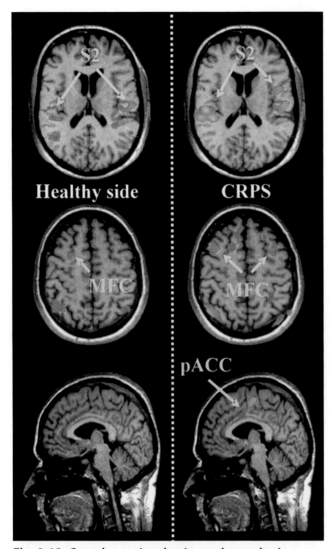

**Fig. 8-12 Complex regional pain syndrome: brain activations (fMRI) during mechanical stimulation.** Left column: brain response during stimulation of the healthy side of the body. Right column: brain response to stimulation of the complex regional pain syndrome–affected side. Stimulation of the CRPS side of the body activates more of the secondary somatosensory cortices (S2) and middle frontal cortices (MFC). Only stimulation of the CRPS side of the body activates the posterior part of the anterior cingulate cortex (pACC). *(With permission from Maihöfner C, Seifert F, Markovic K: Complex Regional Pain Syndromes: new pathophysiological concepts and therapies. Eur J Neurol 17:654, 2010.)*

## Chronic Low Back Pain Syndrome

Compared with people who have subacute low back pain or are pain free, those with chronic low back pain syndrome have more emotional distress and less endurance of abdominal and back muscles (Pathology 8-4).[59] The transition from acute low back pain after injury to chronic low back pain has been characterized by Waddell and associates[60] as a change in pain etiology from tissue damage to a physiologic impairment consisting of the following:

- Muscle guarding
- Abnormal movement
- Disuse syndrome

Subsequent research continues to support these physiologic impairments as significant factors in chronic low back pain syndrome.[61] Figure 8-13 emphasizes the elements contributing to acute (Figure 8-13, *A*) and chronic (Figure 8-13, *B*) low back pain. In discussing chronic low back pain, Waddell[62] cautions that "physical treatment directed to a supposed but unidentified and possibly nonexistent nociceptive source is not only understandably unsuccessful but failed treatment may both reinforce and aggravate pain, distress, disability, and illness behavior." For example, when a person complains of low back pain and magnetic resonance imaging (MRI) shows a bulging intervertebral disk, treatment may be directed toward the disk. However, Jensen and Brant-Zawadzki[63] found that 64% of people *without* low back pain had abnormal findings on MRI of the lower spine, leading to the conclusion that disk bulges or protrusions may be coincidental rather than causative of low back pain. The emotional and cognitive aspects posited by Waddell and colleagues are supported by increasing acceptance of the biopsychosocial model[64] and by the short-term effectiveness of behavioral treatment for chronic low back pain syndrome.[65]

Brain scans show amplified pain signals in patients with idiopathic chronic low back pain. Giesecke and coworkers[66] scanned the low back of patients for signs of musculoskeletal injury and eliminated patients from the study who had signs of disk, ligament, muscle, or joint damage. The pain threshold to blunt pressure on the thumbnail was compared between control and chronic low back pain subjects. At equal levels of pressure, those with chronic low back pain reported significantly greater pain and had more areas of the pain matrix in the brain activated than did control subjects. Only part of the contralateral somatosensory cortex was activated in control subjects. This study also examined fibromyalgia patients and reported similar outcomes to those reported by Gracely and associates.[67] When pain persists, depression, sleep disturbance, preoccupation with pain, decreased activity, and fatigue are common.

In a series of 1172 consecutive people receiving primary care (from general medical practitioners, physical therapists, and chiropractors) for acute low back pain, only 11 people (0.9%) had serious pathology; 8 of these were vertebral fractures. Three red flags were associated with fracture: age over 70 years, significant trauma, and prolonged corticosteroid use. The other three serious pathologies were inflammatory disorders (two people) and cauda equina syndrome (one person).[68] Cauda equina syndrome is covered in Chapter 13. Other red flags that have been advocated previously (by Atlas and Deyo[69]; i.e., unexplained weight loss, no improvement with bed rest, sciatica) were not associated with serious pathology.[68]

> ⊙ **Clinical Pearl**
>
> Chronic low back pain syndrome is a physiologic impairment consisting of pain matrix dysfunction, muscle guarding, abnormal movement, and disuse syndrome.

| PATHOLOGY 8-3 | COMPLEX REGIONAL PAIN SYNDROME |
|---|---|
| Pathology | Increased levels of inflammatory neurochemicals in the periphery, partial denervation of epidermis and upper dermis, impairment of sympathetic regulation of blood flow and sweating, sensitization, and cortical reorganization |
| Etiology | Usually secondary to trauma; genetic predisposition |
| Speed of onset | Chronic |
| Signs and symptoms | |
| Consciousness | Normal |
| Communication and memory | Normal |
| Sensory | Severe, spontaneous pain, often intensified by skin contact, heat, and cold |
| Autonomic | Abnormal sweating, vasodilation in skin, atrophy (due to blood flow changes and disuse) of muscles, joints, and skin |
| Motor | May have paresis, spasms, and tremor; muscle atrophy |
| Region affected | Initially peripheral; as progresses, cortical reorganization occurs |
| Demographics | 2–3 times more frequent in women |
| Incidence | 25.2 per 100,000 people[53] |
| Prognosis | Early intervention has best outcome; intensive physical therapy often required; some cases are intractable[54] |

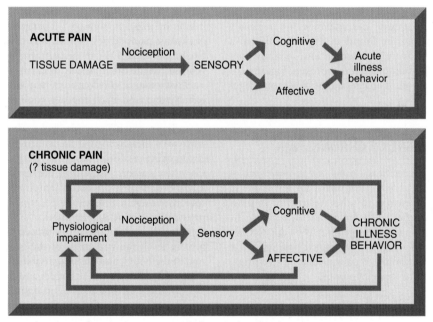

**Fig. 8-13** The differences between factors in acute and chronic low back pain. *(Redrawn with permission from Waddell G, Newton M, Henderson I, et al: A fear-avoidance beliefs questionnaire [FABQ] and the role of fear-avoidance beliefs in chronic low back pain and disability. Pain 52:157–68, 1993.)*

## Medications for Neuropathic Pain, Fibromyalgia, and Chronic Low Back Pain Syndrome

Many different medications are used to treat pain. Tricyclic antidepressants are used at lower doses than for depression, and their action on pain is independent of their antidepressant action (see Table 8-2). Serotonin-norepinephrine reuptake inhibitor (SNRI) antidepressants decrease the reuptake of serotonin and norepinephrine, producing direct inhibition of pain signals in the dorsal horn and brain independent of their antidepressant effects. α2δ calcium channel antagonists belong to the anticonvulsant class of medications. α2δ antagonists bind to and block calcium channels on presynaptic nociceptive terminals, decreasing the release of pain transmitters. Tramadol is

| **PATHOLOGY 8-4** | CHRONIC LOW BACK PAIN SYNDROME |
|---|---|
| Pathology | Decreased endurance of abdominal and back muscles |
| Etiology | Deconditioning, pain matrix dysfunction |
| Speed of onset | Chronic |
| Signs and symptoms | |
| Consciousness | Normal |
| Communication and memory | Normal |
| Sensory | Aching pain |
| Autonomic | Normal |
| Motor | Muscle guarding, disuse, abnormal movement patterns |
| Neural region affected | Central nervous system |
| Incidence | 10,000–15,000 per 100,000 population per year |
| Prevalence | U.S. cumulative lifetime prevalence of low back pain lasting at least 2 weeks of 13.8%[70]; 55% of people with low back pain in outpatient settings had a neuropathic component to their pain[71] |
| Prognosis | Variable |

an opioid agonist that weakly inhibits the reuptake of serotonin and norepinephrine. Cannabinoids are chemicals that activate cannabinoid receptors; cannabinoids are naturally produced in the body and are found in the cannabis sativa plant (marijuana). NSAIDs are nonsteroidal anti-inflammatory drugs, including aspirin, ibuprofen, and naproxen. Figure 8-14 illustrates the sites of action of analgesic (an- = without; algos = pain) drugs.

## SURGICAL TREATMENT OF CHRONIC PAIN

Theoretically, cutting selected dorsal roots *(dorsal rhizotomy)* or the spinothalamic tracts should eliminate pain sensation in people with pain that is resistant to other treatments. In practice, however, both surgeries often fail to alleviate pain. The persistence of pain following these surgeries may be due to CNS changes in response to the original maintained pain or, in the case of spinothalamic tractotomy, to pain-mediating fibers traveling in the dorsal columns (see Chapter 6).

## PSYCHOLOGICAL FACTORS IN CHRONIC PAIN

Expectations, cognition, and emotions powerfully affect the experience of pain. Anxiety, depression, and catastrophizing predict reactions to pain and the ability to cope with pain.[83] Catastrophizing is focusing on the most dreaded possibilities rather than realistic possibilities. Catastrophizing predicts disability, independent of other psychopathologies, including major depression.[84]

How much pain a person expects influences processing in both medial and lateral pain systems, including anterior cingulate cortex, anterior insula, and thalamus.[85] Negative emotions and stress increase pain by augmenting somatosensory attention

to pain, intensifying muscle tension, decreasing role performance, diminishing social participation, and reducing neural inhibition in pain pathways.[86] Therapists must address all 3 D's of chronic pain: distress, disuse, and disability. Neglecting even one of the three D's can cause treatment failure despite intervention for the other aspects of chronic pain.[83]

Psychological interventions may decrease activation of the pain system and may improve coping skills. These therapies include relaxation (breathing and muscle relaxation), biofeedback, imagery, and cognitive-behavioral therapies. Cognitive-behavioral therapy focuses on challenging dysfunctional beliefs, encouraging realistic thoughts, and modifying behaviors.[87] Cognitive factors, including the expectation of pain relief, modify somatosensory cortex, anterior cingulate, and thalamic responses to pain and opioid receptor signaling, affecting both physical and emotional equilibria.[88,89] In rheumatoid arthritis, cognitive-behavioral therapy improved joint stiffness, C-reactive protein levels (an indication of the general level of inflammation in the body), and physical disability; gains were maintained 18 months after treatment ended, and subjects showed reduced anxiety and a further decrease in disability.[90]

Therapists can optimize pain treatment outcomes by using techniques that elicit placebo-associated improvement. Placebo-associated improvement is "any genuine psychological or physiologic effect which is attributable to receiving a substance or undergoing a procedure, but is not due to the inherent powers of that substance or procedure."[91] Therapeutic approaches that mobilize placebo-associated improvement include speaking positively (yet honestly) about the therapy, providing encouragement and education, developing trust, compassion, and empathy, understanding the person as an individual, and creating rituals that provide meaning and expectancy for the person.[92]

The placebo neural mechanism consists of secretion of endogenous opioids in the brain, activating the descending antinociceptive pathway.[93] Dopamine secretion in the nucleus

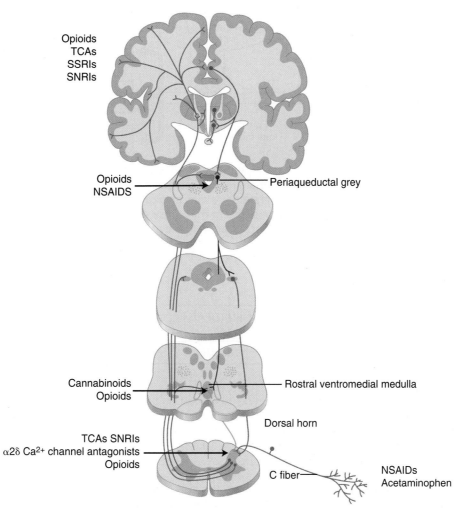

**Fig. 8-14** Sites of action of analgesic drugs. NSAIDs, nonsteroidal anti-inflammatory drugs; SNRIs, serotonin/ norepinephrine reuptake inhibitors; SSRIs, selective serotonin reuptake inhibitors; TCAs, tricyclic antidepressants.

accumbens also correlates with placebo response.[94] Increased anticipatory activity in a frontoparietal network and decreased activity in a posterior insular/temporal network predict placebo analgesia.[95]

> **Clinical Pearl**
>
> In people who respond to placebo, expectations alone activate the same neural pathways and chemicals as drugs. The expectations initiate signals from the prefrontal cortex to the anterior cingulate cortex to the brainstem pain inhibition system.

## CONFLICTS BETWEEN PATIENT AND PROVIDER GOALS

People with chronic pain often want health professionals to acknowledge them as individuals and to have their pain recognized as biologically based.[96] Most patients with pain feel misunderstood and stigmatized by health professionals.[96] Health care providers frequently are more concerned with diagnosis and treatment than with providing biological explanations for chronic pain.[96] In people with chronic pain, the most important factor in achieving a positive patient–physical therapist interaction is the ability of the therapist to explain treatment recommendations in a way that is consistent with the patient's existing beliefs about his or her chronic pain.[96]

## SUMMARY

Pronociception and antinociception can occur in the periphery, dorsal horn, neuronal descending system, hormonal system, and cerebral cortex. Chronic pain may be caused by continuing stimulation of nociceptors, by neuropathic processes, by pain matrix dysfunction, or by chronic pain syndromes. Neuropathic processes include ectopic foci, ephaptic transmission, central sensitization, and structural reorganization. Pain matrix dysfunction causes altered top-down pain modulation (Figure 8-15). Table 8-3 summarizes the differences among various types of chronic somatic pain. Figure 8-16 summarizes the categories and subtypes of chronic somatic pain.

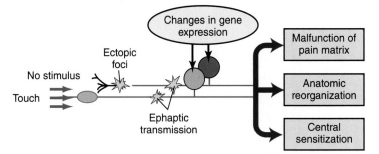

**Fig. 8-15 Mechanisms of neuropathic pain.** Lesions of peripheral nerves cause changes in gene expression of injured neurons, resulting in production of sodium channels that are inserted into the injured membrane, and begin to generate ectopic action potentials. Lesions of peripheral nerves may also cause demyelination, resulting in ephaptic transmission. Pathologic changes in the central nervous system that cause neuropathic pain include changes in gene expression in the primary neuron cell bodies, central sensitization (gene activation in projection neurons), anatomic reorganization, and malfunction of the pain matrix.

**TABLE 8-3** CHRONIC SOMATIC PAIN: NOCICEPTIVE, NEUROPATHIC, MATRIX DYSFUNCTION, AND PAIN SYNDROMES

|  | Mechanism of Pain | Examples | Patient Description of Pain |
|---|---|---|---|
| Nociceptive pain | • Neural activity is normal and appropriate.<br>• Normal transmission of information regarding tissue damage or threat of damage from nociceptors<br>• Pain is a symptom. | • Arthritis pain<br>• Cancer pain<br>• Mechanical low back pain | • Dull, aching, throbbing; rarely sharp<br>• Clinical descriptors: primary hyperalgesia at location of injury |
| Neuropathic pain | • Pathologic neural activity<br>• Pain is a disease, caused by neurochemical, gene expression, and anatomic changes in neurons. | Two types:<br>1. Peripherally generated:<br>  • Painful mononeuropathies<br>  • Nerve entrapment<br>  • Nerve compression<br>2. CNS response to deafferentation<br>  • Avulsion of dorsal roots<br>  • Phantom limb pain<br>  • Central pain:<br>    • Spinal cord injury<br>    • Stroke<br>    • Multiple sclerosis<br>  • Small fiber neuropathy:<br>    • Postherpetic neuralgia<br>    • Diabetic neuropathy<br>    • Guillain-Barré | • Burning, shooting, tingling, electrical, lightning sensations |
| Pain matrix dysfunction | • Dysregulation of pain excitatory and inhibitory mechanisms in CNS | • Fibromyalgia<br>• Episodic tension-type headache<br>• Migraine<br>• Chronic whiplash-associated disorder | • Diffuse deep pain, hyperalgesia, allodynia |
| Pain syndromes | • Pain matrix dysfunction plus autonomic and/or motor dysfunction | • Complex regional pain syndrome (CRPS)<br>• Chronic low back pain (LBP) syndrome | • CRPS: diffuse deep pain, burning, aching, stinging<br>• Chronic LBP syndrome: pain in response to normally nonpainful stimuli, and prickling, itching, burning, or electric shock sensations |

*CNS,* Central nervous system.

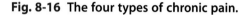

| Nociceptive | Neuropathic | Pain matrix dysfunction | Pain syndromes |
|---|---|---|---|
| Mechanical LBP<br><br>Cancer<br><br>Arthritis<br><br>Burns | Nerve entrapment and compression<br>Avulsion dorsal roots<br>Phantom limb pain<br>Central pain:<br>    Multiple sclerosis<br>    Spinal cord injury<br>    Stroke<br>Small fiber neuropathy:<br>    Diabetic neuropathy<br>    Guillain-Barré<br>    Post-herpetic pain | Fibromyalgia<br><br>Chronic whiplash-<br>associated disorder<br><br>Headache:<br>    Migraine<br>    Episodic<br>      tension-type | Complex regional<br>pain syndrome<br><br>Chronic LBP<br>syndrome |

**Fig. 8-16  The four types of chronic pain.**

## CASE NOTES

### Case 1

A 24-year-old legal secretary was stopped at a traffic signal when her car was struck from behind. X-rays taken 3 hours after the accident were normal. She noted some stiffness of her neck the following day; within a week, her upper back was also stiff and becoming painful. During the next 2 weeks, she was free of pain. Now, 5 weeks after the accident, she is seeking treatment because the neck aching has returned, turning her head while driving is painful, and she has dull headaches. She denies having reinjured her neck but reports stressful deadlines at work.

Tests and measurements:
- She has no motor or sensory loss.
- Active neck range of motion is as follows:
  - 20 degrees forward flexion, 35 degrees extension (30% and 70% of normal values)
  - Lateral flexion: 15 degrees to the left, 24 degrees to the right (38% and 60% of normal)
  - Rotation: 20 degrees to the left, 33 degrees to the right (36% and 60% of normal)

**Question**

What is the probable diagnosis? Why?

### Case 2

C.M., a 42-year-old man, sustained mild soft tissue damage to his right wrist in a fall 2 months ago. While replacing a porch light, he fell approximately 4 feet from a ladder. An x-ray indicated no fracture. The emergency room doctor diagnosed minor wrist sprain. C.M. works as a high school guidance counselor and is right-handed. However, since the injury, C.M. has completely stopped using his right upper limb. He reports that he wears a sling, even while sleeping, and protects his entire right arm as much as possible, and the pain is getting worse. He also reports a constant burning sensation, and that any stimulation, even putting on clothes or a breeze across the skin, evokes sharp pain.

The therapist observes the following abnormalities in his fourth and fifth fingers: excessive sweating; shiny, red skin; and opaque, long fingernails. C.M. states that he cannot tolerate cutting the nails because of pain. When asked to move his right arm, C.M. refuses. He allows passive flexion of the shoulder to 40 degrees. C.M. refuses to allow the therapist to touch his distal arm and refuses to actively move his hand or wrist.

**Question**

What is the most likely diagnosis? Why?

### Case 3

B.J., a 46-year-old woman, has had bilateral pain affecting her neck, upper and lower back, shoulders, and hips for 6 months. She has visited three medical doctors without receiving a diagnosis, and her impression is that the physicians did not believe her pain reports. She is a kidney disease principal investigator at a university research institute, and the pain is interfering with her ability to work. She has taken aspirin and ibuprofen, and neither was effective. B.J. denies feelings of hopelessness or depression. She has found that taking a hot bath temporarily diminishes the pain.

**Questions**

1. Given B.J.'s history, what would be your next step to establish a diagnosis?
2. Assuming that your diagnostic suspicion is confirmed, what would you advise B.J. to do?

## REVIEW QUESTIONS

1. Explain the difference in etiology between nociceptive chronic pain and neuropathic chronic pain.
2. Define *paresthesia* and *dysesthesia*.
3. What self-administered questionnaire can be used to determine whether a patient's pain is neuropathic?
4. What are ectopic foci?
5. What is central sensitization?
6. What happens when novel synapses form between Aβ afferents and central nociceptive neurons?
7. List two examples of painful mononeuropathies.
8. What is phantom limb pain? What causes phantom limb pain? How can phantom limb pain be treated?
9. What common pathology causes pain in diabetic neuropathy, Guillain-Barré, and postherpetic neuralgia?
10. What is the common pathology in fibromyalgia, episodic tension-type headache, migraine, and chronic whiplash-associated disorder?
11. Is fibromyalgia a psychological disorder? Describe the evidence for or against fibromyalgia as a psychological disorder.
12. What medications are ineffective for treating fibromyalgia?
13. What criteria are used to classify a headache as a migraine?
14. What are the three events in migraine without aura?
15. What is the pathology in complex regional pain syndrome?
16. What intervention significantly reduces the incidence of complex regional pain syndrome post stroke?
17. Often, people with chronic low back pain have no identifiable tissue damage. Waddell and associates[55] propose that physiologic changes following acute low back injury may cause chronic pain. What are the changes cited by Waddell's group as responsible for continued pain?

## References

1. Treede RD, Jensen TS, Campbell JN, et al: Redefinition of neuropathic pain and a grading system for clinical use: consensus statement on clinical and research diagnostic criteria. *Neurology* 70:1630–1635, 2008.
2. Diatchenko L, Slade GD, Nackley AG, et al: Genetic basis for individual variations in pain perception and the development of a chronic pain condition. *Hum Mol Genet* 14:135–143, 2005.
3. Lynch ME, Clark AJ, Sawynok J, Sullivan MJ: Topical 2% amitriptyline and 1% ketamine in neuropathic pain syndromes: a randomized, double-blind, placebo-controlled trial. *Anesthesiology* 103:140–146, 2005.
4. Harden RN: Chronic neuropathic pain: mechanisms, diagnosis, and treatment. *Neurologist* 11:111–122, 2005.
5. Arnstein PM: The neuroplastic phenomenon: a physiologic link between chronic pain and learning. *J Neurosci Nurs* 29:179–186, 1997.
6. Willis WD: Long-term potentiation in spinothalamic neurons. *Brain Res Rev* 40:202–214, 2002.
7. Dieleman JP, Kerklaan J, Huygen FJ, et al: Incidence rates and treatment of neuropathic pain conditions in the general population. *Pain* 137:681–688, 2008.
8. Bouhassira D, Lantéri-Minet M, Attal N, et al: Prevalence of chronic pain with neuropathic characteristics in the general population. *Pain* 136:380–387, 2008.
9. Vartiainen N, Kirveskari E, Kallio-Laine K, et al: Cortical reorganization in primary somatosensory cortex in patients with unilateral chronic pain. *J Pain* 10:854–859, 2009.
10. MacIver K, Lloyd DM, Kelly S, et al: Phantom limb pain, cortical reorganization and the therapeutic effect of mental imagery. *Brain* 131:2181–2191, 2008.
11. Moseley GL: Graded motor imagery for pathologic pain: a randomized controlled trial. *Neurology* 67:2129–2134, 2006.
12. Chan BL, Witt R, Charrow AP, et al: Mirror therapy for phantom limb pain. *N Engl J Med* 357:2206–2207, 2007.
13. Griffin R, Fink E, Brenner JG: Functional neuroanatomy of the nociceptive system. In Ballantyne JC, Fishman SM, Rathmell JP, editors: *Bonica's management of pain*, ed 4, Baltimore, 2010, Lippincott Williams & Wilkins.
14. Klit H, Finnerup NB, Jensen TS: Central post-stroke pain: clinical characteristics, pathophysiology, and management. *Lancet Neurol* 8:857–868, 2009.
15. Wasner G: Central pain syndromes. *Curr Pain Headache Rep* 14:489–496, 2010.
16. Martinez V, Fletcher D, Martin F, et al: Small fibre impairment predicts neuropathic pain in Guillain-Barré syndrome. *Pain* 151:53–60, 2010.
17. Scherens A, Maier C, Haussleiter IS, et al: Painful or painless lower limb dysesthesias are highly predictive of peripheral neuropathy: comparison of different diagnostic modalities. *Eur J Pain* 13:711–718, 2009.
18. Bennett GJ, Watson CP: Herpes zoster and postherpetic neuralgia: past, present and future. *Pain Res Manag* 14:275–282, 2009.
19. Geber C, Baumgärtner U, Schwab R, et al: Revised definition of neuropathic pain and its grading system: an open case series illustrating its use in clinical practice. *Am J Med* 122(10 Suppl):S3–12, 2009.
20. Kuchinad A, Schweinhardt P, Seminowicz DA, et al: Accelerated brain gray matter loss in fibromyalgia patients: premature aging of the brain? *J Neurosci* 27:4004–4007, 2007.
21. Jensen KB, Kosek E, Petzke F, et al: Evidence of dysfunctional pain inhibition in fibromyalgia reflected in rACC during provoked pain. *Pain* 144:95–100, 2009.
22. Gracely RH, Geisser ME, Giesecke T, et al: Pain catastrophizing and neural responses to pain among persons with fibromyalgia. *Brain* 127:835–843, 2004.
23. Clauw DJ: The psychophysiology of pain. In Ballantyne JC, Fishman SM, Rathmell JP, editors: *Bonica's management of pain*, ed 4, Baltimore, 2010, Lippincott Williams & Wilkins.
24. Buskila D: Genetics of chronic pain states. *Best Pract Res Clin Rheumatol* 21:535–547, 2007.
25. Xiao Y, He W, Russell IJ: Genetic polymorphisms of the beta2-adrenergic receptor relate to guanosine protein-coupled stimulator receptor dysfunction in fibromyalgia syndrome. *J Rheumatol.* 38(6):1095–1103, 2011.
26. Glass JM: Rheumatologic conditions: Sjögren's syndrome, fibromyalgia, and chronic fatigue syndrome. In Armstrong CL, Morrow L, editors: *Handbook of medical neuropsychology*, New York, 2010, Springer.
27. Weir PT, Harlan GA, Nkoy FL, et al: The incidence of fibromyalgia and its associated comorbidities: a population based retrospective cohort study based on International Classification of

Diseases, 9th Revision codes. *J Clin Rheumatol* 12:124–128, 2006.

28. Lavergne MR, Cole DC, Kerr K, Marshall LM: Functional impairment in chronic fatigue syndrome, fibromyalgia, and multiple chemical sensitivity. *Can Fam Physician* 56:e57–65, 2010.

29. Gormsen L: Depression, anxiety, health-related quality of life and pain in patients with chronic fibromyalgia and neuropathic pain. *Eur J Pain* 14:127, 2010.

30. Culpepper L: Recognizing and diagnosing fibromyalgia. *J Clin Psychiatry* 71:e30, 2010.

31. Carville SF, Arendt-Nielsen S, Bliddal H, et al: EULAR: EULAR evidence-based recommendations for the management of fibromyalgia syndrome. *Ann Rheum Dis* 67:536–541, 2008.

32. Hooten WM, Townsend CO, Sletten CD, et al: Treatment outcomes after multidisciplinary pain rehabilitation with analgesic medication withdrawal for patients with fibromyalgia. *Pain Med* 8:8–16, 2007.

33. Ashina M: Neurobiology of chronic tension-type headache. *Cephalalgia* 24:161–172, 2004.

34. Lyngberg AC, Rasmussen BK, Jørgensen T, Jensen R: Has the prevalence of migraine and tension-type headache changed over a 12-year period? A Danish population survey. *Eur J Epidemiol* 20:243–249, 2005.

35. Ulrich V, Gervil M, Olesen J: The relative influence of environment and genes in episodic tension-type headache. *Neurology* 62:2065–2069, 2004.

36. Woolhouse M: Migraine and tension headache—a complementary and alternative medicine approach. *Aust Fam Physician* 34:647–651, 2005.

37. Goadsby PJ: Migraine pathology. *Headache* 45(Suppl 1):S14–24, 2005.

38. Bartleson JD, Cutrer FM: Migraine update: diagnosis and treatment. *Minn Med* 93:36–41, 2010.

39. Lauritzen M, Dreier JP, Fabricius M, et al: Clinical relevance of cortical spreading depression in neurological disorders: migraine, malignant stroke, subarachnoid and intracranial hemorrhage, and traumatic brain injury. *J Cereb Blood Flow Metab* 31:17–35, 2011.

40. Dodick DW, Gargus JJ: Why migraines strike. *Sci Am* 299:56–63, 2008.

41. D'Andrea G, Leon A: Pathogenesis of migraine: from neurotransmitters to neuromodulators and beyond. *Neurol Sci* 31(Suppl 1):S1–7, 2010.

42. Sprenger T, Goadsby PJ: Migraine pathogenesis and state of pharmacological treatment options. *BMC Med* 7:71, 2009.

43. Joubert J: Diagnosing headache. *Aust Fam Physician* 34:621–625, 2005.

44. Dowson AJ: Casebook: headache. *Practitioner* 247:45–52, 2003.

45. Sobri M, Lamont AC, Alias NA, Win MN: Red flags in patients presenting with headache: clinical indications for neuroimaging. *Br J Radiol* 76:532–535, 2003.

46. Sterling M, Pedler A: A neuropathic pain component is common in acute whiplash and associated with a more complex clinical presentation. *Man Ther* 14:173–179, 2009.

47. Wenzel HG, Mykletun A, Nilsen TI: Symptom profile of persons self-reporting whiplash: a Norwegian population-based study (HUNT 2). *Eur Spine J* 18:1363–1370, 2009.

48. Bruehl S: An update on the pathophysiology of complex regional pain syndrome. *Anesthesiology* 113:713–725, 2010.

49. Maihöfner C, Seifert F, Markovic K: Complex Regional Pain Syndromes: new pathophysiological concepts and therapies. *Eur J Neurol* 17:649–660, 2010.

50. Van Rijn MA, Marinus J, Putter H, et al: Spreading of Complex Regional Pain Syndrome: not a random process. *J Neural Transm* 118:1301–1309, 2011.

51. Güler-Uysal F, Basaran S, Geertzen JH, Göncü K: A 2½-year-old girl with reflex sympathetic dystrophy syndrome (CRPS type I): case report. *Clin Rehabil* 17:224–227, 2003.

52. Harden NR, Bruehl SP: Complex regional pain syndrome. In Ballantyne JC, Fishman SM, Rathmell JP, editors: *Bonica's management of pain*, ed 4, Baltimore, 2010, Lippincott Williams & Wilkins.

53. de Mos M, de Bruijn AG, Huygen FJ, et al: The incidence of Complex Regional Pain Syndrome: a population-based study. *Pain* 129:12–20, 2007.

54. Li Z, Smith BP, Smith TL, Koman LA: Diagnosis and management of Complex Regional Pain Syndrome complicating upper extremity recovery. *J Hand Ther* 18:270–276, 2005.

55. Oerlemans HM, Oostendorp RA, de Boo T, et al: Adjuvant physical therapy versus occupational therapy in patients with reflex sympathetic dystrophy/Complex Regional Pain Syndrome type I. *Arch Phys Med Rehabil* 81:49–56, 2000.

56. Moseley GL: Graded motor imagery is effective for long-standing Complex Regional Pain Syndrome: a randomised controlled trial. *Pain* 108:192–198, 2004.

57. Zollinger PE, Tuinebreijer WE, Breederveld RS, et al: Can vitamin C prevent Complex Regional Pain Syndrome in patients with wrist fractures? A randomized, controlled, multicenter dose-response study. *J Bone Joint Surg Am* 89:1424–1431, 2007.

58. Braus DF, Krauss JK, Strobel J: The shoulder-hand syndrome after stroke: a prospective clinical trial. *Ann Neurol* 36:728–733, 1994.

59. Brox JI, Storheim K, Holm I, et al: Disability, pain, psychological factors and physical performance in healthy controls, patients with sub-acute and chronic low back pain: a case-control study. *J Rehabil Med* 37:95–99, 2005.

60. Waddell G, Newton M, Henderson I, et al: A fear-avoidance beliefs questionnaire (FABQ) and the role of fear-avoidance beliefs in chronic low back pain and disability. *Pain* 52:157–168, 1993.

61. Stewart J, Kempenaar L, Lauchlan D: Rethinking yellow flags. *Man Ther* 16:196–198, 2011.

62. Waddell G: A new clinical model for the treatment of low-back pain. *Spine* 12:632–644, 1987.

63. Jensen MC, Brant-Zawadzki MN: Magnetic resonance imaging of the lumbar spine in people without back pain. *N Engl J Med* 331:69–73, 1994.

64. Weiner BK: Spine update: the biopsychosocial model and spine care. *Spine* 33:219–223, 2008.

65. Henschke N, Ostelo RW, van Tulder MW: Behavioural treatment for chronic low-back pain. *Cochrane Database Syst Rev* (7):CD002014, 2010.

66. Giesecke T, Gracely RH, Grant MA, et al: Evidence of augmented central pain processing in idiopathic chronic low back pain. *Arthritis Rheum* 50:613–623, 2004.

67. Gracely RH, Petzke F, Wolf JM, Clauw DJ: Functional magnetic resonance imaging evidence of augmented pain processing in fibromyalgia. *Arthritis Rheum* 46:1333–1343, 2002.

68. Henschke N, Maher CG, Refshauge KM, et al: Prevalence of and screening for serious spinal pathology in patients presenting to primary care settings with acute low back pain. *Arthritis Rheum* 60:3072–3080, 2009.

69. Atlas SJ, Deyo RA: Evaluating and managing acute low back pain in the primary care setting. *J Gen Intern Med* 16:120–131, 2001.

70. Manchikanti L, Singh V, Datta S, et al: Comprehensive review of epidemiology, scope, and impact of spinal pain. *Pain Physician* 12:E35–70, 2009.

71. El Sissi W, Arnaout A, Chaarani MW: Prevalence of neuropathic pain among patients with chronic low-back pain in the Arabian Gulf Region assessed using the Leeds Assessment of Neuropathic Symptoms and Signs Pain Scale. *J Intern Med Res* 38:2135–2145, 2010.

72. Dworkin RH, O'Connor AB, Backonja M, et al: Pharmacologic management of neuropathic pain: evidence-based recommendations. *Pain* 132:237–251, 2007.

73. Siddall PJ, Cousins MJ, Otte A, et al: Pregabalin in central neuropathic pain associated with spinal cord injury: a placebo-controlled trial. *Neurology* 67:1792–1800, 2006.

74. Ware MA, Wang T, Shapiro S, et al: Smoked cannabis for chronic neuropathic pain: a randomized controlled trial. *CMAJ* 182:E694–701, 2010.

75. Goldenberg DL, Clauw DJ, Palmer RH, et al: Durability of therapeutic response to milnacipran treatment for fibromyalgia: results of a randomized, double-blind, monotherapy 6-month extension study. *Pain Med* 11:180–194, 2010.

76. Mainguy Y: Functional magnetic resonance imagery (fMRI) in fibromyalgia and the response to milnacipran. *Hum Psychopharmacol* 24:S19–23, 2009.

77. Arnold LM, Goldenberg DL, Stanford SB, et al: Gabapentin in the treatment of fibromyalgia: a randomized, double blind, placebo-controlled, multicenter trial. *Arthritis Rheum* 56:1336–1344, 2007.

78. Mease PJ, Russel IJ, Arnold LM, et al: A randomized, double blind, placebo-controlled, phase III trial of pregabalin in the treatment of patients with fibromyalgia. *Nat Clin Pract Rheumatol* 4:514–515, 2008.

79. Kroenke K, Krebs EE, Bair MJ: Pharmacotherapy of chronic pain: a synthesis of recommendations from systematic reviews. *Gen Hosp Psychiatry* 31:206–219, 2009.

80. Saxena A, Solitar BM: Fibromyalgia: knowns, unknowns, and current treatment. *Bull NYU Hosp Jt Dis* 68:157–161, 2010.

81. Skrabek RQ, Galimova L, Ethans K, et al: Nabilone for the treatment of pain in fibromyalgia. *J Pain* 9:164–173, 2008.

82. McGuirk BE, Bogduk N: Chronic low back pain. In Ballantyne JC, Fishman SM, Rathmell JP, editors: *Bonica's management of pain*, ed 4, Baltimore, 2010, Lippincott Williams & Wilkins, pp 1105–1122.

83. Marchand S: The physiology of pain mechanisms: from the periphery to the brain. *Rheum Dis Clin North Am* 34:285–309, 2008.

84. Wasan AD, Sullivan MD, Clark MR: Psychiatric illness, depression, anxiety, and somatoform pain disorders. In Ballantyne JC, Fishman SM, Rathmell JP, editors: *Bonica's management of pain*, ed 4, Baltimore, 2010, Lippincott Williams & Wilkins.

85. Atlas LY, Bolger N, Lindquist MA, et al: Brain mediators of predictive cue effects on perceived pain. *J Neurosci* 30:12964–12977, 2010.

86. Keefe FJ, Somers TJ: Psychological approaches to understanding and treating arthritis pain. *Nat Rev Rheumatol* 6:210–216, 2010.

87. Gulur P, Soldinger SM, Acquadro MA: Concepts in pain management. *Clin Podiatr Med Surg* 24:333–351, 2007.

88. Bingel U, Tracey I: Imaging CNS modulation of pain in humans. *Physiology* 23:371–380, 2008.

89. Pollo A, Benedetti F: Placebo response: relevance to the rheumatic diseases. *Rheum Dis Clin N Am* 34:331–349, 2008.

90. Keefe FJ, Somers TJ, Martire LM: Psychologic interventions and lifestyle modifications for arthritis pain management. *Rheum Dis Clin North Am* 34:351–368, 2008.

91. Stewart-Williams S, Podd J: The placebo effect: dissolving the expectancy versus conditioning debate. *Psychol Bull* 130:324–340, 2004.

92. Barrett B, Muller D, Rakel D, et al: Placebo, meaning and health. *Perspect Biol Med* 49:178–198, 2006.

93. Qiu YH, Wu XY, Xu H, et al: Neuroimaging study of placebo analgesia in humans. *Neurosci Bull* 25:277–282, 2009.

94. Scott DJ, Stohler CS, Egnatuk CM, et al: Individual differences in reward responding explain placebo-induced expectations and effects. *Neuron* 55:325–336, 2007.

95. Wager TD, Atlas LY, Leotti LA, et al: Predicting individual differences in placebo analgesia: contributions of brain activity during anticipation and pain experience. *J Neurosci* 31:439–452, 2011.

96. Frantsve LM, Kerns RD: Patient-provider interactions in the management of chronic pain: current findings within the context of shared medical decision making. *Pain Med* 8:25–35, 2007.

# 9 Autonomic Nervous System

Laurie Lundy-Ekman, PhD, PT

The *autonomic nervous system* is critical for the survival of the individual and the species because it regulates homeostasis and reproduction. *Homeostasis* is the maintenance of an optimal internal environment, including body temperature and chemical composition of tissues and fluids. The autonomic nervous system maintains homeostasis by regulating the activity of internal organs and vasculature. Thus, the autonomic nervous system regulates circulation, respiration, digestion, metabolism, secretions, body temperature, and reproduction. The aspects of the autonomic nervous system considered in this chapter include receptors, afferent pathways, central regulation, and efferent pathways to the effectors (Figure 9-1). The autonomic efferent pathways are the sympathetic and parasympathetic divisions of the nervous system.

---

⊚ *Clinical Pearl*

The autonomic system regulates the viscera, vasculature, and glands.

---

## RECEPTORS

Receptors of the autonomic system include mechanoreceptors, chemoreceptors, nociceptors, and thermoreceptors. The *mechanoreceptors* respond to pressure and to stretch. Pressure receptors are found in the aortic baroreceptors, carotid sinuses, and lungs. Stretch receptors respond to distention of the veins, bladder, or intestines.

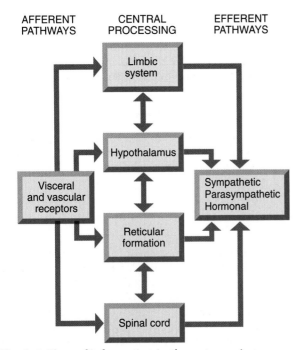

**Fig. 9-1** Flow of information in the autonomic nervous system.

*Chemoreceptors* sensitive to chemical concentrations in the blood are located in the carotid and aortic bodies (respond to oxygen), medulla (respond to hydrogen ions and carbon dioxide), and hypothalamus (respond to blood glucose levels and to concentrations of electrolytes). Chemoreceptors in the stomach, taste buds, and olfactory bulbs also respond to chemical concentrations.

*Nociceptors,* found throughout the viscera and in the walls of arteries, are typically most responsive to stretch and ischemia. Visceral nociceptors are also sensitive to irritating chemicals.

*Thermoreceptors* in the hypothalamus respond to very small changes in the temperature of circulating blood, and cutaneous thermoreceptors respond to external temperature changes.

---

## AFFERENT PATHWAYS

Information from visceral receptors enters the central nervous system by two routes: into the spinal cord via the dorsal roots, and into the brainstem via cranial nerves (Figure 9-2). Cranial nerves conveying autonomic afferent information include the facial (VII), glossopharyngeal (IX), and vagus nerves (X). All three of these cranial nerves transmit taste information, and the glossopharyngeal and vagus nerves transmit information from the viscera.

---

## CENTRAL REGULATION OF VISCERAL FUNCTION

Most visceral information entering the brainstem via cranial nerves converges in the *solitary nucleus,* the main visceral sensory nucleus (Figure 9-3). In turn, information from the solitary nucleus is relayed to visceral control areas in the pons and medulla, and to modulatory areas in the hypothalamus, thalamus, and limbic system. Modulatory areas regulate the activity of areas that directly control a particular function. For example, the limbic system does not directly control respiratory rate but instead influences the activity of respiratory control areas in the pons and medulla.

Visceral afferents entering the spinal cord synapse with visceral efferents (autonomic reflexes; see Chapter 13) and with neurons that ascend to regions of the brainstem, hypothalamus, and thalamus. Visceral nociceptive afferents have additional connections with the following:

- Somatosensory nociceptive tract neurons, contributing to referred pain (see Chapter 7)
- Somatic efferents, to produce muscle guarding (protective contraction of skeletal muscles)

Figure 9-4 illustrates the activity in these pathways during acute appendicitis.

---

⊚ *Clinical Pearl*

Afferent autonomic information is processed in the solitary nucleus, spinal cord, and areas of the brainstem, hypothalamus, and thalamus.

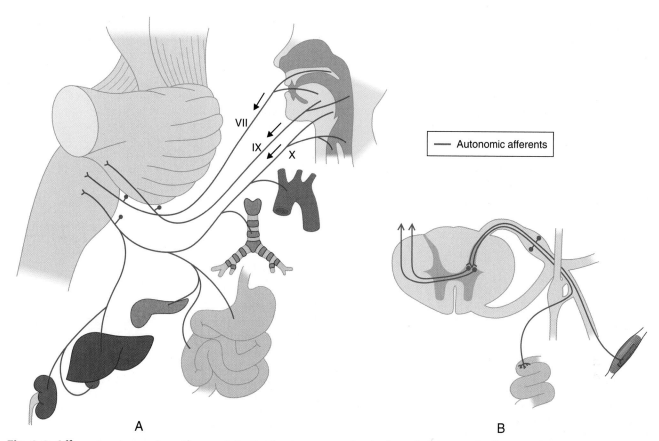

**Fig. 9-2 Afferent autonomic pathways into the brainstem and spinal cord. A,** Visceral afferent information from the tongue and soft palate enters the brainstem through cranial nerves VII and IX. Information from the larynx and thoracic and abdominal viscera reaches the brainstem via cranial nerve X. **B,** Stretch of blood vessels in the periphery is registered by free nerve endings in the vessel walls. This information is conveyed via fibers in peripheral nerves into the spinal cord. Information from stretch receptors in the gastrointestinal tract passes through an autonomic ganglion, without synapsing, before entering the spinal cord.

## Control of Autonomic Functions by the Medulla and Pons

Areas within the medulla regulate heart rate, respiration, vasoconstriction, and vasodilation via signals to autonomic efferent neurons in the spinal cord and by signals conveyed in the vagus nerve. Areas in the pons are also involved in regulating respiration.

## Role of the Hypothalamus, Thalamus, and Limbic System in Autonomic Regulation

The hypothalamus, thalamus, and limbic system modulate brainstem autonomic control. Visceral information reaching the hypothalamus, the master controller of homeostasis, is used to maintain equilibrium in the interior of the body. The hypothalamus influences cardiorespiratory, metabolic, water reabsorption, and digestive activity by acting on the pituitary gland, control centers in the brainstem, and spinal cord. Visceral information reaching the thalamus is projected mainly to the limbic system, a collection of cerebral areas involved in emotions, moods, and motivation. Activation of limbic areas can produce

autonomic responses; examples include increased heart rate due to anxiety, blushing with embarrassment, and crying.[1]

> ◎ *Clinical Pearl*
>
> Vital functions are controlled by areas in the medulla and pons. The hypothalamus, thalamus, and limbic system modulate brainstem control.

## Integration of Information

Autonomic regulation is often achieved by integrating information from peripheral afferents with information from receptors within the central nervous system. For example, if peripheral chemoreceptors in the carotid body signal a drop in oxygen content in the blood, the information is conveyed to the solitary nucleus (in the medulla) by the glossopharyngeal nerve. Then signals are sent to autonomic control areas to increase the depth and rate of respiration. If a specific group of neurons in the medulla, directly sensitive to the concentration of carbon

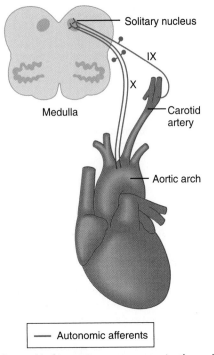

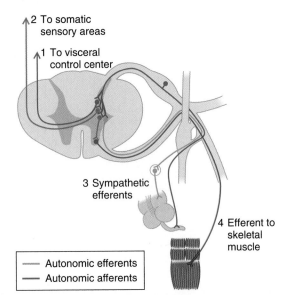

**Fig. 9-3** Visceral information converges in the solitary nucleus of the brainstem. An example is the convergence of blood pressure and blood chemical composition information, monitored by pressure and chemoreceptors in the carotid artery and the aortic arch. The information is transmitted to the solitary nucleus in the medulla.

**Fig. 9-4 Pathways of afferent autonomic information in the spinal cord.** The early stage of acute appendicitis is shown: nociceptive signals enter the T10 spinal segment. Connections with

1. Autonomic tract fibers convey the information to areas in the brainstem, hypothalamus, and limbic system
2. Stimulation of nociceptive second-order neurons results in pain sensation referred to the umbilical region
3. Sympathetic efferents inhibit peristalsis in the intestine
4. Somatic efferents elicit contraction of abdominal muscles

dioxide and to hydrogen ions (pH) in the blood, sense deviations from the optimum physiologic range, respiration is adjusted.

## EFFERENT PATHWAYS

Autonomic efferent neurons are classified as sympathetic and parasympathetic. In general, the connections from the central nervous system to autonomic effectors use a two-neuron pathway, with the two neurons synapsing in a peripheral ganglion. The neuron extending from the central nervous system to the ganglion is called *preganglionic;* the neuron connecting the ganglion with the effector organ is called *postganglionic.*

### Differences Between the Somatic Motor System and the Autonomic Efferent System

All central nervous system output is delivered by somatic or autonomic efferent neurons. Somatic efferents innervate only skeletal muscle, and their activation is frequently voluntary. Autonomic efferents supply all other parts of the body that are innervated. The autonomic system is different from the somatic nervous system in three major ways:

1. Unlike the somatic nervous system, regulation of autonomic functions is typically nonconscious and can be exerted by hormones.
2. Unlike skeletal muscle, many internal organs can function independently of central nervous system input. Examples

include independent activity of the heart and the gastrointestinal tract. The heart can continue to beat without neural connections. The gastrointestinal tract is unique in having an intrinsic nervous system, the enteric nervous system, so capable of operating independently of the central nervous system that the system has been called the *abdominal brain.*[2] This system of ganglia and sensory and motor neurons is located entirely within the walls of the digestive system. Because its function is purely digestive, further discussion of the enteric nervous system is beyond the scope of this text.

3. Somatic efferent pathways use one neuron; autonomic efferent pathways usually use two neurons, with a synapse outside the central nervous system.

### Neurotransmitters Used by the Autonomic Efferent System

Autonomic neurons secrete the neurotransmitter acetylcholine, norepinephrine, or epinephrine. Neurons that secrete acetylcholine are called *cholinergic.* Neurons that secrete norepinephrine or epinephrine are called *adrenergic.*

### Cholinergic Neurons and Receptors

Autonomic neurons that secrete acetylcholine include the following (Figure 9-5):

SYMPATHETIC

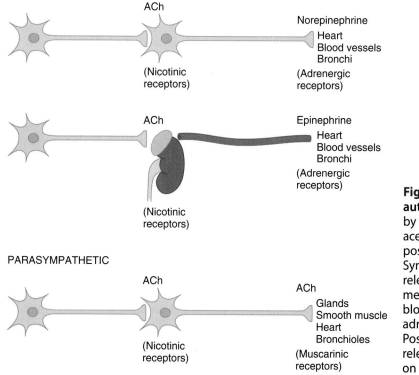

**Fig. 9-5 Neurochemicals secreted by autonomic neurons.** The chemical released by all presynaptic autonomic neurons is acetylcholine (ACh). Receptors on all postganglionic neurons are nicotinic. Sympathetic postganglionic neurons release norepinephrine (NE). The adrenal medulla releases epinephrine into the bloodstream. Both NE and epinephrine bind to adrenergic receptors on their target organs. Postganglionic parasympathetic neurons release ACh that binds to muscarinic receptors on their target organs.

- All preganglionic neurons in the autonomic nervous system
- Postganglionic neurons of the parasympathetic system

The effect of a neurotransmitter depends on the types of receptors activated by the transmitter. This is of particular importance in the autonomic nervous system, where differences in types of receptors are the key to the distinct physiologic effects of different drugs. Based on their ability to bind certain drugs, two groups of *cholinergic receptors* have been identified: muscarinic and nicotinic.

Muscarine, a poison derived from mushrooms, activates only *muscarinic receptors* in the membranes of effectors. Acetylcholine binding to muscarinic receptors initiates a G-protein–mediated response, which can be an excitatory postsynaptic potential (EPSP) or an inhibitory postsynaptic potential (IPSP). Parasympathetic muscarinic acetylcholine receptors regulate glands, smooth muscles, and heart rate.

Nicotine, derived from tobacco, activates only the *nicotinic acetylcholine receptors.* Acetylcholine binding to nicotinic autonomic receptors, located on all postsynaptic autonomic neurons and the adrenal medulla, causes a fast EPSP in the postsynaptic membrane. In addition to effects on the autonomic system, nicotine activates acetylcholine receptors on skeletal muscle membrane and in limbic areas of the brain. Nicotine action in the limbic system induces feelings of alertness and arousal[3] and leads to addiction.[4] Nicotine improves performance on tasks that require careful observation and intense attention.[5] In nonsmoking women, inhaling nicotine improves mood and induces a feeling of calmness by increasing levels of dopamine in neural pathways that induce a feeling of pleasure and reduce anxiety. File and colleagues speculate that women may begin regular smoking as a form of stress self-medication. However, in nonsmoking males, nicotine enhances aggressive mood.[6]

### Adrenergic Neurons and Receptors

The transmitter released by most sympathetic postganglionic neurons is norepinephrine. The adrenal medulla, a part of the sympathetic system, is specialized to release epinephrine and norepinephrine directly into the blood. Receptors that bind norepinephrine or epinephrine are called *adrenergic receptors.* There are two groups of adrenergic receptors, designated $\alpha$ and $\beta$; each of these has subtypes, indicated by subscripts: $\alpha_1$, $\alpha_2$, $\beta_1$, and $\beta_2$.

> **Clinical Pearl**
>
> Cholinergic neurons secrete acetylcholine. Nicotine and muscarine are exogenous chemicals that bind with subtypes of acetylcholine receptors. Adrenergic neurons secrete norepinephrine. Adrenergic receptors are classified as $\alpha$ or $\beta$.

## SYMPATHETIC NERVOUS SYSTEM

### Sympathetic Efferent Neurons

Cell bodies of the sympathetic preganglionic neurons are in the lateral horn of the spinal cord gray matter (Figure 9-6). Because the cell bodies are located from T1 to L2 levels, the sympathetic

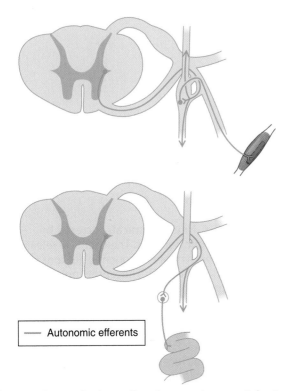

— Autonomic efferents

**Fig. 9-6** Sympathetic outflow innervating arterioles in skeletal muscle and in the walls of viscera.

nervous system is often called the *thoracolumbar outflow.* Sympathetic efferent neurons innervate the adrenal medulla, vasculature, sweat glands, erectors of hair cells, and the viscera.

### Sympathetic Efferents to the Adrenal Medulla

Direct connections are provided from the spinal cord to the adrenal medulla (Figure 9-7, *A*). The adrenal medulla can be considered a specialized sympathetic ganglion that secretes epinephrine and norepinephrine into the bloodstream.

### Sympathetic Efferents to the Periphery and Thoracic Viscera

Sympathetic efferents to the limbs, face, body wall, heart, and lungs synapse in ganglia alongside the vertebral column, called *paravertebral ganglia* (Figure 9-7, *B*). The paravertebral ganglia are interconnected, forming sympathetic trunks. Preganglionic sympathetic axons leave the spinal cord through the ventral root, join the spinal nerve, and then travel in a very short connecting branch to the paravertebral ganglia. The connecting branch, called the *white ramus communicans* (shown in Figure 9-6), is composed of sympathetic axons transferring from the spinal nerve to the paravertebral ganglion. The preganglionic axons may synapse in the paravertebral ganglion or may travel up or down the sympathetic chain before synapsing in a ganglion.

The cell body of the postganglionic neuron is in the paravertebral ganglion. The postganglionic axon enters a peripheral nerve via a connecting branch, the *gray ramus communicans* (see Figure 9-6), then travels in the ventral or dorsal ramus to the periphery.

Given that the head, except for the face, and most of the upper limbs are innervated by cervical spinal cord segments, and preganglionic sympathetic fibers arise only from thoracolumbar segments, how do sympathetic signals reach the head and upper limbs? Cervical paravertebral ganglia are supplied by preganglionic fibers that ascend from the upper thoracic cord. The cervical ganglia are named *superior, middle,* and *cervicothoracic* (see Figure 9-7). The cervicothoracic ganglion, often called the *stellate ganglion* because of its star shape, is formed by the fusion of the inferior cervical ganglion and the first thoracic ganglion. Postganglionic fibers from the superior and stellate ganglia innervate arteries of the face, dilate the pupil of the eye, and assist in elevating the upper eyelid. Other fibers from the cervicothoracic ganglion descend with fibers from the middle cervical ganglion to supply the heart and the blood vessels of the upper limb.

The lower lumbar and the sacral paravertebral ganglia are supplied by preganglionic fibers that descend from the upper lumbar cord. Postganglionic neurons from the lower lumbar and parasacral paravertebral ganglia innervate blood vessels in the lower limbs.

### Sympathetic Efferents to Abdominal and Pelvic Organs

The preganglionic sympathetic axons to abdominal and pelvic organs pass through the sympathetic ganglia without synapsing, then synapse in outlying ganglia near the organs (see Figure 9-7, *C*). The preganglionic neurons travel in splanchnic nerves, which are peripheral nerves that innervate the viscera. Sympathetic signals to the gastrointestinal tract slow or stop peristalsis, reduce glandular secretions, and constrict sphincters within the digestive system.

### Functions of the Sympathetic Nervous System

The primary role of the sympathetic nervous system is to maintain optimal blood supply in the organs. Normally, moderate activity of the sympathetic system stimulates smooth muscle in the walls of blood vessels, maintaining some contraction of the vessel walls. Generally, increasing sympathetic activity further constricts the vessels, and decreasing sympathetic activity allows vasodilation. For example, when a person rises from supine to standing, blood pressure needs to be increased to prevent fainting. Firing of certain sympathetic efferents stimulates vasoconstriction in skeletal muscles, thus maintaining blood flow to the brain.

The role of the sympathetic nervous system is often illustrated by describing the physiologic responses to fear. When a person feels threatened, the sympathetic nervous system prepares for vigorous muscle activity, that is, for fight or flight. Vasoconstriction in the skin and gut increases blood flow to active muscles. Blood glucose levels increase, bronchi and coronary vessels dilate, and blood pressure and heart rate increase. Simultaneously, sympathetic firing reduces activity in the digestive system.

### Regulation of Body Temperature

Sympathetic activity regulates body temperature through effects on metabolism and on effectors in the skin. Epinephrine released by the adrenal medulla increases the metabolic rate

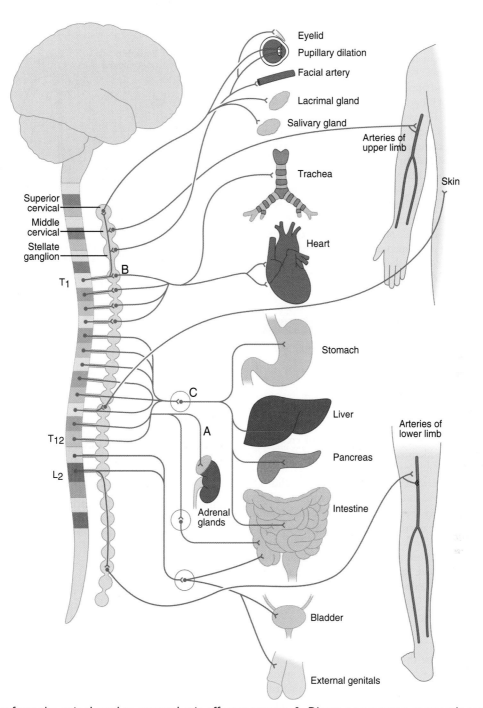

**Fig. 9-7** Efferents from the spinal cord to sympathetic effector organs. **A,** Direct, one-neuron connections to the adrenal medulla. **B,** Two-neuron pathways to the periphery and thoracic viscera, with synapses in paravertebral ganglia. **C,** Two-neuron pathways to the abdominal and pelvic organs, with synapses in outlying ganglia. Note that all sympathetic presynaptic neurons originate in the thoracic cord *(blue)* and the lumbar cord *(pink)*.

throughout the body. In the skin, sympathetic signals control the diameter of the blood vessels, secretion of the sweat glands, and erection of hairs. Blood flow in the skin is controlled by α-adrenergic receptors in the smooth muscles of arterioles. Norepinephrine binding to α-adrenergic receptors in skin arterioles also stimulates precapillary sphincters to contract, forcing blood to bypass the capillaries and decreasing the radiation of heat from the skin. When the precapillary sphincters relax, blood enters the capillaries, and heat radiates from the skin. Sweating also helps dissipate heat. Sweating occurs when adrenergic receptors on sweat glands are activated. In humans, erection of hair cells probably contributes little to the retention of body heat.

## Regulation of Blood Flow in Skeletal Muscle

Control of blood flow in skeletal muscle is more complex than in the skin. Skeletal muscle veins and venules are called *capacitance vessels* because blood pools in these vessels when their walls are relaxed. If pooling of blood in the lower limbs and abdomen is not prevented when a person assumes an upright position, the resulting drop in blood pressure can deprive the brain of adequate blood supply, causing *syncope* (fainting). Normally, the pooling of blood is prevented by vasoconstriction of the capacitance vessels, before the change in position. This is accomplished by the release of norepinephrine to bind with $\alpha$-adrenergic receptors in the walls of skeletal muscle venules and veins, causing vasoconstriction.

Arteriole walls in skeletal muscle contain $\alpha$-adrenergic receptors. The action of norepinephrine on $\alpha$-adrenergic receptors causes vasoconstriction of skeletal muscle arterioles. Local blood chemistry also affects the diameter of arterioles.[7]

> ◎ *Clinical Pearl*
>
> Sympathetic activity constricts arterioles supplying skeletal muscle, skin, and the digestive system.

## Sympathetic Control in the Head

Sympathetic effects on blood flow, sweating, and erection of hair cells of the head are identical to sympathetic actions in the remainder of the body. In addition, sympathetic signals dilate the pupil of the eye and assist in elevating the upper eyelid. The levator palpebrae superioris muscle consists of both smooth and skeletal muscle fibers; only the smooth muscle fibers are innervated by the sympathetic nervous system. The skeletal muscle fibers are innervated by the facial cranial nerve. The sympathetic innervation of the head is shown in Figure 9-8. Sympathetic fibers also innervate salivary glands; their activation causes secretion of thick saliva, which causes a sensation of dryness in the mouth.

## Regulation of the Viscera

Sympathetic effects on the thoracic viscera include increasing heart rate and contractility when $\beta_1$-adrenergic receptors are activated in cardiac muscle and dilation of the bronchial tree when $\beta_2$-adrenergic receptors are activated in the respiratory tract. The distribution of adrenergic receptor types is illustrated in Figure 9-9.

Drugs that bind with a receptor but do not activate the receptor are called *blockers*. Drugs that activate receptors are called *agonists*. $\alpha$-Blockers are used to decrease high blood pressure by blocking the action of norepinephrine on receptors in blood vessels, producing vasodilation. Differences between receptor subtypes (i.e., $\beta_1$ and $\beta_2$) allow the design of drugs that bind with one subtype of receptor and not another. $\beta_1$-Blockers decrease heart rate and contractility without affecting the airways.[8] $\beta_2$-Agonists prevent constriction of the airways and thus are used to treat asthma and chronic obstructive pulmonary disease. However, the heart also has some $\beta_2$ receptors, so $\beta_2$-agonists may cause dangerous side effects on cardiac

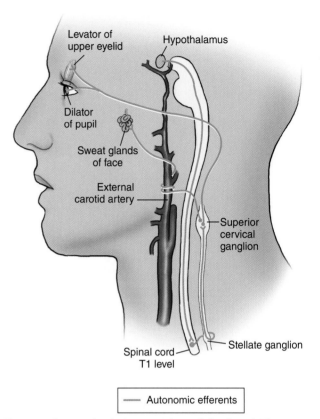

**Fig. 9-8 Sympathetic innervation of the head.** The neural circuit begins in the hypothalamus, then synapses in the upper thoracic spinal cord and the superior cervical ganglion. Axons from the superior cervical ganglion innervate facial sweat glands, the vasculature of the face, the pupillary dilator muscle, the accessory levator muscle of the upper eyelid, and the lacrimal gland.

function; heart ischemia, congestive heart failure, arrhythmias, and sudden death.[9]

In the gastrointestinal tract, sympathetic signals contract sphincters and decrease blood flow, peristalsis, and secretions. Sympathetic stimulation also inhibits contraction of the bladder and bowel walls and contracts internal sphincters.

## Metabolism

When the adrenal medulla releases epinephrine into the bloodstream, the most significant effect is stimulation of metabolism in cells throughout the entire body. Epinephrine release usually coincides with a generalized release of norepinephrine from sympathetic postganglionic neurons because the sympathetic system is often activated as a whole. In addition to its effects on metabolism, epinephrine reinforces the effects of norepinephrine on most target organs.

> ◎ *Clinical Pearl*
>
> The sympathetic nervous system optimizes blood flow to the organs, regulates body temperature and metabolic rate, and regulates the activity of viscera.

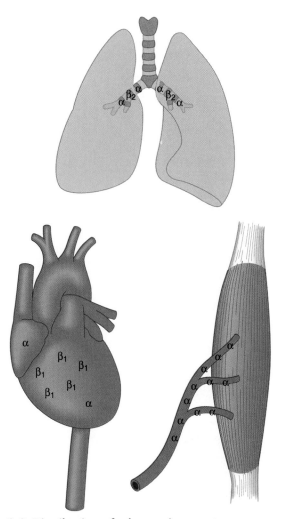

**Fig. 9-9 Distribution of adrenergic receptors.** α-Adrenergic receptors are most abundant in arterioles of peripheral smooth muscle but are also found in the heart and bronchial smooth muscle. $\beta_1$-Adrenergic receptors are found primarily in the heart. $\beta_2$-Adrenergic receptors are most numerous in bronchial smooth muscle. The sympathetic nervous system optimizes blood flow to the organs, regulates body temperature and metabolic rate, and regulates the activity of viscera.

## PARASYMPATHETIC NERVOUS SYSTEM

The parasympathetic nervous system uses a two-neuron pathway from the spinal cord to the effectors. Because preganglionic cell bodies are found in nuclei of the brainstem and the sacral spinal cord, this system is often called the *craniosacral outflow* (Figure 9-10). The ganglia of the parasympathetic nervous system are separate, unlike the interconnected ganglia of the sympathetic trunk. Parasympathetic ganglia are located near or in target organs.

Parasympathetic information from the brainstem travels in cranial nerves to outlying ganglia. Parasympathetic fibers are distributed in cranial nerves III, VII, IX, and X. Fibers in cranial nerve III, the oculomotor nerve, constrict the pupil and increase

the convexity of the lens of the eye for focusing on close objects. Fibers in cranial nerves VII and IX, the facial and glossopharyngeal nerves, innervate salivary glands. Other fibers in cranial nerve VII innervate the lacrimal gland, providing tears to moisten the cornea and for crying. Seventy-five percent of the parasympathetic fibers in cranial nerves travel in cranial nerve X, the vagus nerve.

Parasympathetic fibers arising in the sacral spinal cord have cell bodies in the lateral horn of sacral levels S2-S4. Their axons travel in pelvic splanchnic nerves, distributed to the lower colon, bladder, and external genitalia. In contrast to the sympathetic nervous system, the parasympathetic system does not innervate the limbs or body wall. The sacral parasympathetic efferents regulate emptying of the bowels and bladder and erection of the penis or clitoris. Specific autonomic reflexes are discussed in the context of various regions of the nervous system. For example, reflexive control of the pupil is discussed in Chapter 14, and bladder and bowel reflexes are covered in Chapter 13.

The principal function of the parasympathetic nervous system is energy conservation and storage. Efferent fibers in the vagus nerve innervate the heart and smooth muscle of the lungs and digestive system. Vagus nerve activity to the heart can produce bradycardia (slowing of the heart rate) or decreased cardiac contraction force. Vagus stimulation in the respiratory system causes bronchoconstriction and increases secretion of mucus. In the digestive system, vagus activity increases peristalsis, glycogen synthesis in the liver, and glandular secretions.

---

**◎ Clinical Pearl**

Parasympathetic activity decreases cardiac activity; facilitates digestion; increases secretions in the lungs, eyes, and mouth; controls convexity of the lens in the eye; constricts the pupil; controls voiding of the bowels and bladder; and controls the erection of sexual organs.

---

## COMPARISON OF SYMPATHETIC AND PARASYMPATHETIC FUNCTIONS

In actions on the thoracic and abdominal viscera, the bladder and bowels, and the pupil of the eye, the effects of sympathetic and parasympathetic activity are synergistic: their opposing actions are balanced to provide optimal organ function. For example, immediately before a person begins to exercise, sympathetic signals increase heart rate and contractility, while parasympathetic signals that would slow heart rate decrease. Figure 9-11 illustrates the autonomic areas and pathways that regulate heart rate.

The autonomic efferent systems also have separate, unopposed effects: the sympathetic roles involved in regulating effectors in the limbs, face, and body wall and in assisting elevation of the upper eyelid are not countered by parasympathetic innervation to these effectors. The role of the parasympathetic system in increasing the convexity of the lens of the eye is also unopposed. Tables 9-1 and 9-2 list the actions of the autonomic

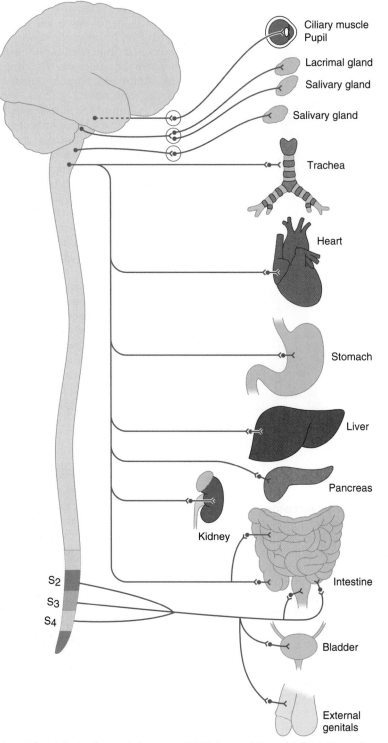

**Fig. 9-10** Parasympathetic outflow through cranial nerves III, VII, IX, and X and S2-S4. Note that all parasympathetic preganglionic neurons originate in the brainstem or the sacral spinal cord.

**TABLE 9-1**  EFFECT OF SYMPATHETIC ACTIVITY ON BLOOD VESSELS

| Organ | Neurochemical | Receptor | Effect on Vessel Wall | Purpose |
|---|---|---|---|---|
| Skin | Adrenergic | $\alpha$ | Vasoconstriction of arterioles | ↓ Radiation of heat from skin |
| Skeletal muscle | Adrenergic | $\alpha$ | Vasoconstriction of venules and veins | ↑ Peripheral vascular resistance<br>↑ Blood pressure |
| Heart | Adrenergic | $\beta_1$ | Dilation | More blood available to the heart |

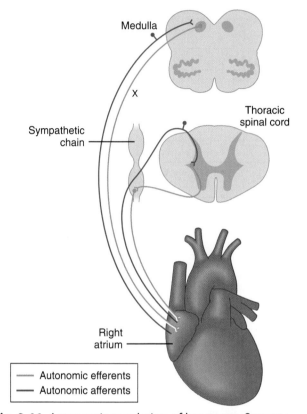

**Fig. 9-11** Autonomic regulation of heart rate. Sensory information enters both the medulla and the spinal cord. Regulation is achieved by parasympathetic fibers in the vagus nerve and by sympathetic fibers from the thoracic spinal cord.

efferent systems. Table 9-3 and Figure 9-12 summarize the distribution of neurotransmitters and receptors in the autonomic efferent systems.

## CLINICAL CORRELATIONS

### Horner's Syndrome

If a lesion affects the sympathetic pathway to the head, sympathetic activity on one side of the head is decreased. This leads to ipsilateral drooping of the upper eyelid, constriction of the pupil, and skin vasodilation, with absence of sweating on the ipsilateral face and neck. This constellation of signs is called *Horner's syndrome* (Figure 9-13) and occurs with lesions of the descending sympathetic tract, upper thoracic spinal cord,

brachial plexus, or cervical sympathetic chain (see Figure 9-8). Interruption of blood supply, trauma, tumor, cluster headache, or stellate ganglion block may cause Horner's syndrome.[10,11] Cluster headache is a severe headache on one side of the head that lasts a few minutes to 3 hours and occurs as a series of headaches.

In early stage complex regional pain syndrome, the stellate ganglion is sometimes therapeutically blocked to temporarily decrease pain in the upper limb,[12] allowing occupational and physical therapy to be more effective. The sympathetic ganglion block decreases adrenergic excitation of sensitized nociceptors in the upper limb with CRPS.[13] Horner's syndrome is a side effect of the block, because the ascending neurons in the cervical ganglia are temporarily prevented from depolarizing.

### Peripheral Region

If a peripheral nerve is severed, interruption of sympathetic efferents causes loss of vascular control, temperature regulation, and sweating in the region supplied by the peripheral nerve. These losses may lead to trophic changes in the skin.

### Spinal Region

A complete spinal cord lesion interrupts all communication between the cord below the lesion and the brain, disrupting ascending and descending autonomic signals at the level of the lesion. The severity of autonomic dysfunction depends on how much of the cord is isolated from the brain. Lower-level lesions allow the brain to influence more of the cord; higher-level lesions isolate more of the cord. Complete lesions above the lumbar level obstruct voluntary control of bladder, bowel, and genital function. Complete lesions above the midthoracic level isolate much of the cord from control by the brain, jeopardizing homeostasis by interfering with blood pressure regulation and the ability to adjust core body temperature. The autonomic consequences of spinal cord injury are discussed more fully in Chapter 13.

### Brainstem Region

Lesions in the brainstem region may interfere with descending control of heart rate, blood pressure, and respiration. Brainstem lesions may also affect cranial nerve nuclei, interfering with constriction of the pupil, production of tears, salivation, or regulation of thoracic and abdominal viscera.

### Cerebral Region

Damage to certain nuclei in the hypothalamus disrupts homeostasis, with consequent metabolic and behavioral dysfunctions. Obesity, anorexia, hyperthermia, hypothermia, and

**TABLE 9-2    COMPARISON OF SYMPATHETIC AND PARASYMPATHETIC EFFECTS ON ORGAN FUNCTION**

| Organ | Function | Sympathetic Effect | Parasympathetic Effect |
|---|---|---|---|
| Eye | Diameter of pupil | ↑ | ↓ |
| | Curvature of lens | | ↑ |
| Heart | Contraction rate | ↑ | ↓ |
| | Force of contraction | ↑ | |
| Blood vessels | See Table 9-1 | | |
| Lungs | Diameter of bronchi | ↑ | ↓ |
| | Diameter of blood vessels | ↑ | |
| | Secretions | | ↑ |
| Sweat glands | Production of sweat | ↑ | |
| Salivary glands | Thick secretion | ↑ | |
| | Thin, profuse secretion | | ↑ |
| Lacrimal glands | Production of tears | | ↑ |
| | Vasomotor to blood vessels in lacrimal gland | ↑ | |
| Adrenal medulla | Secretion of epinephrine | ↑ | |
| Gastrointestinal tract | Peristalsis | ↓ | ↑ |
| | Secretions | ↓ | ↑ |
| Liver | Glucose release | ↑ | |
| | Glycogen synthesis | | ↑ |
| Pancreas | Secretions | ↓ | ↑ |
| Bowel and bladder | Emptying | ↓ | ↑ |
| External genitalia | Erection of penis or clitoris | | ↑ |

**TABLE 9-3    NEUROCHEMICALS AND RECEPTORS IN THE AUTONOMIC NERVOUS SYSTEM***

| Neurochemical | Site of Neurochemical Release | Receptor Type |
|---|---|---|
| Acetylcholine | Synapse between preganglionic and postganglionic neurons (both sympathetic and parasympathetic) | Nicotinic |
| | Parasympathetic postganglionic to smooth muscles and glands | Muscarinic |
| Norepinephrine | Sympathetic postganglionic to constrict blood vessels in skeletal muscles, skin, and viscera, and to dilate pupil | α |
| | Sympathetic postganglionic to dilate bronchi, decrease gastrointestinal activity, accelerate heart rate | β |
| Epinephrine | Adrenal medulla: release transmitter into bloodstream | α and β |

*Norepinephrine has a greater effect on α-adrenergic receptors than on β; epinephrine is equally effective in activating both α and β.

emotional displays dissociated from feelings can occur. Activity in other limbic (emotional) areas can also interfere with homeostasis. For example, the response to perceived threat includes sympathetic activity that increases blood flow to skeletal muscles by accelerating cardiac rate, strengthening cardiac contraction, and decreasing blood flow to skin, kidneys, and digestive tract.

## Syncope

*Syncope* (fainting) is a brief loss of consciousness due to inadequate blood flow to the brain. If the cause of the syncope is powerful emotions, the attack is called *vasodepressor syncope* or

*neurogenic shock.* Strong emotion can initiate sudden, active vasodilation of intramuscular arterioles, causing a precipitous fall in blood pressure. Blood flow to the head is temporarily reduced, leading to loss of consciousness and paleness of the face. Blood flow to the head is restored when the person is horizontal.

In some cases, particularly when syncope occurs in response to painful stimuli or on standing after prolonged bed rest, vagal stimulation to the heart follows the intramuscular vasodilation. Vagal activity slows the heart, further decreasing blood pressure, and elicits nausea, salivation, and increased perspiration. When vagal signs occur with vasodepressor syncope, called a *vasovagal attack,* excessive activity is occurring in both the sympathetic and parasympathetic systems.[14]

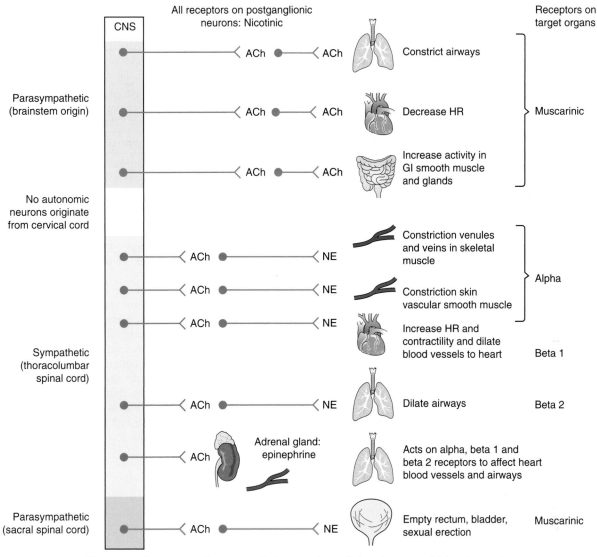

**Fig. 9-12** Summary of autonomic innervation of the viscera and blood vessels.

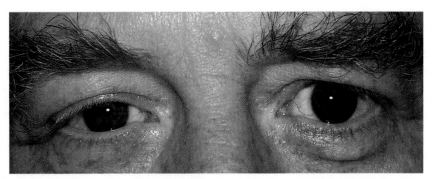

**Fig. 9-13** Horner's syndrome affecting the right side of the face. A lesion of the sympathetic pathway (illustrated in Figure 9-8) to the face results in a drooping eyelid, pupil constriction, and dry, red skin of the face. Normally, activity in this sympathetic pathway dilates the pupil, constricts blood vessels in the face, activates sweat glands of the face and neck, and assists the levator palpebrae muscle in elevating the upper eyelid. *(From Parsons M, Johnson M: Diagnosis in color: neurology, Edinburgh, 2001, Mosby.)*

**TABLE 9-4**   NORMAL RESPONSE TO THE VALSALVA TEST

| Phase | Event | Mechanism |
|---|---|---|
| 1 | Start: 1 to 3 second increase in blood pressure | Mechanical compression of great vessels |
| 2 | Early: systolic and pulse pressures decline<br>Late: BP recovery, HR increase | Peripheral venous pressure increases<br>Peripheral sympathetic vasoconstriction; autonomic increase in heart rate and heart contractility |
| 3 | Pressure release: 1 to 3 second fall in BP | Release of mechanical compression increases venous return |
| 4 | Sustained BP overshoot | Increased stroke volume forced into a constricted arterial system causes increased arterial pressure |

Adapted from Weimer LH: Autonomic testing: common techniques and clinical applications. *The Neurologist* 16:215–222, 2010.

Although vasodepressor syncope is the most common type of syncope, many different causes can produce syncope. As mentioned earlier in this chapter, assuming an upright posture can cause pooling of blood in the lower body, resulting in syncope. Other causes include insufficient cardiac output, hypoxia, and hypoglycemia.

### Orthostatic Hypotension

*Orthostatic hypotension* is a decrease of at least 20 mm Hg systolic blood pressure or 10 mm Hg diastolic pressure during the first 3 minutes of standing. The mechanism is a gravity-induced pooling of blood in the lower limbs, compromising venous return and cardiac output that cause a decrease in arterial pressure. Normally the baroreceptor reflex compensates for the blood pressure drop by eliciting lower extremity vasoconstriction. Symptoms of orthostatic hypotension include dizziness, lightheadedness, feeling as if about to faint, and fainting. A decreased amount of blood in the body from bleeding, drugs (most commonly vasodilators or diuretics), or dehydration can cause orthostatic hypotension.

Neurogenic orthostatic hypotension occurs in people with spinal cord disorders, autonomic degenerative disorders, and peripheral neuropathies. In spinal cord disorders, interruption of signals descending from the medulla to sympathetic preganglionic neurons prevents the vasomotor center from triggering vasoconstriction. In autonomic degenerative disorders, nervous system disease damages the sympathetic nervous system. Autonomic degenerative disorders include pure autonomic failure, Parkinson's disease, and Parkinson-Plus diseases (discussed in Chapter 11). Peripheral neuropathies are dysfunctions of the peripheral nerves that interfere with signals from the spinal cord to target organs including blood vessels. Peripheral neuropathy can cause orthostatic hypotension in people with diabetes, alcoholism, exposure to toxins, high levels of urea in the blood due to kidney failure, and nutritional deficiencies.

### Tests of Autonomic Function

The ability of the sympathetic nervous system to regulate blood pressure can be evaluated by measuring the person's blood pressure in the supine position, having the person stand, and measuring the blood pressure 2 minutes later. Abnormal responses include a drop of more than 30 mm Hg in systolic blood pressure or more than 15 mm Hg in diastolic blood pressure.

Sympathetic regulation of the skin can be tested by the sweat test or the hand vasomotor test. For the sweat test, sweat is absorbed by small pieces of filter paper placed on the skin, and then the filter paper is weighed to determine the amount of sweat. For the vasomotor test, skin temperature is measured before and after the hands are immersed in cold water. This test is used to assess the amount of vasoconstriction.

The *Valsalva test* provides information on both sympathetic and parasympathetic function. The subject blows into a closed tube that has a small leak for 30 seconds, maintaining 40 mm Hg pressure. The test has four phases listed in Table 9-4.

## SUMMARY

The autonomic nervous system regulates circulation, respiration, digestion, metabolism, secretions, body temperature, and reproduction. Receptors include mechanoreceptors, chemoreceptors, nociceptors, and thermoreceptors. Signals from the receptors travel via spinal nerves and cranial nerves VII, IX, and X into the central nervous system. Areas within the medulla and pons regulate vital functions (heart rate, respiration, and blood flow). The hypothalamus serves as the master controller of homeostasis via actions on the pituitary, brainstem centers, and the spinal cord.

The efferent pathways of the autonomic system are the sympathetic and parasympathetic systems. The sympathetic system regulates cardiac muscle, blood vessels, viscera, and sweat glands by activating adrenergic receptors on effectors. Sympathetic outflow arises in spinal segments T1-L2. Control of sympathetic functions in the head and neck is attained via cephalic extension of the sympathetic chain into the stellate, middle cervical, and superior cervical ganglia. Control of lower limb vasculature occurs via the caudal extension of the sympathetic ganglia. The parasympathetic nervous system regulates glands, viscera cardiac muscle and external genitalia via muscarinic receptors on effectors. Parasympathetic outflow is provided through cranial nerves III, VII, IX, and X, and spinal cord segments S2-S4.

## CLINICAL NOTES

### Case 1

R.D. is a 23-year-old professional basketball player. While waiting to play in a championship game, he collapsed on the sidelines. His pulse could not be palpated, his blood pressure was 60/45 mm Hg, breathing was almost imperceptible, his pupils were dilated, and his face was pale. He was unconscious for about 15 seconds; then color began to return to his face, and his breathing and pulse quickly returned to normal. R.D. regained his awareness of the environment on regaining consciousness. He reported feeling fine, although he felt weak; no headache or confusion followed the attack.

#### Question

What is the most likely diagnosis?

### Case 2

B.H., a 47-year-old man, had a myocardial infarction 3 weeks ago. He has been referred to physical therapy for cardiac rehabilitation. He is taking propranolol, a β-blocker.

#### Questions

1. What effect does blocking β-adrenergic receptors have on cardiovascular function?
2. Given that aerobic exercise prescriptions are based on a percentage of predicted age-related maximal heart rate, how will the β-blocker effects impact your exercise prescription?

## REVIEW QUESTIONS

1. As a cardiac rehabilitation client begins treadmill exercise, which of his visceral and vascular sensory receptors would register changes? To what stimuli would the receptors be responding?
2. What is the function of visceral afferents?
3. What areas of the brain directly control autonomic function? What areas modulate activity in the autonomic control centers?
4. What are the differences between the autonomic and somatic efferent systems?
5. What are the sympathetic trunks? How do sympathetic fibers that leave the paravertebral ganglia reach effectors in the periphery, for example, blood vessels in skeletal muscle and in the skin?
6. What are splanchnic nerves?
7. What is the primary function of the sympathetic nervous system?
8. What are capacitance vessels, and what is their significance? How is the blood flow in skeletal muscle arterioles controlled?
9. What would happen if the sympathetic fibers to the levator palpebrae superioris muscle and the pupil of the eye did not function?
10. What functions does the sympathetic nervous system regulate?
11. What functions are controlled by the parasympathetic nervous system?
12. A patient with CRPS (complex regional pain syndrome; see Chapter 8) arrives for an appointment with the following signs affecting the left side of the face: bright red dry skin, drooping of the eyelid, and a constricted pupil. What is your interpretation of these signs?

## References

1. Morgane PJ, Galler JR, Mokler DJ: A review of systems and networks of the limbic forebrain/limbic midbrain. *Prog Neurobiol* 75:143–160, 2005.
2. Holzer P, Schicho R, Holzer-Petsche U, Lippe IT: The gut as a neurological organ. *Wien Klin Wochenschr* 113:647–660, 2001.
3. Trimmel M, Wittberger S: Effects of transdermally administered nicotine on aspects of attention, task load, and mood in women and men. *Pharmacol Biochem Behav* 78:639–645, 2004.
4. Sharma G, Vijayaraghavan S: Nicotinic receptors: role in addiction and other disorders of the brain. *Subst Abuse* 2008:81, 2008.
5. Hahn B, Ross TJ, Wolkenberg FA, et al: Performance effects of nicotine during selective attention, divided attention, and simple stimulus detection: an fMRI study. *Cereb Cortex* 19:1990–2000, 2009.
6. File SE, Fluck E, Leahy A: Nicotine has calming effects on stress-induced mood changes in females, but enhances aggressive mood in males. *Int J Neuropsychopharmacol* 4:371–376, 2001.
7. Thomas GD, Segal SS: Neural control of muscle blood flow during exercise. *J Appl Physiol* 97:731–738, 2004.

8. Salpeter SR, Ormiston TM, Salpeter EE, et al: Cardioselective beta-blockers for chronic obstructive pulmonary disease: a meta-analysis. *Respir Med* 97:1094–1101, 2003.

9. Salpeter SR, Ormiston TM, Salpeter EE: Cardiovascular effects of beta-agonists in patients with asthma and COPD: a meta-analysis. *Chest* 125:2309–2321, 2004.

10. Almog Y, Gepstein, R, Kesler A: Diagnostic value of imaging in Horner syndrome in adults. *J Neuroophthalmol* 30:7–11, 2010.

11. George A, Haydar AA, Adams WM: Imaging of Horner's syndrome. *Clin Radiol* 63:499–505, 2008.

12. Drummond PD: Sensory disturbances in complex regional pain syndrome: clinical observations, autonomic interactions, and possible mechanisms. *Pain Med* 11(8):1257–1266, 2010.

13. Yucel I, Demiraran Y, Ozturan K, Degirmenci E: Complex regional pain syndrome type I: efficacy of stellate ganglion blockade. *J Orthop Traumatol* 10(4):179–183, 2009.

14. Tan MP, Duncan GW, Parry SW: Head-up tilt table testing: a state-of-the-art review. *Minerva Med* 100:329–338, 2009.

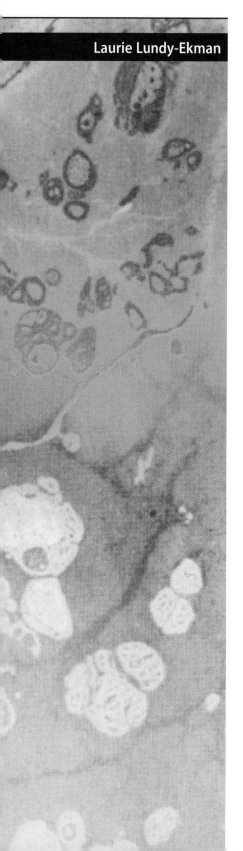

# 10 The Motor System: Motor Neurons

Laurie Lundy-Ekman

On July 4, almost 2 years ago, I had served a brunch for family and friends. Everything seemed fine. After our guests left, my husband found me collapsed on the floor. I don't remember anything about July that year. An aneurysm burst and took away some parts of my life. I had surgery to repair the aneurysm on July 5 and another surgery on August 3 to insert a shunt. I remember things since the second surgery. I had 3 weeks of rehabilitation in the hospital and then physical and occupational therapy twice a week for almost a year.

Now my movements are still too slow; everything takes me twice as long as before. I can't move my right foot, so I wear a brace to keep from turning my ankle or tripping. I used to bicycle long distances. Now I can't bicycle independently, so I ride a tandem bicycle. I can move my right arm from the wrist up but can't move my right hand. Writing is almost impossible because I was right-handed. I can type on the computer keyboard using my left hand only. Cooking takes me a long time, and I have trouble lifting things out of the oven. I enjoy traveling, but it's hard to get around in other countries. Many places don't have stair railings, and that makes it tough to go up or down stairs. I have minimal problems with language; my mouth works slower, and sometimes I forget parts of what I want to say.

I've made a lot of progress since the aneurysm burst. At first I could barely speak; trying to figure out the words was too difficult. I had to use a wheelchair because my balance was so bad. Now I can walk long distances, and I am completely independent.

In therapy we worked on walking, strengthening, balance, and stretching. I used an electrical stimulator to help contract the muscles that lift the front of the foot up, but that didn't seem to help. I haven't taken any medications for my condition.

—*Jane Lebens*

**An aneurysm is a balloon-like swelling of a weak section of an arterial wall. Because the wall of an aneurysm is stretched thin, aneurysms tend to rupture. Bleeding from a burst aneurysm in the brain is one of the causes of stroke. In Jane's case, the stroke affected the left middle cerebral artery, which supplies blood to the somatosensory and motor areas of the left cerebral cortex. The stroke killed neurons that communicate with the right side of the body and lower face, thus she has permanent paralysis of the right hand and foot and weakness that affects the muscles she can voluntarily contract on the right side of the body. The left middle cerebral artery also supplies the cortical area that processes language in right-handed people. Because many neurons in the language area survived, once extravascular blood and damaged tissue were removed during the healing process, most of her language skills returned. This chapter covers the motor neurons that control contraction of skeletal muscles; language is discussed in Chapters 17 and 18.**

Every action we perform requires the motor system. Movement—which allows us to read, talk, walk, prepare dinner, and play musical instruments—is orchestrated by the coordinated action of the peripheral, spinal, brainstem/cerebellar, and cerebral regions, shaped by a specific context, and directed by our intentions. Consider how movement strategies change when we walk on an icy sidewalk: our cadence, step length, and posture adjust to the differences. A young child may choose to sit and scoot rather than risk falling. We select these alternatives based on sensory information. As we saw in the example of Rothwell's patient (severe peripheral neuropathy, Chapter 7), normal motor performance and sensation are interdependent. Sensory information required varies with the task and is often used to prepare for movement, in addition to providing information during and after movement.

## SENSORY CONTRIBUTION TO MOVEMENT CONTROL

The anticipatory use of sensory information to prepare for movement is referred to as *feedforward*. An example of feedforward is the increase in hamstring activity before joint loading in people who have had an anterior cruciate ligament rupture.[1] Increased hamstring contraction prevents anterior tibial translation during acceptance of the load. *Feedback* is the use of sensory information during or after movement to make corrections to the ongoing movement or to future movements. Feedback from proprioceptors, skin, vision, hearing, and vestibular receptors continually adapts walking to environmental constraints.[2]

Somatosensory information is important for motor learning. Disrupting somatosensory cortex function by repetitive transcranial magnetic stimulation (rTMS) over the somatosensory cortex impairs motor learning.[3]

Proprioceptive information is analyzed to predict interaction torques and to plan synchronization of multijoint movements. In people with normal nervous systems, joint movements are synchronized and the kinematics of most movements is the same, regardless of whether the movements are performed slowly, at natural speed, or quickly. In people with complete loss of somatosensation below the neck, joint movements are not well synchronized, and fast movements are decomposed. In movement decomposition, only one joint is moved at a time, to simplify control by eliminating interaction torques. For example, the person will keep the elbow joint in a fixed position and will move only the shoulder.[4]

Well-learned movements, including walking, eating, and driving, normally require little conscious attention. The smoothness of these practiced movements is remarkable, given the complexity of simultaneously coordinating the interacting torques produced by muscle actions with environmental conditions. The seeming effortlessness of automatic movement requires continuous integration of visual, somatosensory, and vestibular information with motor processing.

Loss of any of the three senses integral to automatic movement interferes with ease and gracefulness. In the absence of vision, the act of reaching depends on somatosensation and proprioception to locate objects. Compared with visually guided reaching, movements without vision require more time and are less accurate. Loss of somatosensation in people with complete deafferentation disrupts positioning of limbs.[5]

Complete, bilateral vestibular loss interferes with balance, yet visual or touch information from a stable surface can significantly improve balance despite complete absence of vestibular information.[6] Smooth, accurate movement requires visual, somatosensory, and gravitational information.

## PATIENT-CONTROLLED MOVEMENTS

My first experience as a therapist teaching wheelchair-to-car transfers to a person with quadriplegia (C7 level; complete paralysis below shoulder level except for the biceps brachii) underscores the complexity of movement. Despite my attempt to instruct him, he didn't move from the wheelchair. He asked if he could try it his way, so I guarded as he placed his forehead on the dashboard, threw his forearm onto the roof using biceps brachii, momentum, and gravity, and then, by contracting neck and elbow flexors, lifted himself into the car. Paralysis prevented a conventional car transfer, but he used biomechanics and environmental resources to solve the movement problem. As in most normal movements, he initiated and controlled the action; the movement was not in response to any external stimulus.

## THE MOTOR SYSTEM

Even a simple motor act, such as picking up a pen, involves a complex sequence of events (Figure 10-1). Neural activity begins with a decision made in the anterior part of the frontal lobe. Next, motor planning areas are activated, followed by control circuits. Control circuits, consisting of the cerebellum and the basal ganglia, regulate the activity in upper motor neuron tracts. Upper motor neuron tracts deliver signals to spinal interneurons and lower motor neurons. Lower motor neurons transmit signals directly to skeletal muscles, eliciting contraction of muscle fibers that move the upper limb and fingers.

Voluntary movement is controlled from the top down (brain to spinal cord to muscle). However, because understanding the function of higher levels depends on knowledge of lower levels, the following discussion begins with lower levels and progresses to higher levels of the nervous system.

In the spinal cord, interactions among neurons determine the information conveyed by lower motor neurons (LMNs) to muscles. Descending upper motor neuron (UMN) tracts deliver movement information from the brain to motor neurons in the spinal cord or brainstem. UMN tracts are classified as postural/gross movement tracts, fine movement tracts, and nonspecific tracts. Postural/gross movement tracts control automatic skeletal muscle activity, fine movement tracts control fractionated movements of the limbs and face, and nonspecific UMNs facilitate all motor neurons. Fractionated movements are independent contractions of single muscles. Fractionated movements allow us to flex only the index finger when typing or playing the piano, without the other fingers simultaneously flexing, and to target specific muscle groups when weight lifting.

The control circuits adjust activity in the descending tracts, resulting in excitation or inhibition of motor neurons. Thus, control circuits partially determine muscle contraction. In all

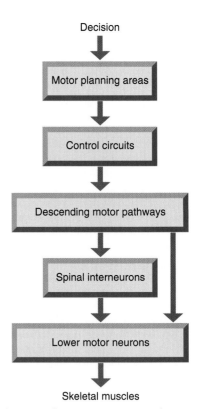

**Fig. 10-1** The neural structures required to produce normal movements. Although sensory information influences each of the neural structures involved in generating movements, the sensory connections have been omitted for simplicity.

regions of the central nervous system, sensory information adjusts motor activity. Therefore, the contribution of sensation to movement will be covered with each motor section.

> **◎ Clinical Pearl**
>
> Lower motor neurons have their cell bodies in the spinal cord or brainstem and synapse with skeletal muscle fibers. Synapses in the spinal cord or brainstem determine the activity of lower motor neurons. In contrast, UMNs arise in the cerebral cortex or brainstem, and their axons travel in descending tracts to synapse with lower motor neurons and/or interneurons in the brainstem or spinal cord. Control circuits adjust the activity of the upper motor neurons.

## SKELETAL MUSCLE STRUCTURE AND FUNCTION

Skeletal muscle is excitable, contractile, extensile, and elastic. To understand these properties, the structure and function of skeletal muscle must be considered. The membrane of a muscle cell has projections that extend into the muscle, called *T (transverse) tubules*. Adjacent to the T tubules is the sarcoplasmic reticulum, a series of storage sacs for $Ca^{2+}$ ions. When

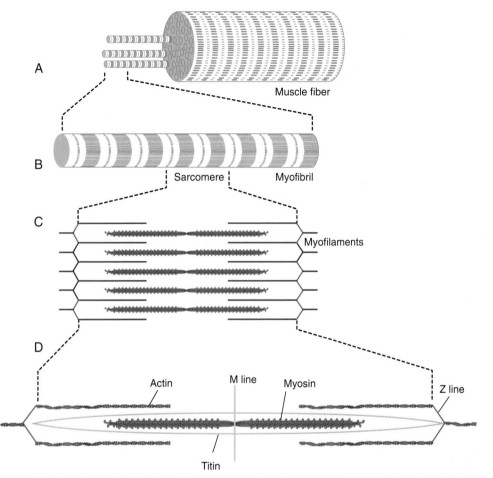

**Fig. 10-2** **Structure of skeletal muscle. A,** Muscle fiber, consisting of many myofibrils. **B,** Myofibril. The section of a myofibril between two Z lines is a sarcomere. **C,** Sarcomere. A sarcomere is composed of myofilaments, including actin and myosin. **D,** Proteins in a sarcomere. Actin is the thin filament, attached to the Z line. Myosin is the thick filament, attached to the M line. Titin is the elastic filament that anchors the M line to the Z line.

acetylcholine (ACh) from an LMN binds with receptors on the muscle membrane, the membrane depolarizes, inducing depolarization of the T tubules. This change in electrical potential elicits the release of $Ca^{2+}$ ions from their storage sacs in the sarcoplasmic reticulum. The $Ca^{2+}$ ions bind to receptors inside muscle fibers, initiating muscle contraction.

Individual muscle fibers consist of *myofibrils* arranged parallel to the long axis of the muscle fiber (Figure 10-2). Myofibrils consist of proteins arranged in *sarcomeres*. Sarcomeres are the functional units of muscle. Sarcomeres are composed of two types of proteins: structural and contractile. Proteins that provide structure to the sarcomere include the Z line, M line, and titin. The Z line is a fibrous structure at each end of the sarcomere. The M line anchors the fibers in the center of the sarcomere. Titin, a large elastic protein in muscle, connects the Z line with the M line. Titin maintains the position of myosin relative to actin and prevents the sarcomere from being pulled apart (Figure 10-3).

Myosin, actin, tropomyosin, and troponin are the proteins involved in muscle contraction. Myosin filaments have specialized projections called *cross-bridges,* ending in myosin heads. These heads are capable of binding with active sites on actin.

Actin filaments are anchored at each end of the sarcomere to Z lines.

## Contraction

Muscle contraction is produced when actin slides relative to myosin. This sliding is initiated when $Ca^{2+}$ binds to troponin, and a conformational change in troponin induces movement of the tropomyosin to uncover active sites on actin. This allows myosin heads to attach to these exposed active sites (Figure 10-4). Then the myosin heads swivel, pulling actin toward the center of the sarcomere. Repeated attachment, swiveling, and detachment of myosin heads produces contraction of the muscle (Figure 10-5).

## Total Muscle Resistance to Stretch

Muscles behave somewhat like springs: the resistance to stretch muscles generated depends on their length. A stretched spring generates more resistance to stretch than the same spring when it is shortened. Active contraction, titin, and weak actin-myosin bonds determine the total resistance to muscle stretch

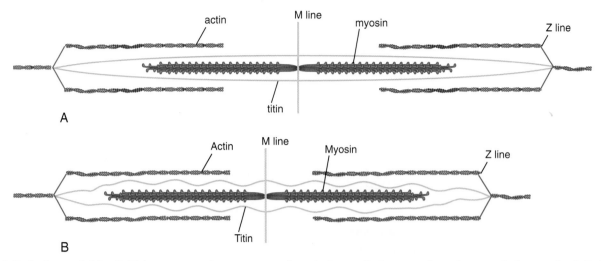

**Fig. 10-3  Actions of titin. A,** Titin prevents the sarcomere from being pulled apart when the muscle is stretched. **B,** At normal sarcomere lengths, titin maintains the position of myosin in the center of the sarcomere.

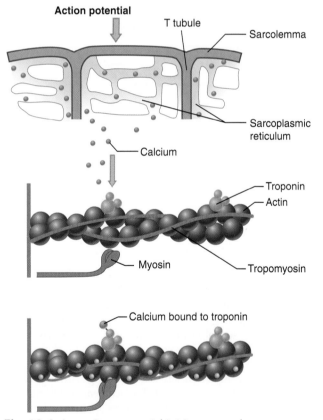

**Fig. 10-4** An action potential initiates muscle contraction. When an action potential depolarizes the muscle membrane, the depolarization spreads to the T tubules. This causes the sarcoplasmic reticulum to release $Ca^{2+}$ into the sarcoplasm. The $Ca^{2+}$ binds to troponin, and the tropomyosin moves to expose binding sites on actin. Myosin cross-bridges bind to the sites on actin.

(Figures 10-6 and 10-7). Weak actin-myosin bonds are discussed in the next section.

## Muscle Tone: Resistance to Passive Stretch

Muscle tone is the resistance to stretch in resting muscle. Clinically, passive range of motion is used to assess muscle tone. When muscle tone is normal, resistance to passive stretch is minimal. Normal resting muscle tone is provided by titin and weak actin-myosin bonds.

Weak actin-myosin bonds are formed when myosin attaches to actin but the myosin heads do not swivel, so there is no power stroke. Thus no muscle contraction occurs, yet mild resistance to stretch is generated by these bonds (Figure 10-8). This weak binding between actin and myosin is somewhat similar to loosely attached Velcro strips, where relatively little force is required to separate the strips. In the relaxed state, when muscles are stretched slowly, individual cross-bridges detach before generating large resistance to stretch. However, during fast stretches, cross-bridges do not have the opportunity to detach, making the muscle more resistant to stretch.[7] An example is the hamstring tightness experienced when one stands up after prolonged sitting on an airplane. If a muscle remains immobile, weak actin-myosin bonds continually form; these bonds are easily broken by stretching the muscle. Even in people with intact neuromuscular systems, resistance to stretch of forearm muscles increases significantly during a few minutes of rest,[8] owing to weak actin-myosin bonds. Thus, if a muscle is stretched following a prolonged period of immobility, the resistance of the muscle to stretch is increased. Also, in normally innervated muscle, resistance to stretch increases briefly following a prolonged contraction. Weak actin-myosin bonds are an important factor in standing ankle stability.[9] In relaxed standing, humans rely primarily on loading of the skeleton, ligamentous structures, titin, and weak actin-myosin bonds; muscles are only slightly active or become active intermittently when sway exceeds tolerable limits.[10]

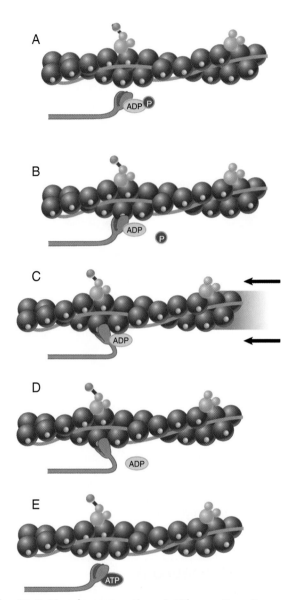

**Fig. 10-5 Muscle contraction. A,** When active sites are exposed on actin, the myosin head is activated by splitting of the attached ATP into ADP + P (i.e., adenosine triphosphate → adenosine diphosphate and phosphate). **B,** The myosin head binds to actin, and P is released from the myosin head. **C,** The cross-bridge swivels, causing the actin to slide relative to the myosin. **D,** ADP detaches from the myosin head. **E,** A new ATP molecule binds to the myosin head, breaking the bond with actin.

Healthy muscle resistance to stretch has frequently been attributed to stretch reflexes and connective tissue. A stretch reflex is muscle contraction elicited by stretch of the spindle. However, the minimal change in muscle membrane electrical activity during slow stretch of relaxed muscle[14] eliminates reflexes as a possible contributor to resting muscle tone, because if the muscle membrane is not depolarizing, the muscle does not contract.

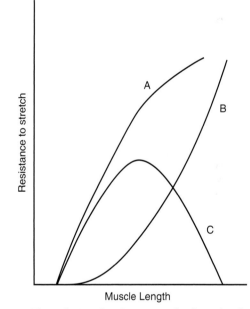

**Fig. 10-6** The relationship between the length of a muscle and the resistance to stretch generated by the muscle. A, Total resistance. B, Weak actin-myosin bonds and titin. C, Active contraction.

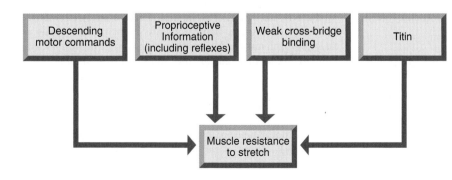

**Fig. 10-7** Summary of factors that contribute to muscle resistance to stretch.

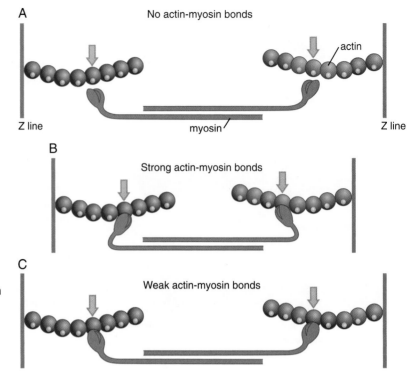

**Fig. 10-8 Actin and myosin bonds. A,** Actin and myosin are dissociated (no actin-myosin bonds). **B,** Strong bonds between actin and myosin. When a strong bond is formed, the myosin heads swivel, pulling the actin (and the attached Z lines) closer together. This active contraction shortens the sarcomere. **C,** Weak actin-myosin bonds. Actin and myosin are attached, but because the myosin heads do not swivel, the sarcomere length is unchanged. However, a muscle with many weak actin-myosin bonds will produce greater resistance to stretch than a muscle with fewer actin-myosin bonds.

## Number of Sarcomeres Adapts to Muscle Length

When healthy, innervated muscle is continuously immobilized in a shortened position for a prolonged period of time, sarcomeres disappear from the ends of myofibrils. For example, if the elbow is maintained at 90 degrees of flexion by a cast for 2 months, the biceps will lose sarcomeres. Figures 10-9 and 10-10 illustrate contracture, the changes in muscle structure that occur secondary to prolonged muscle shortening. This loss of sarcomeres is a structural adaptation to the shortened position,[11] so that the muscle can generate optimal force at the new resting length. When a structurally shortened muscle is stretched, it will quickly reach the limits of its elasticity and therefore will be very resistant to stretch, that is, the decreased amount of titin available to be stretched will limit the extensibility of the muscle. Conversely, if muscle is immobilized in a lengthened position, the muscle will add new sarcomeres.[12] Chronic loading of muscle, as in physical training, stimulates mechanoreceptors that switch on genes for producing collagen and extracellular matrix to improve the muscle's tensile strength.[13]

## Joint Resistance to Movement and Cocontraction

Both elastic and contractile forces of muscles that act on a joint determine the joint's resistance to movement. This resistance can be increased by *cocontraction,* the simultaneous contraction of antagonist muscles. Cocontraction stabilizes joints. In the upper limbs, this enables precise movements. An example is threading a needle. In the lower limbs, cocontraction allows a person to stand on an unstable surface, as on the deck of a ship or a moving bus. People frequently use cocontraction when learning a new movement skill.[15]

## LOWER MOTOR NEURONS

Lower motor neurons are the only neurons that convey signals to extrafusal and intrafusal skeletal muscle fibers. There are two types of lower motor neurons: alpha and gamma. Both types have cell bodies in the ventral horn of the spinal cord. Their axons leave the spinal cord via the ventral root, travel through the spinal nerve, and then travel through the peripheral nerve to reach skeletal muscle.

### Alpha Motor Neurons

Alpha motor neurons have large cell bodies and large, myelinated axons. The axons of alpha motor neurons project to extrafusal skeletal muscle, branching into numerous terminals as they approach muscle. Normally an alpha motor neuron releases enough ACh that all of the muscle fibers it innervates contract.

### Gamma Motor Neurons

Gamma motor neurons have medium-sized myelinated axons (Table 10-1). Axons of gamma motor neurons project to intrafusal fibers in the muscle spindle (see Chapter 6).

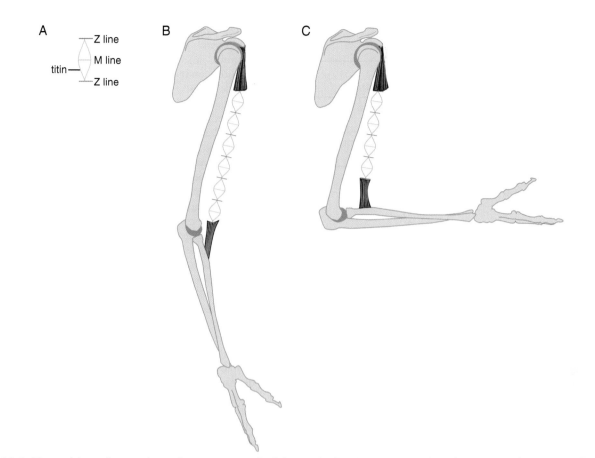

**Fig. 10-9 Normal-length muscle and contracture. A,** Schematic drawing representing the structural proteins of a sarcomere. **B,** A muscle of normal length, represented by six sarcomeres. This muscle can easily be stretched to achieve full range of motion at the joint. **C,** Contracture, structurally shortened muscle, represented by four sarcomeres. This muscle cannot be stretched to a full range of motion without rupturing.

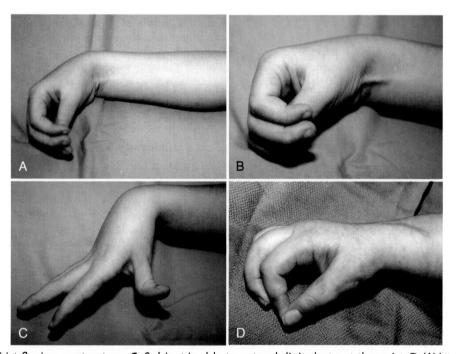

**Fig. 10-10 A–C** Wrist flexion contracture. **C,** Subject is able to extend digits but not the wrist. **D,** Wrist extension post surgery. *(From Canale ST, Beaty JH. Campbell's Operative Orthopaedics, ed 11. Philadelphia, 2007, Mosby.)*

**TABLE 10-1    CHARACTERISTICS OF MOTOR NEURONS**

| Axon Size and Myelination | Axon Type | Innervates |
|---|---|---|
| Large myelinated | Aα | Extrafusal muscle fibers |
| Medium myelinated | Aγ | Intrafusal muscle fibers |

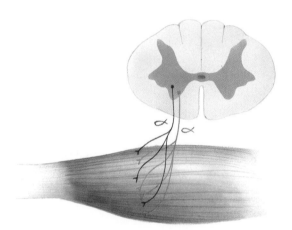

**Fig. 10-11** A motor unit consists of an alpha motor neuron and the muscle fibers it innervates. Two motor units are illustrated to show that muscle fibers innervated by a single neuron are distributed throughout the muscle.

## Alpha-Gamma Coactivation

During most movements, the alpha and gamma motor neuron systems function simultaneously. This pattern, called *alpha-gamma coactivation,* maintains the stretch on the central region of the muscle spindle intrafusal fibers when the muscle actively contracts. Excitatory signals sufficient to stimulate alpha motor neurons also stimulate gamma motor neurons to spindle fibers in the same muscle. Alpha-gamma coactivation occurs because most sources of input to alpha motor neurons have collaterals that project to gamma motor neurons, and because gamma motor neurons, with their smaller cell bodies, require less excitation to reach threshold than do alpha motor neurons.

Activation of alpha and gamma motor neurons depends on sensory information, spinal circuitry, and descending commands.

## Motor Units

An alpha motor neuron and the muscle fibers it innervates are called a *motor unit* (Figure 10-11). Whenever an alpha motor neuron is active, the neurotransmitter ACh is released at all of its neuromuscular junctions, and all muscle fibers innervated by that neuron contract. Motor units are classified as slow twitch or fast twitch, depending on the speed of muscle contraction in response to a single electrical shock. The neuron

innervating the muscle determines the twitch characteristics of the muscle fibers. Smaller-diameter, slower-conducting alpha motor neurons innervate slow twitch muscle fibers; larger-diameter, faster-conducting alpha motor neurons innervate fast twitch muscle fibers.

Slow twitch fibers constitute the majority of muscle fibers in postural and slowly contracting muscles. For example, the soleus muscle has primarily slow twitch fibers and is tonically active in standing and phasically active in walking. The gastrocnemius muscle has more fast twitch muscle fibers than the soleus. Phasic contraction of the gastrocnemius produces fast, powerful movements, like sprinting. In most movements, slow twitch muscle fibers are activated first because the small cell bodies of the slow-conducting alpha motor neurons depolarize before the cell bodies of the larger alpha motor neurons do. Slow twitch muscle fibers typically continue to contribute during faster actions as fast twitch units are recruited. The order of recruitment from smaller to larger alpha motor neurons is called *Henneman's size principle.* However, the order of recruitment is modified depending on the task and phase during human walking and running.[16]

Motor units also vary in the number of muscle fibers innervated by a single neuron. The human gastrocnemius muscle has approximately 2000 muscle fibers innervated by each alpha motor neuron. In contrast, the lateral extraocular muscle averages 2.5 muscle fibers per alpha motor neuron because precise control of eye movements is required.[17]

---

⊙ *Clinical Pearl*

A motor unit is a single alpha motor neuron and the muscle fibers the alpha motor neuron innervates.

---

The activity of a motor unit depends on the convergence of information from peripheral sensors, spinal connections, and descending tracts onto the cell body and dendrites of the alpha motor neuron. Next we will consider how spinal region circuitry contributes to spinal region coordination and to spinal reflexes (simple movement responses to peripheral inputs).

## SPINAL REGION

Movements are generated when somatosensory information is integrated with descending motor commands in the spinal cord. Networks of spinal interneurons act flexibly to elicit coordinated muscle contractions. As noted in Chapter 5, a group of muscles innervated by a single spinal nerve is called a *myotome.* Movements associated with specific myotomes are listed in Table 10-2. See Tables 13-1 and 13-2 for lists of specific muscles innervated by spinal nerves.

### Lower Motor Neuron Pools in the Spinal Cord

Lower motor neuron pools are groups of cell bodies in the spinal cord whose axons project to a single muscle. Lower motor neuron pools are located in the ventral horn. The actions of these pools correlate with their anatomic position: medially

**TABLE 10-2  MOVEMENTS ASSOCIATED WITH SPECIFIC MYOTOMES**

| Myotome | Movements Produced |
|---------|--------------------|
| C5 | Elbow flexion |
| C6 | Wrist extension |
| C7 | Elbow extension |
| C8 | Flexion of tip of middle finger |
| T1 | Finger abduction |
| L2 | Hip flexion |
| L3 | Knee flexion |
| L4 | Ankle dorsiflexion |
| L5 | Great toe extension |
| S1 | Ankle plantarflexion |

located pools innervate axial and proximal muscles, and laterally located pools innervate distal muscles. Anteriorly located pools innervate extensors, whereas more posterior pools (still within the ventral horn) innervate flexors (Figure 10-12). Axons of descending pathways from the brain are grouped according to their termination in the medial or lateral cord.

## Spinal Region Coordination

Neuronal connections within the spinal cord contribute to coordination of movement. Reciprocal inhibition, muscle synergies, proprioceptive input, and stepping pattern generators are mechanisms that organize and synchronize muscle contractions to achieve smooth, flowing, effective movements.

## Reciprocal Inhibition

*Reciprocal inhibition,* the inhibition of antagonist muscles during agonist contraction, is achieved by interneurons in the spinal cord that link lower motor neurons into functional groups. This process is used extensively during voluntary motion to prevent antagonist opposition to the movement. For example, reciprocal inhibition prevents hamstring muscle firing when the quadriceps femoris contracts (Figure 10-13). Reciprocal inhibition also prevents activation of antagonist muscles when an agonist is reflexively activated: a reflex hammer tap on the biceps tendon causes shortening of the biceps and abruptly stretches the triceps. Without a mechanism to prevent a triceps stretch reflex, the biceps contraction would be opposed by contraction of the antagonist muscle. To avert an antagonist stretch reflex, activity in collateral branches from type Ia afferents stimulates interneurons to inhibit the alpha efferent to the antagonist. A more complex example of spinal coordination is the activation of muscle synergies by type II afferents.

## Muscle Synergies

*Muscle synergy* is coordinated muscular action. We use muscle synergies constantly. When we eat, finger and elbow flexion combine with supination of the forearm to bring food to the mouth. Type II afferents contribute to synergies by delivering information to spinal cord neurons from tonic receptors in

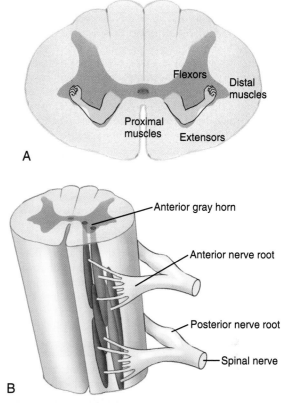

A

B

**Fig. 10-12 The cell bodies of lower motor neurons are arranged in groups corresponding to each muscle innervated. A,** The upper limb superimposed on the left anterior horn shows the arrangement of lower motor neuron pools. Medially located pools innervate axial and girdle muscles. Laterally located pools innervate distal limb muscles. Posterior pools (within the anterior horn) innervate flexor muscles. Anterior pools innervate extensor muscles. **B,** The pools may extend several spinal cord segments.

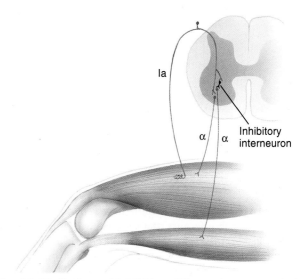

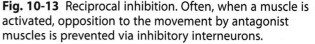

**Fig. 10-13** Reciprocal inhibition. Often, when a muscle is activated, opposition to the movement by antagonist muscles is prevented via inhibitory interneurons.

muscle spindles, certain joint receptors, and cutaneous and subcutaneous touch and pressure receptors. Interneurons excited by type II afferents project to lower motor neurons of muscles acting at other joints, providing a spinal region basis for muscle synergies. Motor control researchers typically use the term *synergy* to describe the activity of muscles that are often activated together by a normal nervous system. Clinicians often restrict use of the term to pathologic synergies, for example, when a person with a UMN lesion (due to head injury or stroke) cannot flex the shoulder without simultaneous, obligatory flexion of the elbow.

## Proprioceptive Body Schema

The spinal cord creates a complete proprioceptive model, called a *schema,* of the body in time and space. This nonconscious schema is used to plan and adapt movements.[18,19] For example, to hit a tennis ball, one must know the initial position of the arm to plan whether to move the racket hand up or down. Joint capsule and ligament receptors, muscle spindle receptors, and Golgi tendon organs provide the proprioceptive input required to generate the body schema.

> ### ◎ Clinical Pearl
>
> The spinal cord interprets proprioceptive information as a whole, and computes a complete proprioceptive image (schema) of the body in time and space. This schema is essential for adapting movements to the environment, based on proprioceptive feedback.

## Role of Golgi Tendon Organs in Movement

Golgi tendon organs (GTOs) contribute to proprioception by registering tendon tension. This information is conveyed by type Ib afferents to the spinal cord, stimulating interneurons that excite or inhibit lower motor neurons to synergists and the muscle of origin (Figure 10-14). For example, stimulation of

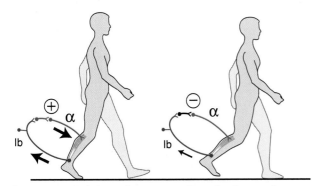

**Fig. 10-14 Golgi tendon organ.** Stretch of a tendon activates type Ib afferents that synapse with interneurons. Depending on the task, Golgi tendon organ (GTO) input facilitates or inhibits lower motor neuron (LMN) firing. For example, during the stance phase of gait, GTO input facilitates LMNs to lower limb extensor muscles. During the swing phase, GTO input inhibits lower motor neurons to the same muscles.

tendon organs in certain extensor muscles during weight bearing elicits autogenic excitation of the muscles of origin.[20] Interneurons that receive signals from GTOs also receive signals from muscle spindles, cutaneous afferents, joint afferents, and descending pathways. In vivo, GTO signals are never isolated from the input of other proprioceptors, and GTO signals do not elicit responses independently from the responses to other proprioceptors. The role of GTOs in movement is to adjust muscle contraction, in concert with other proprioceptive signals and UMN control.

Until recently, signals from GTOs were believed to protect muscles from excess loading injury by reflexively preventing excessive muscle contraction. However, the effect of GTO input is not powerful enough to inhibit voluntary muscle contraction. Maximal GTO activity occurs before 50% of maximal voluntary contraction.[21] Therefore, GTO activation cannot elicit sufficient inhibition to cause reflexive relaxation of overloaded muscle.[21] Decreased muscle contraction when muscles are severely overloaded may instead be a response to integrated afferent information from musculoskeletal receptors, or may be a volitional response. Nor can GTO inhibition explain muscle relaxation following maximal muscle contraction, because when the muscle stops contracting, the GTO firing rate decreases.

## Spinal Control of Walking: Stepping Pattern Generators

When a person is walking, each lower limb alternately flexes and extends. *Stepping pattern generators (SPGs)* are adaptable networks of spinal interneurons that activate lower motor neurons to elicit alternating flexion and extension of the hips and knees. Each lower limb has a dedicated SPG.[22] The cycles of the two SPGs are coordinated by signals conveyed in the anterior commissure of the spinal cord,[23] so that when one leg flexes, the other extends. In addition to generating repetitive cycles, SPGs receive and interpret proprioception and predict the appropriate sequences of actions throughout the step cycle.[24,25]

However, the alternating flexion/extension elicited by SPG activity is not the only mechanism responsible for walking. Postural control, cortical control of dorsiflexion,[26] and afferent information are also essential for human locomotion. Afferent input adjusts timing, facilitates the transition from stance to swing phase of gait, and reinforces muscle activation.[25]

> ### ◎ Clinical Pearl
>
> Stepping pattern generators in the spinal cord contribute to walking in humans. However, descending input is normally required to activate SPGs, and the SPGs provide only bilaterally coordinated reciprocal hip and knee flexion/extension. Cortical control is essential for directing ankle dorsiflexion, and UMN signals from the brainstem are required to maintain postural control during walking.

## Spinal Region Reflexes

Most movement is automatic or voluntary and anticipatory—not reflexive. When a person decides to reach for a book, there is no external stimulus; this movement does not arise from

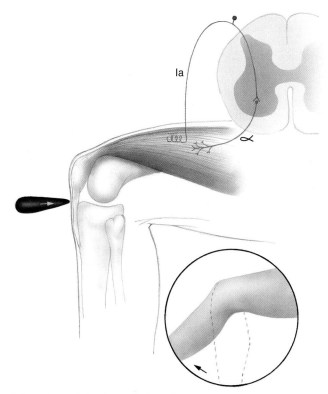

**Fig. 10-15 Phasic stretch reflex.** Quick stretch of a muscle, elicited by striking the muscle's tendon, stimulates type Ia afferents from the muscle spindle. Activity of type Ia afferents causes monosynaptic excitation of alpha motor neurons to the stretched muscle, resulting in abrupt contraction of muscle fibers.

reflex. However, clinical examination of reflexes provides important information about the peripheral and spinal circuits and the level of background excitation in the spinal cord. Spinal region reflexes require sensory receptors, primary afferents, synapses between primary afferents and lower motor neurons, and muscles. Spinal region reflexes can operate without brain input; however, signals from the brain normally influence spinal reflexes by adjusting the background level of neural activity in the spinal cord. In this section, stretch reflexes and cutaneous reflexes are discussed.

### Stretch Reflexes: Muscle Spindles

There are two types of stretch reflexes: phasic and tonic. The term *phasic* indicates that the response to the stimulus is brief. *Tonic* refers to responses that last as long as the stimulus is maintained. Muscle contraction in response to quick stretch is called the *phasic stretch reflex*. A brisk tap with a reflex hammer on the quadriceps tendon elicits a reflexive contraction of the quadriceps muscle, because quick stretch activates neural connections between muscle spindles and alpha motor neurons to the same muscle (Figure 10-15). Tapping the tendon delivers a quick stretch to the muscle and the spindles embedded parallel to the muscle fibers. The primary endings of the spindles are stimulated by the quick stretch. Type Ia afferents then transmit action potentials to the spinal cord and release

neurotransmitters at synapses with alpha motor neurons. The alpha motor neurons depolarize, action potentials are propagated to the neuromuscular junctions, ACh is released and binds with muscle receptors, the muscle membrane depolarizes, and the muscle fibers contract. There is only one synapse between the afferent and efferent neurons; thus the quick response to stretch is a monosynaptic reflex. The terms *myotatic reflex, muscle stretch reflex,* and *deep tendon reflex* are synonymous with *phasic stretch reflex.*

At velocities of stretch used clinically to test muscle resistance to stretch, the *tonic stretch reflex* is present only following UMN lesions.[27] In contrast to the phasic stretch reflex, the tonic stretch reflex continues as long as the stretch is maintained. Receptors for the tonic stretch reflex are primary and secondary endings in the muscle spindle. Maintained stretch of the central region fires the spindle sensory endings, type Ia and II afferents conduct excitation into the spinal cord, and multiple interneurons link the afferent fiber terminals with lower motor neurons (Figure 10-16). Following UMN lesions, loss of presynaptic inhibition allows slow or sustained stretch of the central spindle to elicit continual muscle contraction. In intact nervous systems, the information conveyed by type Ia and II afferents regarding sustained stretch is used to adjust muscle activity but does not elicit reflexive contraction because presynaptic inhibition and other inputs also influence the lower motor neurons.

### Cutaneous Reflexes: Withdrawal Reflexes

Cutaneous stimulation can also elicit reflexive movements. If a person steps on a tack, the withdrawal reflex automatically lifts the foot by flexing the lower limb, even before the person is consciously aware of pain (Figure 10-17). The circuitry responsible for the withdrawal reflex is located within the spinal cord. The withdrawal reflex and related reactions will be described in Chapter 13, Spinal Region.

---

> **◎ *Clinical Pearl***
>
> Activation of the Golgi tendon organ can inhibit or facilitate activity of the corresponding muscle. Reflexes can be elicited by stimulation of musculoskeletal or cutaneous receptors. Stimulation of muscle spindle receptors can result in phasic stretch reflexes and, in cases of UMN lesions, tonic stretch reflexes. Noxious cutaneous information can result in a withdrawal reflex.

---

### Relationship Between Reflexive and Voluntary Movement

Classically, reflexes were considered to be responses to particular types of sensory information, exciting only specific, isolated pathways within the spinal cord and resulting in stereotypic output. Voluntary movement was considered entirely separate from reflexes. Research has refuted this division. Most sensory stimuli act in an ensemble fashion, the involved interneurons can vary, and appropriate levels of the central nervous system interact to produce context-dependent movement. For example, changing a person's arousal, or alertness, level can modify the movement response to a tendon tap. If a person is relaxed, a quadriceps tendon tap tends to elicit a small movement. If the

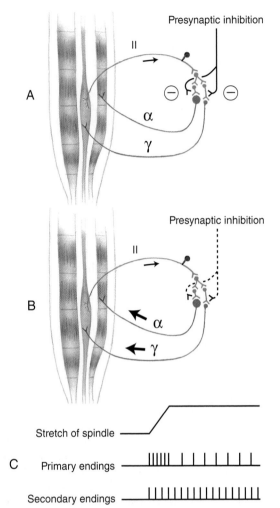

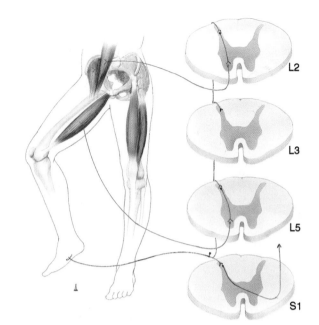

**Fig. 10-17  Withdrawal reflex.** Usually in response to a painful cutaneous stimulus, muscles are activated to move the body part away from the stimulation. This action requires signals at multiple synapses at several levels of the cord because various spinal segments innervate the active muscles.

**Fig. 10-16  Tonic stretch reflex.** At low or moderate velocities of joint rotation (less than 200 degrees per second), this reflex is present only in people with upper motor neuron (UMN) lesions.[28] **A,** In an intact neuromuscular system, a muscle at rest is stretched passively and the stretch is maintained. Although spindle afferents convey signals into the spinal cord, the lower motor neurons (LMNs) do not fire because presynaptic inhibition prevents their activation. **B,** Following a complete spinal cord injury, maintained stretch of the muscle spindle elicits sustained firing of spindle endings. Because presynaptic inhibition is absent, spindle input is sufficient to activate LMNs, eliciting a tonic stretch reflex. For simplicity, the primary spindle endings are omitted from **A** and **B. C,** The firing frequency of primary endings is maximal while the spindle is being stretched, and the firing rate decreases when the spindle is maintained in a stretched position. The secondary endings fire at a high frequency during stretch of the spindle and while the spindle is maintained in a stretched position. In some UMN lesions, loss of presynaptic inhibition allows input from secondary endings to elicit LMN firing and active muscle contraction (tonic stretch reflex). In an intact nervous system, input from secondary endings is used to adjust muscle contraction but does not elicit a tonic stretch reflex unless the velocity of stretch is extremely high.

person is extremely anxious, a tendon tap using the same amount of force probably will elicit much greater movement. Arousal changes the level of descending input to the spinal circuitry. Furthermore, muscle spindle output is modified by sensitivity adjustments and by the recent movements and contractions the muscle has undergone.[29] As a result, muscle spindle output is not linearly related to changes in muscle length or rate of change in length. Spindle information is integrated with other proprioceptive inputs to adjust muscle output.

## H-Reflexes

The H-reflex is a monosynaptic reflex elicited by electrically stimulating a nerve. The purpose is to quantify the level of alpha motor neuron facilitation or inhibition. H-reflex testing substitutes cutaneous electrical stimulation of a peripheral nerve for tendon percussion of the myotatic reflex. For example, a stimulating electrode is placed over the tibial nerve in the popliteal fossa, and a recording electrode is placed on the inferomedial gastrocnemius (Figure 10-18). A weak current, adequate to stimulate only the largest axons (motor axons and type Ia and Ib afferents, which have the lowest electrical thresholds), is administered to the skin over the tibial nerve. Action potentials travel both toward the muscle (via motor axons) and toward the spinal cord (via type Ia and Ib afferents). The electrical stimulation produces two action potentials with different latencies that can be recorded from the skin over the muscle: the M wave and the H-reflex. The shorter-latency M wave is produced by impulses traveling along motor fibers, causing an almost immediate muscle contraction. Afferent fiber activity elicits the H-reflex. Action potentials in the large afferent fibers travel into the spinal cord, resulting in transmission across synapses to

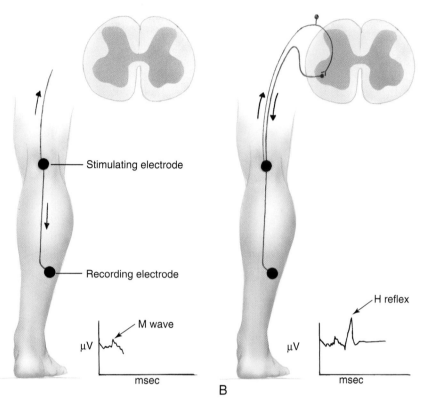

**Fig. 10-18 H-reflex electrode placement for quantifying the level of excitation in tibial nerve alpha motor neurons.**
**A,** Electrical stimulation applied to the skin in the popliteal fossa over the tibial nerve evokes action potentials in both sensory and motor axons. These action potentials are propagated proximally and distally from the site of stimulation. When the action potentials in alpha motor neurons reach the terminals, acetylcholine (ACh) is released and binds with receptors on the muscle membrane, and the muscle membrane depolarizes. The depolarization is recorded as the M wave. **B,** Action potentials evoked in type Ia and Ib fibers are propagated into the spinal cord. Via synaptic activity, alpha motor neurons are stimulated. Then action potentials are propagated toward the muscle, and ACh is released at the neuromuscular junction and binds with receptors on the muscle membrane. When the muscle membrane depolarizes, the H-reflex is recorded.

facilitate alpha motor neurons. If the central excitatory state of the alpha motor neurons is near threshold, activation of the alpha motor neurons will in turn cause depolarization of the calf muscle membranes. The H-reflex is slightly faster (by 10 milliseconds) than the tendon tap reflex because it does not require activation of spindle receptors.

## UPPER MOTOR NEURONS

UMNs provide all of the motor signals from the brain to the spinal cord and from the cerebrum to the cranial nerve lower motor neurons in the brainstem. UMNs project from cortical and brainstem centers to lower motor neurons (alpha and gamma) and to interneurons in the brainstem and spinal cord. UMNs projecting to the spinal cord are classified according to whether they synapse medially, laterally, or throughout the ventral horn (Figure 10-19). Medial UMNs signal lower motor neurons that innervate postural and girdle muscles. Lateral UMNs signal lower motor neurons that innervate muscles used for fractionated movement and muscles in the face and neck. The group ending throughout the ventral horn, the nonspecific UMNs, contributes to background levels of excitation in the cord and facilitates local reflex arcs.

### Postural and Gross Movements: Medial Upper Motor Neurons

UMN activity controlling posture and gross movements usually occurs automatically, without conscious effort. Medial UMN activity can occur before a person is consciously aware of a stimulus. For example, if a loud noise occurs behind a person, the eyes and face turn toward the sound, before the person is consciously aware of the auditory stimulus. These coordinated, involuntary reactions are initiated in the brainstem. From there, medial UMNs convey signals to the appropriate lower motor neurons.

Three tracts from the brainstem* and one from the cerebral cortex deliver signals that control posture and gross movements to medial lower motor neuron pools in the spinal cord. The axons of these tracts are located in the medial white matter of the spinal cord. The tracts include (Figure 10-20) the following:

---

*A fourth tract from the brainstem, the tectospinal tract, is prominent in lower mammals but insignificant in primates.[30] In primates, the reticulospinal tract instead of the tectospinal tract conveys signals from the tectum to the spinal cord.[30] Signals from the superior colliculus to the reticular formation, the source of the reticulospinal tract, are important in neck reflexive responses to visual and auditory input.[31]

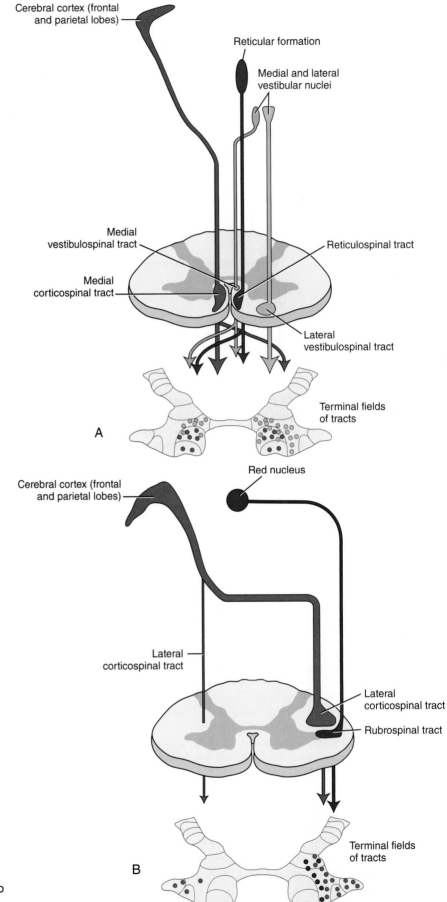

**Fig. 10-19  Medial and lateral upper motor neurons (UMNs) influence different groups of lower motor neurons (LMNs). A,** Medial UMN tracts descend in the anterior column of the spinal cord and synapse with LMNs located in the anteromedial gray matter. These LMNs synapse with axial and gross movement limb muscles. **B,** Lateral UMN tracts descend in the lateral column of the spinal cord and synapse with LMNs located in the anterolateral gray matter. These LMNs synapse with limb muscles.

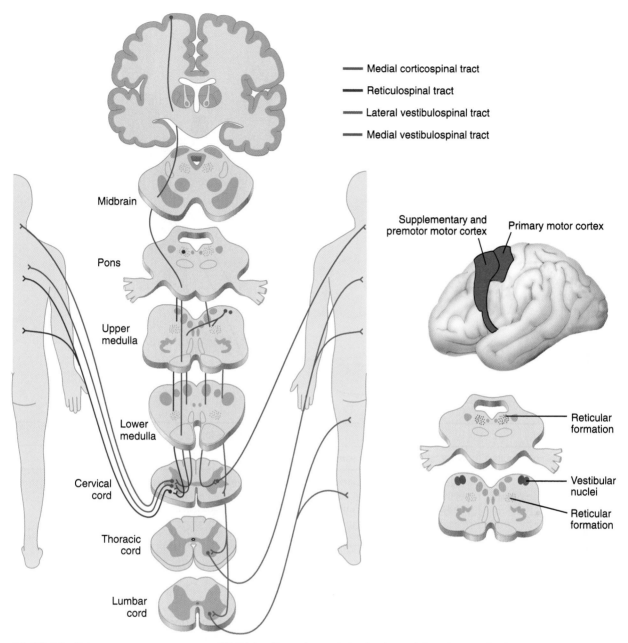

— Medial corticospinal tract
— Reticulospinal tract
— Lateral vestibulospinal tract
— Medial vestibulospinal tract

**Fig. 10-20  Medial upper motor neurons (UMNs) adjust the activity in the axial and gross limb movement muscles.**
**A,** The illustrations on the right show the origins of each of the medial UMN tracts. All sections are horizontal except the coronal section of the cerebrum *(top left)* and the intact cerebrum *(top right).* For the primary motor cortex, only the areas that control trunk, arm, and leg muscles are colored in the drawing at top right, because the areas that control face and distal arm movements do not contribute to control of axial and gross limb movement muscles. The color of the UMN tracts is continued for the LMNs facilitated by each tract.

*Continued*

- Reticulospinal
- Medial and lateral vestibulospinal
- Medial corticospinal

## Medial Upper Motor Neuron Tracts

### Reticulospinal Tract
This tract begins in the reticular formation. Reticulospinal neurons facilitate bilateral lower motor neurons innervating postural and gross limb movement muscles throughout the

entire body. For example, the reticulospinal tracts are essential for coordinating muscular activity of the trunk and the proximal muscles of all four limbs during walking.[32] Reticulospinal neurons are also involved in anticipatory postural adjustments and reaching.[33-35] Figure 10-21 shows a person post stroke attempting to reach upward with both upper limbs. Her right (paretic) arm is unable to combine shoulder flexion with elbow extension. Instead, the attempt at reaching elicits an unwanted combination of movements, called a *flexion synergy*: her shoulder abducts and internally rotates while the elbow and wrist

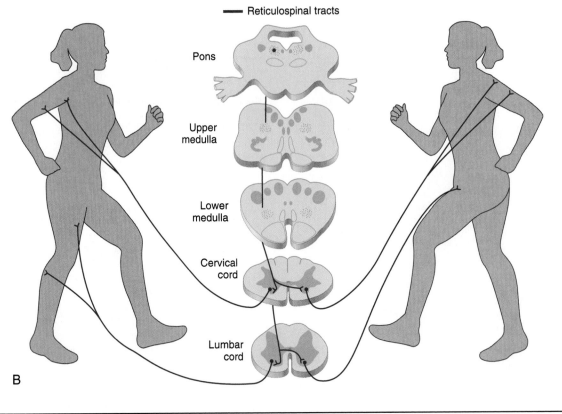

— Reticulospinal tracts

Pons

Upper medulla

Lower medulla

Cervical cord

Lumbar cord

B

| Tract | Facilitates motor neurons to: |
|---|---|
| Medial corticospinal | Neck, shoulder, and trunk muscles |
| Reticulospinal | Bilateral postural muscles (for simplicity, only motor neurons to the right side of the body are shown in panel A) and gross limb movement muscles of entire body (projections of the right reticulospinal tract) are shown in B |
| Lateral vestibulospinal | Postural muscles |
| Medial vestibulospinal | Neck |

**Fig. 10-20, cont'd**

flex. This abnormal synergy is a result of reticulospinal activation without modification by collaterals of the corticospinal tracts.[32] Normally, reticulospinal neurons are influenced by the cerebral cortex and by cerebellar and sensory input to the reticular formation.

Reticulospinal neurons are the UMN pathway for neck reflexes in response to visual or auditory input.[31] When a person automatically turns his or her head on hearing a sound or seeing an object in peripheral vision, the colliculi in the posterior midbrain process the information and signal the reticulospinal neurons to LMNs that innervate neck muscles.

### Medial Vestibulospinal Tract
Medial vestibular nuclei receive information about head movement and position from the vestibular apparatus, located in the inner ear. Axons projecting from the medial vestibular nuclei to the spinal cord, the medial vestibulospinal tracts, project to cervical and thoracic levels and affect activity in lower motor neurons controlling neck and upper back muscles.

### Lateral Vestibulospinal Tract
The lateral vestibular nuclei respond to gravity information from the vestibular apparatus. Pathways from the lateral vestibular nuclei, the lateral vestibulospinal tracts, facilitate lower motor neurons to extensors while inhibiting lower motor neurons to flexors. When a person is upright, the lateral vestibulospinal tracts are continuously active to maintain the center of gravity over the base of support, responding to the slightest destabilization.[36]

### Medial Corticospinal Tract*
A direct connection from the cerebral cortex to the spinal cord, the medial corticospinal tract, descends from the cortex through

---

*Evolving terminology: corticospinal neurons are also known as *corticomotoneuronal.* Historically, *corticospinal* was an appropriate term because the sensory regulation function of some corticospinal neurons was undiscovered; now, *corticospinal* is a somewhat ambiguous term but remains the most commonly used term to describe UMNs that arise in the cerebral cortex and terminate in the spinal cord.

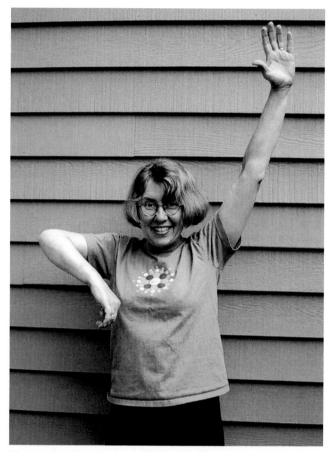

**Fig. 10-21** Person post stroke reaching upward. Her intent is to raise both upper limbs overhead. However, owing to a middle cerebral artery stroke interrupting the left hemisphere corticospinal tracts, she is unable to combine shoulder flexion with elbow extension. Descending signals from the reticulospinal tract activate lower motor neurons to muscles that produce abnormal synergy in the right upper limb.

the internal capsule and the anterior brainstem. Individual medial corticospinal axons project to the ipsilateral, contralateral, and bilateral spinal cord.[37,38] Medial corticospinal neurons synapse with lower motor neurons that control neck, shoulder, and trunk muscles.

---

**◎ Clinical Pearl**

Medial UMNs are involved primarily in control of posture and proximal movements. Medial UMNs include the reticulospinal, medial corticospinal, and medial and lateral vestibulospinal tracts.

---

Most brain control of posture and proximal movement is derived from brainstem centers. Cortical projections probably prepare the postural system for intended movements. In contrast to postural and gross movement control of the medial UMNs, a different group of UMN pathways controls fractionated movements and distal limb movements.

## Fractionated Movements and Distal Limb Movements: Lateral Upper Motor Neurons

*Fractionation* is the ability to activate individual muscles independently of other muscles. Fractionation is essential for normal movement of the hands, enabling us to button a button, press individual piano or computer keyboard keys, and pick up small objects. Without fractionation, the fingers and thumb would act as a single unit, as they do when picking up a water bottle.

The two UMN tracts that descend in the lateral spinal cord and synapse with laterally located lower motor neuron pools in the ventral horn are:
- Rubrospinal
- Lateral corticospinal

Figure 10-22 illustrates these pathways. The function of the lateral UMNs versus the medial UMNs was discovered in a classic experiment: in monkeys, the only long-term deficit caused by severing the lateral corticospinal and rubrospinal tracts was an inability to use the fingers individually to pick small objects out of deep cavities in a board; balance, walking, running, and climbing abilities remained near normal.[39]

In people, the rubrospinal tract is small and makes a minor contribution to control of upper limb distal extensor muscles.[40,41] The tract arises in the red nucleus of the midbrain.

### Lateral Corticospinal Tract

The lateral corticospinal tract is the most important pathway controlling voluntary movement. The unique contribution of the lateral corticospinal tract* is fractionation of movement. The lateral corticospinal tract fractionates by activating inhibitory neurons to prevent unwanted muscles from contracting.[41]

This tract arises in motor planning areas and in the primary motor cortex. From their origin in the cerebral cortex, the axons project downward, passing first through the internal capsule, then the cerebral peduncles, the anterior pons, and the pyramids of the medulla, and finally, the lateral spinal cord, to synapse with lower motor neurons that control fine distal movements (Figure 10-23). The corticospinal tracts in the lower medulla form the pyramids, where, at the junction of the medulla and spinal cord, approximately 88% of lateral corticospinal axons cross to the contralateral side, and most synapse with lower motor neurons in the contralateral spinal cord. Ten percent of neurons in the lateral corticospinal tract travel ipsilaterally in the lateral corticospinal tract; most terminate in the ipsilateral spinal cord.[37,38] Some lateral corticospinal neurons that crossed the midline in the pyramidal decussation cross the

---

*Clinical terminology: historically, the corticospinal tract was considered to be the most important pathway, with other descending motor pathways playing minor supporting roles. Because the lateral corticospinal tract forms the medullary pyramids, this tract was called the *pyramidal system*. The remaining motor tracts were called *extrapyramidal*. The basal ganglia were mistakenly believed to exclusively control the extrapyramidal tracts; thus, in clinical terminology, extrapyramidal became synonymous with basal ganglia. This terminology remains common in clinical use. The division of motor control into pyramidal/extrapyramidal is a false dichotomy because the basal ganglia have a major influence on cortical motor areas and so contribute to control of the pyramidal tract, and because the cerebral cortex and cerebellum have great influence on the descending motor tracts that were formerly called *extrapyramidal*.

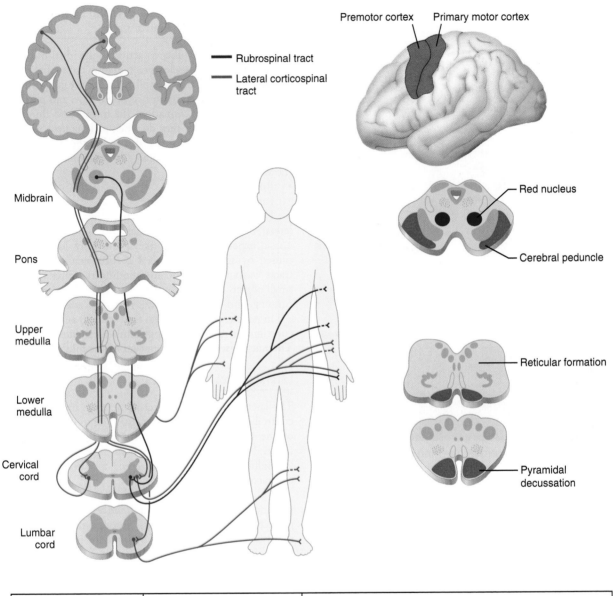

**Fig. 10-22** Lateral upper motor neurons (UMNs) adjust the activity in limb muscles. The illustrations on the right show the origins of each of the lateral UMN tracts and highlight areas of the brainstem *(in red)* that are composed of lateral corticospinal axons.

| Tract | Projection | Facilitates motor neurons to muscles that: |
|---|---|---|
| Lateral corticospinal | Mainly contralateral | Fractionate movements of the distal limbs |
| Rubrospinal | Contralateral upper limb | Extend wrist and fingers |

midline again in the spinal cord, thus terminating ipsilateral to the cortex of origin. The remaining 2% of corticospinal neurons travel in the medial corticospinal tract.[37]

### Origin of Corticospinal Tracts

Lateral corticospinal fibers arise in the primary motor, premotor, and supplementary motor cortex. The primary motor cortex is located anterior to the central sulcus, in the precentral gyrus. This area of cortex provides precise, predominantly contralateral control of movements of the limbs. In contrast, muscles that are frequently activated bilaterally, including muscles of the back, receive signals from both primary motor cortices via the medial corticospinal tract. The corticospinal cell bodies in the primary motor cortex are arranged somatotopically in an inverted homunculus, similar to cortical sensory representation (Figure 10-24).

Two regions anterior to the primary motor cortex are involved in preparing for movement: the lateral premotor area is on the lateral surface of the hemisphere, and the

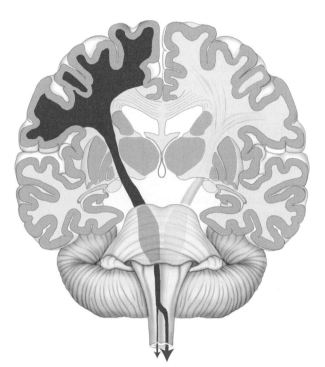

supplementary motor area is on the superior and medial surface (Figure 10-25). The lateral premotor area is named for its position anterior to the primary motor cortex. Stimulation of the lateral premotor area produces muscle activity that spans several joints. Unlike in the lateral premotor cortex, many supplementary motor cortex cells are active before movements that require coordination of both hands (e.g., buttoning a button) and sequential movements that require actions to be accomplished in a specific order (e.g., putting on socks before shoes).[42]

> ### ⊙ *Clinical Pearl*
>
> The lateral UMN tracts that direct limb movements via spinal lower motor neurons are the lateral corticospinal and rubrospinal. The lateral corticospinal tract is unique in providing fractionation of limb movements.

## Control of Muscles of the Face and Tongue, and Some Muscles of the Neck: Corticobrainstem Tracts

Corticobrainstem fibers arise in motor areas of the cerebral cortex, then project to cranial nerve nuclei in the brainstem. These tracts facilitate lower motor neurons innervating the muscles of the face, tongue, pharynx, and larynx, and the trapezius and sternocleidomastoid (Figure 10-26). Lower motor neurons to muscles of the lower face are controlled by contralateral corticobrainstem neurons. Lower motor neurons to muscles of the upper face are bilaterally controlled by corticobrainstem neurons.

**Fig. 10-23 Paths of corticospinal tracts in the brain.** The right corticospinal tract is shown in red. Corticospinal neuron cell bodies are in the cerebral cortex. Their axons travel through the corona radiata, internal capsule, cerebral peduncles, anterior pons, and medullary pyramids before reaching the spinal cord.

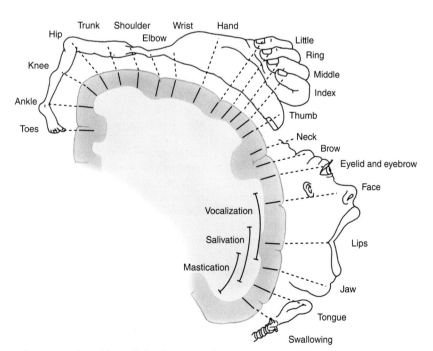

**Fig. 10-24 Motor homunculus.** Map of the functional arrangement of neurons in the primary motor cortex.

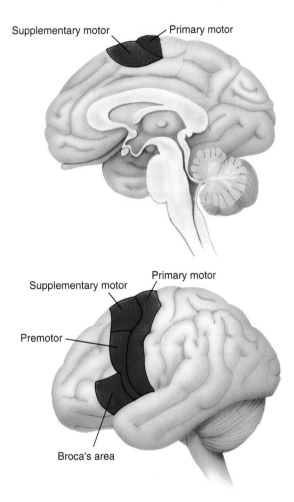

**Fig. 10-25** Location of the primary motor, premotor, and supplementary motor cortices. Broca's area plans the movements of speech.

### Nonspecific Upper Motor Neurons

Tracts descending from two bilateral nuclei in the brainstem enhance the activity of interneurons and lower motor neurons in the spinal cord. The locus coeruleus and raphe nuclei are the sources of the *ceruleospinal* and *raphespinal* tracts (Figure 10-27). The raphespinal tract releases serotonin, modulating the activity of spinal lower motor neurons. The ceruleospinal tract releases norepinephrine, producing tonic facilitation of spinal lower motor neurons.[43] Both of these tracts are activated during excessive limbic activity. Holstege (2009)[43] calls these tracts part of the *emotional motor system.* The motor effects of both tracts are general, are not related to specific movements, and may contribute to poorer motor performance when anxiety is high. For example, climbers on a high wall move more slowly, make

more exploratory movements, and use each hold longer than those on a lower climbing wall, even when the traverse itself is identical.[44] Similarly, in normal young adults, fear of falling (induced by standing at the edge of an elevated platform) reduces the magnitude and rate of postural adjustments.[45]

## SIGNS OF MOTOR NEURON LESIONS

Disorders of the motor system may cause the following:
- Paresis and paralysis
- Muscle atrophy
- Involuntary muscle contractions
- Abnormal muscle tone
- Abnormal reflexes
- Disturbances of movement efficiency and speed (discussed in Chapter 11)
- Impaired postural control (discussed in Chapter 11)

The first four impairments listed are described in the following section. Abnormal reflexes are discussed within the context of specific neurologic disorders.

### Paresis and Paralysis

Decreased ability to generate muscle force and decreased muscle bulk are common consequences of lower motor neuron lesions. Although the terms *paresis* and *paralysis* are often used synonymously, technically, *paralysis* refers to complete loss of voluntary contraction, and *paresis* refers to partial loss. Decreased muscle strength is commonly described by its distribution: *hemiplegia* is weakness affecting one side of the body, *paraplegia* affects the body below the arms, and *tetraplegia* affects all four limbs (Figure 10-28). A complete lesion of a peripheral nerve, interrupting all axons in the nerve, produces paralysis because lower motor neurons are the only pathway from the central nervous system to skeletal muscle. UMN lesions may cause paresis because some of the descending motor tracts may be intact. For example, a stroke may interrupt the corticospinal tract neurons that synapse with lower motor neurons to the right upper limb. The person may retain some voluntary control of right hand movements via the reticulospinal tracts. Figure 10-29 shows paralysis of finger extensors post stroke.

### Muscle Atrophy

*Muscle atrophy* is the loss of muscle bulk. *Disuse atrophy* results from lack of muscle use, and *neurogenic atrophy* is caused by damage to the nervous system. Denervation of skeletal muscle produces the most severe atrophy because frequent neural stimulation, even at a level inadequate to produce muscle contraction, is essential for the health of skeletal muscle. When lower motor neurons no longer provide stimulation that influences genetic expression in muscles, muscle atrophy occurs rapidly, because the pattern of protein production in the muscle changes. Normally innervated skeletal muscle produces 400 proteins. Following denervation, muscle production of 26 proteins decreases, and the production of 6 proteins increases.[46] In UMN lesions, skeletal muscle continues to receive stimulation from intact lower motor neurons, and the rate of atrophy is slower than in LMN lesions.

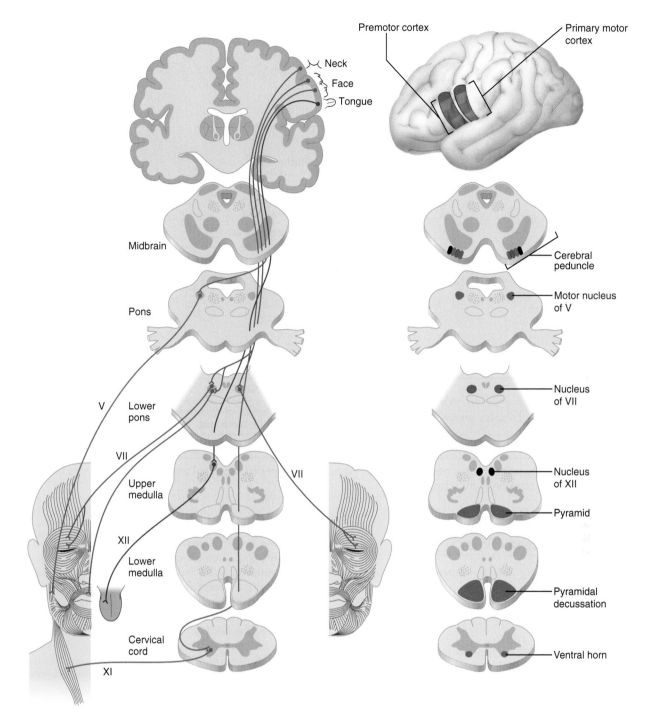

**Fig. 10-26 Corticobrainstem tracts.** Axons from the cerebral cortex transmit information to cranial nerve cell bodies; the cranial nerves project to muscles that control movements of the head and neck. Descending input from the cortex influences all eight cranial nerves that innervate skeletal muscle. For simplicity, only four of the eight cranial nerves that innervate skeletal muscle are illustrated. The illustrations on the right show the origin of the corticobrainstem tracts, areas composed of corticobrainstem axons, and sites of synapse between corticobrainstem neurons and lower motor neurons. The sites of synapse illustrated are the nuclei of cranial nerves V, VII, XI, and XII.

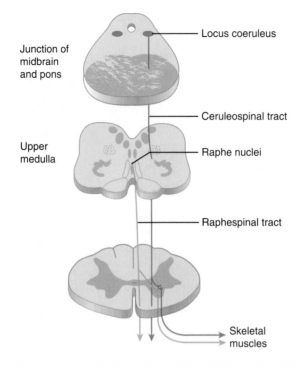

Fig. 10-27 Nonspecific upper motor neurons (UMNs). When active, the ceruleospinal and raphespinal tracts facilitate lower motor neurons to skeletal muscles.

|  | Origin | Function |
|---|---|---|
| Ceruleospinal | Locus coeruleus in the brainstem | Enhances activity of interneurons and motor neurons throughout the spinal cord |
| Raphespinal | Raphe nucleus in the brainstem | Same as ceruleospinal |

## Involuntary Muscle Contractions

Spontaneous involuntary muscle contractions include the following:

- Muscle spasms
- Cramps
- Fasciculations
- Myoclonus
- Tremors
- Fibrillations
- Abnormal movements generated by dysfunctional basal ganglia

Of these involuntary contractions, the first five occasionally occur in a healthy neuromuscular system, or they may be signs of pathology. *Muscle spasms* (sudden, involuntary contractions of muscle) and *cramps* (particularly severe and painful muscle spasms) are common following prolonged exercise, particularly if sweating has led to sodium depletion. *Fasciculations* (quick twitches of muscle fibers of a single motor unit that are visible on the surface of the skin) are responsible for the eyelid twitches that sometimes accompany anxiety. *Myoclonus* (brief, involuntary contractions of a muscle or group of muscles) explains hiccups and the muscle jerks that some people experience when falling asleep. Sleep-onset myoclonus occurs when the wake-sleep transition elicits spinal lower motor neuron activity.[47]

*Tremors* are involuntary, rhythmic movements of a body part. Physiologic tremors can be enhanced by anxiety, stress, fatigue, caffeine, or alcohol withdrawal. Tremors are classified as resting or intention tremors. *Resting tremors* are most visible when the person is not intentionally moving. The most common resting tremors are essential (familial) tremor and Parkinson's tremor (see Chapter 11). Essential tremor affects the head and hands, interfering with using utensils, eating, drinking, and grooming. Autosomal dominant inheritance accounts for about half of essential tremor cases. *Intention tremor* is absent at rest and increases as voluntary movement proceeds. Intention tremor occurs in alcohol intoxication and cerebellar disorders.

Pathologic cramps, spasms, and fasciculations will be discussed within the context of specific lesions. Pathologic myoclonus occurs in epilepsy, brain or spinal cord injury, stroke, and chemical or drug poisoning. *Fibrillations* (brief contractions of single muscle fibers not visible on the surface of the skin) and abnormal movements are always pathologic. Fibrillations can result from UMN or LMN disorders. Abnormal movements due to basal ganglia disorders are considered within that context in Chapter 11.

## Abnormal Muscle Tone

*Muscle tone* is resistance to stretch in resting muscle. *Hypotonia* is abnormally low resistance to passive stretch. *Flaccidity* is lack

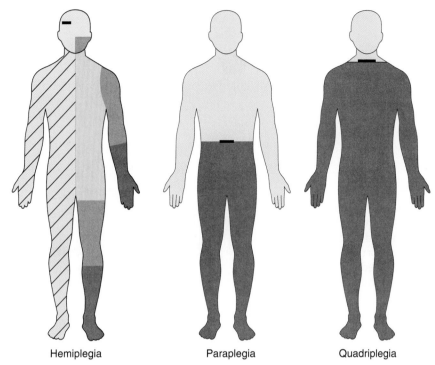

Hemiplegia        Paraplegia        Quadriplegia

**Fig. 10-28 Distribution of paresis or paralysis.** Black indicates the site of the lesion; gray indicates the location of the paretic or paralyzed muscles. Light gray indicates mild paresis; dark gray indicates severe paresis or paralysis; intermediate gray indicates moderate weakness. Hemiplegia is usually caused by interruption of the medial and lateral corticospinal tracts in one cerebral hemisphere. Here the lesion is in the right internal capsule, causing weakness that affects the distal limbs *(darker gray)* more than the trunk and shoulder girdle and hip muscles *(lighter gray)* because lower motor neurons (LMNs) to trunk and girdle muscles receive signals from the uninterrupted reticulospinal and vestibulospinal tracts. The stripes on the ipsilateral side indicate mild paresis due to loss of ipsilateral corticospinal inputs to lower motor neurons (LMNs). The LMNs to distal limb muscles receive signals from the uninterrupted rubrospinal and reticulospinal tracts in addition to ipsilateral lateral corticospinals. Interruption of corticobrainstem tracts to LMNs that control muscles of the lower face causes contralateral paresis of the tongue, muscles that move the face, and sternocleidomastoid and trapezius muscles. Paraplegia and quadriplegia are caused by a lesion affecting the spinal cord.

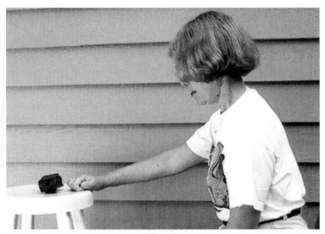

**Fig. 10-29** Person post stroke reaching for a camera. Her right finger extensors are completely paralyzed, so although she is able to reach toward the camera, she cannot pick it up using the right upper limb.

of resistance to passive stretch. Hypotonia or flaccidity can be caused by:

- LMN lesions
- Acute UMN lesions (hypotonia is usually temporary in this case)
- Developmental disorders, usually caused by brain hypoxia/ischemia, intracranial hemorrhage, or genetic or metabolic disorders[48]

*Hypertonia,* abnormally strong resistance to passive stretch, can be caused by:

- Chronic UMN lesions
- Some basal ganglia disorders

There are two types of hypertonia: velocity-dependent and rigid. In velocity-dependent hypertonia, the amount of resistance to passive movement depends on the velocity of movement. Resistance during slow stretch is low, and greater resistance occurs with faster stretch. Both changes in muscle tissue (myoplasticity) and neuromuscular overactivity (spasticity) contribute to velocity-dependent hypertonia. Myoplasticity and spasticity are discussed in the UMN lesion section later in this chapter. In velocity-independent hypertonia, or *rigidity,* resistance to passive movement remains constant, regardless of

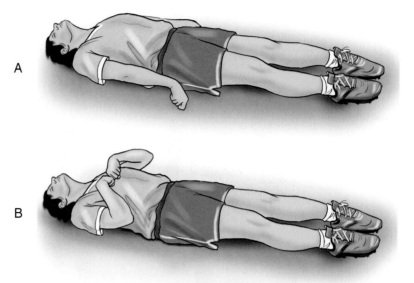

**Fig. 10-30  Rigidity. A,** In decerebrate rigidity, the limbs and the trunk are extended, the upper limbs are internally rotated, and the feet are plantarflexed. **B,** In decorticate rigidity, the upper limbs are flexed and the lower limbs are extended with the feet plantarflexed.

the speed of force application. Thus rigidity is velocity-independent hypertonia. Decerebrate rigidity, caused by severe midbrain lesions, comprises rigid extension of the limbs and trunk, internal rotation of the upper limbs, and plantar flexion (Figure 10-30, *A*). Decorticate rigidity, caused by severe lesions superior to the midbrain, comprises flexed upper limbs, extended neck and lower limbs, and plantarflexion (Figure 10-30, *B*). Table 10-3 summarizes the variations in muscle tone.

When an acute UMN lesion interrupts descending motor commands, the lower motor neurons affected become temporarily inactive owing to loss of descending facilitation and edema affecting the area of the lesion. This condition is called *spinal shock* or *cerebral shock,* depending on the location of the lesion. During nervous system shock, stretch reflexes cannot be elicited, and the muscles are hypotonic, that is, the muscles have abnormally low tone because facilitation of lower motor neurons by UMNs has been lost. Following recovery from central nervous system shock, interneurons and lower motor neurons usually resume activity, although their activity is no longer modulated (or is abnormally modulated) by UMNs. In many cases, during the months following a UMN lesion, muscle tone increases as a result of neural and muscular changes, producing excessive resistance to muscle stretch (see later section on hypertonia). See Chapter 13 for a discussion of spinal shock and recovery of reflexes.

## DISORDERS OF LOWER MOTOR NEURONS

Trauma, infection (poliomyelitis), degenerative or vascular disorders, and tumors can damage lower motor neurons. Interrupting LMN signals to muscle decreases or prevents muscle contraction. If LMN cell bodies and/or axons are destroyed, the affected muscles can undergo:
- Loss of reflexes
- Atrophy
- Flaccid paralysis
- Fibrillations

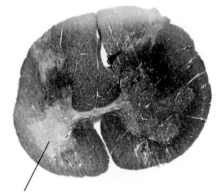

Loss of lower motor neuron cell bodies

**Fig. 10-31** Horizontal section of a spinal cord post polio. The section has been stained for myelin, so that the white matter appears dark. Loss of cell bodies is visible in the anterior horn. *(Courtesy Dr. Melvin J. Ball.)*

Traumatic injuries to lower motor neurons are discussed in Chapter 12. An infection that affects only lower motor neurons is poliovirus, which selectively invades lower motor neurons and destroys some of them (Figure 10-31), denervating some muscle fibers. Polio survivors recover some muscle strength as surviving neurons sprout new terminal axons and reinnervate the muscle fibers (Figure 10-32). In some polio survivors, post polio syndrome occurs years after the acute illness. This syndrome is not due to death of entire lower motor neurons; instead, the overextended surviving neurons cannot support the abnormal number of axonal branches, causing some distal branches to die. Post polio syndrome is the most common lower motor neuron disease in the United States.[49]

Symptoms of post polio syndrome include increasing muscle weakness, joint and muscle pain, fatigue, and breathing problems. People who had polio more than 30 years previously had only 46% of the lower limb isometric strength of

**TABLE 10-3 MUSCLE TONE***

| | Definition | Muscle Resistance During Passive Stretch | EMG Activity During Passive Stretch | Occurs in | Mechanism |
|---|---|---|---|---|---|
| Rigidity | Velocity-independent increase in resistance to stretch | Excess resistance that does not change with speed of stretch | Greater than normal | Basal ganglia disorders (see Chapter 11) and severe lesions affecting the midbrain or structures above the midbrain | Direct upper motor neuron facilitation of alpha motor neurons |
| Hypertonia: Spasticity and/or myoplasticity | Velocity dependent increase in resistance to stretch | Excess resistance that increases with movement | Spasticity, EMG activity greater than normal; myoplasticity: none | Chronic UMN lesions (SCI, spastic CP, stroke, traumatic brain injury, multiple sclerosis) | May be caused by neuromuscular overactivity, contracture, and/or weak actin-myosin bonds |
| Normal | Resistance to stretch in a resting, normally innervated muscle | Normal | None | Normal neuromuscular system | Titin and weak actin-myosin bonds |
| Hypotonia | Abnormally low muscular resistance to passive stretch | Less than normal resistance | None | Developmental disorders (trisomy 21, muscular dystrophy, CP) and temporarily following UMN lesions during neural shock | Decreased descending facilitation resulting in fewer weak actin-myosin bonds; excessive muscle length |
| | | | | LMN disorders | Decreased LMN input to skeletal muscles |
| Flaccidity | Complete loss of muscle tone | No resistance | None | LMN disorders, severe spina bifida, floppy infant syndrome (severe hypotonic CP) | Loss of LMN input to skeletal muscles |

*CP*, Cerebral palsy; *LMN*, lower motor neuron; *SCI*, spinal cord injury; *UMN*, upper motor neuron.
*Note that amount of resistance increases from the bottom of the table to the top, from no resistance (at bottom of table) to strong resistance (at top).

age-matched control subjects and 67% of control values for upper extremity strength when tested using a dynamometer.[50] Despite severe weakness, manual muscle testing scores were normal or near normal (>4 on a 0 to 5 scale) in 75% of subjects. This muscle weakness may be a normal age-related strength decline, more obvious in people who previously had polio because their muscles were previously weakened.

Post polio motor units show signs of ongoing denervation/reinnervation of muscle fibers.[51] No prospective data show that increased physical activity leads to muscle weakness. Exercise recommendations for people post polio are as follows: if strength is near normal and there are no signs of reinnervated motor units, heavy resistance training; if moderate weakness and signs of reinnervation, submaximal endurance training; and if severe paresis, walking, stationary bicycling, and swimming.[51]

## UPPER MOTOR NEURON SYNDROME

UMNs can be damaged by spinal cord injury, spastic cerebral palsy, multiple sclerosis, trauma, or loss of blood supply to part of the brain (stroke). UMN lesions can produce several changes in movement control, including:

1. Paresis or paralysis
2. Loss of fractionation of movement
3. Abnormal reflexes
4. Velocity-dependent hypertonia

Two other signs that typically occur only in specific types of UMN lesions—abnormal cocontraction (usually in spastic cerebral palsy) and abnormal muscle synergies (usually post stroke)—will be discussed later in this chapter.

### Paresis or Paralysis

Paresis occurs in UMN lesions as a consequence of inadequate facilitation of lower motor neurons. Paresis is common following *stroke*, the sudden onset of neurologic deficits due to disruption of the blood supply in the brain (also called *cerebrovascular accident*, or *CVA*). Paresis is also common in spastic cerebral palsy, traumatic brain injury, and incomplete spinal cord injury. In incomplete spinal cord injury, some somatosensory and/or motor function remains intact below the level of the lesion.

Paresis following UMN lesions leads to muscle disuse, causing secondary changes in muscles and the nervous system. Chronic muscle disuse often causes adaptive muscle contracture

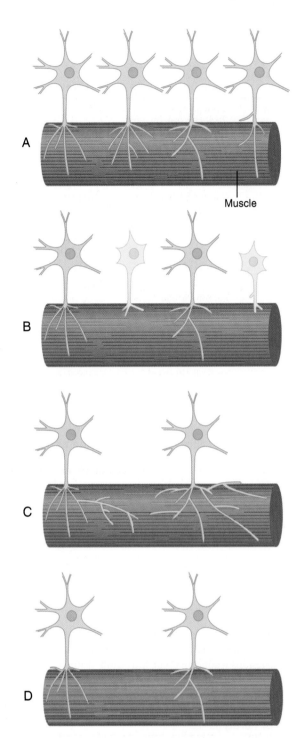

Muscle

**Fig. 10-32 Effects of polio on alpha motor neurons.**
**A,** Healthy motor units with normal innervation. **B,** Acute polio; death of some neurons leading to muscle fiber atrophy. **C,** Recovery; surviving neurons grow new distal branches to reinnervate surviving muscle fibers. **D,** Late post polio; overextended neurons can no longer support the excessive number of distal branches. The newer distal branches atrophy, leaving some muscle fibers denervated.

in addition to atrophy. Disuse also decreases the motor cortex representation of the disused body parts, leading to further paresis.[52]

*Paralysis* is the complete loss of voluntary control of muscles. Paralysis occurs in the muscles innervated by lower motor neurons below the level of a complete spinal cord lesion (loss of all somatosensory and motor function below the lesion). For example, if the spinal cord is completely severed at waist level, the person will have no voluntary control of the muscles below the waist.

## Loss of Fractionation of Movement

As discussed earlier, fractionation is the ability to activate individual muscles independently of other muscles. Interruption of lateral corticospinal signals prevents fractionation, profoundly affecting the ability to use the hand. Loss of fractionation interferes with fine movements, including fastening buttons or picking up coins, because the fingers of the involved hand act as a single unit. In the lower limb, loss of fractionation interferes with dorsiflexing the ankle. Attempts to dorsiflex the ankle produce inversion with plantarflexion instead.

## Abnormal Reflexes

Abnormal reflexes that may occur following UMN lesions include abnormal cutaneous reflexes, muscle stretch hyperreflexia, clonus, and the clasp-knife response.

### Abnormal Cutaneous Reflexes

Changes in cutaneous reflexes include Babinski's sign (Figure 10-33) and muscle spasms that occur in response to normally innocuous stimuli. *Babinski's sign* is extension of the great toe, often accompanied by fanning of the other toes. Firm stroking of the lateral sole of the foot, from the heel to the ball of the foot, then across the ball of the foot, elicits the sign. A key or the end of the handle of a reflex hammer is usually used as the stimulus. In infants until about 7 months of age, Babinski's sign is normal because the corticospinal tracts are not adequately myelinated. Although Babinski's sign is pathognomonic for corticospinal tract damage in people older than 6 months of age, the mechanism is not understood.

In people with spinal cord injury, muscle spasms may occur in response to cutaneous stimuli. These spasms begin after recovery from spinal shock (*spinal shock*, caused by edema at the lesion level and loss of descending facilitation below the lesion, is a temporary suppression of spinal cord function at and below the lesion following spinal cord injury). Following spinal shock, mild cutaneous stimulation, such as a gentle touch on the foot or putting on clothing, may result in abrupt flexion of the lower limb. Occasionally, a touch on one lower limb may elicit bilateral lower limb flexion. In rare cases, the muscle spasms are severe enough to disturb the person's sitting balance, which can cause the person to fall out of a chair.

The following three abnormal reflexes occur most often in people with chronic spinal cord injuries, although these signs may also occur in other types of UMN lesions.

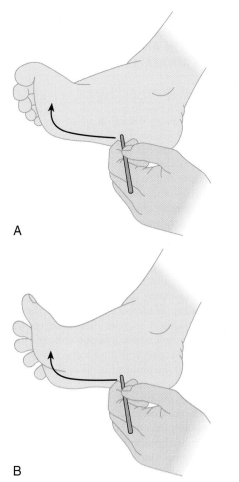

A

B

**Fig. 10-33** Babinski's sign. **A,** Normal. Stroking from the heel to the ball of the foot along the lateral sole, then across the ball of the foot, normally causes the toes to flex. **B,** Developmental or pathologic. Babinski's sign in response to the same stimulus. In people with corticospinal tract lesions or in infants younger than 7 months old, the great toe extends. Although the other toes may fan out, as shown, movement of the toes other than the great toe is not required for Babinski's sign.

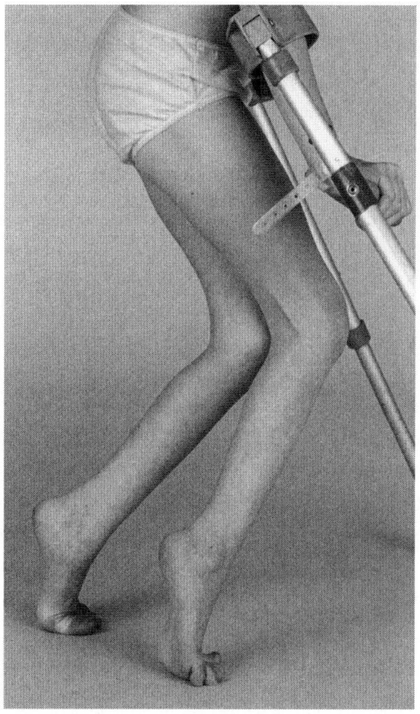

**Fig. 10-34** An 8-year-old with hypertonia of the hip and knee flexors and ankle plantarflexors. *(From Young JL, Rodda J, Selber P, et al: Management of the knee in spastic diplegia: what is the dose? Orthop Clin North Am 41:568, 2010, Figure 4, part A.)*

## Muscle Stretch Hyperreflexia

In muscle stretch hyperreflexia, loss of inhibitory corticospinal input combined with LMN and interneuron development of enhanced excitability results in excessive LMN response to afferent input from stretch receptors. The result is excessive muscle contraction when spindles are stretched, caused by excessive firing of lower motor neurons (see Figure 10-16).

## Clonus

Involuntary, repeating, rhythmic contractions of a single muscle group are called *clonus.* In contrast, tremor involves alternating agonist/antagonist contractions. Muscle stretch, cutaneous and noxious stimuli, and attempts at voluntary movement can induce clonus.[53] Not all clonus is pathologic; rapid passive ankle

dorsiflexion may elicit unsustained clonus in neurologically intact people. Unsustained clonus fades after a few beats, even with maintained muscle stretch.[54] Sustained clonus is always pathologic. Sustained clonus is produced when lack of UMN control allows activation of oscillating neural networks in the spinal cord.[53] In people with chronic spinal cord injury or other UMN lesions, sustained clonus of the soleus muscle may be triggered by placement of a foot on a wheelchair footrest.

## Clasp-Knife Response

Occasionally, when a paretic muscle is slowly and passively stretched, resistance drops at a specific point in the range of motion. This is called the *clasp-knife response* because the change in resistance is similar to opening a pocketknife: initial strong resistance to opening the knife blade gives way to easier movement. When a therapist passively stretches a paretic biceps brachii muscle, resistance to passive movement is initially strong. However, if stretch is steadily applied, often the therapist will encounter an abrupt decrease in resistance. Type II afferents, including some joint capsule receptors and cutaneous and subcutaneous touch and pressure receptors, elicit the clasp-knife response.[55]

## Velocity-Dependent Hypertonia

Velocity-dependent hypertonia limits joint range of motion, interferes with function, and may cause deformity. For example, significant bilateral plantarflexor hypertonia may allow only toe walking, because lack of ankle dorsiflexion prevents the heels from touching the ground (Figure 10-34).

## Myoplasticity and Spasticity

*Myoplasticity* comprises adaptive changes within a muscle in response to changes in neuromuscular activity level and to prolonged positioning. In a person with an intact nervous system, chronic muscle disuse and immobility (e.g., wearing a cast for 6 weeks) result in an increased number of weak actin-myosin bonds, disuse atrophy, and contracture. Similar muscular changes occur following UMN lesions owing to loss of normal neural signals to the muscle. Decreased neuromuscular signals cause both disuse and neurogenic muscle atrophy. Paresis or paralysis leads to immobility that causes contracture. For example, contracture of lower limb muscles contributes to shortening of the soleus and gastrocnemius muscles in people with stroke, traumatic brain injury, spinal cord injury, or spastic cerebral palsy.[56-58] Contractures can make dressing, hygiene, and positioning difficult.

*Spasticity* is neuromuscular overactivity secondary to an UMN lesion. Overactive neural input to muscles causes excessive contraction. Two mechanisms produce neural overactivity: *hyperreflexia* and *brainstem UMN overactivity*. In hyperreflexia, absence of corticospinal inhibition onto LMNs and subsequent development of LMN excessive excitability cause an excessive LMN response to muscle spindle input. Cerebral lesions that disinhibit the reticulospinal and/or vestibulospinal tracts cause brainstem UMN overactivity; this will be discussed further in the sections on developmental spasticity and cerebral spasticity.

Spasticity affects approximately 20% of people with stroke, between 47% and 70% of those with multiple sclerosis, 34% of those with spinal cord injury, more than 90% with cerebral palsy, and 50% of patients with traumatic brain injury.[59] Spasticity is beneficial when the muscle contraction contributes to postural control and mobility, maintains muscle mass and bone mineralization, decreases dependent edema, and prevents deep vein thromboses. Spasticity may require treatment if muscle contractions interfere with function, activities of daily living, and/or sleep, or cause discomfort.[59]

For optimal therapeutic intervention, precise terminology must be used to accurately describe pathology. *Myoplasticity* denotes contracture, atrophy, and weak actin-myosin binding. *Spasticity* is neuromuscular overactivity caused by hyperreflexia and/or brainstem UMN overactivity. *Hyperreflexia* refers to muscle spindle input leading to overactivity in disinhibited and excessively excitable LMNs, resulting in muscle contraction. *Brainstem UMN overactivity* indicates excessive reticulospinal or vestibulospinal tract signals to LMNs. These terms differentiate among factors causing hypertonia.

## MECHANISM OF SPASTICITY DEPENDS UPON SITE OF LESION AND WHETHER LESION OCCURS PERINATALLY

### Developmental Spasticity: Spastic Cerebral Palsy

In spastic cerebral palsy, the lesion affects the corticospinal and corticobrainstem tracts during the perinatal period, interfering with development of the spinal cord and brain. When the nervous system is developing normally, a single corticospinal axon may synapse with spinal LMNs that innervate an agonist muscle, synergists, and antagonists. In normal development, the weaker synapses are eliminated, and by age 4, a corticospinal axon that previously synapsed with LMNs to antagonists and synergists will synapse only with LMNs to agonists. Damage to the corticospinal tracts during development eliminates some competition for synaptic sites during a critical period, causing persistence of inappropriate connections and abnormal development of spinal motor centers. Persistence of inappropriate connections causes *abnormal cocontraction*, the simultaneous activation of antagonist muscles that interferes with task performance. For example, when a person attempts to contract the biceps brachii, synergists and the triceps also contract. Loss of corticospinal input disinhibits LMNs in the spinal cord, resulting in hyperreflexia.

Loss of cortical inhibition to the brainstem allows overactivity of neck reflexes (collicular signals to reticulospinal tracts) and the vestibulospinal tracts, producing changes in posture with changes in head position (see Figure 11-22). Disinhibition of the reticulospinal tract also produces abnormal synergies. Thus developmental spasticity is caused predominantly by cocontraction, hyperreflexia, and brainstem UMN overactivity affecting the vestibulospinal and reticulospinal tracts.

### Adult-Onset Cerebral Spasticity: Reticulospinal Overactivity

Typical stroke (affecting the middle cerebral artery) interrupts the corticospinal and corticoreticular tracts on one side of the brain. Because stroke usually affects the adult nervous system, unilateral loss of corticospinal and corticoreticular tracts is imposed on a nervous system that has completed development. Corticoreticular lesions diminish cortical inhibition of the reticulospinal tract that originates in the brainstem. The disinhibition increases reticulospinal tract signals to spinal lower motor neurons, causing excessive muscle contraction.[32] Thus reticulospinal tract overactivity is the primary cause of stroke spasticity. An example is involuntary flexion of the paretic upper limb fingers and elbow when the person walks (Figure 10-35). This exaggerated interlimb neural coupling occurs as a result of disinhibited reticulospinal tract activity and subsequent concurrent activation of muscles in upper and lower extremities.[60] Similar patterns of cerebral spasticity occur with lesions of the corticoreticular tract in multiple sclerosis and traumatic brain injury.

### Spinal Spasticity: Primarily Hyperreflexia

In spinal cord injury, corticobrainstem activity is normal. When UMN tracts are severed in the spinal cord, disinhibited interneurons and lower motor neurons below the lesion develop enhanced excitability; this causes hyperreflexia.[61] When normal somatosensory signals reach the spinal cord below the lesion, the interneurons and lower motor neurons overreact. In people with complete spinal cord injury, hyperreflexia can elicit contraction of muscles that cannot voluntarily contract.

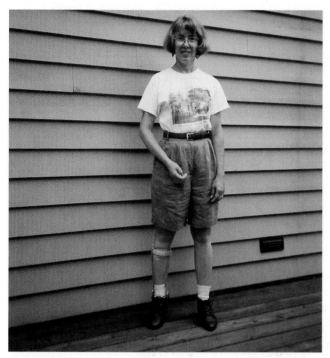

**Fig. 10-35** Person post stroke after walking. Note the right elbow flexion that persists after walking, caused by increased reticulospinal tract activity during walking. The flexion is temporary, is not caused by hyperreflexia, and does not cause further loss of upper limb function.

Hyperreflexia can contribute to movement dysfunction in people with chronic incomplete spinal cord injury (iSCI). Excessive phasic stretch reflex activity may occur during both passive muscle stretch and active movements in people with iSCI.[62] For example, passive range of motion that normally would not elicit muscle contraction may trigger a vigorous muscle contraction, strong enough to propel a person out of a chair. Hyperreflexia may also limit walking speed, as antagonist muscles contract in response to stretch during the gait cycle. In addition, hyperreflexia can interfere with positioning, mobility, hygiene, comfort, and sleep. However, there are positive aspects to hyperreflexia. People can intentionally trigger hyperreflexia to elicit involuntary muscle contraction during transfers, and muscle contractions triggered by hyperreflexia help maintain muscle mass (prevent atrophy) and assist venous return.

Contracture also affects muscles in spinal cord injury (SCI). In some people with incomplete spinal cord injury (iSCI), gastrocnemius muscle electromyographic (EMG) activity during gait is minimal, yet the force exerted on the Achilles tendon exerted by muscle contracture is excessive (Figure 10-36).

Clinical signs of spinal spasticity include a velocity-dependent increase in tonic stretch reflexes, brisk deep tendon reflexes, exaggerated cutaneous reflexes, involuntary flexor and extensor spasms, and clonus. The last three signs listed occur much more frequently in spinal spasticity than in other UMN lesions.

Table 10-4 summarizes the terms used to describe common impairments in UMN lesions.

Figure 10-37 lists the factors that contribute to hypertonia.

## MEASURING HYPERTONIA

EMG recordings and the Ashworth Scale are often used to assess hypertonia. Surface EMG can be used to reveal the mechanisms of hypertonia and to assess effects of interventions on tone and motor impairment. Passive testing provides little

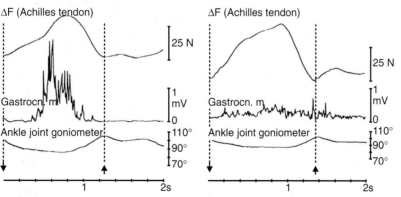

**Fig. 10-36** Averaged recordings (30 steps) of a step cycle during slow gait of a normal subject *(left)* and a subject with paraparesis *(right)* due to a spinal cord lesion. From top to bottom in each recording, changes in tension recorded from the Achilles tendon, a gastrocnemius electromyogram (EMG), and a goniometer signal from the ankle joint. Rectified EMG recordings are shown. In the normal subject, an increase in Achilles tendon tension correlates with an increase in gastrocnemius EMG activity. In the paraparetic subject, the increase in Achilles tendon tension does not correlate with an increase in EMG. Instead, the increase in Achilles tendon tension coincides with stretch of the triceps surae during passive dorsiflexion of the foot in the stance phase. Down arrow, foot strike; up arrow, toe off. *(From Dietz V, Berger W: Normal and impaired regulation of muscle stiffness in gait: a new hypothesis about muscle hypertonia. Exp Neurol 79:680-7, 1983.)*

**TABLE 10-4**    TERMS DESCRIBING IMPAIRMENTS COMMON IN UPPER MOTOR NEURON LESIONS*

| Term | Definition and Comments |
|---|---|
| Abnormal synergy | Abnormal coupling of movements at adjacent joints due to stereotyped coactivation of muscles. An example is shoulder abduction and external rotation combined with elbow flexion when the person is attempting to reach forward. Mechanism: loss of cortical inhibition of reticulospinal tracts |
| Abnormal cocontraction | Temporal overlap of agonist and antagonist muscle contraction. Cocontraction is normal when learning a new motor skill and when stability is required. Cocontraction is abnormal only when it interferes with achieving the movement goal. Abnormal cocontraction is prevalent in spastic cerebral palsy, due to persistence of developmental corticospinal inputs to agonist, synergist, and antagonist muscles. |
| Hyperreflexia | Excessive reflex response to muscle stretch. Hyperreflexia is caused by reduced descending inhibition of lower motor neurons (LMNs) and the subsequent development of LMN excessive excitability. Hyperreflexia often contributes to movement disorders post spinal cord injury and in spastic cerebral palsy. Hyperreflexia usually does not interfere with active movement post stroke. |
| Muscle contracture | Adaptive shortening of muscle, caused by the muscle remaining in a shortened position for prolonged periods of time. The decrease in length is caused by loss of sarcomeres. |
| Hypertonia | Excessive resistance to muscle stretch regardless of whether the stretch is active or passive. Produced by neural input to muscles (overactive stretch reflex or overactivity of reticulospinal and/or vestibulospinal tracts resulting in active muscle contraction) and/or by changes within the muscle (myoplasticity: contracture and weak actin-myosin bonding). |
| Muscle overactivity | Muscle contraction that is excessive for the task. Caused by excess neural input to the muscle(s). May be due to reticulospinal tract overactivity,[32,60] vestibulospinal tract overactivity, pain, anxiety, or lack of skill in task performance |
| Muscle tone | Amount of tension in resting muscle. Muscle tone is examined passively and is not an indicator of ability to move actively. |
| Myoplasticity | Changes within muscle secondary to an upper motor neuron (UMN) lesion and/or prolonged positioning. Produced by contracture and increased weak actin-myosin bonding. |
| Paresis | Decreased ability to generate the level of force required for a task. Occurs in all UMN lesions. |
| Spasticity | Neuromuscular overactivity secondary to UMN lesion. |

*Note: Some of these terms are also used to describe impairments resulting from pathologies other than UMN lesions.

| | Neural factors | | | Myoplastic factors | | |
|---|---|---|---|---|---|---|
| | Brainstem UMN overactivity | Tonic stretch hyperreflexia | Abnormal cocontraction | Contracture | Increased # weak actin-myosin bonds | Abnormal muscle development |
| Cerebral spasticity (stroke, MS, traumatic brain injury) | Primarily reticulospinal | No | Primarily affects finger movements (lack of fractionation) | ✓ | ✓ | No |
| Developmental cerebral spasticity (spastic cerebral palsy) | Vestibulospinal and reticulospinal | ✓ | ✓ | ✓ | ✓ | ✓ |
| Spinal spasticity (complete spinal cord injury, MS) | No | ✓ | No | ✓ | ✓ | No |

**Fig. 10-37  Factors contributing to hypertonia during active movements.** In people post stroke or with spastic cerebral palsy, reticulospinal tract overactivity, contracture, and increased number of weak actin-myosin bonds contribute to hypertonia. Note that post stroke, hyperreflexia typically does not contribute to hypertonia during active movements. After spinal cord injury, tonic stretch hyperreflexia contributes to the increased resistance to stretch. If the spinal cord injury is motor incomplete, then upper motor neuron (UMN) overactivity contributes to the hypertonia (not shown). In spastic cerebral palsy, the unique contributors to hypertonia are vestibulospinal tract overactivity and abnormal muscle development.

information about how a person performs actively, regardless of whether the person is neurologically intact or has a neurologic deficit.

EMG recordings and muscle resistance to stretch should be considered within the context of functional tasks. Therefore, clinically pertinent information can be obtained by using surface EMG to determine which of the following factors is contributing to movement impairment:

- Contracture
- Hyperreflexia
- Cocontraction
- Inappropriate timing of muscle activity

Contracture, adaptive shortening of muscle, produces decreased passive range of motion without increased EMG output.

Phasic stretch hyperreflexia is indicated by excessive EMG amplitude occurring 30 to 50 msec after the initiation of muscle stretch; tonic stretch hyperreflexia produces excessive EMG amplitude 80 to 100 msec after initiation of muscle stretch (Figure 10-38). Loss of inhibitory corticospinal input results in excessive lower motor neuron response to afferent input from stretch receptors. The excessive lower motor neuron signals depolarize the muscle membrane causing increased muscle contraction that interferes with the desired movement. Increased muscle membrane depolarization registers as increased amplitude on EMG.

Cocontraction produces temporal overlap of EMG activity in antagonist muscles (Figure 10-39). Cocontraction and increased muscle resistance to stretch are abnormal only if they interfere with achieving the goal of the task; people with intact

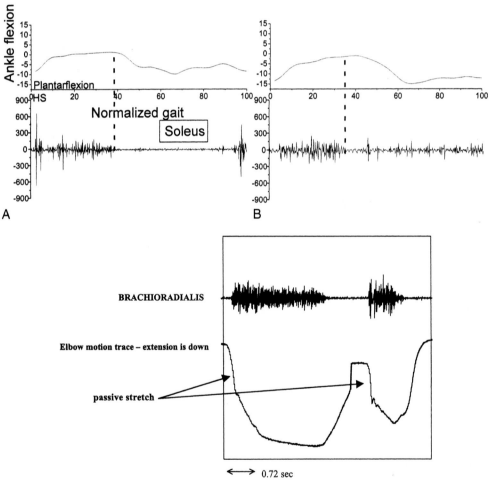

**Fig. 10-38 Hyperreflexia. A,** Phasic stretch hyperreflexia. Electomyogram (EMG) of soleus muscle activity during gait in a 31-year-old subject with spastic cerebral palsy. When the foot begins to bear weight, soleus muscle stretch elicits a spike in EMG activity. **B,** After drug treatment (intrathecal baclofen) to reduce spasticity, phasic stretch hyperreflexia is absent. **C,** Tonic stretch hyperreflexia. Abnormal EMG activity continues for the duration of the muscle stretch. *(**A** and **B** modified from Rémy-Néris O, Tiffreau V, Bouilland S, Bussel B: Intrathecal baclofen in subjects with spastic hemiplegia: assessment of the antispastic effect during gait. Arch Phys Med Rehabil 84:643-650, 2003, Figure 4, p 647. **C** from Mayer NH, Esquenazi A: Muscle overactivity and movement dysfunction in the upper motoneuron syndrome. Phys Med Rehabil Clin North Am 14:855-83, 2003.)*

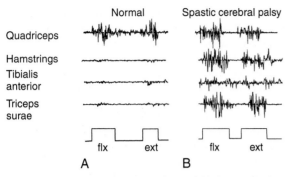

**Fig. 10-39 Electromyograms of gait-like lower limb movements in supine children. A,** Normal motor control; quadriceps muscle is contracting, and the other muscles are relatively inactive. **B,** Spastic cerebral palsy; abnormal cocontraction. Quadriceps, hamstrings, tibialis anterior, and triceps surae are cocontracting during lower limb movements. Electromyographic (EMG) data were selected specifically to show abnormal cocontraction, the simultaneous contraction of agonists and antagonists that interferes with performing tasks. Not all children with spastic cerebral palsy have abnormal cocontraction; in many cases, paresis or hyperreflexia causes the gait abnormalities. *(From Wong AM, Chen CL, Hong WH, et al: Motor control assessment for rhizotomy in cerebral palsy. Am J Phys Med Rehabil 79:441-450, 2000.)*

**TABLE 10-5  MODIFIED ASHWORTH SCALE: MUSCLE RESISTANCE TO PASSIVE STRETCH**

| Grade | Description |
|---|---|
| 0 | No increase in muscle tone |
| 1 | Slight increase in muscle tone, manifested by a catch or by minimal resistance at the end of the range of motion (ROM) when the affected part(s) is moved in flexion or extension |
| 1+ | Slight increase in muscle tone, manifested by a catch, followed by minimal resistance throughout the remainder (less than half) of ROM |
| 2 | More marked increase in muscle tone through most of ROM, but affected part(s) easily moved |
| 3 | Considerable increase in muscle tone; passive movement difficult |
| 4 | Affected part(s) rigid in flexion or extension |

From Bohannon RW, Smith MB: Interrater reliability of a modified Ashworth scale of muscle spasticity. Phys Ther 67:206-7, 1987.

neuromuscular systems often use cocontraction and increased muscle resistance to stretch when learning a new movement or for stability.[63]

Inappropriate timing of muscle activity (e.g., premature, prolonged, delayed, absent, out of phase during gait[64-67]) may interfere with movement in patients with upper motor neuron syndrome.

Paresis, decreased ability to generate appropriate force for a functional movement, is often an important contributor to movement impairment. However, paresis cannot be assessed accurately with the use of EMG because functional tasks involve multiple muscles, and the force generated at a specific joint depends on the contributions of agonists, antagonists, and synergists. Assessing only the contribution of the agonist may be misleading because antagonists and synergists may be deficient in providing stability or in reinforcing or opposing the agonist's activity at the appropriate time. Two technical problems are associated with using EMG to assess paresis. First, EMG amplitude must be normalized by comparing the EMG elicited by a maximal electrical stimulus to the motor nerve with the EMG elicited by a maximum voluntary contraction of the muscle. People with central paresis cannot completely activate their LMN pools; therefore, normalization cannot be accomplished. Second, more general, because muscles slide under the skin and electrical signals spread from adjacent muscles, there is no way to ascertain that the amplitude of EMG activity recorded from the skin above a particular muscle is produced only by that muscle.

The Ashworth Scale is a subjective clinical assessment of resistance to passive stretch. For example, the evaluator passively stretches the biceps and assesses whether the resistance to stretch is normal or greater than normal. Although the Ashworth Scale

and the Modified Ashworth Scale (the modified Ashworth adds the 1+ score, the scales are otherwise the same; Table 10-5) are purported to measure spasticity, these scales do not actually measure spasticity because information from this test cannot be used to distinguish between contracture and hyperreflexia.[68,69] Further, no direct relationship exists between changes in the Ashworth score and improvements or declines in functional activity. High scores on the Ashworth Scale are associated with contracture, not spasticity.[70] Ashworth scores assigned by an experienced neurologist correlate poorly with EMG recording during passive stretching using a motor that controls the velocity of muscle stretch.[71] The reliability and validity of the Ashworth Scale are inadequate to recommend its use as a measure of spasticity.[69,72]

Given that myoplasticity, hyperreflexia, and brainstem UMN overactivity are independent of each other, it is not surprising that little correlation has been found among clinical measures of spasticity using the Modified Ashworth Scale, a strain gauge, and EMG activity. Although measurement techniques vary, their validity is questionable. Scores on these measurements do not correlate well, and most measures do not differentiate among the three causes of hypertonia. Lack of consistent results caused by using several different measures of spasticity on the same individuals has been confirmed by Malhotra and associates.[73] Researchers tested resistance to passive wrist extension using a strain gauge, the Modified Ashworth Scale, and EMG activity. Even though only passive evaluation techniques were used, the degree of spasticity was not consistently assessed.

A new five-step clinical assessment of spasticity has been proposed.[74] This assessment measures passive range of motion (PROM), angle of catch or clonus on fast passive stretch, active range of motion, maximal frequency of rapid alternating movements, and active function. The authors suggest that unacceptably limited PROM alerts the clinician to consider lengthening interventions or blocking injections into the shortened muscles. The catch angle indicates whether phasic hyperreflexia is a movement limiting factor; active ROM limitations indicate that strengthening should be emphasized; maximal frequency of rapid alternating movements may also indicate strengthening intervention; and active function tests indicate the task-specific movements that need intervention.[74] Although the reliability of this assessment has not been evaluated, different aspects of myoplasticity and spasticity are included.

## TYPES OF UPPER MOTOR NEURON LESIONS

This section discusses spastic cerebral palsy, stroke, and spinal cord injury. Although head trauma, tumors, and multiple sclerosis can damage UMNs, affected structures and clinical outcomes are so variable that a discussion of motor effects is beyond the scope of this text.

### Spastic Cerebral Palsy

In spastic cerebral palsy (CP), abnormal supraspinal influences, failure of normal neuronal selection, and consequent aberrant muscle development lead to movement dysfunction. Motor disorders in spastic CP include problems with coordination, abnormal tonic stretch reflexes during rest and active movement, reflex irradiation (spread of reflex activity; e.g., tapping the biceps tendon causes finger flexor contraction in addition to biceps contraction), lack of postural preparation prior to movement, and abnormal cocontraction of muscles.

Adults with spastic CP typically have adequate strength for upper limb activities despite being able to generate only half of the force that age-matched controls can generate.[75] Their upper limb function is impaired by poor coordination, hyperreflexia, and contracture.[75] Lower limb strength correlates well with motor function and with gait. Spasticity does not contribute significantly to gait and gross motor dysfunction.[76] Lower limb strength in ambulatory children with spastic cerebral palsy ranges from 43% to 90% of control values.[77]

### Stroke, Middle Cerebral Artery (MCA)

Stroke most frequently affects the middle cerebral artery (see Chapters 1, 18, and 19), damaging corticospinal, corticoticular and corticobrainstem neurons and thus disrupting cortical connections with the spinal cord, brainstem, and cerebellum, in addition to intracortical connections. In this chapter, only middle cerebral artery stroke (Pathology 10-1) is discussed; other locations of stroke have different effects and are considered in Chapters 15, 18, and 19. Post–MCA stroke changes in communication among neurons within the cerebrum are illustrated in Figure 10-40. Because lateral corticospinal neurons are

| PATHOLOGY 10-1 | STROKE, MIDDLE CEREBRAL ARTERY |
|---|---|
| Pathology | Interruption of blood supply |
| Etiology | Occlusion or hemorrhage |
| Speed of onset | Acute |
| Signs and symptoms | |
| Consciousness | May be temporarily impaired |
| Affect (emotional expression), mood | Affect: emotional lability (abnormal, uncontrolled expression of emotions, often pathological laughter or crying; see Chapter 18). Mood: depression, anxiety disorder, apathy; rarely mania |
| Communication and memory | May be impaired (see Chapter 18) |
| Sensory | Usually impaired contralateral to the lesion |
| Autonomic | May be impaired |
| Language | May be impaired (see Chapter 18) |
| Motor | Contralateral to the lesion: paresis, muscle atrophy, contracture, loss of fractionation of movement, decreased movement speed and efficiency, impaired postural control, spasticity, Babinski's sign; ipsilesion: mild paresis; may have difficulty eating, speaking |
| Region affected | Cerebrum: corticospinal, corticoreticular, and corticobrainstem tracts |
| Demographics | Males affected more frequently than females |
| Incidence | First CVA (any artery): 198 per 100,000 population per year[80] |
| Prevalence | 2.6% of population[81] |
| Recurrence | Cumulative risk of stroke recurrence at 1 year, 5 years, and 10 years: 7.1%, 16.2%, and 24.5%[82] |
| Prognosis: ischemic stroke | About 20% die from stroke within the first 30 days; a total of 31% die within the first year post stroke, with cardiovascular disease the most common cause of death[83] |

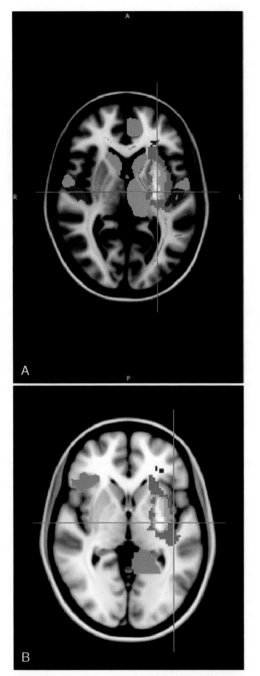

**Fig. 10-40 Changes in neural communication post stroke.** Location of stroke lesions shown in red to white. Lesions are in the area of the internal capsule/basal ganglia. **A,** Gray matter regions with reduced communications in patients relative to controls *(light blue shows significant differences, dark blue area shows trends).* Pink indicates white matter areas with reduced communication. **B,** Gray matter areas with increased communication relative to controls are colored green. *(From Crofts JJ, Higham DJ, Bosnell R, et al: Network analysis detects changes in the contralesional hemisphere following stroke. Neuroimage 54:161-9, 2011.)*

frequently affected, the impairments that most often limit activities of daily living are paresis and decreased fractionation of movement in both the upper and lower limbs contralateral to the lesion.[78,79] However, because 10% of the lateral corticospinal tract projects ipsilaterally, the function of the ipsilateral limbs is also impaired (see later section).

## Myoplasticity Post Stroke

After a stroke, paretic muscles exert excessive resistance to muscle stretch. Excessive resistance during active movement is due primarily to changes within the muscles (myoplasticity). These changes include:

1. Contracture
2. Increased weak binding of actin and myosin

Contracture is normal in muscles maintained in shortened positions. When muscles are paretic, immobility often leads to structural shortening of specific muscles. For example, people who have had strokes may tend to rest their paretic arm for long periods in their lap when sitting.[84] This sustained positioning, with the arm comfortable and somewhat protected, may predispose the elbow flexor muscles to contracture.[85] This adaptive muscle shortening prevents normal range of motion at involved joints. Similarly, impairment of hand function following stroke is associated with wrist flexion contractures, not with spasticity (spasticity measured with EMG during passive movement).[86]

In any resting muscle (normal or paretic), weak bonds between actin and myosin produce resistance to stretch. These bonds produce the initial resistance that arises when muscle is stretched. *Weak actin-myosin bonds* continue to form as long as the muscle remains immobile. Because paretic muscles seldom contract, prolonged immobility occurs frequently. Immobility allows excessive numbers of weak actin-myosin bonds to form, producing increased resistance to stretch.

Post stroke, force generation in the nonparetic leg correlates with the level of EMG activity (as it does in people with intact neuromuscular systems). This correlation occurs because LMN signals depolarize the muscle membrane before muscle contraction. Greater intensity of neural signals causes greater muscle membrane depolarization (muscle membrane depolarization is recorded by EMG) and increased muscle contraction. However, in the paretic leg, high levels of force generation are simultaneous with low levels of EMG activity. This indicates that motor neurons are less active than normal in the paretic limb.[87,88] If neural signals were contributing to hypertonia, EMG activity recorded from depolarizing muscle membranes would increase with increased muscle force output. Contracture causes increased resistance to stretch. EMG, force, and goniometric readings comparing data from the paretic and the nonparetic leg of a person with hemiplegia are shown in Figure 10-41. The ability to produce high levels of force with little neural input to the muscles is beneficial; it allows weight bearing on a paretic lower limb that would collapse without contracture because the paretic muscle could not support body weight.[89] However, loss of neural control prevents fast movements and adjustments to uneven surfaces, and may cause knee hyperextension, because the ankle cannot dorsiflex during mid- to late stance phases of gait. Development of hypertonia post stroke is summarized in Figure 10-42.

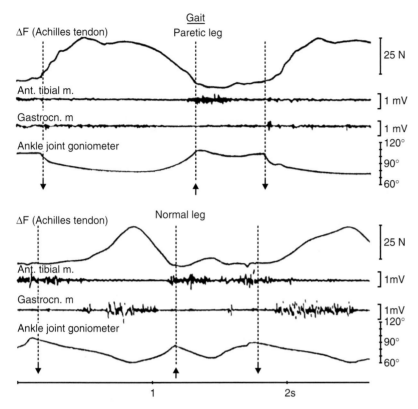

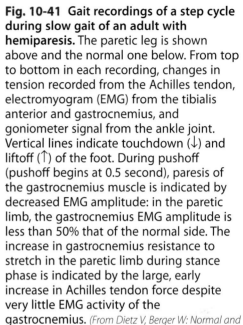

**Fig. 10-41 Gait recordings of a step cycle during slow gait of an adult with hemiparesis.** The paretic leg is shown above and the normal one below. From top to bottom in each recording, changes in tension recorded from the Achilles tendon, electromyogram (EMG) from the tibialis anterior and gastrocnemius, and goniometer signal from the ankle joint. Vertical lines indicate touchdown (↓) and liftoff (↑) of the foot. During pushoff (pushoff begins at 0.5 second), paresis of the gastrocnemius muscle is indicated by decreased EMG amplitude: in the paretic limb, the gastrocnemius EMG amplitude is less than 50% that of the normal side. The increase in gastrocnemius resistance to stretch in the paretic limb during stance phase is indicated by the large, early increase in Achilles tendon force despite very little EMG activity of the gastrocnemius. *(From Dietz V, Berger W: Normal and impaired regulation of muscle stiffness in gait: a new hypothesis about muscle hypertonia. Exp Neurol 79:680-7, 1983.)*

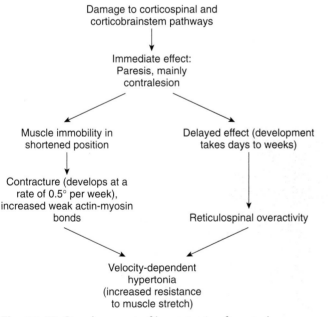

**Fig. 10-42** Development of hypertonia after stroke. Immobility leads to contracture; spasticity does not affect the development of contracture post stroke. *(Rate of development of contracture post stroke is from Malhotra S, Pandyan AD, Rosewilliam S, et al: Spasticity and contractures at the wrist after stroke: time course of development and their association with functional recovery of the upper limb. Clin Rehabil 25(2):184-91, 2011.)*

Becher and colleagues[90] demonstrated the dissociation of myoplasticity from neural influence. They found that people post stroke had excessive resistance to stretch in the triceps surae muscles. Following local anesthesia of the tibial nerve to prevent neural activation of the muscle, there was no change in muscle resistance to stretch, demonstrating that hypertonia was due to changes within the muscle and is independent from hyperreflexia. Consistent with this concept, in the upper limbs of people post stroke, the stretch reflex amplitude of the bicep muscle is reduced compared with normal, despite continued excessive bicep muscle resistance to stretch.[91]

Rarely, following a stroke, phasic stretch hyperreflexia occurs when sufficient force can be generated quickly enough to produce sufficient type Ia afferent activity. However, phasic stretch hyperreflexia during active movement is rare because most paretic muscles cannot generate sufficient force quickly enough to rapidly stretch antagonist muscles. Phasic stretch hyperreflexia is a far less important factor in movement impairment post stroke than paresis, decreased fractionation of movement, abnormal timing of muscle contraction, and muscular changes, are, because people can avoid phasic stretch hyperreflexia by simply moving slowly. In summary, when poststroke paretic muscle is stretched, the initial, strong resistance to stretch is produced by weak actin-myosin bonds. The resistance encountered as the stretch continues through the range of motion is due to contracture. During active movements on the paretic side, hyperreflexia typically does not contribute to resistance to movement.

## Paresis and Voluntary Movement Post Stroke

Contrary to a common misconception, neither contracture nor hyperreflexia of elbow flexors contributes significantly to activity limitations in the poststroke upper limb. After stroke, the only factor that limits upper limb activity is weakness.[92] Weakness is due to both voluntary activation failure (inability to send adequate signals to specific muscles[88]) and muscle atrophy.[93]

The reticulospinal tract provides voluntary control of paretic limb muscles post stroke.[32] Reticulospinal voluntary control consists of abnormal synergies that mainly affect the proximal joints. In the upper limb, the flexion synergy comprises shoulder abduction and internal rotation, elbow flexion, and forearm pronation. Lower limb flexion synergy consists of hip external rotation, abduction, flexion, knee flexion, and ankle flexion. In the lower limb, the extensor synergy is as follows: hip internal rotation, adduction, extension, knee extension, and ankle extension and inversion. The effect of reticulospinal overactivity on LMNs that innervate elbow flexors during walking is mainly a cosmetic problem. Excessive elbow flexion during walking contributes to an abnormal appearance but has little influence on function. Reticulospinal overactivity to LMNs that innervate hip and knee muscles in the lower limb initiates and regulates gait.[32]

## Ipsilateral Upper Limb Impairment Post Stroke

In adults with unilateral stroke, maximum recovery of the ipsilesional upper limb was reached approximately 1 month post stroke; however, the ipsilesional side did not completely recover upper limb function to age-matched control levels.[94] Shoulder movements recovered to near-normal levels, but hand function ipsilateral to the lesion remained impaired.[94] The proximal upper limb recovery can be explained by bilateral control from medial UMNs to LMNs that innervate proximal muscles. The hand recovers less because loss of ipsilesional lateral corticospinal tract input to LMNs partially deprives the ipsilateral hand of control of fractionated movements.

> ### ◉ Clinical Pearl
>
> Movement disorders post middle cerebral artery stroke are the consequences of paresis, decreased fractionation of movement, and myoplasticity. Rarely does hyperreflexia contribute significantly to movement limitations. The reticulospinal tract provides control of voluntary movement of the paretic limbs.

## Spinal Cord Injury

A person with a complete SCI loses all descending neuronal control below the level of the lesion. In iSCI, the function of some ascending and/or descending fibers is preserved within the spinal cord. The following conditions occur following SCI:

1. Phasic stretch reflexes and the withdrawal reflex involving intact spinal segments below the lesion can still be elicited.[89]
2. The amount of contracture significantly correlates with the amount of resistance to muscle stretch.[58]
3. Type IIb muscle fibers predominate and the number of type I muscle fibers is reduced.[95]

In incomplete spinal cord injury, excessive soleus muscle stretch reflexes occur during midstance and the swing phase of gait.[62] In iSCI, hyperreflexia is a major contributor to excess muscle contraction, and resistance to stretch increases significantly at end range, probably owing to contracture.[96]

> ### ◉ Clinical Pearl
>
> Following spinal cord injury, excessive stretch reflexes, muscle contracture, and increased cross-bridge binding produce excessive resistance to muscle stretch. In people with iSCI, paresis, hyperreflexia and contracture limit active movement.

## Common Characteristics of Upper Motor Neuron Lesions

Muscle resistance to stretch is produced by weak actin-myosin bonds, the amount of titin, and active factors (contractile). In people with chronic UMN lesions, weak actin-myosin bonds, contracture, and spasticity cause increased resistance to muscle stretch. Figure 10-43 summarizes the differences in hypertonia in stroke and complete spinal cord injury. Emotional agitation and pain lead to excessive muscle force in people with CVA, spastic cerebral palsy, and iSCI via limbic action on motor cortical areas and via nonspecific UMNs to lower motor neurons.

In summary, common signs of UMN lesions include paresis, abnormal timing of muscle activity, Babinski's sign, and myoplasticity. Hyperreflexia of the phasic stretch reflex, clonus, abnormal cutaneous reflexes (withdrawal reflex, Babinski's sign), and the clasp-knife phenomenon occur most commonly in chronic spinal cord injury. Reflex irradiation and abnormal cocontraction of antagonist muscles typically do not occur with damage to the mature nervous system (which includes most strokes and spinal cord injuries); these signs typically accompany UMN syndromes that arise during nervous system development (e.g., spastic cerebral palsy). Reciprocal inhibition is preserved in adult CVA and in most spinal cord injuries because damage occurs to a mature nervous system.

## INTERVENTIONS FOR IMPAIRMENTS SECONDARY TO UPPER MOTOR NEURON LESIONS

### Spastic Cerebral Palsy

Paresis, loss of fractionation of movement, abnormal cocontraction, and hyperreflexia affect the ability of people with spastic cerebral palsy to perform desired actions. Paresis of agonist postural muscles is the primary impairment that interferes with balance recovery in children with spastic CP.[98] However, lower limb strengthening in children with spastic CP does not improve gait, nor does it have any effect on spasticity.[99,100] Spasticity (assessed during varying velocities of passive muscle stretch) is not a significant contributor to lower limb dysfunction in children with spastic CP.[76,101]

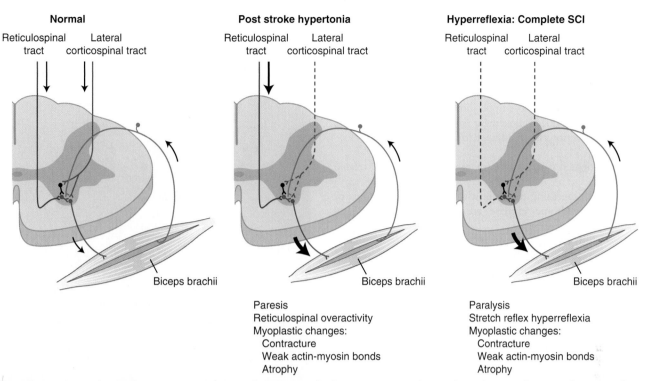

**Fig. 10-43 Normal muscle resistance to stretch, post stroke hypertonia, and spinal cord injury hyperreflexia.** In the biceps brachii, the long dark pink structure is the muscle spindle. The receptor in the muscle spindle is a secondary ending. Note the biceps muscle atrophy in **B** and **C. A,** Normal. **B,** Post stroke, the lateral corticospinal tract is interrupted. Contracture, weak actin-myosin bonds, and reticulospinal tract overactivity cause hypertonia. **C,** In a complete spinal cord injury (SCI), the upper motor neurons (UMNs) are interrupted and normal muscle stretch input to the lower motor neurons elicits a greater than normal reflexive muscle contraction. Dotted lines indicate nonfunctioning tracts. The green interneuron is excitatory, and the black interneuron is inhibitory. The thin arrows indicate normal signaling, and the thick arrows indicate excessive neural signaling.

Until recently, many therapists regarded increased muscle tone as the primary problem in people with spastic CP. These therapists attempted to normalize muscle tone with therapy, assuming that hypertonia was produced by involuntary muscle contraction, and that motor control would be normalized if excessive active muscle contraction was successfully reduced. These assumptions have been thoroughly disproved. Tedroff and coworkers (2011)[97] demonstrated that surgical reduction of hyperreflexia by dorsal rhizotomy in children with spastic cerebral palsy does not improve long-term function (children were followed for 10 years post surgery). In dorsal rhizotomy, muscles are stretched while exposed dorsal roots are electrically stimulated. If dorsal root electrical stimulation elicits muscle contraction, that dorsal root is cut. If dorsal root electrical stimulation does not elicit muscle contraction, that dorsal root is left intact to provide sensation from its dermatome. Although selective dorsal rhizotomy alone does not improve function, the surgery is beneficial in some children when combined with therapy (see next paragraph).

Task-oriented gait training improves gait more effectively than therapy that focuses on normalizing muscle tone and facilitating movements.[102] Selective dorsal rhizotomy in carefully selected young children, when combined with physical therapy, improves performance of functional skills and activities and increases independence in self-care and mobility for at least 5 years after surgery.[103]

Constraint-induced movement therapy (discussed in Chapter 4) is beneficial in hemiplegic CP. The less affected upper limb is restrained during sessions that demand use of the paretic upper limb. Following therapy, the paretic upper limb is spontaneously used more frequently.[104]

In some cases, botulinum toxin (Botox) is injected directly into the muscles that produce excessive force during active muscle contraction. Botox inhibits the release of ACh at the neuromuscular junction, preventing active muscle contraction. This allows the clinician to specifically target particular muscles without interfering with the contraction of other muscles. Botox does not affect contracture or muscle atrophy. For the upper limb, Botox in combination with occupational therapy improves goal achievement and activity levels and reduces impairment in children with spastic CP.[105] Occupational therapy alone is less effective than the combination of therapy and Botox, and Botox alone is not effective.[105] For the lower limb, Botox is effective in decreasing plantarflexion, adduction, and inversion of the distal limb.[106]

## Stroke

Laidler (1994)[107] advocates avoiding effortful movements while using paretic muscles, claiming that these movements reinforce abnormal patterns of movement and increase spasticity. Contrary to Laidler's contentions, research has consistently demonstrated that forceful movement is beneficial in adults following stroke[108] and does not increase spasticity.[92,109] Paresis and lack of fractionation are the two most important factors limiting function. Improved movement in people post stroke has been demonstrated with a variety of therapies, including:

- Hand and finger movements against resistance
- Robotic therapy for the upper limb
- Constraint-induced movement (see Chapter 4)
- Botox injections as an adjunct to therapy
- Cycling
- Task-oriented gait training (practicing gait and gait-related tasks[110])
- Gait training using treadmill with body weight support or progressive home exercise administered by a physical therapist

In a study comparing the effects of treatments for hand function in adults with hemiparesis, Butefisch and associates (1995)[111] report that techniques focusing on muscle tone reduction (techniques developed by Bobath [1977][112]) instead of on active movement produce no significant improvement in motor capabilities of the hand. In contrast, training of finger and hand flexion and extension against resistance result in significant improvement in grip strength, hand extension force, and other indicators of hand function.

Robotic therapy can also improve upper limb function post stroke. For active movement training, subjects reached toward a target on a computer monitor. A robot assisted or resisted the movement depending on the amount of force generated by the subject. The robotic assistance/resistance was adjusted so that moving was challenging yet not discouraging. Visual feedback informed subjects about the initiation, speed, coordination, and range of their movements. Three months after the end of robotic therapy, scores on shoulder movements improved 48% compared with baseline.[113] Another research group reported gains in a variety of hand function tests ranging from 12% to 25% 1 month post robotic therapy.[114] This contrasts with the small amount of hand function recovery typical for people receiving conventional therapy.[115]

In some cases, Botox is a useful adjunct to occupational and physical therapy. In the upper limb, Botox injection facilitates hygiene and dressing but does not improve the ability to actively use the arm.[116] Botox injection into calf muscles produces improvements in gait velocity, self-ratings of pain and gait function, manual muscle tests, and ankle clonus post stroke.[117] However, the authors of a meta-analysis of studies using Botox injection in calf muscles reported that the increased speed probably is not clinically significant because the speed after Botox treatment remained at less than half the speed required for walking in the community.[118] The long-term effects of Botox treatment have not been evaluated. If contracture and atrophy occur secondary to paresis, then increasing paresis by using Botox may have harmful long-term effects.

Brown and Kautz (1998)[119] demonstrated that people with poststroke hemiplegia were able to ride a stationary bike with high workloads without generating increased inappropriate muscle activity or any change in abnormal movements. In another group of people post stroke, muscle tone decreased in the more paretic lower limb after cycling.[120]

Treadmill training with body weight support, an intervention for walking, is shown in Figure 10-44. Participants wear a

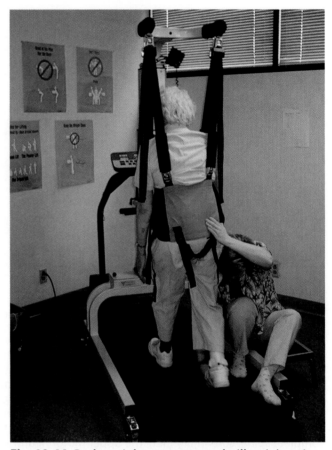

**Fig. 10-44 Body weight support treadmill training.** A harness, mounted overhead, supports part of the person's weigh while the individual walks on a treadmill with a therapist assisting movements of the paretic lower limb.

harness that partially supports their body weight while walking on a treadmill with therapist assistance. However, a meta-analysis of the research on this technique found no difference in walking outcomes for treadmill training without body weight support, treadmill training with body weight support, and other interventions for walking post stroke.[121] A prospective study comparing treadmill training with body weight support (begun at 2 months or 6 months post stroke) versus a home exercise program provided by a physical therapist found that all three groups improved equally in motor recovery, walking speed, balance, function, and quality of life. The home exercise program emphasized range of motion, limb strengthening, coordination, balance, and daily walking[122] (see Chapter 4 for more information on task specificity and repetition as essential elements promoting motor function post stroke).

## Spinal Cord Injury

For people with SCI, activity-based therapy consists of rehabilitation that activates the neuromuscular system below the level of the lesion. Examples include treadmill training with body weight support and functional electrical stimulation.

Somatosensory input to the spinal cord during treadmill training with body weight support elicits neuromuscular activation that does not occur during overground walking. Even in people with complete SCI, appropriate stimulation (body weight support, weight bearing on treadmill, therapist-assisted lower limb movement) can activate stepping pattern generators and elicit a walking EMG pattern at the hips and knees if the lower thoracic and lumbar spinal cord is intact below the lesion. Robotic walking therapy, which uses a treadmill and body weight support with motors providing control of paretic or paralyzed lower limbs, is not currently as effective as therapist-guided gait training.[123] Functional electrical stimulation (FES) is provided via implanted or skin surface electrodes. If FES promotes recovery of neuromuscular function, FES can be withdrawn and walking will continue to be possible. If continued FES is required for walking, FES is acting as a neuroprosthesis.[124]

For the upper limb, FES combined with active movement is effective in improving hand function and sensation in people with quadriplegia.[123] In animal studies, FES significantly improved spontaneous regeneration of cells after spinal cord injury.[125] Activity-based therapy optimizes the use-dependent plasticity of the spinal cord below the lesion and reorganizes circuits within the spinal cord.

The use of drugs to control SCI spasticity has been common practice; however, with changing understanding of spasticity, this use is being questioned. Baclofen is frequently used to decrease excessive muscle resistance to stretch produced by hyperreflexia following spinal cord injury. Baclofen is administered systemically, either orally or via an implanted pump that delivers the drug into the subarachnoid or subdural space. Baclofen causes inhibition in spinal cord stretch reflex pathways (by decreasing calcium influx into the presynaptic terminals of primary afferent fibers[126] and by stabilizing the postsynaptic membrane).[127] Baclofen therefore inhibits hyperreflexia but does not have an effect on myoplasticity. However, baclofen may cause a decrease in function if reflexive muscle contraction is used functionally. For example, hyperreflexia may enable a person who is otherwise unable to sit upright to be stable in sitting, and baclofen would prevent this functionally beneficial use. Recent research indicates that baclofen interferes with cell proliferation, differentiation, and survival in spinal cord injury.[128]

Neural stem cell implants into the injured spinal cord are promising because stem cells can replace damaged cells, provide neuroprotection, or make the spinal cord more capable of regenerating cells. However, many questions about stem cell therapy are currently unresolved: what types of stem cells should be used, how soon after injury should stem cells be implanted, how safe are stem cell implants and associated promoters, and what is the long-term safety of immune suppression[129] and stem cell therapy? These issues are discussed at the end of Chapter 2.

> **◎ Clinical Pearl**
>
> Voluntary movement training and botox injections as an adjunct to training are effective in spastic cerebral palsy and post MCA stroke. For SCI, treadmill training with body weight support and functional electrical stimulation are effective.

## Medications for Spasticity

Spasticity is caused by hyperreflexia or brainstem UMN overactivity, so medications that interfere with either of these mechanisms decrease spasticity. Table 10-6 lists the actions, disadvantages, and side effects of drugs commonly prescribed for spasticity. According to a systematic review of 101 randomized trials, no trial was rated as having good quality.[130] The

## TABLE 10-6   MEDICATIONS FOR SPASTICITY

| Medication | Action | Disadvantages/Side Effects |
|---|---|---|
| Baclofen, oral | Interferes with excitatory transmission in spinal cord | CNS depressant: causes drowsiness, fatigue, confusion, headache |
| Diazepam | Increases inhibition in reticular formation (brainstem) and spinal cord | CNS depressant: causes drowsiness, fatigue; impairs: intellect, attention, memory, motor coordination |
| Dantrolene sodium | Interferes with $Ca^{2+}$ release from skeletal muscle sarcoplasmic reticulum (directly interferes with muscle contraction) | Generalized skeletal muscle weakness; liver toxicity |
| Tizanidine | Inhibits excitatory neurons throughout CNS | Dry mouth, dizziness, sedation |
| Baclofen, intrathecal (delivered by implanted pump) | Interferes with excitatory transmission in spinal cord | Complications with pump: infection, dislocation of catheter, pump malfunction. Pump failure can cause withdrawal signs. Pump overdose can depress breathing and heart function, and cause coma |
| Botulinum toxin injection | Prevents lower motor neurons from releasing acetylcholine (ACh) | Effects begin 2 to 5 days post injection and last 2 to 6 months; repeated injections necessary. Total amount of toxin that can be injected is limited by risk of respiratory depression. |

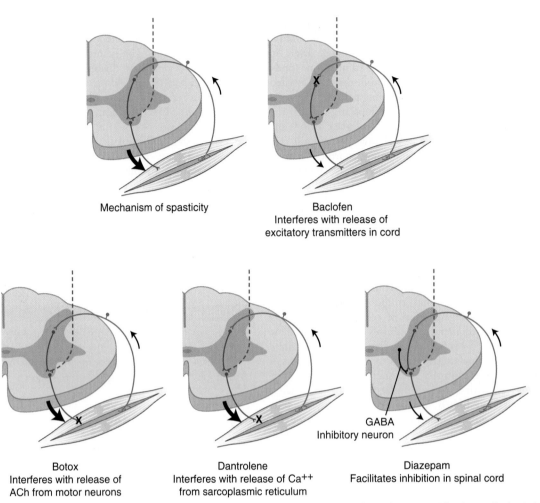

Mechanism of spasticity

Baclofen
Interferes with release of
excitatory transmitters in cord

Botox
Interferes with release of
ACh from motor neurons

Dantrolene
Interferes with release of Ca++
from sarcoplasmic reticulum

GABA
Inhibitory neuron

Diazepam
Facilitates inhibition in spinal cord

**Fig. 10-45 Action of medications used to treat spasticity secondary to spinal cord injury.** The long dark pink structure inside the muscle is the muscle spindle, and the receptor in the spindle is a secondary ending. After spinal cord injury, spinal interneurons and lower motor neurons below the lesion develop enhanced excitability. The thin arrows indicate normal signaling, and the thick arrows indicate excessive neural signaling.

authors concluded that fair evidence suggests that baclofen, tizanidine, and dantrolene are more effective than placebo in people with spasticity, primarily those with multiple sclerosis.[130] Figure 10-45 illustrates the effects of antispasticity medications.

### Stretching Is Ineffective for Contracture Treatment in People With Neurologic Conditions

Unfortunately, stretching does not prevent or reverse contracture, regardless of whether the subjects were at risk of developing contractures or had contractures. This conclusion is based on a systematic review and meta-analysis of 24 studies with a total of 782 participants with neurologic conditions, including spastic cerebral palsy, stroke, spinal cord injury, traumatic brain injury, and hereditary peripheral nerve disease. Stretching methods included self-stretch, manual stretch by therapists, splinting, positioning programs, and serial casts (casts changed at regular intervals). Stretch was performed for up to 7 months. Despite the diversity of methods, no clinically important difference in joint range of motion, pain, spasticity, activity limitation, participation restriction, or quality of life occurred over the short term (1 to 7 days) or the long term (more than 1 week

after last stretch).[131] In people with normal neuromuscular systems, regular 30 minute hamstring stretching for 6 weeks does not improve muscle extensibility.[132] In normal neuromuscular systems, apparent increases in extensibility are due to increased tolerance to discomfort during stretch.[132-134]

## AMYOTROPHIC LATERAL SCLEROSIS

Amyotrophic lateral sclerosis (ALS) is a disease that destroys only somatic motor neurons. ALS destroys UMNs and brainstem and spinal cord lower motor neurons bilaterally (Figure 10-46), resulting in both UMN and LMN signs. The disease leads to paresis, myoplasticity, hyperreflexia, Babinski's sign, atrophy, fasciculations, and fibrillations. Loss of lower motor neurons in cranial nerves causes difficulty with breathing, swallowing, and speaking. Nearly 50% of people with ALS experience pathologic laughter or crying (uncontrollable laughing or crying that may not be congruent with the person's emotional state). Approximately 90% of cases are idiopathic, although the gene responsible for the familial type of ALS has been identified. In ALS, astrocytes fail to clean up excessive glutamate, causing excitotoxicity.[135,136] Recent research indicates that brief

| **PATHOLOGY 10-2** AMYOTROPHIC LATERAL SCLEROSIS | |
|---|---|
| Pathology | Bilateral degeneration of lower motor neurons and upper motor neurons; usually some degeneration in frontal cerebral cortex |
| Etiology | Excessive levels of glutamate[135,136] |
| Speed of onset | Chronic |
| Signs and symptoms | |
| Cognitive function | Decision making often impaired[135] |
| Consciousness | Normal |
| Communication and memory | Memory normal; language and verbal fluency may be impaired |
| Affect (emotional expression) | Emotional lability (abnormal, uncontrolled expression of emotions, often pathological laughter or crying; see Chapter 18) |
| Sensory | Normal |
| Autonomic | Normal |
| Motor | Paresis, spasticity, clonus, Babinski's sign, hyperreflexia or hyporeflexia, fasciculations, fibrillations, muscle atrophy; difficulty with breathing, swallowing, speaking |
| Region affected | Upper motor neurons in cerebrum, brainstem, and spinal cord; lower motor neurons in brainstem, spinal and peripheral regions, frontal cerebral cortex |
| Demographics | Onset is usually >50 years old; males outnumber females by 3:2 |
| Incidence | 2.2 cases per 100,000 population per year[135] |
| Prevalence | 0.05 case per 1000 people |
| Prognosis | Progressive; average life span after diagnosis = 3 years; rarely live >20 years; death usually from respiratory complications[136] |

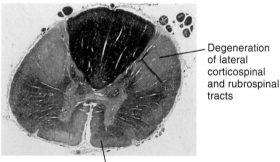

Degeneration of lateral corticospinal and rubrospinal tracts

Degeneration of medial activating pathways

**Fig. 10-46** Spinal cord section, stained for myelin, showing loss of upper motor neurons (UMNs) in amyotrophic lateral sclerosis (ALS). The loss is visible dorsolaterally, where the lateral corticospinal and rubrospinal axons should be, and ventromedially, where the medial UMNs should be. *(Courtesy Dr. Melvin J. Ball.)*

exercise of low to moderate intensity is beneficial for muscles that are not profoundly weak.[137] People with ALS usually die of respiratory complications (Pathology 10-2).

## SUMMARY

For normal movement, motor planning areas, control circuits, and descending tracts must act together with sensory information to provide instructions to lower motor neurons. Only lower motor neurons deliver signals from the central nervous system to the skeletal muscles that generate movement. UMNs convey signals from the brain to lower motor neurons and interneurons. The locations of selected motor system lesions are illustrated in Figure 10-47.

To treat patients, a therapist must understand normal and impaired skeletal muscles and motor neurons. Because research regularly reveals new information about motor neurons and the effectiveness of different treatments, therapists should keep up-to-date with developments in this field.

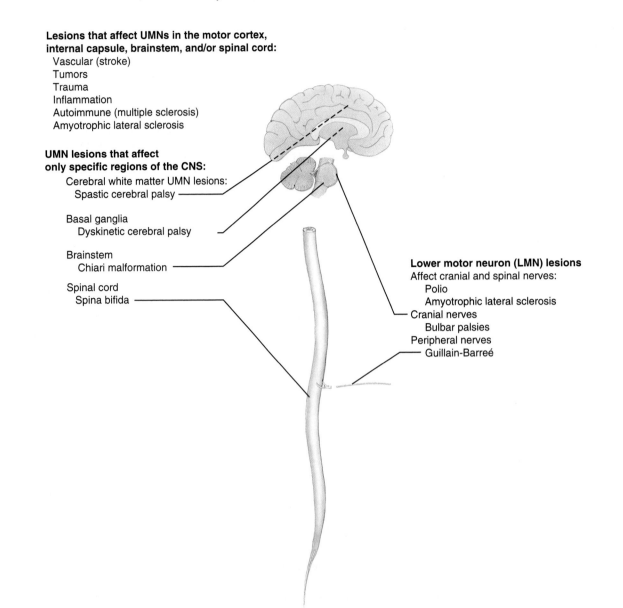

**Lesions that affect UMNs in the motor cortex, internal capsule, brainstem, and/or spinal cord:**
Vascular (stroke)
Tumors
Trauma
Inflammation
Autoimmune (multiple sclerosis)
Amyotrophic lateral sclerosis

**UMN lesions that affect only specific regions of the CNS:**
Cerebral white matter UMN lesions:
Spastic cerebral palsy

Basal ganglia
Dyskinetic cerebral palsy

Brainstem
Chiari malformation

Spinal cord
Spina bifida

**Lower motor neuron (LMN) lesions**
Affect cranial and spinal nerves:
Polio
Amyotrophic lateral sclerosis
Cranial nerves
Bulbar palsies
Peripheral nerves
Guillain-Barreé

**Fig. 10-47** Locations and types of upper motor neuron (UMN) lesions are shown on the left. Locations and types of lower motor neuron (LMN) lesions are indicated on the right.

## CLINICAL NOTES

### Case 1

H.J., a 17-year-old student, sustained a head injury when he hit a tree while snowboarding 4 months ago. After a 2 day coma, he received inpatient occupational and physical therapy for 4 weeks. At discharge, he had full function of the left side of his body but was severely hemiparetic on the right. When discharged, he was independent in ambulation with a cane and was able to voluntarily move his right arm in an abnormal synergy pattern (attempts at shoulder flexion resulted in elbow flexion and shoulder abduction). One week ago, he returned to occupational therapy for treatment of his right arm. He still has no hand function. He complained of pain produced by the pressure of his fisted hand pressing on his chest when his right elbow flexes involuntarily, especially when he walks.

## CLINICAL NOTES—cont'd

- Passive elbow extension was limited to –90 degrees from full extension. Biceps and brachioradialis surface EMG showed strong activity during sustained passive stretch (normally surface EMG should be silent during sustained passive stretch).
- The therapist decided to use serial casts to increase elbow extension and referred H.J. to a physician with experience in nerve and motor point blocks for blocks to decrease hyperreflexia before casting.
- The physician blocked the musculocutaneous nerve and was able to gain an additional 10 degrees of elbow extension. An hour after the brachioradialis motor point was blocked, elbow PROM was –55 degrees from full extension. Surface EMG during sustained stretch was reduced to nearly silent. However, the resting position of the elbow was flexed 75 degrees.

### Questions

1. Why does elbow flexion involuntarily increase when H.J. is walking?
2. What factors were limiting passive elbow extension before the nerve and motor point blocks?
3. Why did the therapist want the patient to have nerve and motor point blocks before casting the elbow?
4. Why is there a difference between the "resting" position of the elbow and the maximum passive range following motor point blocks?

### Case 2

M.V. is a 62-year-old man. While eating breakfast, he suddenly lost control of the left side of his body and face. He fell to the floor but did not lose consciousness. Now, 2 weeks later, he is examined in the hospital. Results are as follows:
- He has complete loss of sensation and voluntary movement of his left side.
- He requires assistance to move from supine to sitting and from sitting to standing.
- He cannot sit or stand independently.
- He has difficulty speaking because of lack of sensation and reduced control of the oral and pharyngeal muscles on the left side. The nursing staff reports that he also has difficulty eating.
- Babinski's sign is present on the left side.

### Question

What is the location of the lesion and its probable etiology?

### Case 3

A.F. is a 15-year-old girl who was thrown from a horse. She sustained fractures of the humerus and the C5 vertebra. Her coma lasted 2 days. Examination reveals:
- Mentation and consciousness are normal.
- Except for the distal right upper limb, sensation, autonomic function, and movement are normal.
- Sensation and sweating are absent in the little finger, the medial half of the ring finger, and the adjacent palm of the right hand. The skin is warm and red in the same distribution.
- Wrist flexion on the ulnar side and ulnar deviation are impaired. She cannot flex the distal interphalangeal joints in the fourth and fifth digits.

### Question

What is the location of the lesion and its probable cause?

### Case 4

P.A. is a 39-year-old woman, 1 month post injury sustained from a 30 foot fall while mountain climbing. She suffered multiple injuries, most prominently fractures of the right femur, right fibula, and T10 vertebra.
- The right lower limb is in a cast, restricting evaluation, but sensation is absent in the L1 dermatome above the cast and in the toes. No voluntary movement of the right quadriceps or toes can be elicited.
- Sensation is absent throughout the left lower limb and bilaterally in the trunk below the top of the pelvis.
- No voluntary movement can be elicited in the left lower limb.
- The Achilles tendon reflex and Babinski's sign are present bilaterally.

### Question

What is the location of the lesion and its probable etiology?

*Continued*

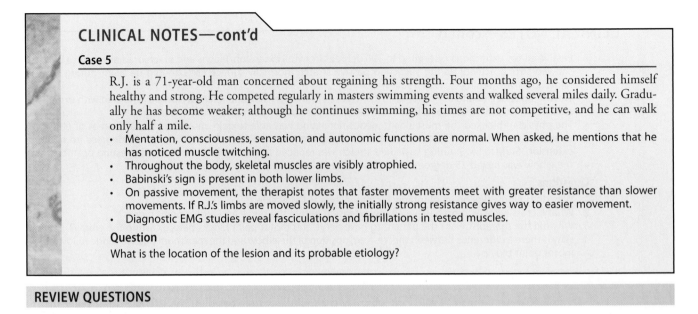

**CLINICAL NOTES—cont'd**

**Case 5**

R.J. is a 71-year-old man concerned about regaining his strength. Four months ago, he considered himself healthy and strong. He competed regularly in masters swimming events and walked several miles daily. Gradually he has become weaker; although he continues swimming, his times are not competitive, and he can walk only half a mile.

- Mentation, consciousness, sensation, and autonomic functions are normal. When asked, he mentions that he has noticed muscle twitching.
- Throughout the body, skeletal muscles are visibly atrophied.
- Babinski's sign is present in both lower limbs.
- On passive movement, the therapist notes that faster movements meet with greater resistance than slower movements. If R.J.'s limbs are moved slowly, the initially strong resistance gives way to easier movement.
- Diagnostic EMG studies reveal fasciculations and fibrillations in tested muscles.

**Question**

What is the location of the lesion and its probable etiology?

## REVIEW QUESTIONS

1. List the factors that contribute to muscle resistance to stretch in an intact neuromuscular system.
2. Why do your hamstrings feel stiff when you stand after sitting for several hours?
3. When a person with an intact neuromuscular system is anxious, muscle resistance to stretch increases. What produces this increase in resistance to stretch?
4. What is the difference between an LMN and a UMN?
5. What is the general function of control circuits?
6. Why are slow twitch muscle fibers usually activated before fast twitch muscle fibers?
7. What is alpha-gamma coactivation?
8. What factors determine the activity of a motor unit?
9. What are the differences between phasic and tonic stretch reflexes?
10. What roles does the information from a Golgi tendon organ play in movement control?
11. How does changing a person's arousal level alter the response to a quadriceps tendon tap?
12. How is an H-reflex produced? What information does an H-reflex give?
13. What is the function of reciprocal inhibition?
14. How does use of the term *synergy* differ between clinicians and motor control researchers?
15. What is a stepping pattern generator?
16. In an intact nervous system, how is the stepping pattern generator activated?
17. List each medial UMN tract and its function. Which medial UMN tract regulates LMN to muscles throughout the body, except distal limb muscles?
18. List each lateral UMN tract and its function.
19. What does the corticobrainstem tract do?

20. What is hemiplegia?
21. Which of the following signs always indicates pathology? Muscle spasms, cramps, fasciculations, fibrillations, abnormal movements.
22. What is hypertonia? What are the differences among the types of hypertonia? How is hypertonia produced?
23. What is spinal shock?
24. If a person has loss of reflexes, muscle atrophy, flaccid paralysis, and fibrillations, what is the location of the lesion?
25. What does Babinski's sign in an adult indicate?
26. What is the location of a lesion that produces abnormal cutaneous reflexes, abnormal timing of muscle activation, paresis, and hypertonia?
27. What factors contribute to hypertonia post stroke?
28. Following a UMN lesion, if there is excessive resistance to active dorsiflexion yet very little EMG activity in the ankle plantar flexors, what is the source of the hypertonia?
29. What is clonus?
30. Post stroke, is hypertonia caused primarily by hyperreflexia?
31. How can cocontraction, myoplasticity, and hyperreflexia be quantified using surface EMG?
32. What is the difference in effects on lower motor neurons between a complete spinal cord lesion and a typical middle cerebral artery stroke?
33. What motor signs occur in spastic cerebral palsy that are not also seen in adult-onset UMN lesions?
34. What types of therapy have been shown to improve function in people post stroke? What do all of these types of therapy have in common?
35. What parts of the nervous system does ALS destroy?

## References

1. Riemann BL, Lephart SM: The sensorimotor system, Part II. The role of proprioception in motor control and functional joint stability. *J Athl Train* 37:80–84, 2002.
2. Rossignol S, Dubuc R, Gossard JP: Dynamic sensorimotor interactions in locomotion. *Physiol Rev* 86:89–154, 2006.
3. Vidoni ED, Acerra NE, Dao E, et al: Role of the primary somatosensory cortex in motor learning: an rTMS study. *Neurobiol Learn Mem* 93:532–539, 2010.
4. Messier J, Adamovich S, Berkinblit M, et al: Influence of movement speed on accuracy and coordination of reaching

movements to memorized targets in three-dimensional space in a deafferented subject. *Exp Brain Res* 150:399–416, 2003.

5. Medina J, Jax SA, Brown MJ, et al: Contributions of efference copy to limb localization: evidence from deafferentation. *Brain Res* 1355:104–111, 2010.

6. Horak FB, Buchanan J, Creath R, Jeka J: Vestibulospinal control of posture. *Adv Exp Med Biol* 508:139–145, 2002.

7. Nichols TR, Cope TC: Cross-bridge mechanisms underlying the history-dependent properties of muscle spindles and stretch reflexes. *Can J Physiol Pharmacol* 82:569–576, 2004.

8. Axelson HW, Hagbarth K-E: Human motor control consequences of thixotropic changes in muscular short-range stiffness. *J Physiol* 535:279–288, 2001.

9. Casadio M, Morasso PG, Sanguineti V: Direct measurement of ankle stiffness during quiet standing: implications for control modelling and clinical application. *Gait Posture* 21:410–424, 2005.

10. Loram ID, Maganaris CN, Lakie M: The passive, human calf muscles in relation to standing: the non-linear decrease from short range to long range stiffness. *J Physiol* 584:661–675, 2007.

11. Coutinho EL, Gomes AR, França CN, et al: Effect of passive stretching on the immobilized soleus muscle fiber morphology. *Braz J Med Biol Res* 37:1853–1861, 2004.

12. Caiozzo VJ, Utkan A, Chou R, et al: Effects of distraction on muscle length: mechanisms involved in sarcomerogenesis. *Clin Orthop Relat Res* 403(Suppl):S133–145, 2002.

13. Kjaer M: Role of extracellular matrix in adaptation of tendon and skeletal muscle to mechanical loading. *Physiol Rev* 84:649–698, 2004.

14. Gajdosik RL, Vander Linden DW, McNair PJ, et al: Slow passive stretch and release characteristics of the calf muscles of older women with limited dorsiflexion range of motion. *Clin Biomech (Bristol, Avon)* 19:398–406, 2004.

15. Darainy M, Ostry DJ: Muscle cocontraction following dynamics learning. *Exp Brain Res* 190:153–163, 2008.

16. Wakeling JM: Motor units are recruited in a task-dependent fashion during locomotion. *J Exp Biol* 207:3883–3890, 2004.

17. Shall MS, Dimitrova DM, Goldberg SJ: Extraocular motor unit and whole-muscle contractile properties in the squirrel monkey: summation of forces and fiber morphology. *Exp Brain Res* 151:338–345, 2003.

18. Longo MR, Haggard P: An implicit body representation underlying human position sense. *Proc Natl Acad Sci U S A* 107:11727–11732, 2010.

19. Shenton JT, Schwoebel J, Coslett HB: Mental motor imagery and the body schema, evidence for proprioceptive dominance. *Neurosci Lett* 370:19–24, 2004.

20. Grey MJ, Nielsen JB, Mazzaro N, et al: Positive force feedback in human walking. *J Physiol* 581:99–105, 2007.

21. Pratt CA: Evidence of positive force feedback among hindlimb extensors in the intact standing cat. *J Neurophysiol* 73:2578–2583, 1995.

22. Yang JF, Lamont EV, Pang MY: Split-belt treadmill stepping in infants suggests autonomous pattern generators for the left and right leg in humans. *J Neurosci* 25:6869–6876, 2005.

23. Tazerart S: The persistent sodium current generates pacemaker activities in the central pattern generator for locomotion and regulates the locomotor rhythm. *J Neurosci* 28:8577–8589, 2008.

24. Edgerton VR, Tillakaratne NJ, Bigbee JA, et al: Plasticity of the spinal neural circuitry after injury. *Annu Rev Neurosci* 27:145–167, 2004.

25. Knikou M: Neural control of locomotion and training-induced plasticity after spinal and cerebral lesions. *Clin Neurophysiol* 121:1655–1668, 2010.

26. Giesebrecht S, Martin PG, Martin Gandevia SC, et al: Facilitation and inhibition of tibialis anterior responses to corticospinal stimulation after maximal voluntary contractions. *J Neurophysiol* 103:1350–1356, 2010.

27. Chou SW, Abraham LD, Huang IS, et al: Starting position and stretching velocity effects on the reflex threshold angle of stretch reflex in the soleus muscle of normal and spastic subjects. *J Formos Med Assoc* 104:493–501, 2005.

28. Thilmann AF, Fellows SJ, Garms E: The mechanism of spastic muscle hypertonus: variation in reflex gain over the time course of spasticity. *Brain* 114:233–244, 1991.

29. Windhorst U: Muscle proprioceptive feedback and spinal networks. *Brain Res Bull* 73:155–202, 2007.

30. Riddle CN, Baker SN: Interneurons descending pathways onto macaque cervical spinal convergence of pyramidal and medial brain stem. *J Neurophysiol* 103:2821–2832, 2010.

31. Perkins E, Warren S, May PJ: The mesencephalic reticular formation as a conduit for primate collicular gaze control: tectal inputs to neurons targeting the spinal cord and medulla. *Anat Rec (Hoboken)* 292:1162–1181, 2009.

32. Buford JA: Reticulospinal system. In Squire L, et al, editors: *The encyclopedia of neuroscience*, London, 2009, Elsevier, pp 151–158.

33. Herbert WJ, Davidson AG, Buford JA: Measuring the motor output of the pontomedullary reticular formation in the monkey: do stimulus-triggered averaging and stimulus trains produce comparable results in the upper limbs? *Exp Brain Res* 203:271–283, 2010.

34. Riddle CN, Edgley SA, Baker SN: Direct and indirect connections with upper limb motoneurons from the primate reticulospinal tract. *J Neurosci* 29:4993–4999, 2009.

35. Sakai ST, Davidson AG, Buford JA: Reticulospinal neurons in the pontomedullary reticular formation of the monkey *(Macaca fascicularis)*. *Neuroscience* 163:1158–1170, 2009.

36. Kennedy PM, Cresswell AG, Chua R, Inglis JT: Vestibulospinal influences on lower limb motoneurons. *Can J Physiol Pharmacol* 82:675–681, 2004.

37. Lacroix S, Havton LA, McKay H, et al: Bilateral corticospinal projections arise from each motor cortex in the macaque monkey: a quantitative study. *J Comp Neurol* 473:147–161, 2004.

38. Rosenzweig ES, Brock JH, Culbertson MD, et al: Extensive spinal decussation and bilateral termination of cervical corticospinal projections in rhesus monkeys. *J Comp Neurol* 513:151–163, 2009.

39. Lawrence D, Kuypers H: The functional organization of the motor system in the monkey: I. The effects of bilateral pyramidal lesions. II. The effects of lesions of the descending brainstem pathways. *Brain* 91:1–36, 1968.

40. Miller LE, Gibson AR: Red nucleus. In Squire L, et al, editors: *The encyclopedia of neuroscience*, London, 2009, Elsevier, pp 55–62.

41. Schieber MH: Comparative anatomy and physiology of the corticospinal system. *Handb Clin Neurol* 82:15–37, 2007.

42. Chouinard PA, Paus T: What have we learned from "perturbing" the human cortical motor system with transcranial magnetic stimulation? *Front Hum Neurosci* 4:173, 2010.

43. Holstege G: The mesopontine rostromedial tegmental nucleus and the emotional motor system: role in basic survival behavior. *J Comp Neurol* 513:559–565, 2009.

44. Pijpers JR, Oudejans RR, Bakker FC: Anxiety-induced changes in movement behaviour during the execution of a complex whole-body task. *Q J Exp Psychol A* 58:421–445, 2005.

45. Adkin AL, Frank JS, Carpenter MG, Peysar GW: Fear of falling modifies anticipatory postural control. *Exp Brain Res* 143:160–170, 2002.

46. Jia L, Xu L, Jiang M, et al: Protein abnormality in denervated skeletal muscles from patients with brachial injury. *Microsurgery* 25:316–321, 2005.

47. Montagna P, Provini F, Vetrugno R: Propriospinal myoclonus at sleep onset. *Neurophysiol Clin* 36:351–355, 2006.

48. Laugel V: Diagnostic approach to neonatal hypotonia: retrospective study on 144 neonates. *Eur J Pediatr* 167:517–523, 2008.

49. Trojan DA, Cashman NR: Post-poliomyelitis syndrome. *Muscle Nerve* 31:6–19, 2005.

50. Lygren H, Jones K, Grenstad T, et al: Perceived disability, fatigue, pain and measured isometric muscle strength in patients with post-polio symptoms. *Physiother Res Int* 12:39–49, 2007.

51. Gonzalez H, Olsson T, Borg K: Management of postpolio syndrome. *Lancet Neurol* 9:634–642, 2010.

52. Gracies JM: Pathophysiology of spastic paresis: I. Paresis and soft tissue changes. *Muscle Nerve* 31:535–551, 2005.

53. Beres-Jones JA, Johnson TD, Harkema SJ: Clonus after human spinal cord injury cannot be attributed solely to recurrent muscle-tendon stretch. *Exp Brain Res* 149:222–236, 2003.

54. Campbell WW: *In DeJong's the neurologic examination*, Philadelphia, 2005, Lippincott Williams & Wilkins.

55. Ivanhoe CB, Reistetter TA: Spasticity: the misunderstood part of the upper motor neuron syndrome. *Am J Phys Med Rehabil* 83(10 Suppl):S3–9, 2004.

56. Gao F, Zhang L-Q: Altered contractile properties of the gastrocnemius muscle post stroke. *J Appl Physiol* 105:1802–1808, 2008.

57. Malaiya R, McNee AE, Fry NR, et al: The morphology of the medial gastrocnemius in typically developing children and children with spastic hemiplegic cerebral palsy. *J Electromyogr Kinesiol* 17:657–663, 2007.

58. McDonald MF, Kevin Garrison M, Schmit BD: Length-tension properties of ankle muscles in chronic human spinal cord injury. *J Biomech* 38:2344–2353, 2005.

59. Kennedy KA: Focal spasticity. In Ferri FR, editor: *Ferri's clinical advisor*, ed 1, St Louis, 2011, Mosby.

60. Kline TL, Schmit BD, Kamper DG: Exaggerated interlimb neural coupling following stroke. *Brain* 130:159–169, 2007.

61. Elbasiouny SM, Moroz D, Bakr MM, et al: Management of spasticity after spinal cord injury: current techniques and future directions. *Neurorehabil Neural Repair* 24:23–33, 2010.

62. Phadke CP, Thompson FJ, Kukulka CG, et al: Soleus H-reflex modulation after motor incomplete spinal cord injury: effects of body position and walking speed. *J Spinal Cord Med* 33:371–378, 2010.

63. Hautier CA, Arsac LM, Deghdegh K, et al: Influence of fatigue on EMG/force ratio and cocontraction in cycling. *Med Sci Sports Exerc* 32:839–843, 2000.

64. Fowler EG, Goldberg EJ: The effect of lower extremity selective voluntary motor control on interjoint coordination during gait in children with spastic diplegic cerebral palsy. *Gait Posture* 29:102–107, 2009.

65. Melzer I, Goldring M, Melzer Y, et al: Voluntary stepping behavior under single- and dual-task conditions in chronic stroke survivors: a comparison between the involved and uninvolved legs. *J Electromyogr Kinesiol* 20:1082–1087, 2010.

66. Prosser LA, Lee SC, VanSant AF, et al: Trunk and hip muscle activation patterns are different during walking in young children with and without cerebral palsy. *Phys Ther* 90:986–997, 2010.

67. Policy JF, Torburn L, Rinsky LA, et al: Electromyographic test to differentiate mild diplegic cerebral palsy and idiopathic toe-walking. *J Pediatr Orthop* 21:784–789, 2001.

68. Alhusaini AA, Dean CM, Crosbie J, et al: Evaluation of spasticity in children with cerebral palsy using Ashworth and Tardieu Scales compared with laboratory measures. *J Child Neurol* 25:1242–1247, 2010.

69. Fleuren JF, Voerman GE, Erren-Wolters CV, et al: Stop using the Ashworth Scale for the assessment of spasticity. *J Neurol Neurosurg Psychiatry* 81:46–52, 2010.

70. Cooper A, Musa IM, van Deursen R, Wiles CM: Electromyography characterization of stretch responses in hemiparetic stroke patients and their relationship with the Modified Ashworth scale. *Clin Rehabil* 19:760–766, 2005.

71. Lorentzen J, Grey MJ, Crone C, et al: Distinguishing active from passive components of ankle plantar flexor stiffness in stroke, spinal cord injury and multiple sclerosis. *Clin Neurophysiol* 121:1939–1951, 2010.

72. Platz T, Eickhof C, Nuyens G, et al: Clinical scales for the assessment of spasticity, associated phenomena, and function: a systematic review of the literature. *Disabil Rehabil* 7:7–18, 2005.

73. Malhotra S, Cousins E, Ward A, et al: An investigation into the agreement between clinical, biomechanical and neurophysiological measures of spasticity. *Clin Rehabil* 22:1105–1115, 2008.

74. Gracies JM, Bayle N, Vinti M, et al: Five-step clinical assessment in spastic paresis. *Eur J Phys Rehabil Med* 46:411–421, 2010.

75. Chiu HC, Ada L, Butler J, et al: Relative contribution of motor impairments to limitations in activity and restrictions in participation in adults with hemiplegic cerebral palsy. *Clin Rehabil* 24:454–462, 2010.

76. Ross SA, Engsberg JR: Relationships between spasticity, strength, gait, and the GMFM-66 in persons with spastic diplegia cerebral palsy. *Arch Phys Med Rehabil* 88:1114–1120, 2007.

77. Thompson N, Stebbins J, Seniorou M, et al: Muscle strength and walking ability in diplegic cerebral palsy: implications for assessment and management. *Gait Posture* 33:321–325, 2011.

78. Clark DJ, Ting LH, Zajac FE, et al: Merging of healthy motor modules predicts reduced locomotor performance and muscle coordination complexity post-stroke. *J Neurophysiol* 103:844–857, 2010.

79. Schieber MH, Lang CE, Reilly KT, et al: Selective activation of human finger muscles after stroke or amputation. *Adv Exp Med Biol* 629:559–575, 2009.

80. Ovbiagele B: National sex-specific trends in hospital-based stroke rates. *J Stroke Cerebrovasc Dis* 2010 Aug 17. [Epub ahead of print]

81. Rosamond W, Flegal K, Friday G, et al: Heart disease and stroke statistics—2007 update: a report from the American Heart Association Statistics Committee and Stroke Statistics Subcommittee. *Circulation* 115:e69–171, 2007.

82. Mohan KM, Crichton SL, Grieve AP, et al: Frequency and predictors for the risk of stroke recurrence up to 10 years after stroke: the South London Stroke Register. *J Neurol Neurosurg Psychiatry* 80:1012–1018, 2009.

83. Fonarow GC, Smith EE, Reeves MJ, et al: Hospital-level variation in mortality and rehospitalization for Medicare beneficiaries with acute ischemic stroke. *Stroke* 42:159–166, 2011.

84. Ada L, Canning C: Anticipating and avoiding muscle shortening. In Ada L, Canning C, editors: *Key issues in neurological physiotherapy*, Oxford, 1990, Butterworth Heinemann, pp 219–236.

85. O'Dwyer NJ, Ada L, Neilson PD: Spasticity and muscle contracture following stroke. *Brain* 119:1737–1749, 1996.

86. Malhotra S, Pandyan AD, Rosewilliam S, et al: Spasticity and contractures at the wrist after stroke: time course of development and their association with functional recovery of the upper limb. *Clin Rehabil* 25:184–191, 2011.

87. Dietz V, Berger W: Normal and impaired regulation of muscle stiffness in gait: a new hypothesis about muscle hypertonia. *Exp Neurol* 79:680–687, 1983.

88. Klein CS, Brooks D, Richardson D, et al: Voluntary activation failure contributes more to plantar flexor weakness than antagonist coactivation and muscle atrophy in chronic stroke survivors. *J Appl Physiol* 109:1337–1346, 2010.

89. Dietz V: Behavior of spinal neurons deprived of supraspinal input. *Nat Rev Neurol* 6:167–174, 2010.

90. Becher JG, Harlaar J, Lankhorst GJ, Vogelaar TW: Measurement of impaired muscle function of the gastrocnemius, soleus, and tibialis anterior muscles in spastic hemiplegia: a preliminary study. *J Rehabil Res Dev* 35:314–326, 1998.

91. Salazar-Torres Jde J, Pandyan AD, Price CI, et al: Does spasticity result from hyperactive stretch reflexes? Preliminary findings from a stretch reflex characterization study. *Disabil Rehabil* 26:756–760, 2004.

92. Ada L, O'Dwyer N, O'Neill E: Relation between spasticity, weakness and contracture of the elbow flexors and upper limb activity after stroke: an observational study. *Disabil Rehabil* 28:891–897, 2006.

93. English C, McLennan H, Thoirs K, et al: Loss of skeletal muscle mass after stroke: a systematic review. *Int J Stroke* 5:395–402, 2010.

94. Jung HY, Yoon JS, Park BS: Recovery of proximal and distal arm weakness in the ipsilateral upper limb after stroke. *NeuroRehabilitation* 17:153–159, 2002.

95. Biering-Sørensen B, Kristensen IB, Kjaer M, et al: Muscle after spinal cord injury. *Muscle Nerve* 40:499–519, 2009.

96. Mirbagheri MM, Barbeau H, Ladouceur M, Kearney RE: Intrinsic and reflex stiffness in normal and spastic, spinal cord injured subjects. *Exp Brain Res* 141:446–459, 2001.

97. Tedroff K, Löwing K, Jacobson DN, et al: Does loss of spasticity matter? A 10-year follow-up after selective dorsal rhizotomy in cerebral palsy. *Dev Med Child Neurol* 53:724–729, 2010.

98. Roncesvalles MN, Woollacott MW, Burtner PA: Neural factors underlying reduced postural adaptability in children with cerebral palsy. *Neuroreport* 13:2407–2410, 2002.

99. Scholtes VA, Becher JG, Comuth A, et al: Effectiveness of functional progressive resistance exercise strength training on muscle strength and mobility in children with cerebral palsy: a randomized controlled trial. *Dev Med Child Neurol* 52:e107–113, 2010.

100. Scianni A, Butler JM, Ada L, et al: Muscle strengthening is not effective in children and adolescents with cerebral palsy: a systematic review. *Aust J Physiother* 55:81–87, 2009.

101. Gorter JW, Verschuren O, van Riel L, et al: The relationship between spasticity in young children (18 months of age) with cerebral palsy and their gross motor function development. *BMC Musculoskelet Disord* 10:108, 2009.

102. Salem Y, Godwin EM: Effects of task-oriented training on mobility function in children with cerebral palsy. *NeuroRehabilitation* 24:307–313, 2009.

103. Nordmark E, Josenby AL, Lagergren J, et al: Long-term outcomes five years after selective dorsal rhizotomy. *BMC Pediatr* 8:54, 2008.

104. Huang HH, Fetters L, Hale J, et al: Bound for success: a systematic review of constraint-induced movement therapy in children with cerebral palsy supports improved arm and hand use. *Phys Ther* 89:1126–1141, 2009.

105. Hoare BJ, Wallen MA, Imms C, et al: Botulinum toxin A as an adjunct to treatment in the management of the upper limb in children with spastic cerebral palsy (UPDATE). *Cochrane Database Syst Rev* (1):CD003469, 2010.

106. Lukban MB, Rosales RL, Dressler D: Effectiveness of botulinum toxin A for upper and lower limb spasticity in children with cerebral palsy: a summary of evidence. *J Neural Transm* 116:319–331, 2009.

107. Laidler P: *Stroke rehabilitation: structure and strategy*, San Diego, Calif, 1994, Singular.

108. Van Peppen RP, Kwakkel G, Wood-Dauphinee S, et al: The impact of physical therapy on functional outcomes after stroke: what's the evidence? *Clin Rehabil* 18:833–862, 2004.

109. Pak S, Patten C: Strengthening to promote functional recovery poststroke: an evidence-based review. *Top Stroke Rehabil* 15(3):177–199, 2008.

110. Wevers L, van de Port I, Vermue M, et al: Effects of task-oriented circuit class training on walking competency after stroke: a systematic review. *Stroke* 40:2450–2459, 2009.

111. Butefisch C, Hummelsheim H, Denzler P, Mauritz KH: Repetitive training of isolated movements improves the outcome of motor rehabilitation of the centrally paretic hand. *J Neurol Sci* 130:59–68, 1995.

112. Bobath B: Treatment of adult hemiplegia. *Physiotherapy* 63:310–313, 1977.

113. Hogan N, Krebs HI, Rohrer B, et al: Motions or muscles? Some behavioral factors underlying robotic assistance of motor recovery. *J Rehabil Res Dev* 43:605–618, 2006.

114. Takahashi CD, Der-Yeghiaian L, Le V, et al: Robot-based hand motor therapy after stroke. *Brain* 131:425–437, 2008.

115. Lang CE, DeJong SL, Beebe JA: Recovery of thumb and finger extension and its relation to grasp performance after stroke. *J Neurophysiol* 102:451–459, 2009.

116. Shaw LC, Price CI, van Wijck FM, et al: Botulinum toxin for the upper limb after stroke (BoTULS) trial: effect on impairment, activity limitation, and pain. *Stroke* 2011 Mar 17. [Epub ahead of print]

117. Mancini F, Sandrini G, Moglia A, et al: A randomised, double-blind, dose-ranging study to evaluate efficacy and safety of three doses of botulinum toxin type A (Botox) for the treatment of spastic foot. *Neurol Sci* 26:26–31, 2005.

118. Foley N, Murie-Fernandez M, Speechley M, et al: Does the treatment of spastic equinovarus deformity following stroke with botulinum toxin increase gait velocity? A systematic review and meta-analysis. *Eur J Neurol* 17:1419–1427, 2010.

119. Brown DA, Kautz SA: Increased workload enhances force output during pedaling exercise in persons with poststroke hemiplegia. *Stroke* 29:598–606, 1998.

120. Yeh CY, Tsai KH, Su FC, et al: Effect of a bout of leg cycling with electrical stimulation on reduction of hypertonia in patients with stroke. *Arch Phys Med Rehabil* 91:1731–1736, 2010.

121. Moseley AM, Stark A, Cameron ID, et al: Treadmill training and body weight support for walking after stroke. *Cochrane Database Syst Rev* (4):CD002840, 2005.

122. Duncan PW, Sullivan KJ, Behrman AL, et al: Body-weight-supported treadmill rehabilitation after stroke. *N Engl J Med* 364:2026–2036, 2005.

123. Sadowsky CL, McDonald JW: Activity-based restorative therapies: concepts and applications in spinal cord injury-related neurorehabilitation. *Dev Disabil Res Rev* 15:112–116, 2009.

124. Behrman AL, Harkema SJ: Physical rehabilitation as an agent for recovery after spinal cord injury. *Phys Med Rehabil Clin N Am* 18:183–202, 2007.

125. Becker D, Gary DS, Rosenzweig ES, et al: Functional electrical stimulation helps replenish progenitor cells in the injured spinal cord of adult rats. *Exp Neurol* 222:211–218, 2010.

126. Sakaba T, Neher E: Direct modulation of synaptic vesicle priming by GABA(B) receptor activation at a glutamatergic synapse. *Nature* 424:775–778, 2003.

127. Fairfax BP, Pitcher JA, Scott MG, et al: Phosphorylation and chronic agonist treatment atypically modulate GABAB receptor cell surface stability. *J Biol Chem* 279:12565–12573, 2004.

128. Belegu V, Oudega M, Gary DS, et al: Restoring function after spinal cord injury: promoting spontaneous regeneration with stem cells and activity-based therapies. *Neurosurg Clin N Am* 18:143–168, 2007.

129. Zhang N, Wimmer J, Qian SJ, et al: Stem cells: current approach and future prospects in spinal cord injury repair. *Anat Rec (Hoboken)* 293:519–530, 2010.

130. Chou R, Peterson K, Helfand M: Comparative efficacy and safety of skeletal muscle relaxants for spasticity and musculoskeletal conditions: a systematic review. *J Pain Symptom Manage* 28:140–175, 2004.

131. Katalinic OM, Harvey LA, Herbert RD, et al: Stretch for the treatment and prevention of contractures. *Cochrane Database Syst Rev* (9):CD007455, 2010.

132. Ben M, Harvey LA: Regular stretch does not increase muscle extensibility: a randomized controlled trial. *Scand J Med Sci Sports* 20:136–144, 2010.

133. Folpp H, Deall S, Harvey LA, et al: Can apparent increases in muscle extensibility with regular stretch be explained by changes in tolerance to stretch? *Aust J Physiother* 52:45–50, 2006.

134. Law RYW, Harvey LA, Nicholas MK, et al: Stretch exercises increase tolerance to stretch in patients with chronic musculo-skeletal pain: a randomized controlled trial. *Phys Ther* 89:1016–1026, 2009.

135. Kiernan MC, Vucic S, Cheah BC, et al: Amyotrophic lateral sclerosis. *Lancet* 377:942–955, 2011.

136. Philips T, Robberecht W: Neuroinflammation in amyotrophic lateral sclerosis: role of glial activation in motor neuron disease. *Lancet Neurol* 10:253–263, 2011.

137. Simmons Z: Management strategies for patients with amyotrophic lateral sclerosis from diagnosis through death. *The Neurologist* 11:257–270, 2005.

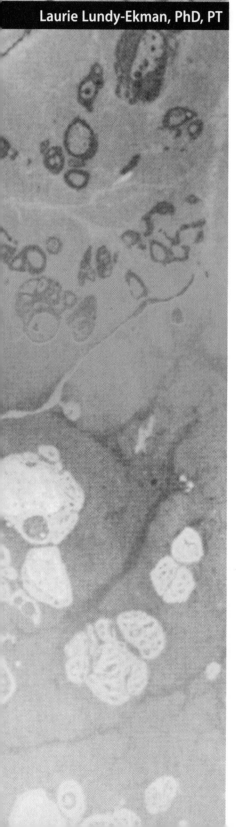

# 11

# Basal Ganglia, Cerebellum, and Movement

Laurie Lundy-Ekman, PhD, PT

## Chapter Outline

The basal ganglia and the cerebellum adjust activity in the descending upper motor neurons (UMNs), despite lack of direct connections with lower motor neurons (LMNs). The basal ganglia and the cerebellum influence movement via different pathways through the thalamus to motor areas of the cerebral cortex and by connections with UMNs. In this chapter, basal ganglia motor and nonmotor functions and their clinical disorders will be discussed first, the cerebellum and clinical disorders affecting the cerebellum will be covered second, and the chapter will conclude with a summary of normal motor control and the three fundamental types of movements.

## BASAL GANGLIA

The basal ganglia predict the effects of various actions, then make and execute action plans.[1]

The basal ganglia include the following nuclei (Figure 11-1):

- Caudate
- Putamen
- Globus pallidus
- Subthalamic nucleus
- Substantia nigra

The caudate, putamen, and globus pallidus are located within the cerebrum. Based on anatomic proximity, the cerebral basal ganglia have joint names: the globus pallidus and putamen together form the *lentiform nucleus;* the caudate and putamen together are the *striatum.* The lentiform nucleus is shaped like a broad, solid cone, with the putamen lateral (wide end of cone) and the globus pallidus medial (point of cone). The globus pallidus has an internus (medial) section and an externus (lateral) section. The caudate is joined with the putamen anteriorly. Their junction is called the *ventral striatum* (see Figure 11-1). The *nucleus accumbens* is part of the ventral striatum.

During brain development, the caudate assumes a C shape adjacent to the lateral ventricle (see Chapter 5). The large, anterior part of the caudate is the head, the adjacent section is the body, and the part on the edge of the inferior horn of the lateral ventricle is the tail of the caudate.

The *subthalamic nucleus* is located inferior to the thalamus and lateral to the hypothalamus (Figure 11-2). The *substantia nigra* is a nucleus in the midbrain named for the color of its cells. Some substantia nigra cells contain melanin, making the

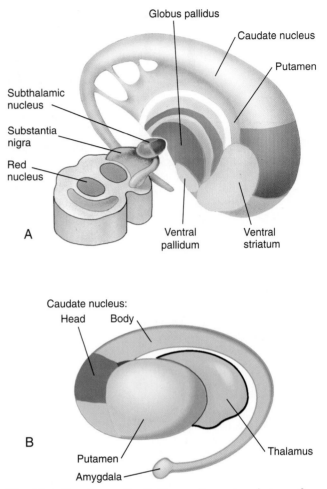

**Fig. 11-1 Basal ganglia. A,** Three-dimensional view of the midbrain and the left caudate, putamen, and globus pallidus. Anterior is to the right. The basal ganglia include the caudate, putamen, globus pallidus, substantia nigra, and subthalamic nucleus. The red nucleus, shown for anatomic reference, is not part of the basal ganglia. **B,** Lateral view of the left caudate and putamen, showing their anatomic relationships with the amygdala (part of the limbic system) and the thalamus. Anterior is to the left. *(A modified with permission from Hendelman WJ: Student's atlas of neuroanatomy, Philadelphia, 1994, WB Saunders, p 39.)*

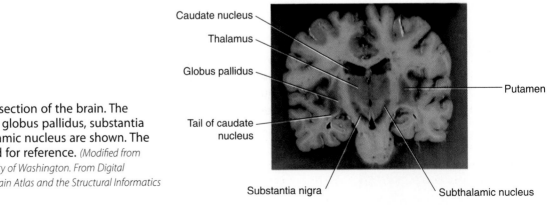

**Fig. 11-2** Coronal section of the brain. The caudate, putamen, globus pallidus, substantia nigra, and subthalamic nucleus are shown. The thalamus is labeled for reference. *(Modified from copyright 1994, University of Washington. From Digital Anatomist Interactive Brain Atlas and the Structural Informatics Group.)*

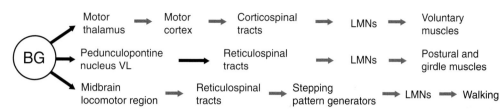

**Fig. 11-3 Simplified summary of the role of the basal ganglia in movement.** The basal ganglia inhibit the motor thalamus, contributing to a normal level of activity in the motor cortex. Therefore the corticospinal tracts provide a normal level of facilitation to the lower motor neurons that innervate voluntary muscles. Output from the basal ganglia also inhibits the ventrolateral pedunculopontine nucleus (VL indicates ventrolateral part of the nucleus). The vlPPN inhibits the reticulospinal tracts, which, in turn, provide the normal level of facilitation to lower motor neurons that innervate postural and girdle muscles, thus controlling muscle tone.[2,3] The basal ganglia inhibit the midbrain locomotor region (cuneiform nucleus and dorsal pedunculopontine nucleus [PPN]). The midbrain locomotor region stimulates reticulospinal neurons that activate stepping pattern generators, facilitating walking or running. Red arrows indicate facilitation; black arrows indicate inhibition.

nucleus appear black. The substantia nigra has two parts: compacta and reticularis. The substantia nigra compacta provides essential dopamine to the striatum.

The *substantia nigra reticularis* and the *globus pallidus internus* are the output nuclei of the basal ganglia system.

## Neurotransmitters in the Basal Ganglia Circuit

Of the many neurotransmitters and neuromodulators active in the basal ganglia motor circuitry, the actions of only a few are well understood. The cortical motor areas produce excitation of the striatum by delivering the transmitter glutamate. Dopamine from the substantia nigra to the striatum adjusts signals to the output nuclei, so the output nuclei provide the appropriate level of inhibition to their target nuclei.

## BASAL GANGLIA MOTOR CIRCUIT

The output of the basal ganglia motor circuit regulates muscle contraction, muscle force, multijoint movements, and sequencing of movements via the pathways shown in Figure 11-3. The basal ganglia motor circuit includes cerebral cortex motor areas, putamen, subthalamic nucleus, globus pallidus internus, and motor areas of the thalamus (dark pink boxes in Figure 11-4).

Although the basal ganglia have profound effects on movement, they have no direct output to LMNs. The motor control exerted by the basal ganglia is transmitted to LMNs by three routes. One is via the thalamus and then to UMN tracts whose cell bodies are in the cerebral cortex (the corticospinal, corticopontine, and corticobrainstem tracts). The second is via the *pedunculopontine nucleus* (PPN) to reticulospinal tracts. The third is via the midbrain locomotor region to reticulospinal tracts. Stimulation of the PPN regulates contraction of postural and girdle muscles via reticulospinal neurons acting on inhibitory spinal interneurons.[3,4] Stimulation of the *midbrain locomotor region* elicits rhythmic lower limb movements similar to walking or running via stimulation of reticulospinal neurons.[3,5]

The globus pallidus internus provides the output of the basal ganglia motor circuit, inhibiting the motor thalamus, the PPN, and the midbrain locomotor region (Table 11-1).

| TABLE 11-1 | BASAL GANGLIA MOTOR CIRCUIT |
|---|---|
| **Role** | **Structure** |
| Receive input from premotor and motor cortex | Putamen |
| Process information within the basal ganglia circuit | Subthalamic nucleus<br>Substantia nigra compacta |
| Send output to motor areas of the cerebral cortex (via the motor thalamus), PPN, and midbrain locomotor region | Globus pallidus internus |

*PPN,* Pedunculopontine nucleus.

## BASAL GANGLIA EXECUTIVE, SOCIAL, BEHAVIORAL, AND EMOTIONAL FUNCTIONS

Traditionally, the basal ganglia were considered devoted to motor control. However, in the striatum, only the putamen and the body of the caudate participate in motor control. The role of the putamen in control of movements has been discussed. The basal ganglia are critical parts of four additional separate, parallel cortico-basal ganglia-thalamic loops: oculomotor, executive, behavioral flexibility and control, and limbic. The motor, executive, behavioral, and limbic loops are shown in Figure 11-5. All five loops contribute to predicting future events, selecting desired behaviors and preventing undesired behaviors, motor learning, shifting attention, and spatial working memory.[6]

The body of the caudate is part of an oculomotor loop that makes decisions about eye movements and spatial attention. The caudate body loop determines whether fast eye movements occur.[7,8] The oculomotor loop runs parallel to the motor loop, linking cortical frontal and supplementary motor eye fields, caudate body, substantia nigra reticularis, and thalamic nuclei, and returns to the cortical motor eye fields.

The ventral striatum and the caudate head are not directly involved in controlling movements. The ventral striatum is part of the limbic system and participates in emotions and motivation. The ventral striatum acts as a link between the limbic, cognitive, and motor systems.[9] The role of the ventral striatum in the reward circuit and addiction is discussed in Chapter 18.

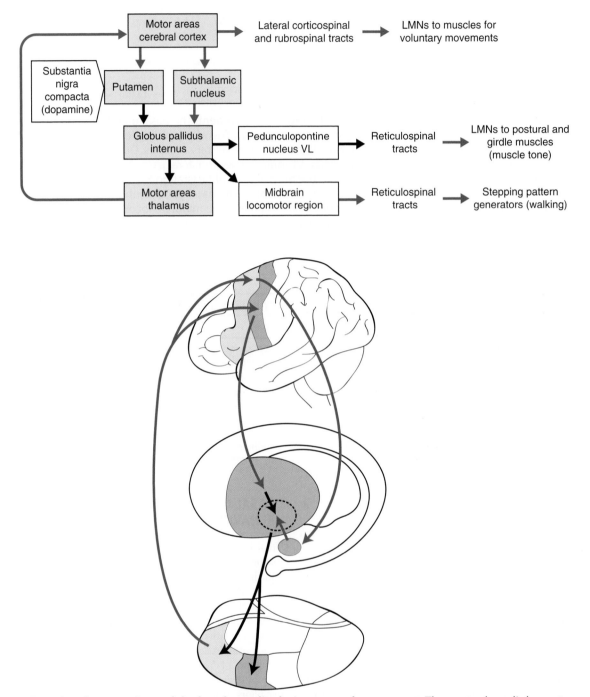

**Fig. 11-4 Functional connections of the basal ganglia during normal movement.** The motor loop links motor areas of the cerebral cortex with the putamen, subthalamic nucleus, globus pallidus internus, and motor areas of the thalamus. The substantia nigra compacta supplies dopamine to the putamen. Red arrows are excitatory; black arrows are inhibitory. *(Developed from Karachi C, Grabli D, Bernard FA, et al: Cholinergic mesencephalic neurons are involved in gait and postural disorders in Parkinson disease. J Clin Invest 120(8):2745–2755, 2010; Matsumura M: The pedunculopontine tegmental nucleus and experimental parkinsonism. A review. J Neurol 252 Suppl 4:IV5–IV12, 2005.)*

The head of the caudate is part of a decision-making loop that participates in goal-directed behavior, including evaluating information for making perceptual decisions, planning, and choosing actions in context[10-13]; the head of the caudate is not involved in controlling movements.[14-16] Imagine you are driving to a job interview and are running late. A green traffic light turns yellow. Your caudate head evaluates how heavy the traffic is, how much time you have, and whether to risk running the light as it turns red. Once the decision is made by the executive, decision-making loop (including the caudate head), the motor loop (including the putamen) initiates hitting the brakes or accelerating. Now imagine a different context: you are driving to the grocery store, without time constraints, and are feeling relaxed; at the same intersection, the light turns yellow. The

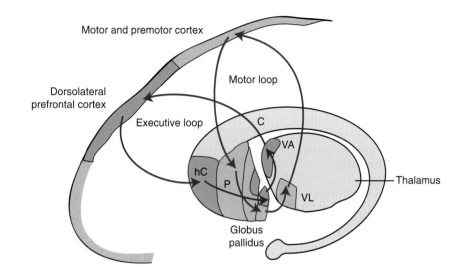

| | Cerebral cortex | Basal ganglia | Thalamic nuclei |
|---|---|---|---|
| Motor loop | Motor and premotor cortex | Putamen, globus pallidus | Ventral lateral |
| Executive loop | Dorsolateral prefrontal cortex | Head of caudate, globus pallidus | Ventral anterior |
| Behavioral flexibility and control loop | Ventrolateral prefrontal and lateral orbital cortex | Head of caudate, substantia nigra reticularis | Mediodorsal |
| Limbic | Medial orbital and medial prefrontal cortex | Ventral striatum, ventral pallidum | |

A

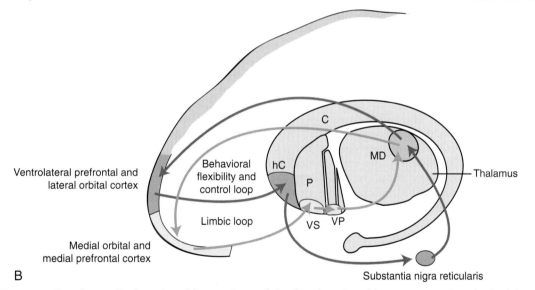

B

**Fig. 11-5  Basal ganglia functional loops.** Four of the five functional loops connecting the basal ganglia with the cerebral cortex and thalamus. The posterior two-thirds of the lentiform nucleus has been cut away so the entire thalamus is visible. The oculomotor loop is omitted for simplicity. The basal ganglia and thalamic components of the loops are as follows: Part A: the motor loop includes putamen (P), globus pallidus, and ventral lateral (VL) nucleus of the thalamus. The executive loop includes the head of the caudate (hC), the globus pallidus, and the ventral anterior (VA) nucleus of the thalamus. Part B: The behavioral flexibility and control loop includes the head of the caudate, the substantia nigra reticularis, and the mediodorsal (MD) thalamic nucleus. The limbic loop includes the ventral striatum (VS), the ventral pallidum (VP), and the mediodorsal thalamic nucleus. *(Developed from Cohen MX, Frank MJ: Neurocomputational models of basal ganglia function in learning, memory and choice. Behav Brain Res 199(1):141–156, 2009; Middleton FA, Strick PL: A Revised Neuroanatomy of Frontal-Subcortical Circuits. In Uchle, J, editor: Frontal-Subcortical Circuits In Psychiatric and Neurological Disorders, JL Cummings, New York, 2001 by Guilford Publications. Inc, pp 44–58; R Nieuwenhuys, J Voogd, C van Huijzen, Telencephalon: the basal ganglia. In: The human central nervous system, Springer, 2008, Berlin, pp 427–489; Roelofs K, Minelli A, Mars RB et al: On the neural control of social emotional behavior. Soc Cogn Affect Neurosci. 4(1):50–58, 2009.)*

**TABLE 11-2    FUNCTION OF THE FIVE BASAL GANGLIA LOOPS**

| Name of Loop | Role |
|---|---|
| Motor | Movement selection and action |
| Oculomotor | Decisions about eye movements and spatial attention; initiation of fast eye movements |
| Executive[18] | Goal-directed behavior; makes perceptual decisions, plans, and decides upon actions in context |
| Behavioral flexibility and control[14,22] | Recognition of social disapproval, self-regulatory control, selecting relevant knowledge from irrelevant,[23] maintaining attention, stimulus-response learning |
| Limbic | Links limbic, cognitive, and motor systems; identifies value of stimuli; involved in reward-guided behaviors; monitors errors in predictions; concerned with seeking pleasure[24,25,26] |

Data from DeLong M, Wichmann TL: Changing views of basal ganglia circuits and circuit disorders. *Clin EEG Neurosci* 41:61–67, 2010; Middleton FA, Strick PL: A revised neuroanatomy of frontal subcortical circuits. In Lichter DG, Cummings JL, editors: *Frontal-subcortical circuits in psychiatry and neurology*, New York, 2000, Guilford Publishing, pp 44–58.

caudate head evaluates the full context and selects an appropriate action.

The head of the caudate is also active in learning and changes its activity before the cortex when reward contingencies are reversed.[1,17] For example, if an experimenter repeatedly rewards a monkey when it picks up a cube and not a cylinder, and then the experimenter suddenly rewards picking up the cylinder and not the cube, the caudate head is the first neural area to learn the new contingency. The link between the action chosen by the caudate head and the selected movement occurs primarily in the thalamus.[18,19]

A case report of a 55-year-old woman who had bilateral discrete caudate head infarctions clarifies the function of the caudate head: she had *executive function* (decision-making) deficits including inattention, distractibility, disorientation, poor concentration, and short-term memory. There was no movement disorder.[20] A second case study of isolated bilateral caudate head lesions reports extreme behavior changes in a 25-year-old woman. Previous to the lesions, she was employed full time and had been academically successful in high school. After the lesions, she became impulsive, prone to frustration over minor issues, violent, indifferent, and hypersexual, shoplifting, exposing herself, and experiencing urinary incontinence. No motor abnormalities were present.[21]

Table 11-2 summarizes the functions of the basal ganglia loops. The executive, behavioral flexibility and control, and limbic loops are discussed more extensively in Chapters 17 and 18.

## BASAL GANGLIA MOVEMENT DISORDERS

Movement disorders in basal ganglia dysfunction range from hypokinetic disorders (too little movement) to hyperkinetic disorders (excessive movement). Differences in abnormal movements are due to dysfunction in specific parts of the basal ganglia–thalamocortical motor circuit and in basal ganglia–PPN and midbrain locomotor region (MLR) output. The basal ganglia inhibit the motor thalamus, the PPN, and the MLR; excessive inhibition results in hypokinetic disorders, and inadequate inhibition results in hyperkinetic disorders.

## Hypokinetic Disorders

### Parkinson's Disease

The most common basal ganglia motor disorder is Parkinson's disease. Parkinson's disease has three subtypes: akinetic/rigid, tremor-dominant, and mixed.[27] A study in California reported prevalence of the subtypes as akinetic/rigid 50%, tremor-dominant 40%, and mixed 10%.[28] Akinetic/rigid Parkinson's will be discussed first, then tremor-dominant. Mixed subtype will not be discussed further because it is simply a combination of the akinetic/rigid and tremor-dominant types.

#### Akinetic/Rigid Parkinson's Disease

This form of Parkinson's disease is characterized by muscular rigidity, shuffling gait, drooping posture, rhythmic muscular tremors, and a mask-like facial expression. Parkinson's disease interferes with both voluntary and automatic movements. People with akinetic/rigid subtype have difficulty coming to standing from sitting, and their gait is characterized by a flexed posture, shuffling of the feet, and decreased or absent arm swing. Distinctive signs of akinetic/rigid disease include the following:

- Akinesia/hypokinesia
- Rigidity
- "Freezing" during movement
- Visuoperceptive impairments
- Postural instability
- Resting tremor
- Nonmotor signs: depression, psychosis, Parkinson's dementia, autonomic dysfunction

*Rigidity* is increased resistance to movement in all muscles. In contrast to spasticity, rigidity results from direct upper motor neuron facilitation of alpha motor neurons. Thus, in rigidity, output from the nervous system causes active muscle contraction, directly increasing resistance to movement. The rigidity is present during sleep.[29]

Akinesia, strictly defined, is the absence of movement. However, in clinical use, the term *akinesia* is used as a synonym for hypokinesia, to describe decreased movement. *Hypokinesia* is manifested in decreased ranges of active motion and in lack of automatic movements, including facial expression and normal arm swing during walking. Hypokinesia may be related to decreased ability to control the force output of muscles. Compared to people with intact neuromuscular systems, people with Parkinson's disease have less control over the amount of force their muscles produce.[30] People with akinetic/rigid Parkinson's disease are prone to falls because of their inability to generate adequate muscle force quickly. Their postural corrections may be too slow to be useful.

People with akinetic/rigid Parkinson's disease often have episodes when their walking abruptly ceases, called *freezing of gait*. Excessive basal ganglia inhibition of the midbrain locomotor region contributes to this phenomenon.[3]

**TABLE 11-3** STAGES OF AKINETIC/RIGID PARKINSON'S DISEASE

| Stage | Characteristics |
|---|---|
| Stage 1 | Unilateral signs and symptoms, typically mild tremor of one limb |
| Stage 2 | Bilateral signs, posture and gait affected, minimal disability |
| Stage 3 | Moderately severe generalized dysfunction, significant slowing of body movements, early impairment of equilibrium on walking or standing |
| Stage 4 | Severe signs; able to walk to limited extent; rigidity, bradykinesia; unable to live alone |
| Stage 5 | Extreme weight loss, cannot stand or walk, requires constant nursing care |

From Hoehn MM, Yahr MD: Parkinsonism: onset, progression and mortality. *Neurology* 17:427–442, 1967.

*Visuoperceptive impairments* are deficits in using visual information to guide movement. Visuoperceptive impairments produce impediments to action. For example, a walker, intended to assist a person with ambulation, may create a visual block, and movement ceases. A therapist standing near the person may also unwittingly interfere with the person's ability to move. People with Parkinson's disease frequently report difficulties moving past visual movement blocks, like doorways; if a marker is placed on the floor, the person can use the marker as a cue for getting through the doorway. Why the marker does not serve as an additional visual block is unknown. Visuoperceptive impairments in Parkinson's disease are associated with abnormal processing in the temporal lobe visual identification pathway.[31]

*Postural instability,* secondary to extreme stiffness of postural flexors and extensors, becomes a severe problem as akinetic/rigid Parkinson's progresses. Motor progression of Parkinson's disease occurs in predictable stages (Table 11-3). Clinical diagnosis of Parkinson's disease requires hypokinesia affecting the upper body combined with rigidity and/or resting tremor.[32]

In contrast to the hypokinetic signs, a hyperkinetic sign of Parkinson's disease is resting tremor. *Resting tremor* is involuntary, rhythmic shaking movements of the limbs produced by contractions of antagonist muscles. Resting tremor of the hands consists of rhythmic movement that appears as though the thumb is rolling a pill along the fingertips (pill-rolling tremor); the tremor is prominent when the hand is at rest and diminishes during voluntary movement. Resting tremor has a frequency of three to six tremors per second. Tremor may persist during sleep.[35] In akinetic/rigid Parkinson's, tremor is often absent; even when present, it does not contribute significantly to activity limitations.

Given that a significant proportion of the basal ganglia are devoted to *nonmotor functions,* deficits affecting nonmotor systems in Parkinson's disease should be anticipated. Akinetic/rigid Parkinson's is associated with psychopathology. Often depression, *psychosis* (usually visual hallucinations), *Parkinson's dementia,* and *autonomic dysfunction* (constipation, orthostatic

hypotension) further decrease the person's independence. Dementia is deterioration of intellectual function. Parkinson's dementia is different from Alzheimer's dementia. Alzheimer's dementia primarily affects memory. Parkinson's dementia interferes with the ability to plan, to maintain goal orientation, and to make decisions.[34] Tremor-dominant type is not associated with psychological disorders.[33]

### Tremor-Dominant Parkinson's Disease

In tremor-dominant Parkinson's, the most disabling feature is the presence of both action and resting tremors. Action tremors occur during voluntary movements. Examples include tremors while getting dressed and during eating. In the tremor-dominant subtype, rigidity and slowing of movement are relatively mild, and tremors are the primary factor interfering with daily activities.[36] Rhythmic firing of neuron groups in the subthalamic nucleus is correlated with tremor in Parkinson's disease.[37]

### Pathology in Parkinson's Disease

The pathology in Parkinson's disease is the death of dopamine-producing cells in the substantia nigra compacta (see Figure 11-5) and acetylcholine-producing cells in the PPN. Oxidative stress, mitochondrial dysfunction, and programmed cell death kill the cells.[38] Cell death occurs long before clinical signs of Parkinson's disease become evident; about 80% of dopamine-producing cells die before signs of the disease appear.[39] Loss of dopamine to the putamen reduces activity in motor areas of the cerebral cortex, decreasing voluntary movements. Loss of pedunculopontine cells, combined with increased inhibition of the PPN, disinhibits the reticulospinal tracts, producing excessive contraction of postural muscles (Figure 11-6). Figure 11-7 compares the locations and effects of upper motor neuron lesions with the locations and effects of Parkinson's disease (Pathology 11-1).

### Treatments for Parkinson's Disease

Drugs, invasive procedures, and physical and occupational therapy are used to treat Parkinson's disease. Because Parkinson's disease involves loss of dopamine-producing cells in the substantia nigra, drug therapy that replaces dopamine (L-dopa) is initially effective in reducing signs of the disease. However, tolerance to L-dopa, side effects (including hallucinations, delusions, psychosis, and dyskinesia), and progression of the disease with involvement of other cells and neurotransmitters limit the effectiveness of L-dopa therapy. *Dyskinesia* is involuntary movement that resembles chorea (brisk, jerky movements) and/or dystonia (involuntary sustained postures or repetitive movements). Even with L-dopa therapy, people with Parkinson's disease may experience periods of near-normal mobility alternating with periods of immobility. This is called the *on-off phenomenon.* The duration of "on" times tends to decrease with continued use of L-dopa. Moreover, motor performance often varies at different times of the day regardless of the medication.

Invasive procedures, including deep-brain stimulation (DBS), neuronal transplantation, and destructive surgery, may be used to treat the dyskinesia, tremors, and hypokinesia associated with Parkinson's disease. For selected patients, DBS is an effective adjunct to drug therapy. DBS requires surgical implantation of a stimulator and electrodes. Typically, the stimulator is implanted inferior to the clavicle. To treat tremors, electrodes are implanted into the thalamus.[42] Continuous high-frequency

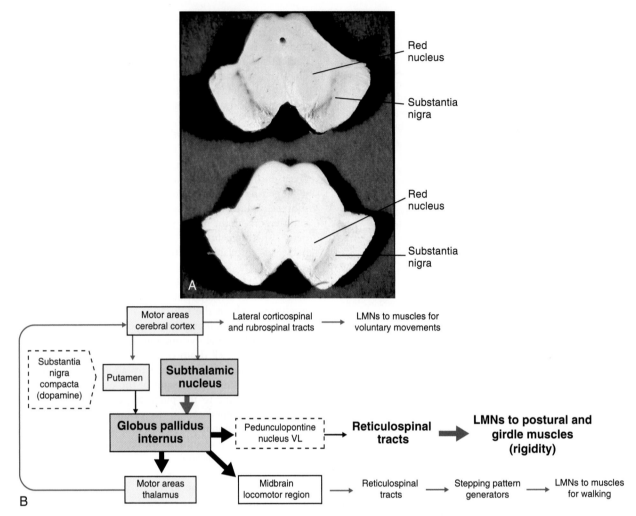

**Fig. 11-6 Parkinson's disease A,** Horizontal sections of the midbrain. The upper section is normal, with darkly pigmented cells in the substantia nigra. The lower section is from a person with Parkinson's disease, with the characteristic loss of darkly pigmented, dopamine-producing cells. *(Courtesy Dr. Melvin J. Ball.)* **B,** Changes in neural activity in Parkinson's disease. Compare this with normal basal ganglia activity in Figure 11-4. Red arrows indicate that the connection is excitatory. Black arrows indicate that the connection is inhibitory. The sizes of the arrows, boxes, and letters symbolize the amount of activity in pathways and structures. Thick arrows represent increased neural activity, and thin arrows represent decreased neural activity. Dark pink boxes indicate normal level of activity in the structure. Light pink boxes represent decreased activity. A dotted outline surrounding a structure indicates the death of neurons within that structure. In Parkinson's disease, neurons die in the substantia nigra compacta and the pedunculopontine nucleus. The subthalamic nucleus output increases because globus pallidus externus inhibition decreases (not shown). VL: ventrolateral. Decreased dopamine from the substantia nigra compacta is the primary change leading to excessive activity of the globus pallidus internus (GPi). The GPi inhibits the following:

|  | This causes: | Resulting in: |
|---|---|---|
| 1. Motor thalamus | Decreased activity of cerebral cortex motor areas to the lateral group of UMNs | Less activity of the lateral group of UMNs, impairing voluntary movement |
| 2. Midbrain locomotor region | Decreased signals from the reticular formation to spinal stepping pattern generators | Loss of automatic gait |
| 3. Pedunculopontine nucleus | Disinhibition of the reticulospinal tracts, activating LMNs | Rigidity of postural and girdle muscles |

*(Developed from Karachi C, Grabli D, Bernard FA, et al: Cholinergic mesencephalic neurons are involved in gait and postural disorders in Parkinson disease. J Clin Invest 120(8):2745–2755, 2010, Matsumura M: The pedunculopontine tegmental nucleus and experimental parkinsonism. A review. J Neurol 252 Suppl 4:IV5–IV12, 2005. Takakusaki K, Tomita N, Yano M: Substrates for normal gait and pathophysiology of gait disturbances with respect to the basal ganglia dysfunction. J Neurol 255 Suppl 4:19–29, 2008.)*

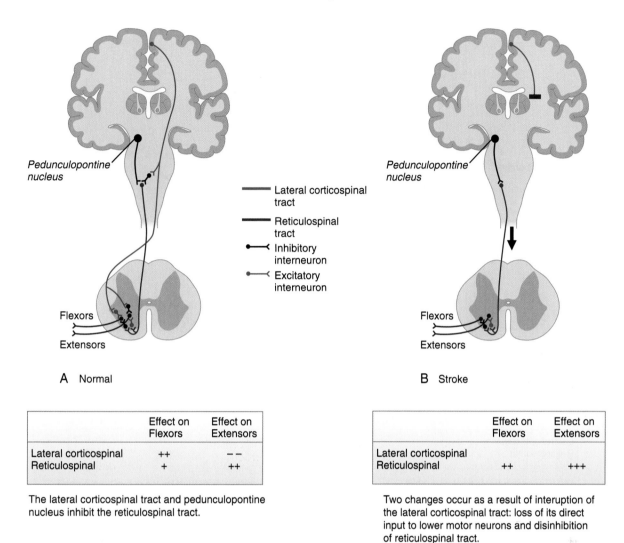

| | Effect on Flexors | Effect on Extensors |
|---|---|---|
| Lateral corticospinal | ++ | – – |
| Reticulospinal | + | ++ |

The lateral corticospinal tract and pedunculopontine nucleus inhibit the reticulospinal tract.

**A  Normal**

| | Effect on Flexors | Effect on Extensors |
|---|---|---|
| Lateral corticospinal Reticulospinal | ++ | +++ |

Two changes occur as a result of interuption of the lateral corticospinal tract: loss of its direct input to lower motor neurons and disinhibition of reticulospinal tract.

**B  Stroke**

**Fig. 11-7  A** through **D,** Comparison of the effects of stroke, complete spinal cord injury, and Parkinson's disease on activity in descending activating tracts and resulting activity levels in skeletal muscles. Black interneurons are inhibitory; green interneurons are excitatory. The spinal cord section is a lumbar segment. In each table, a "+" sign indicates facilitation and a "–" sign indicates inhibition. Thus, in an intact nervous system, the lateral corticospinal tract moderately facilitates lower motor neurons to flexor muscles and inhibits lower motor neurons to extensors.

*Continued*

electrical stimulation inhibits the firing of overactive thalamic neurons. Bilateral subthalamic nucleus DBS improves speed of movement, rigidity, gait, and postural stability and allows decreased L-dopa dosage.[43] However, subthalamic nucleus DBS is appropriate only for relatively healthy, young, cognitively intact patients who are on optimal medications and have severe fluctuations of motor signs.[44] Globus pallidus internus stimulation is effective for reducing dyskinesias and can be used in older patients.[44] Long-term follow up demonstrates that thalamic DBS is safe and effective for reducing tremors,[45] and stimulation of the subthalamic nucleus provides sustained improvement in motor function.[46] DBS slightly posterior to the PPN is most effective for improving gait and postural reflexes.[43,47] In a study of 255 patients with advanced Parkinson's disease, bilateral DBS was more effective than best medical therapy in

improving motor function, quality of life, and time without dyskinesias. However, the DBS group had 39 adverse events related to the surgery.[48]

Researchers have also used neuronal transplantation to treat Parkinson's disease, placing fetal-donor dopamine-producing cells in the basal ganglia. This approach is based on the hypothesis that if transplanted cells thrive in the brain environment, they will become internal sources of dopamine. However, to optimize transplantation, problems with culturing and delivering the cells and selecting locations need to be overcome.[49]

Some specialized treatment centers perform destructive surgery for the treatment of severe tremor and akinesia associated with Parkinson's disease.[42] In these surgeries, called *thalamotomy* and *pallidotomy,* surgery destroys a small, precise region of cells in the thalamus (for the treatment of tremor) or in the

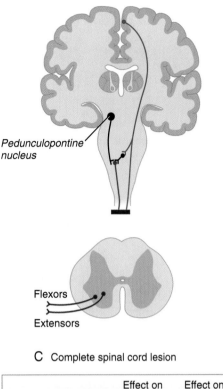

Pedunculopontine
nucleus

Flexors

Extensors

C   Complete spinal cord lesion

|                      | Effect on Flexors | Effect on Extensors |
|----------------------|-------------------|---------------------|
| Lateral corticospinal Reticulospinal |                   |                     |

All descending tracts are interrupted.

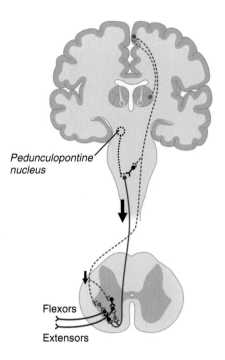

Pedunculopontine
nucleus

Flexors

Extensors

D   Parkinson's disease

|                      | Effect on Flexors | Effect on Extensors |
|----------------------|-------------------|---------------------|
| Lateral corticospinal | +                 | –                   |
| Reticulospinal        | +++               | +++                 |

The lateral corticospinal tract is less active than normal
due to increased globus pallidus inhibition of motor
thalamus. The reticulospinal tract is overactive due to
reduced inhibition (from both the lateral corticospinal
tract and pedunculopontine nucleus). Excessive
reticulospinal signals elicit lower motor neuron
overactivity to postural and proximal limb muscles,
causing trunk and proximal limb muscle rigidity.

**Fig. 11-7, cont'd**

globus pallidus of the basal ganglia (for the treatment of akinesia). Destruction of these cells, which are thought to be overactive in the disease process, may result in functional improvement.
However, unlike DBS, destructive surgery and neural transplantation are not reversible. DBS, destructive surgery, and
neural transplantation are also used to treat other movement
disorders and for intractable chronic pain.

Physical and occupational therapy improve mobility and
functional status in people with Parkinson's disease.[50,51] Intense
resistance training produces greater muscle hypertrophy and
functional gains than are produced by standard exercise.[52]

### Parkinson-Plus Syndromes

Other disorders cause signs similar to Parkinson's disease and
must be distinguished from true idiopathic Parkinson's. Red
flags indicating a diagnosis other than Parkinson's disease
include early postural instability, rapid progression, respiratory
dysfunction, abnormal postures, uncontrollable inappropriate
laughter or crying,[53] and signs of cerebellar, corticospinal, or
voluntary gaze dysfunction. Parkinson-Plus syndrome is the
collective name for primary neurodegenerative diseases that
cause motor signs similar to Parkinson's disease.

| PATHOLOGY 11-1 | AKINETIC/RIGID PARKINSON'S DISEASE |
|---|---|
| Pathology | Death of dopaminergic neurons in substantia nigra compacta and in pedunculopontine nucleus (PPN) |
| Etiology | Oxidative stress, mitochondrial dysfunction, and programmed cell death |
| Speed of onset | Chronic |
| Signs and symptoms | |
|    Psychological | Depression is common |
|    Cognition | Dementia and psychosis (hallucinations) late in the disease |
|    Consciousness | Alterations in sleep/wake cycles cause excessive daytime sleepiness |
|    Communication and memory | Normal; dementia may occur in late stages |
|    Sensory/perceptual | Visuoperceptive blocks: movement slows or stops in response to nearby visual stimuli, including doorways, other objects, or people |
|    Autonomic | Constipation, orthostatic hypotension, thermal dysregulation, bladder and sexual dysfunction |
|    Motor | Hypokinesia; rigidity; stooped posture; shuffling gait; difficulty initiating movements, turning, and stopping; resting tremor; visuoperceptive movement blocks; freezing during movements; decreased postural control |
| Region affected | Basal ganglia nuclei in cerebrum and midbrain |
| Demographics | Onset typically between 50 and 65 years of age; men and women affected equally |
|    Incidence | 8–18 cases per 100,000 population per year[40] |
|    Lifetime prevalence | 3 cases per 1000 population[40] |
| Prognosis | Progressive; mean age at death 75 years old[41]; death usually by heart disease or infection |

The term *primary neurodegenerative disease* indicates that the cause is idiopathic or genetic. Parkinson-Plus syndromes include progressive supranuclear palsy, dementia with Lewy bodies, and multiple system atrophy. The most common cause of death in people with Parkinson-Plus syndromes is pneumonia. Approximately 25% of people with Parkinson-Plus syndromes are initially misdiagnosed as having Parkinson's disease.[54]

*Progressive supranuclear palsy* (PSP) is characterized by early onset of gait instability with a tendency to fall backward, axial rigidity, freezing of gait, depression, psychosis, and rage attacks, plus supranuclear gaze palsy. *Supranuclear* refers to loss of descending neurons that synapse in the cranial nerve nuclei controlling eye movement. In supranuclear gaze palsy, the patient is unable to voluntarily control gaze. Vertical gaze is usually affected before horizontal gaze, so initially the patient may be unable to look downward or upward. Reflexive eye movements remain normal. The pathology is neurodegeneration with tauopathy (abnormal accumulation of the structural protein tau within neurons). The cause of PSP is unknown. PSP prevalence is 2 to 7 cases per 100,000 person-years.[55]

*Dementia with Lewy bodies* causes early, generalized cognitive decline, visual hallucinations, and motor signs indistinguishable from akinetic/rigid Parkinson's disease. Lewy bodies are abnormal accumulations of proteins (tau and alpha-synuclein) within neurons. Unlike Alzheimer's disease, memory is not disproportionately impaired compared with other cognitive functions. Prevalence estimates range from 0% to 5%, and incidence is 0.1% per year.[56]

*Multiple system atrophy* (MSA) is a progressive degenerative disease that affects the basal ganglia, cerebellar, and autonomic systems; the peripheral nervous system; and the cerebral cortex (Pathology 11-2).

MSA is characterized by:
- Akinetic/rigid syndrome
- Cerebellar signs
- Autonomic dysfunction
- Corticospinal tract dysfunction

The Parkinson-like features of MSA include slow movements and rigidity. Cerebellar aspects are *dysarthria* (uncoordinated speech) and truncal and gait ataxia. *Ataxia* is lack of coordination. The gait ataxia in MSA is not typical of cerebellar gait ataxia, because the ataxic gait in MSA is narrow-based. Autonomic features include postural hypotension, bladder and bowel incontinence, abnormal respiration, decreased sweating, tears, and saliva, and, in men, impotence. A decrease in goal-oriented cognitive ability and difficulty with directing attention have been reported.[58] In women, the first sign of MSA is usually difficulty urinating. In men, the first sign is usually impotence.

The diagnosis requires differentiating MSA from Parkinson's disease, secondary parkinsonism (see next section), and pure autonomic failure. The distinction between MSA and Parkinson's disease or parkinsonism is made by exclusion; if no autonomic or cerebellar signs are present, the disorder is Parkinson's disease or parkinsonism. In pure autonomic failure, orthostatic hypotension and other autonomic signs occur without signs of basal ganglia or cerebellar involvement. Another distinguishing feature is that pure autonomic failure primarily affects the postganglionic neurons of the sympathetic system, whereas MSA affects both preganglionic and

| **PATHOLOGY 11-2**    MULTIPLE SYSTEM ATROPHY | |
|---|---|
| Pathology | Progressive degenerative disease affecting the basal ganglia, cerebellar, and autonomic systems and the cerebral cortex |
| Etiology | Unknown; associated with accumulation of alpha-synuclein in both neurons and oligodendrocytes |
| Speed of onset | Chronic |
| Signs and symptoms | |
| Consciousness | Decreased goal-oriented cognition and difficulty with attention; may have dementia late in the disease process |
| Communication and memory | May be impaired late in the disease process |
| Sensory | May have polyneuropathy that includes sensory fibers |
| Autonomic | Postural hypotension; hypotension after eating; bladder and bowel incontinence; abnormal respiration; decreased sweating, tears, and saliva; male impotence |
| Motor | Slow movements, rigidity, dysarthria, truncal ataxia, narrow-based gait ataxia, Babinski's signs, and hyperreflexia |
| Region affected | Basal ganglia, cerebellum, autonomic systems and the cerebral cortex |
| Demographics | |
| Prevalence | 2 to 7 cases per 100,000 population per year[55]; males affected approximately twice as frequently as females |
| Prognosis | Progressive; average life span after diagnosis is approximately 8 years[57] |

postganglionic neurons in the sympathetic and parasympathetic systems. In MSA, autonomic neurons are lost from brainstem nuclei, including the vagus, and from the spinal cord. Signs indicating that MSA is a more likely diagnosis than Parkinson's disease include a poor response to L-dopa (Sinemet, a drug that is effective in Parkinson's disease), orthostatic hypotension, difficulty with urination, rapid progression of functional limitations, loud breathing, and impotence.

Subtypes of MSA have been named for the structures predominantly affected or for the physicians who first described the disorder. Thus, three names are synonymous with MSA: olivopontocerebellar atrophy, striatonigral degeneration, and Shy-Drager syndrome. When the initial signs of MSA are incoordination, dysarthria, and balance deficits, the disorder is often called *olivopontocerebellar atrophy*. When the most prominent signs initially are rigidity and bradykinesia, the disease may be called *striatonigral degeneration*. When the first signs are autonomic dysfunction, the disorder may be called *Shy-Drager syndrome*.

The cause of MSA is unknown. Treatment is symptomatic: fludrocortisone and midodrine to increase blood pressure, and pergolide, bromocriptine, and anticholinergic drugs to improve the movement disorder. Therapists advise people with MSA on methods to decrease orthostatic hypotension (slow position changes, avoiding prolonged standing, eating smaller meals, increasing consumption of salt and caffeine, using elastic garments, avoiding warm temperatures) and on exercise programs to maintain strength and physiologic fitness as long as possible.

## Parkinsonism

Parkinsonism encompasses disorders with signs that mimic Parkinson's disease, but the origin is known to be toxic, infectious, or traumatic. Lesions of the lentiform nucleus are associated

with parkinsonism. Parkinsonism is often a side effect of drugs that treat psychosis or digestive problems. Phenothiazine, thioxanthine, antiemetics, and other drugs that block central nervous system dopamine receptors may cause parkinsonism; nearly 40% of people treated with antipsychotic medications develop parkinsonism.[59] *Drug-induced parkinsonism* frequently leads to misdiagnosis and unnecessary treatment for Parkinson's disease in the elderly.[59] Signs that parkinsonism may be drug-induced include subacute, bilateral onset with rapid progression; early postural tremor; and involuntary movements of the face and mouth.

*Chronic traumatic encephalopathy* (CTE) is characterized by parkinsonism, disordered thinking, depression, memory loss, executive dysfunction, and disinhibition. A history of multiple incidents of head trauma and the accumulation of tau protein in the basal ganglia, diencephalon, brainstem, and focal areas of the frontal, temporal, and insular cerebral cortex are required for diagnosis. CTE has been documented in American football players, professional wrestlers, soccer and hockey players, people subjected to physical abuse, and those with epilepsy or head banging behavior.[60]

## Hyperkinetic Disorders

Abnormal involuntary movements are characteristic of Huntington's disease, dystonia, Tourette's disorder, and dyskinetic cerebral palsy.

## Huntington's Disease

*Chorea,* consisting of involuntary, jerky, rapid movements, and dementia are the signs of Huntington's disease. This autosomal dominant hereditary disorder causes degeneration in many areas of the brain, most prominently in the striatum and

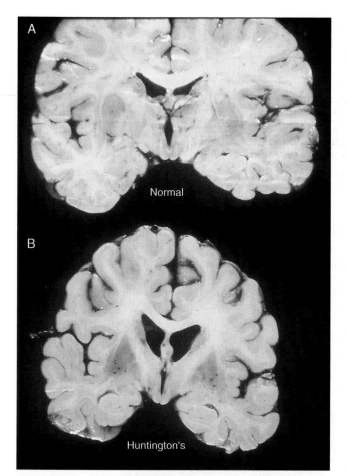

**Fig. 11-8 A,** Coronal section of a normal cerebrum. Compare the size of the caudate nucleus and the overall size of the cerebrum versus **B,** a cerebrum from a person with Huntington's disease. Atrophy of the caudate nucleus produces enlargement of the lateral ventricles.
*(Courtesy Dr. Melvin J. Ball.)*

**TABLE 11-4    TYPES OF FOCAL DYSTONIA**

| | Body Region Affected | Differential Diagnosis |
|---|---|---|
| Cervical dystonia (spasmodic torticollis) | Neck | Congenital muscular torticollis; torticollis caused by inflammatory, ocular, other neurologic, and orthopedic disorders |
| Blepharospasm (involuntary closure of eyes) | Orbicularis oculi muscles | Irritation or inflammation of eyes or eyelids |
| Occupational dystonia: musician's cramp, writer's cramp | Upper limb | Carpal tunnel syndrome, apraxia |
| Oromandibular | Lower facial, masticatory, and tongue muscles | Dental problems, teeth grinding, drug side effect |
| Spasmodic dysphonia | Laryngeal muscles | Inflammatory conditions, vocal misuse, nodules, tumors, psychological factors |

cerebral cortex (Figure 11-8). The degeneration decreases signals from the basal ganglia output nuclei, resulting in disinhibition of the motor thalamus and PPN. The result is excessive output from the motor areas of the cerebral cortex (Figure 11-9). Although the chorea decreases during sleep, people with Huntington's disease move more frequently and forcefully while sleeping than those without the disease.[61] Onset is typically between 40 and 50 years of age, and the disease is progressive, resulting in death about 15 years after signs first appear. The prevalence of Huntington's disease is 7 cases per 100,000 people.[62]

## Dystonia

Dystonias are genetic, usually nonprogressive, movement disorders characterized by involuntary sustained muscle contractions causing abnormal postures or twisting, repetitive movements (Figure 11-10). Dystonia often increases during activity and emotional stress and vanishes completely during sleep.[63] Tremor is frequently associated with dystonia.[64] Abnormal proteins in the pedunculopontine nucleus occur in one severe type of dystonia.[2]

Focal dystonias are the most common, limited to one part of the body (Table 11-4 and Figure 11-11). An example of focal dystonia is spasmodic torticollis (also known as *cervical dystonia*). Torticollis is involuntary, asymmetric contraction of neck muscles, causing abnormal position of the head. Not all torticollis is caused by dystonia: torticollis can also be caused by inflammatory, ocular, congenital, orthopedic, and other neurologic disorders. Focal hand dystonias usually occur only during a specific task. For example, writer's cramp is deterioration in handwriting due to involuntary muscle contractions in the upper limb. Similarly, musician's cramp most often involves the fourth and fifth fingers flexing involuntarily, interfering with the ability to play an instrument (Pathology 11-3). A sports-specific movement disorder, the yips in golf, can be caused by focal dystonia or by performance anxiety. Yips are abrupt, involuntary wrist movements that interfere with putting.[65]

Byl (2000)[67] demonstrated that focal dystonia can be produced in some monkeys by requiring them to open and close one hand hundreds of times every day for several weeks. However, some monkeys spontaneously took breaks and performed the task more slowly than the other monkeys; these monkeys did not develop dystonia. In the monkeys that developed dystonia, neuronal activity in the primary somatosensory cortex was mapped. Receptive fields for the cortical neurons were 10 to 1000 times larger than normal, and many multiple receptive fields were documented.

In humans with focal dystonia, magnetic resonance imaging shows somatotopic degradation in the somatosensory cortex and in the somatosensory part of the thalamus.[67,68] Thus loss of fractionation of movement results from maladaptive neural plasticity. Proprioception and stereognosis are impaired.[69] A treatment protocol for musician's dystonia developed by Byl consists of cessation of abnormal movements, avoidance of

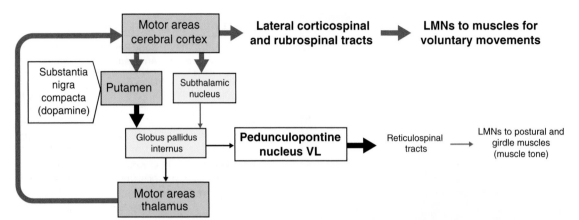

**Fig. 11-9  Changes in neural activity in Huntington's disease.** Compare with normal basal ganglia activity in Figure 11-4. Red arrows indicate that the connection is excitatory. Black arrows indicate that the connection is inhibitory. Thick arrows represent increased neural activity, and thin arrows represent decreased neural activity. Dark pink boxes indicate normal level of activity in the structure. Light pink boxes represent decreased activity. Huntington's disease is characterized by excessive direct inhibition of the globus pallidus internus by the putamen. Thus the inhibitory output of the globus pallidus internus is inadequate, producing disinhibition of the motor thalamus and the pedunculopontine nucleus. This results in excessive activity of the motor areas of the cerebral cortex, producing hyperkinesias, combined with excessive output from the pedunculopontine nucleus, causing insufficient activity in reticulospinal tracts to girdle and postural muscles. The midbrain locomotor region is omitted from this figure because no data are available on its function in Huntington's disease (Medline search, January 2011). Subthalamic nucleus output is decreased due to enhanced inhibition by globus pallidus externus (not shown). VL: ventrolateral.

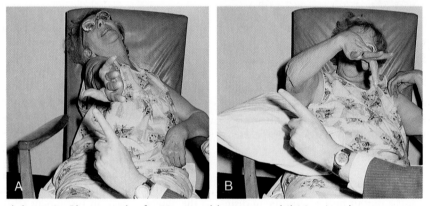

**Fig. 11-10**  Generalized dystonia. Photograph of a 70-year-old woman exhibiting involuntary movements, including shoulder flexion, elbow extension, lateral flexion and extension of the neck, and trunk extension. *(Reproduced with permission from Parsons M, Johnson M:* Diagnosis in color neurology, *St Louis, 2011, Mosby.)*

heavy gripping of instruments (pens, musical instruments), sensory retraining, and mental rehearsal of the target movement without overt body movement. After completing the protocol, all subjects in Byl's study showed improvement in strength, stereognosis, motor control, and other clinical measures. Improvement in motor control was accompanied by improvement in the organization of the somatosensory cortex.[67] Focal dystonia of the hand is frequently misdiagnosed as carpal tunnel syndrome, tennis elbow, strain, or a psychogenic disorder. Because the muscle contractions are caused by basal ganglia dysfunction, attempts at treating the disorder by stretching the muscles are ineffective. Heat, cold, and exercise may be helpful to relieve pain and/or spasms. Severe dystonia can be alleviated by surgical destruction of part of the motor thalamus or by injection of botulinum toxin into the affected muscles.

Generalized dystonia causes involuntary twisting postures of the limbs and trunk. Unlike other dystonias, generalized dystonia is often progressive. Typically, generalized dystonia begins with inversion and plantarflexion of the foot while walking. Occasionally, the prolonged muscle contractions can be relieved by tactile stimulation applied to or near the affected body part. Medications that affect acetylcholine (ACh), gamma-aminobutyric acid (GABA), and/or dopamine levels are effective in some cases. A very rare disorder, Segawa's dystonia, interferes with walking and may mimic the appearance of cerebral palsy; however, Segawa's dystonia progresses slowly and can be effectively treated with medications.

## Tourette's Disorder

Tourette's disorder causes vocal and motor tics. The tics are abrupt, repetitive, stereotyped movements including repeating

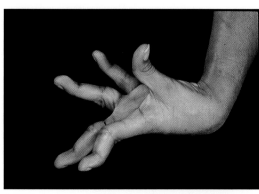

**A**

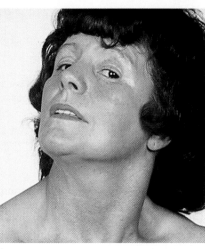

**B**

**Fig. 11-11 Focal dystonia. A,** Sustained involuntary muscle contraction of the hand. **B,** Spasmodic torticollis. Involuntary contraction of neck muscles causes abnormal head posture. *(Reproduced with permission from Perkin GD: Mosby's colour atlas and text of neurology, ed 2, Edinburgh, 2002, Mosby.)*

syllables, words, or phrases; coughing; clearing the throat; twitching; and eye blinking. Onset is during childhood. Many people with the disorder are aware of nearly irresistible sensory urges that precede tics. Stress, emotional excitement, and fatigue exacerbate tics. Tics can be temporarily voluntarily suppressed, but the urge to tic builds during suppression. Motor, limbic, and behavioral cortico-basal ganglia-thalamic circuits are implicated in Tourette's, as are abnormalities of dopamine and norepinephrine transmission.[70]

### Dyskinetic Cerebral Palsy

Abnormal involuntary movements are also observed in people with dyskinetic cerebral palsy (the other major types of cerebral palsy are spastic and ataxic; see Chapter 5). In dyskinetic cerebral palsy, muscle tone and posture are abnormal and involuntary movements occur. Dystonia (involuntary sustained muscle contractions) causes the abnormal posture. The involuntary movements are choreoathetosis; the term chorea indicates abrupt, jerky movements, and the term athetosis identifies slow, writhing, purposeless movements. Dyskinetic cerebral palsy is associated with lesions involving both the basal ganglia and the ventrolateral thalamus.[71]

## CEREBELLUM

The cerebellum coordinates movement and postural control by comparing actual motor output with the intended movement and then adjusting movement as necessary. Information regarding intended movements is delivered to the cerebellum by corticopontine fibers that synapse in the pontine nuclei. Axons from the pontine nuclei project to the cerebellum. The cerebellum also receives information regarding activity in spinal interneurons via internal feedback tracts (anterior spinocerebellar and rostrospinocerebellar tracts; see Chapter 6). Information about the actual movement is provided by information from muscle spindles, Golgi tendon organs, and cutaneous mechanoreceptors (posterior spinocerebellar and cuneocerebellar tracts; see Chapter 6). The cerebellum integrates information from these sources and adjusts the activity of upper motor neurons. The cerebellum is also involved in learning the timing and rhythm of movements and the synchronization of movements, and in learning to correct motor errors.[72,73]

Massive amounts of sensory information enter the cerebellum, and cerebellar output is vital for normal movement. However, severe damage to the cerebellum does not interfere with sensory perception or with muscle strength. Instead, coordination of movement and postural control are degraded.

### Anatomy of the Cerebellum

The outer layer of the cerebellum is gray matter, consisting of three cortical layers (Figure 11-12). The outer and inner layers contain interneurons (granule, Golgi, stellate, and basket cells), and the middle layer contains Purkinje cell bodies.

Deep to the cortex is white matter, and within the white matter are the cerebellar nuclei. Axons from the cerebellar nuclei project to vestibular, reticular, and red nuclei, and to the motor thalamus. Motor thalamus neurons project to motor areas of the cerebral cortex.

Purkinje cells are the output cells from the cerebellar cortex; their projections inhibit the cerebellar nuclei and the vestibular nuclei. Two types of afferents enter the cerebellar cortex: mossy

| **PATHOLOGY 11-3**   FOCAL HAND DYSTONIA | |
|---|---|
| Pathology | Basal ganglia dysfunction |
| Etiology | Genetic predisposition combined with highly repetitive movement patterns |
| Speed of onset | Chronic |
| Signs and symptoms | |
| Consciousness | Normal |
| Communication and memory | Normal |
| Sensory | Impaired proprioception and stereognosis; degradation of the somatic representation in somatosensory cortex |
| Autonomic | Normal |
| Motor | Involuntary, sustained muscle contractions |
| Region affected | Cerebrum: basal ganglia |
| Demographics | Average age at onset 45 years old; males and females affected equally |
| Incidence | Of hand dystonia: unknown. Focal dystonias including hand dystonia: 30 cases per 100,000 population per year.[63] Musician's dystonia affects approximately 1% of professional musicians and usually terminates their career.[66] |
| Prognosis | Normal life span |

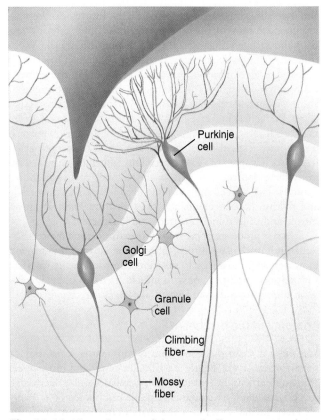

**Fig. 11-12 Three layers of the cerebellar cortex.** In the middle layer are cell bodies of Purkinje cells, the output neurons of the cerebellar cortex. Climbing and mossy fibers are the input fibers to the cerebellar cortex. Most climbing fibers arise from the inferior olivary nucleus. Mossy fibers originate in the spinal cord (spinocerebellar tracts) and in the brainstem.

fibers, from the spinal cord, reticular formation, vestibular system, and pontine nuclei; and climbing fibers, from the inferior olivary nucleus in the medulla. The mossy fibers convey somatosensory, arousal, equilibrium, and cerebral cortex motor information to the cerebellum. The climbing fibers convey information regarding movement errors to the cerebellum. Climbing fibers synapse with Purkinje dendrites. Mossy fibers synapse with interneurons that convey information to Purkinje cells.

Three lobes form the cerebellum (Figure 11-13):
- Anterior
- Posterior
- Flocculonodular

The anterior lobe is superior and is separated from the larger posterior lobe by the primary fissure. The inferior part of the posterior lobe is called the *cerebellar tonsil*. The cerebellar tonsils are clinically significant because increased intracranial pressure can force the tonsils into the foramen magnum, compressing vital brainstem structures that regulate breathing and cardiovascular activity. Tucked underneath the posterior lobe, touching the brainstem, is the small flocculonodular lobe.

Vertically, the cerebellum can be divided into sections (Figure 11-13, *E*):
- Midline vermis
- Paravermal hemisphere
- Lateral hemisphere

Each of the vertical sections is associated with a specific class of movements, as we will see later. Each vertical section projects to specific cerebellar nuclei or to vestibular nuclei. The cerebellar nuclei, from medial to lateral, are the fastigial, globose, emboliform, and dentate nuclei.

Fibers connecting the cerebellum with the brainstem form three cerebellar peduncles on each side of the brainstem. The superior cerebellar peduncle connects to the midbrain and contains most of the cerebellar efferent fibers. Fibers from the cerebral cortex synapse in the pons, and the information then

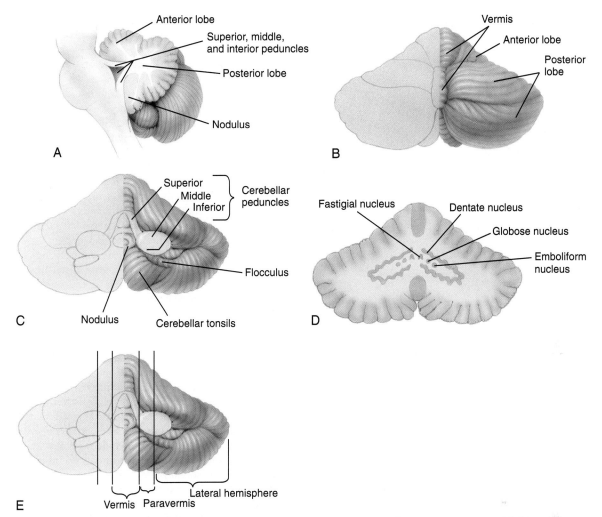

**Fig. 11-13 Anatomy of the cerebellum. A,** Midsagittal section showing cerebellar peduncles and lobes of the cerebellum. **B,** Posterior view of cerebellum. **C,** Anterior view of cerebellum with the brainstem removed. **D,** Coronal section of cerebellum, revealing the cerebellar nuclei. **E,** Vertical divisions of the cerebellum.

travels via axons in the middle peduncle into the cerebellum. The inferior peduncle brings afferent information from the brainstem and spinal cord into the cerebellum and sends efferents from the cerebellum to the vestibular nuclei and reticular nuclei in the brainstem.

### Clinical Pearl

Input to the cerebellum is received from the cerebral cortex (via pontine nuclei), the vestibular apparatus, vestibular and auditory nuclei, and the spinal cord, via high-fidelity pathways (proprioceptive information) and internal feedback tracts (information regarding activity in spinal interneurons and in descending motor tracts). The output of the cerebellum is provided via connections that influence vestibulospinal, reticulospinal, rubrospinal, corticobrainstem, and corticospinal tracts.

## Functional Regions of the Cerebellum

Human movements can be categorized into three broad classes:
* Equilibrium
* Gross movements of the limbs
* Fine, distal, voluntary movements

The cerebellum has specialized regions for controlling each of these classes of movement. The vestibulocerebellum, named for its reciprocal links with the vestibular system, regulates equilibrium. The spinocerebellum, named for its extensive connections with the spinal cord, coordinates gross limb movements. The cerebrocerebellum, named for its connections with the cerebral cortex, coordinates distal limb voluntary movements (Figure 11-14).

When a person reaches for a book from a high shelf, the vestibulocerebellum provides anticipatory contraction of lower limb and back muscles to prevent loss of balance. Otherwise, as the upper limb moves, altering the position of the body's center of mass, the person would fall forward. The upper limb reaching movement is coordinated by the spinocerebellum. Without the spinocerebellar contribution, the reach would be jerky and inaccurate. The cerebrocerebellum coordinates finger and thumb movements to grasp the book.

*Vestibulocerebellum* is the functional name for the flocculonodular lobe because this area receives information directly from vestibular receptors and connects reciprocally with the vestibular nuclei. The vestibulocerebellum also receives information from

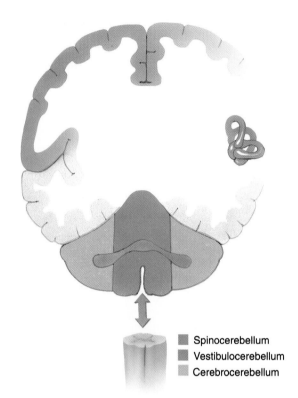

■ Spinocerebellum
■ Vestibulocerebellum
■ Cerebrocerebellum

**Fig. 11-14 Conceptual diagram of the three functional divisions of the cerebellum and their connections.** The purple part of the cerebellum is the flocculonodular lobe, the location of the vestibulocerebellum. The purple structure with three rings *(on the right side)* is the vestibular apparatus, the sensory organ that detects head position relative to gravity and detects movement of the head. Much of the information processed by the vestibulocerebellum is from the vestibular apparatus. The blue part of the cerebellum is the spinocerebellum, and correspondingly the spinal cord is also blue. The green part of the cerebellum is the cerebrocerebellum, and correspondingly the cerebral cortex is also green.

visual areas of the brain. Via connections with vestibular nuclei, the vestibulocerebellum influences eye movements and postural muscles.

*Spinocerebellum* is the functional name for the vermis and the paravermal region because of extensive connections with the spinal cord. Somatosensory information, internal feedback from spinal interneurons, and sensorimotor cortex information converge in the spinocerebellum. This information is used to control ongoing movement via brainstem descending tracts.

The vermal section of the spinocerebellum adjusts activity in the medial upper motor neurons by direct action on brainstem nuclei and indirectly on the cerebral cortex via the motor thalamus. The paravermal area influences the lateral upper motor neurons by action on brainstem nuclei and by projecting to the cerebral cortex via the motor thalamus.

The lateral cerebellar hemispheres connect indirectly with areas of the cerebral cortex that control distal limb muscles; thus this section of the cerebellum is the *cerebrocerebellum*. Input to the cerebrocerebellum is received from cerebral cortex (somatosensory and motor areas) fibers that synapse with neurons in the pons. Axons of the pontine neurons project to the cerebrocerebellum. Efferents from the lateral cerebellar hemispheres project to the dentate nucleus. The dentate is involved in motor planning. Before voluntary movements, alterations in dentate neural activity precede changes in activity in motor areas of the cerebral cortex. Efferents from the dentate nucleus project to the motor thalamus, then efferents from the motor thalamus project to the cerebral cortex. Functions of the cerebrocerebellum and dentate include the following:

• Coordination of voluntary movements via influence on corticospinal, corticobrainstem, and rubrospinal tracts
• Planning of movements
• Timing[74]

The connections of functional divisions of the cerebellum are listed in Table 11-5 and are illustrated in Figures 11-15 and 11-16.

**TABLE 11-5    NEURAL CONNECTIONS OF THE CEREBELLAR FUNCTIONAL DIVISIONS**

| Functional Division (Anatomic Location) | Receives Input From: | Sends Output to: | Output Reaches Lower Motor Neurons Via |
|---|---|---|---|
| Vestibulocerebellum (flocculonodular lobe) | Vestibular apparatus Vestibular nuclei | Vestibular nuclei | Vestibulospinal tracts and tracts that coordinate eye and head movements (see Chapter 15) |
| Spinocerebellum | | | |
| • Vermal section | Spinal cord (from trunk) Vestibular nuclei Auditory and vestibular information (via brainstem nuclei) | Vestibular nuclei Reticular nuclei Motor cortex (via thalamus) | Vestibulospinal tracts Reticulospinal tracts Medial corticospinal tract |
| • Paravermal section | Spinal cord (from limbs) | Red nucleus Motor cortex (via thalamus) | Rubrospinal tract Lateral corticospinal tract |
| Cerebrocerebellum (lateral cerebellar hemispheres) | Cerebral cortex (via pontine nuclei) | Motor and premotor cortices (via dentate nucleus and motor thalamus) Red nucleus | Lateral corticospinal and corticobrainstem tracts Rubrospinal tract |

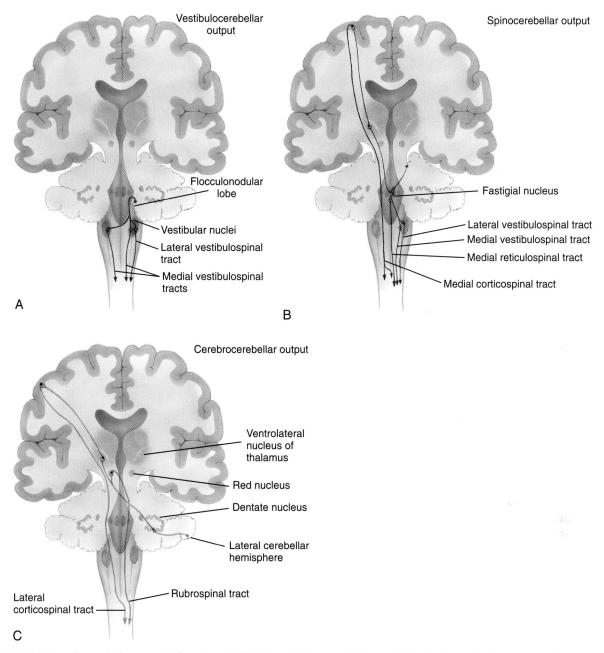

**Fig. 11-15 The efferents from each functional division of the cerebellum. A,** Vestibulocerebellar output. For simplicity, the tracts that transmit signals for eye and head movements are omitted. **B,** Spinocerebellar output. The connections with the red nucleus and the rubrospinal tract are omitted for simplicity. The red nucleus and the rubrospinal tract are illustrated in part **C. C,** Cerebrocerebellar output. The corticobrainstem tracts are omitted for simplicity.

## Cerebellar Clinical Disorders

Unilateral lesions of the cerebellum affect the same side of the body. The cerebellar signs are ipsilateral because cerebellar efferents to the medial descending tracts remain ipsilateral, and because cerebellar efferents project to the contralateral cerebral cortex and red nucleus, whose descending tracts cross the midline (see Figure 11-15).

*Ataxia* is the movement disorder common to all lesions of the cerebellum. Ataxia describes uncoordinated voluntary movements: the movements are normal-strength, jerky, inaccurate, and not caused by spasticity or contracture. Vermal and flocculonodular lobe cerebellar lesions result in truncal ataxia, paravermal lesions result in gait and limb ataxia, and lateral cerebellar lesions cause hand ataxia. Consequences of lesions in each of the functional regions of the cerebellum follow.

Lesions involving the vestibulocerebellum cause *nystagmus* (abnormal eye movements; see Chapter 16), dysequilibrium, and difficulty maintaining sitting and standing balance (truncal ataxia). Paravermal and cerebrocerebellar lesions result in

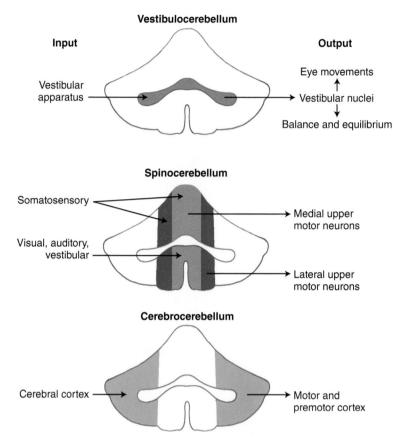

**Fig. 11-16** The inputs and outputs of the three functional divisions of the cerebellum.

*dysarthria*—slurred, poorly articulated speech.[75] Dysfunction of the spinocerebellum results in ataxic gait—a wide-based, unsteady, staggering, veering gait. In *chronic alcoholism,* the anterior lobe section of the spinocerebellum is often damaged because of malnutrition, resulting in the characteristic ataxic gait.

Spinocerebellar lesions result in limb ataxia, with the following manifestations:

- *Dysdiadochokinesia:* inability to rapidly alternate movements (e.g., inability to rapidly pronate and supinate the forearm, inability to rapidly alternate toe tapping)
- *Dysmetria:* inability to accurately move an intended distance
- *Action tremor:* shaking of the limb during voluntary movement

Action tremor may arise because onset and offset of muscle activity are delayed. Thus, in a rapid movement, the agonist burst is prolonged, and onset of braking by the antagonist is delayed, causing overshoot of the target. As correction of the movement is attempted, the same dysfunctions lead to repeated overshoot.[76] People with cerebellar lesions often compensate for limb ataxia by using movement decomposition. This decomposition consists of maintaining a fixed position of one joint while another joint is moving. For example, when ascending a 30 degree incline, people with cerebellar lesions tend to maintain the ankle joint in a fixed position during early stance phase. In contrast, people with intact neuromuscular control extend the knee and flex the ankle simultaneously during early stance phase (Figure 11-17).

Cerebrocerebellar lesions interfere with coordination of fine finger movements. This ataxia affects the ability to play musical instruments, fasten buttons, and type on a keyboard.

A 39-year-old patient of mine sustained a stroke that partially deprived the cerebellum of blood supply. The first 2 days post stroke, he was so severely ataxic that he was unable to sit on a firm surface without back and arm support. He required assistance eating, grooming, and dressing because jerky uncoordinated movements of his arm prevented him from being able to bring food to his mouth, use a comb or razor, wash, or dress. Five days post stroke he was able to walk with two people maximally assisting him for balance. His gait was wide based, irregular, and stumbling. At discharge from the hospital, 3 weeks later, he was fully independent, and his gait was near normal. This nearly complete recovery is common among people who have ischemic cerebellar stroke.[77]

## Differentiating Cerebellar From Somatosensory Ataxia

Not all ataxia is caused by cerebellar lesions. Interference with the transmission of somatosensory information to the cerebellum, by lesions of the spinocerebellar tracts or by peripheral neuropathy, may also produce ataxia. Ataxia in the lower limbs may be caused by sensory deficits or by paravermal cerebellar lesions. To differentiate between the two possibilities, use the Romberg test[78] and test proprioception, vibration sense, and ankle reflexes. The Romberg tests the ability to use proprioceptive information for standing balance. The

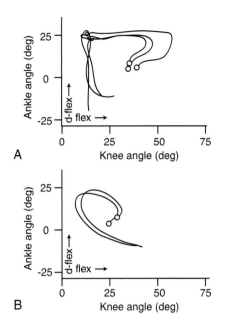

**Fig. 11-17 Movement decomposition.** Plots of ankle angle versus knee angle during stance while walking up a 30 degree incline. Heel strike is indicated by a circle and is the starting point of the plot. **A,** Subject with a superior cerebellar artery infarct demonstrating movement decomposition. The horizontal line indicates that the ankle angle is maintained at approximately 25 degrees dorsiflexion as the knee extends from 60 degrees flexion to 15 degrees. The vertical line indicates that the knee angle remains fixed at 15 degrees, and the ankle plantarflexes from 25 to −25 degrees. **B,** Normal movement composition. In a subject with normal neuromuscular control, ankle and knee joints move simultaneously. During early stance, the knee extends while the ankle dorsiflexes; then during late stance, the knee flexes while the ankle plantarflexes. *(Modified with permission from Earhart GM, Bastian AJ: Selection and coordination of human locomotor forms following cerebellar damage.* J Neurophysiol *85:759–769, 2001.)*

Romberg test criteria and interpretation are discussed in Table 11-7 at the end of the chapter.

## MOTOR CONTROL DISORDERS

Characteristics of the major types of motor control disorders are compared in Table 11-6.

## MOVEMENT

### Summary of Normal Motor Control

For normal movement, the motor planning areas, control circuits, and descending tracts must act in concert with sensory information to provide instructions to lower motor neurons.

The basal ganglia receive most of their input from the cerebral cortex, and their influence on movement is provided via the cerebral cortex, PPN, and reticular formation. In contrast, the cerebellum receives copious information from the spinal cord, vestibular system, and brainstem. The cerebellum influences movement via motor areas of the cerebral cortex and extensive connections with upper motor neurons that arise in the brainstem. Only lower motor neurons deliver signals from the central nervous system to the skeletal muscles that generate movement. Figures 11-18 and 11-19 summarize the complex neural activity required to generate movement.

### Three Fundamental Types of Movements

Movements can be classified into three types:
- Postural
- Ambulatory
- Reaching/grasping

Posture is controlled primarily by brainstem mechanisms, ambulation by brainstem and spinal regions, and reaching/grasping by the cerebral cortex; however, all regions of the nervous system contribute to each type of movement.

The contributions of each region of the central nervous system to an externally imposed movement can be assessed by surface electromyography (EMG) (Figure 11-20). Electrodes on the skin record the electrical activity produced by underlying skeletal muscles. For example, a subject is asked to support a light weight and to maintain a constant position of the elbow (flexion at 90 degrees). Then additional weight is added unexpectedly, resulting in displacement of the forearm and the hand downward. After about one tenth of a second, biceps contraction begins to restore the elbow angle to 90 degrees. The EMG response to displacement shows three distinct increases in activity occurring at 30 milliseconds, 50 to 80 milliseconds, and 80 to 120 milliseconds after the imposed biceps stretch.

The shortest latency response, M1, is the monosynaptic stretch reflex; this reflex does not generate enough force to restore the elbow position. The second response, M2, is the long loop response; this response generates enough force to begin to move the hand upward. The subject's intentions influence M2: if instructions to the subject are to "let go" when the extra weight is added, the M2 response is attenuated or disappears. The final response, which is voluntary, completes return of the elbow angle to 90 degrees. Latencies provide clues to the central nervous system region involved in each response. The 30 millisecond latency of M1 is just enough time for the afferent conduction, transmission across one synapse in the spinal cord, and efferent conduction to activate the biceps. Fifty to eighty milliseconds allows enough time for transmission involving brainstem connections. The 120 millisecond response requires synapses in the cerebral cortex.

### Postural Control

Postural control provides orientation and balance (equilibrium). Orientation is the adjustment of the body and head to vertical, and balance is the ability to maintain the center of mass relative to the base of support. Postural control is achieved by central commands to lower motor neurons; the central output

**TABLE 11-6    CHARACTERISTICS OF MAJOR TYPES OF MOTOR CONTROL DISORDERS**

| Characteristic | Complete Severance of Peripheral Nerve (Lower Motor Neuron Lesions) | Upper Motor Neuron Lesions | Parkinson's Disease | Huntington's Disease | Cerebellar Lesions |
|---|---|---|---|---|---|
| Muscle strength | Absent (paralysis) | Decreased (paresis) | Normal | Normal | Normal |
| Muscle bulk | Severe atrophy | Variable atrophy | Normal | Normal | Normal |
| Involuntary muscle contraction | Fibrillations | Fibrillations | Resting tremor | Chorea | None |
| Muscle tone* | Decreased | In spinal cord injury or spastic cerebral palsy: velocity-dependent increase (spasticity and myoplasticity) | Velocity-independent increase (rigidity) | Variable | Normal |
| Movement speed and efficiency | Absent | Decreased | Decreased | Abnormal | Ataxic |
| Postural control | Normal | Decreased or normal, depending on location of lesion | Excessive | Abnormal | Depends on location of lesion |

*Muscle tone ratings are compared with muscle tone ratings in an alert person. Thus, muscle tone in a person with a complete peripheral nerve lesion would be similar to muscle tone in a completely relaxed person with an intact nervous system because titin would be the primary source of resistance to stretch in both cases.

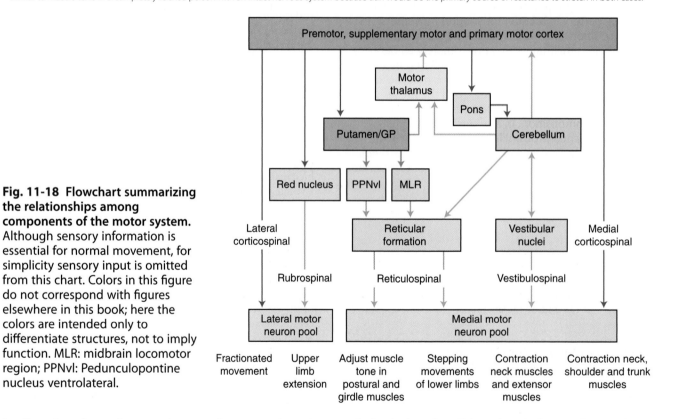

**Fig. 11-18 Flowchart summarizing the relationships among components of the motor system.** Although sensory information is essential for normal movement, for simplicity sensory input is omitted from this chart. Colors in this figure do not correspond with figures elsewhere in this book; here the colors are intended only to differentiate structures, not to imply function. MLR: midbrain locomotor region; PPNvl: Pedunculopontine nucleus ventrolateral.

is adjusted to the environmental context by sensory input.* Central commands are mediated by the reticulospinal, vestibulospinal, and medial corticospinal tracts. Sensory input is used in both feedback and feedforward mechanisms. Feedback is information about the state of the system. For example, if I slip while walking on ice, I get feedback from proprioceptors, vestibular receptors, and vision that elicits equilibrium adjustments. Feedforward consists of anticipatory motor impulses that prepare the body for movement. Feedforward control involves prediction and anticipation to prepare for upcoming hazards to stability. Before I lift my arms forward, I

*Historical note: An earlier theory of postural control posited three separate control mechanisms: reflexive, reactive, and voluntary. The theory proposed that during development, reflexes and reactions were inhibited by the voluntary system; in the mature nervous system, the voluntary system controlled all normal movements. However, as noted in the text, reflexes and reactions help to restore stability before the voluntary system is aware of possible loss of balance and participate extensively in mature motor control.

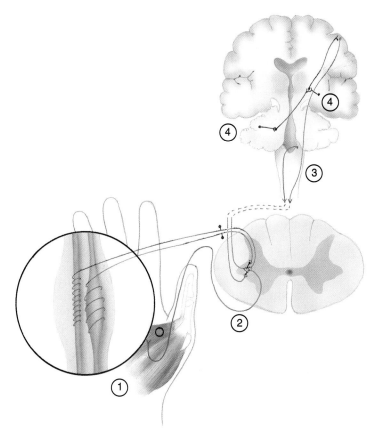

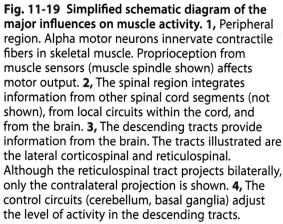

**Fig. 11-19 Simplified schematic diagram of the major influences on muscle activity. 1,** Peripheral region. Alpha motor neurons innervate contractile fibers in skeletal muscle. Proprioception from muscle sensors (muscle spindle shown) affects motor output. **2,** The spinal region integrates information from other spinal cord segments (not shown), from local circuits within the cord, and from the brain. **3,** The descending tracts provide information from the brain. The tracts illustrated are the lateral corticospinal and reticulospinal. Although the reticulospinal tract projects bilaterally, only the contralateral projection is shown. **4,** The control circuits (cerebellum, basal ganglia) adjust the level of activity in the descending tracts.

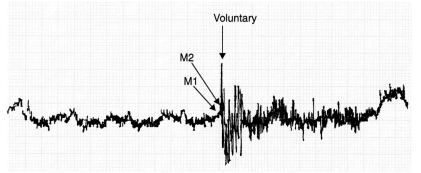

**Fig. 11-20** Surface electromyographic (EMG) responses to displacement when the subject is instructed to maintain 90 degrees of elbow flexion; then a weight is placed in the subject's hand. The first response, called M1, occurs 25 to 30 msec after the weight is added. M1 is the EMG activity produced by the monosynaptic stretch reflex. The second response, called M2, or the long latency response, occurs 50 to 80 msec after the weight is added. Production of M2 requires brainstem connections. The third response, the voluntary response, occurs 80 to 120 msec after the weight is added.

contract my gastrocnemii to prevent the change in center of gravity from causing me to lose my balance.

To orient in the world, we use three senses:
- Somatosensation
- Vision
- Vestibular

Somatosensation provides information about weight bearing and the relative positions of body parts. Vision provides information about movement and cues for judging upright. Vestibular input from receptors in the inner ear informs us about head position relative to gravity and about head movement. Visual and somatosensory information can predict destabilization; all three sensations can be used to shape the motor reaction to instability (Figure 11-21).

Head position in reference to gravity, to the neck, and to the visual world affects muscular activation. Head position in space is signaled by neck proprioception and vestibular and visual information (visual aspects will be covered in Chapter 16). In normal infants and in children and adults with extensive cerebral lesions, neck and vestibular reflexes can be elicited by neck movements or by head position changes. In children and adults with intact nervous systems, the same stimuli do not produce obvious responses.

Activity of cervical joint receptors and neck muscle stretch receptors elicits neck reflexes. The *asymmetric tonic neck reflex* is elicited by head rotation to the right or left; limbs on the nose side extend, and limbs on the skull side flex (Figure 11-22, *A*). The *symmetric tonic neck reflex* results in flexion of the upper

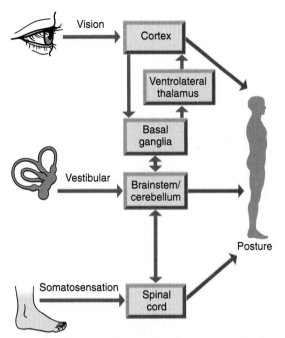

**Fig. 11-21** Sensory influences on postural control.

limbs and extension of the lower limbs when the neck is flexed and the opposite pattern in the limbs when the neck is extended (Figure 11-22, *B*).

When the head is tilted, information from vestibular gravity receptors is used to right the head by contraction of neck muscles. Vestibular gravity receptors also influence limb muscle activity in a manner opposite to the neck reflexes; for instance, tilting the head back causes flexion of the upper limbs and extension of the lower limbs if the position of the head relative to the neck is unchanged (eliminating the influence of neck reflexes). Because vestibular receptors for gravity are in the labyrinthine part of the inner ear, the reflex is called the *tonic labyrinthine reflex* (Figure 11-22, *C*). Because vestibular and neck reflexes oppose each other, and normally head and neck movements occur together, the reflexes usually counteract each other. By canceling out these two reflexes, our limbs are not compelled to move when we turn or nod or shake our heads.

During stance, we sway continuously; to prevent falling, the postural control system makes adjustments to maintain upright posture. Sometimes inappropriate sensory information is selected, as when we rely on visual information regarding movement and a large object nearby moves. A person standing next to a bus that unexpectedly moves can misinterpret the moving visual information and make inappropriate postural adjustments to compensate for the illusory movement. The person's goal is to maintain upright posture, but reacting to deceptive sensory information leads to instability.

Posturography can be used to determine sensory organization (which sensory stimuli a person relies on preferentially) and muscle coordination (how postural adjustments are coordinated). The subject stands on a force platform, and surface EMGs are recorded from specific muscles. As indicated in Figure 11-23, six sensory conditions can be tested.[79] In the sensory conflict conditions, vision and/or proprioception is rendered inaccurate by having the visual field and/or the support surface move with the subject as the subject sways. Thus subjects have the visual and/or proprioceptive illusion that they are not swaying when in fact they are moving; under these conditions, a person without vestibular function will fall. Results of posturography can be compared with norms for different diagnostic groups. For example, the postural responses of an individual can be compared with those of people with Parkinson's disease and other disorders.

Posturography can also test motor coordination. If the platform moves forward, the subject sways backward; the normal response is contraction of the tibialis anterior, then quadriceps, then abdominal muscles to return the subject to upright (Figure 11-24). If the platform moves backward, the gastrocnemius, then hamstrings, then back muscles contract to restore the person to upright. In both cases, distal-to-proximal muscle activation normally occurs.

When the platform moves backward, the subject's forward lean stretches the gastrocnemius muscle. An equivalent stretch of the gastrocnemius can be provided by dorsiflexing the subject's ankles by tilting the platform so that the anterior edge of the platform is higher than the posterior edge. However, in the platform tilt situation, contracting the gastrocnemius further destabilizes the subject. Because the subject's ankles are dorsiflexed, contracting the gastrocnemius pushes the person posteriorly. After a few trials, healthy subjects learn to reduce the response of the gastrocnemius, thus preserving their balance.

People with intact nervous systems respond to movement of the supporting platform differently depending on instructions.[81] If asked to maintain stance when the platform moves, the first response is to sway forward or backward. If asked to step when the platform moves, the first response is to weight shift laterally. This ability to switch motor response to identical stimuli demonstrates the importance of both instructions and the subject's intentions in sculpting motor output.

Although sophisticated, moving platform posturography is similar to the clinical practice of pushing a person off balance to test the equilibrium response. Both tests assess the ability to respond to externally imposed displacements; in daily life, these displacements are uncommon. The continual challenge in everyday posture is to anticipate and adjust for voluntary destabilization. For example, before a forward reach when a person is standing, the muscles of the opposite leg and back contract to provide stability before the deltoid contracts.[80] If a standing person decides to walk, anticipatory adjustments must prepare for movement of the center of mass. Posturography can also be used to assess these active conditions. A complete postural evaluation includes sensory and motor assessment under three conditions: imposed displacement, active reaching, and ambulation.

Certain nervous system dysfunctions produce recognizable postural abnormalities. People with Parkinson's disease have muscle rigidity and reduced central control. This combination of deficits results in flexed posture, lack of protective reactions, and weak anticipatory postural adjustments. The postural effects of cerebellar lesions depend on the cerebellar region involved. As noted earlier, cerebrocerebellar lesions have little effect on posture, spinocerebellar lesions result in gait and stance ataxia, and vestibulocerebellar lesions result in truncal ataxia. The sequence of muscle activation is normal in people with spinocerebellar lesions, but the duration and amplitude of

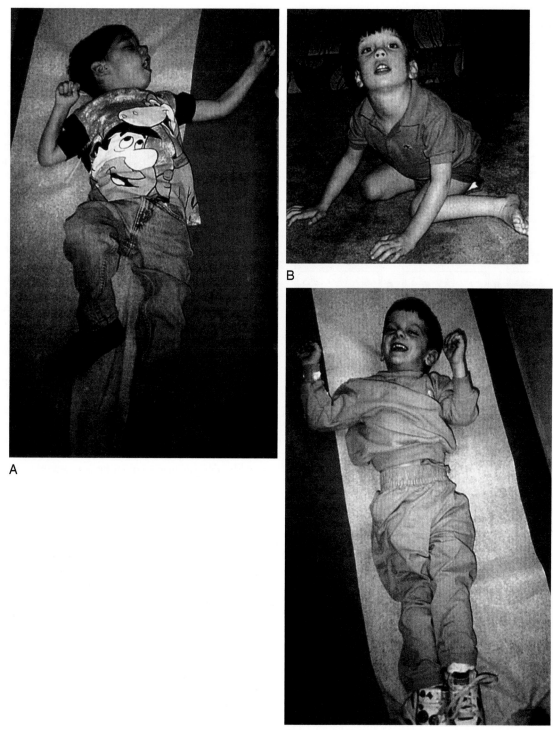

**Fig. 11-22 Neck and vestibular reflexes. A,** Asymmetric tonic neck reflex: when the head is rotated right or left, the limbs move into the fencer's position. **B,** Symmetric tonic neck reflex: when the neck is extended, the upper limbs extend and the lower limbs flex. **C,** Tonic labyrinthine reflex: when the head is tilted back, upper limbs flex and lower limbs extend. These reflexes may be elicited with head and neck movements in infants with intact neuromuscular systems. The reflexes are obligatory only in people with cerebral damage. *(Reproduced with permission from Braddom RL: Physical medicine and rehabilitation, ed 2, Philadelphia, 2001, Saunders.)*

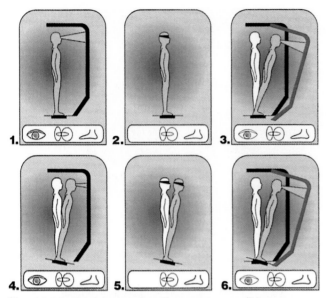

**Fig. 11-23 Posturography.** Six sensory conditions are used to evaluate the relative contributions of vision, vestibular, and somatosensory input to balance function. The icons at the bottom of each figure indicate the eyes, vestibular system, and foot and ankle proprioceptors. If the eye icon is red, this indicates that the visual surround sways with the person's postural sway. In conditions 3 and 6, if the person sways forward, movement of the visual field matches the person's sway; this creates the visual illusion of lack of movement. If the foot icon is red, this indicates that the support surface moves with the person's postural sway, providing inaccurate information about orientation. In conditions 4 through 6, if the person sways forward, the support surface under the toes tilts downward, so proprioception from the distal lower limbs does not give accurate orientation information. *(Courtesy Neurocom International Inc., Clackamas, Ore.)*

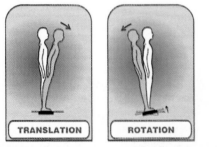

**Fig. 11-24** The gastrocnemius can be passively stretched by moving the support surface backward (translation) or by tilting the support surface to raise the toes (rotation). Illustration shows the body position at the end of platform movement in gray and the return to upright in white. If the support surface moves backward, the long latency stretch reflex helps return the body to upright. If platform rotation causes ankle dorsiflexion, the long latency stretch reflex will plantarflex the ankle, resulting in loss of balance backward. With repeated trials, the long latency reflex decreases as the nervous system learns to maintain posture efficiently when the platform tilts.

*(Courtesy Neurocom International Inc., Clackamas, Ore.)*

postural adjustments are larger than normal, and anticipatory adjustments for predictable conditions are lacking.

### Ambulation

All regions of the nervous system are required for normal human ambulation. The cerebral cortex provides goal orientation and control of ankle movements, the basal ganglia govern generation of force, and the cerebellum provides timing, coordination, and error correction. Brainstem descending tracts (reticulospinal) adjust the strength of muscle contractions by two mechanisms: direct connections with lower motor neurons and adjusted transmission in spinal reflex pathways. In the spinal cord, stepping pattern generators are neural networks that control the pattern of lower limb muscle activation during walking or running (see Chapter 13). Sensory information is used to adapt motor output appropriately for environmental conditions.

During normal gait initiation, the swing limb first pushes downward and backward against the support surface. This pattern of force results in movement of the center of mass forward and onto the stance leg in preparation for foot-off and increases the magnitude of the subsequent movement. However, if an adult with hemiplegia initiates gait using the nonimpaired limb as the swing limb, the preparatory movement center of mass does not occur, interfering with gait initiation.[82] If the same adult initiates gait using the paretic limb, the initial movement of the center of mass is nearly normal.[82] People with Parkinson's disease also fail to adequately move the center of mass before attempting stepping,[83] leading to inability to initiate gait.

Although gait may seem automatic, attention is required.[84] The attention required is determined by studying gait with dual tasks, that is, by carrying out an additional task while walking. A commonly used clinical test is to ask the person to walk while serially subtracting sevens from 100. Adults without neurologic deficits often show decreased gait speed when performing dual tasks. Dual tasks cause additional decrements in walking in people with neurologic disorders. People with Alzheimer's disease, traumatic brain injury, Parkinson's disease, and idiopathic falling all demonstrate slower gait speed, shorter step length, increased double support time, and increased gait variability during dual tasks.[84]

### Reaching and Grasping

Vision and somatosensation are essential for normal reaching and grasping. Vision provides information for locating the object in space, as well as for assessing the shape and size of the object. Preparation for movement (feedforward) is the primary role of visual information; if the movement is inaccurate, vision also guides corrections (feedback). The stream of visual information used for movement ("action stream"[85]) flows from the visual cortex to the posterior parietal cortex (Figure 11-25). The posterior parietal cortex contains neurons associated with both sensation and movement; these neurons project to premotor cortical areas that control reaching, grasping, and eye movements. The premotor cortical areas for each action are somewhat distinct, with the result that reaching, grasping, and eye movements are controlled separately but coordinated by connections among the areas. Information from sensory and

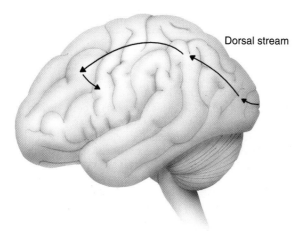

**Fig. 11-25** Visual action stream. Visual information traveling from occipital to parietal to premotor cortex helps control movement.

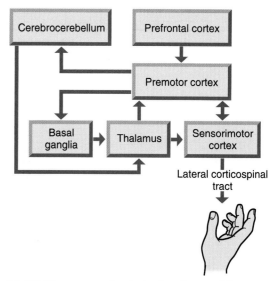

**Fig. 11-26** The motor circuit for fractionated finger movements.

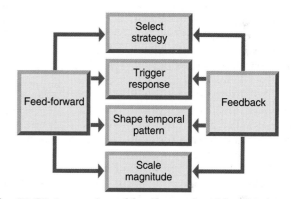

**Fig. 11-27** Interaction of feedforward and feedback in determining movements. *(Modified with permission from Horak FB: Somatosensory experience in adapting postural coordination. Presented at Sensory Mechanisms in Motor Coordination: Implications for Motor Control and Rehabilitation Symposium, Society for Neuroscience, November 13, 1994.)*

planning areas of the cerebral cortex projects to the basal ganglia and cerebellum, then via the thalamus to the sensorimotor cortex, the origin of the corticospinal tract. Proprioception is used similarly to vision, to prepare for movement and to provide information regarding movement errors. Proprioceptive and cutaneous information also triggers changes in movement, as when contact with an object triggers the fingers to close around the object.

Before one can reach accurately, visual grasp (fixing the object in central vision) and proprioceptive information about upper limb position are required. This information allows successful prediction of task dynamics and control for the first phase of reaching: fast approach to the object, which is primarily a feedforward process. The second phase of reaching is homing in—a slower, corrective adjustment to achieve contact with the target. Visual guidance (feedback) is necessary for homing in.[86] In contrast to classic concepts of proximal-to-distal muscle activation during reaching, proximal muscles move the hand toward the target; the muscles are controlled by the medial upper motor neurons. Simultaneously, distal muscles orient and preshape the hand for grasp; these actions are controlled primarily by feedforward mechanisms via the lateral upper motor neurons. If fractionated movements are used, as in picking up a coin with the index finger and thumb, neural activity that begins in the prefrontal cortex eventually activates the lateral corticospinal tract (Figure 11-26).

Grasping is coordinated with activity of the eyes, head, proximal upper limb, and trunk; orientation and postural preparation are integral to the movement. When the object is contacted, grip force adjusts quickly, indicating feedforward control. After the object is grasped, somatosensory information corrects any error in grip force. Somatosensory information is also used to trigger shifts in movement, for example, to switch from touch to grasp or from grasp to lift.[87]

During development, normal infants grasp objects before they can control their posture, and the ability of infants to manipulate objects in their hands does not depend on proximal control.[88] In fact, early manual activity may be important in developing normal proximal control.[89]

Adults with parietal lobe damage have abnormal timing of reaching and grasp, lack anticipatory adjustments of the fingers, and use a palmar, rather than pincer, grasp.[90] Pincer grasp requires corticospinal control. The lack of proprioceptive input to the corticospinal tract explains why adults with parietal lobe damage use a palmar grasp. Infants use the palmar grasp before myelination of the corticospinal tracts is complete.

In normal actions, feedforward and feedback interact to create movement. Preparation for movement (feedforward) is based on prediction, and movement is adjusted according to the resulting sensory information (feedback) (Figure 11-27). The source of the signal to initiate movements is unknown.

## Testing the Motor System

An evaluation of the motor system assesses strength, muscle bulk, muscle tone, reflexes, movement efficiency and speed, postural control, and abnormal movements (Table 11-7).

**TABLE 11-7    EVALUATION OF THE MOTOR SYSTEM**

| | Test | Procedure and Interpretation |
|---|---|---|
| Strength | Quick screening | Resist abduction, adduction, flexion, and extension at the shoulder, elbow, fingers, hip, and ankle. Resist flexion and extension at the elbow and knee. Paresis or paralysis usually indicates a lower or upper motor neuron lesion. |
| | Manual muscle test | Position patient appropriately; see Kendall and colleagues (2005)[91] or Hislop and Montgomery (2002)[92]; apply manual resistance to patient's movement. |
| | Pronator drift | Patient flexes both shoulders 90 degrees, extends elbows, fully supinates both forearms, and closes eyes. Inability to maintain this position for 30 seconds, with gradual pronation and downward drift of one arm, indicates an upper motor neuron lesion. |
| | Muscle bulk | Visually inspect for disparity in muscle size. Measure the circumference of the limbs if a difference is suspected. More severe atrophy typically indicates a lower motor neuron lesion. Less severe atrophy indicates an upper motor neuron lesion or disuse. |
| Muscle resistance to stretch | Passive ROM | Passively flex and extend patient's elbow, wrist, knee, ankle, and neck; note resistance to movement. Less resistance than normal may indicate a lower motor neuron lesion. Excessive resistance to stretch may be a sign of upper motor neuron or basal ganglia lesion. Velocity-dependent resistance to stretch indicates an upper motor neuron lesion. Excessive resistance that does not vary with the speed of the stretch, *rigidity,* is characteristic of Parkinson's disease, Parkinson-Plus syndromes, and parkinsonism. Muscle guarding or contracture may also cause decreased passive ROM. |
| Reflexes | Phasic stretch reflex (also called deep tendon reflex, muscle stretch reflex, and tendon jerk) | Use a reflex hammer to tap the tendon of a relaxed muscle; muscle should contract. Indicates whether the reflex loop (spindle, afferents, spinal segment, efferent, and muscle) is functioning. Biceps, triceps, quadriceps, and triceps surae tendons are most commonly tested. The response of each muscle is compared with the response of the same muscle on the other side of the body. Asymmetric hyperreflexia may indicate an upper motor neuron lesion. Asymmetric hyporeflexia (or absence of reflex) indicates a peripheral or spinal region lesion. Sometimes no reflexes can be elicited even in people with intact nervous systems. The presence of more than four beats of clonus is always an abnormal sign. |
| | Babinski's sign | Extend the patient's knee, then firmly stroke the outer edge of the patient's foot with the handle of a reflex hammer. Babinski's sign is present if the great toe extends; other toes may spread apart. Babinski's sign indicates an upper motor neuron lesion. The response is normal if no response occurs or all toes curl. |
| | H-reflex* | Electrically stimulates skin over large fiber afferents; a reflexive contraction of muscle should occur. Indicates excitability of alpha motor neurons. |
| Movement efficiency and speed | Rapid alternating movements | Patient taps both index fingers or both feet, then pronates and supinates forearms; note speed, smoothness, symmetry, and rhythm of movements. If patient has difficulty with these movements in the absence of weakness, cerebellar or proprioceptive dysfunction is indicated. |
| | Accuracy and smoothness of movement | Patient performs the following movements several times: <br>(1) Finger-to-nose test—patient laterally abducts the arm with the elbow extended, then touches own nose; 2–3 repetitions with eyes open then 2–3 attempts with eyes closed. <br>(2) Finger-to-finger test—patient abducts the arm with the elbow extended, then touches examiner's fingertip; 2–3 repetitions with eyes open then 2–3 attempts with eyes closed. <br>(3) Heel-to-shin test—patient places heel on knee of opposite leg and slides the heel down the shin to the ankle while maintaining contact with the tibial crest; 2–3 repetitions with eyes open then 2–3 attempts with eyes closed. <br>(4) Walking heel-to-toe with eyes open and with eyes closed. <br>Normal performance: all movements are smooth and precise. For example, the patient slows the finger movements as the finger approaches the target and stops the movement accurately. Observe for jerky movements (ataxia), tremor worsening with movement (action tremor), and inability to move the precise distance required (dysmetria). Difficulty indicates cerebellar or proprioceptive dysfunction. |
| | Transcranial magnetic stimulation* | Currently experimental, not used clinically. Investigates possible upper motor neuron lesions by inducing magnetic activation of cortical neurons; the effect on movement is observed. |

**TABLE 11-7   EVALUATION OF THE MOTOR SYSTEM—cont'd**

| | Test | Procedure and Interpretation |
|---|---|---|
| Surface EMG to test neural activation of muscle | During active movement<br>• Hyperreflexia | Increase in EMG activity during passive muscle lengthening (lengthening occurs due to active contraction of antagonist muscles) indicates hyperreflexia. |
| | • Cocontraction | Measure the amount of time antagonist muscles are contracting simultaneously. Cocontraction is abnormal only if it interferes with movement goals. |
| | During passive muscle stretch | If EMG does not increase during stretch despite limitation in ROM, restriction is due to non-neural factors (i.e., intrinsic changes in the muscle). If EMG increases, neural factors are contributing to decreased ROM. |
| Postural control | Romberg test | Patient stands with arms folded across chest, feet together. Time how long patient can maintain balance with eyes open (maximum of 30 seconds), then with eyes closed (maximum of 30 seconds). The Romberg is scored pass/fail; criteria for failure include moving the arms or feet to maintain balance, opening the eyes during the eyes closed section, beginning to fall, and requiring assistance. If patient has difficulty maintaining balance with eyes open and eyes closed, a cerebellar problem is indicated; vibratory sense, proprioception, and ankle reflexes are normal in cerebellar ataxia. A proprioceptive problem (sensory ataxia) exists if the person is able to maintain balance with eyes open for 30 seconds but balance is impaired when eyes are closed. Sensory ataxia is confirmed by impaired conscious proprioception and vibratory sense and diminished or absent ankle reflexes. |
| | Sharpened Romberg | Same as Romberg test, but with one foot in front of the other foot. Stop test if time exceeds 1 minute. Interpretation is the same as for Romberg test. |
| | Tinetti balance scale[93] | Balance in sitting, standing, moving from sit to stand and stand to sit, and turning 360 degrees, and in response to push on sternum is assessed. Score is used to predict likelihood of falls. |
| | Clinical test for sensory interaction in balance | Three visual conditions—eyes opened, eyes closed, and vision altered by a dome covering the face—are combined with standing on firm surface or on foam. See Shumway-Cook and Horak (1986)[94] for interpretation. |
| | Functional reach | Patient stands with feet together, shoulders flexed 90 degrees, then patient reaches as far forward as possible.[95] Distance reached is recorded. Score is used to predict likelihood of falls. |
| | Computerized balance testing | Stationary posturography: patient stands on force platform; variations in force exerted are recorded. May incorporate EMG recording and different sensory conditions (see text). May vary foot position and eyes open, closed. Moving platform posturography: as previously noted, with movement of platform. |
| | Postural muscle EMG | During three conditions: external displacement (push on shoulder), before voluntary limb movement, during walking. |
| Stability | Abnormal involuntary movements | Patient sits quietly; note any of the following: athetosis, chorea, dystonia. These involuntary movements indicate basal ganglia disorders. A more sensitive test is to have patient stand with eyes closed, arms stretched forward, forearms pronated, and fingers abducted; note any involuntary movements. |

*EMG*, Electromyography; *ROM*, range of motion.
*Indicates a test used by researchers but not routinely used by therapists.

## Electrodiagnostic Studies

Frequently the purpose of nerve conduction studies in motor disorders is to differentiate among three possible sites of dysfunction: nerve, neuromuscular junction, and muscle. In nerve conduction studies examining motor nerve, the skin over a nerve is electrically stimulated, and potentials are recorded from the skin overlying an innervated muscle. In surface EMG, the electrical activity of muscle is recorded from the skin overlying the muscle. Diagnostic EMG, using a needle electrode inserted into muscle, is commonly used to distinguish between denervated muscle and myopathy. *Myopathy* is an abnormality or disease intrinsic to muscle tissue. The electrical activity of a muscle is recorded using an oscilloscope and a loudspeaker.

### Motor Nerve Conduction Studies

The function of motor fibers in the median nerve can be tested by electrically stimulating the median nerve at the wrist while recording from electrodes over the abductor pollicis brevis muscle and then stimulating at the elbow while recording from the same site. The depolarization of the muscle is recorded as a muscle action potential (MAP). The nerve conduction velocity equals the distance between the proximal and distal stimulation sites, divided by the difference between the latencies. MAP

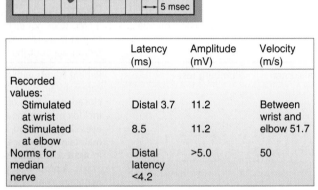

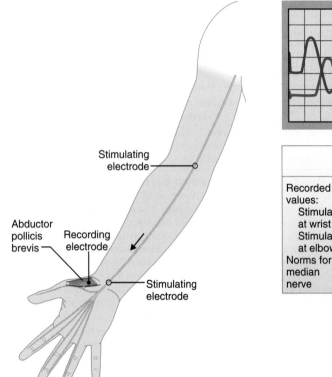

| | Latency (ms) | Amplitude (mV) | Velocity (m/s) |
|---|---|---|---|
| Recorded values: | | | |
| Stimulated at wrist | Distal 3.7 | 11.2 | Between wrist and |
| Stimulated at elbow | 8.5 | 11.2 | elbow 51.7 |
| Norms for median nerve | Distal latency <4.2 | >5.0 | 50 |

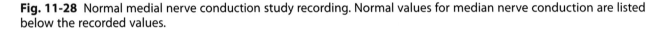

**Fig. 11-28** Normal medial nerve conduction study recording. Normal values for median nerve conduction are listed below the recorded values.

amplitude indicates the function of the neuromuscular junction and muscle fibers, in addition to the conduction ability of the alpha motor neurons (Figure 11-28).

### Electromyography

Diagnostic EMG requires inserting an electrode directly into muscle. Muscle electrical activity is recorded during four conditions: on insertion of the needle into the muscle (insertional activity), during rest, during minimal voluntary contraction, and during maximal voluntary contraction. Normal response to needle insertion is a brief interval of depolarization that is due to mechanical irritation of muscle fibers. At rest, normal muscle is electrically silent. Minimal voluntary contraction elicits single motor unit action potentials. Increasing voluntary contraction generates a full interference pattern, created by the asynchronous discharge of many muscle fibers.

If a muscle membrane is unstable owing to denervation, trauma, electrolyte imbalance, or an upper motor neuron lesion, its fibers become hypersensitive to ACh, and fibrillation (random, spontaneous contraction of individual muscle fibers) ensues. Fibrillation occurs when the subject intends the muscle to be at rest. If muscle is reinnervated, larger than normal amplitude muscle potentials are recorded owing to axons innervating a greater than normal number of muscle fibers. In primary disease of muscle (myopathy), axons innervate fewer than normal numbers of muscle fibers, resulting in a small-amplitude MAP. Myopathy is indicated by short-duration, low-amplitude potentials during voluntary contraction, lack of

spontaneous muscle activity (fasciculations, fibrillations), and absence of sensory involvement.

> **◎ Clinical Pearl**
>
> Nerve conduction studies differentiate among nerve, neuromuscular junction, and muscle disorders. Diagnostic EMG distinguishes between denervated muscle and myopathy.

## SUMMARY

The basal ganglia are a group of interconnected nuclei located in the cerebrum and midbrain. Together these nuclei regulate muscle force, muscle contraction, multijoint movements, and movement sequencing. Basal ganglia pathology causes a spectrum of movement disorders, ranging from the hypokinesia of Parkinson's disease to the hyperkinesia of dytonia.

The cerebellum coordinates movement and postural control. Cerebellar dysfunctions can cause ataxia, nystagmus, and dysarthria.

Although all regions of the nervous system have some involvement in control of posture, ambulation, and reaching/grasping, specific neural areas provide the primary control for each of these fundamental types of movements. Posture is controlled predominantly by brainstem mechanisms, ambulation by brainstem and spinal circuits, and reaching/grasping by the cerebral cortex.

## CLINICAL NOTES

### Case 1

K.L. is a 73-year-old woman recently admitted to long-term care because she is unable to care for herself. Ten years ago, she developed tremor in both hands; the tremor has gotten progressively worse. Her current status is as follows:

- Consciousness and sensation are intact.
- About once a week she is observed having conversations with people who are not present (hallucinations).
- Autonomic dysfunctions: orthostatic hypotension, difficulty regulating body temperature, constipation, excessive urinary urgency and frequency (caused by involuntary contraction of the bladder wall).
- The tremor is worse when her hands are resting and improves when she is using her hands.
- She tends to remain in the position the staff leaves her in. She does not move spontaneously.
- She cannot independently change from sitting to standing, nor can she initiate walking. However, if someone assists her by leaning her forward, she can walk with a shuffling gait.
- During passive range of motion, all muscles show increased resistance compared with normal, regardless of the velocity of muscle stretch.

#### Question

What is the location of the lesion and the probable diagnosis?

### Case 2

L.F. is a 67-year-old retired man. During the past 5 years, he has complained of gradual onset of balance and gait problems, including dizziness when standing, difficulty with sit-to-stand, difficulty initiating gait, and frequent tripping and falling. Autonomic complaints include erectile dysfunction, urinary retention, chronic constipation, and occasional incontinence.

- Consciousness, mentation, and sensation are normal.
- Facial expression is lacking.
- Posture: trunk and head are flexed forward.
- Strength is normal throughout the body.
- During passive range of motion, all muscles show increased resistance compared with normal.
- Cranial nerve function is normal.
- Babinski's sign: bilateral upgoing toe signs.
- Coordination: lower limb ataxia; equal ataxia in supine, standing, and sitting positions. Dysmetria bilaterally (finger-to-nose and heel-shin test). Bilateral dysdiadochokinesis.
- Narrow-based ataxic gait. Able to heel walk and toe walk with assistance. Unable to tandem walk.

#### Question

What is the location of the lesions and the probable diagnosis?

### Case 3

B.F. is a 52-year-old accountant. His only complaints are right forearm muscle pain and cramping when writing.

- Normal right upper limb cutaneous sensation and autonomic function, except cannot distinguish between closely spaced tactile stimuli on fingertips and thumb pad, poor stereognosis, and impaired proprioception in the digits of the right hand.
- When the therapist palpates the muscles of the forearm, B.F. reports no pain in the wrist extensor muscles, and deep, aching pain on palpation of the wrist and finger flexor muscles.
- Active range of motion is normal throughout the right upper limb.
- When B.F. is asked to write, after 2 minutes his forearm and finger flexor muscles cramp. To continue writing, he must use an abnormal upper limb position with the shoulder abducted 60 degrees.

#### Question

What is the location of the lesion and the probable diagnosis?

### Case 4

R.L., a 57-year-old man, complains of increasing right-sided clumsiness and shaking. Onset has been gradual, beginning 4 months ago.

- Somatosensation, autonomic function, and muscle strength are normal throughout the entire body.
- Coordination tests are normal in the left upper and lower limbs.
- On the right side: attempts at rapid alternating movements are slow and uncoordinated; action (intention) tremor occurs during finger-to-nose and heel-to-shin tests; dysmetria on finger-to-nose test.
- Abnormal involuntary eye movements.

#### Question

What is the location of the lesion and the probable diagnosis?

## REVIEW QUESTIONS

1. What are the three routes for information from the basal ganglia output nuclei to the lower motor neurons?
2. List the nuclei that form the basal ganglia.
3. What are the basic functions of the basal ganglia as a group?
4. What disease is characterized by rigidity, hypokinesia, resting tremor, and visuoperceptive impairments? Cell death in which nuclei produce this disease?
5. What disease is characterized by parkinsonism, cerebellar and corticospinal signs, and autonomic dysfunction?
6. List three disorders that cause hyperkinesia.
7. Involuntary abnormal postures and repetitive twisting movements are signs of what disorder?
8. What is the major function of the cerebellum?
9. What are the major sources of input to the cerebellum?
10. Which part of the cerebellum coordinates individual finger movements? Gross limb movements? Postural adjustments?
11. Ataxic gait indicates damage to what part of the cerebellum?
12. What is movement decomposition? Where is a lesion that produces movement decomposition?
13. List and define the signs of spinocerebellar lesions.
14. What is a long loop response?
15. What is an asymmetric tonic neck reflex?
16. What information can posturography provide?
17. Give an example of a preparatory postural adjustment.
18. Give an example of identical stimuli eliciting different responses depending on instructions given to a person.
19. If a person with hemiplegia is having difficulty initiating gait, what simple adjustment might make gait initiation easier?
20. What are the two phases of reaching?
21. Diagnostic EMG is used for what purpose?
22. What is the difference in purpose between motor nerve conduction velocity studies and movement analysis by surface EMG tests?

## References

1. Graybiel AM, Mink JW: The basal ganglia and cognition. In Gazzaniga M, editor: *The cognitive neurosciences IV*, Cambridge, Mass, 2009, MIT Press.
2. McNaught KS, Kapustin A, Jackson T, et al: Brainstem pathology in DYT1 primary torsion dystonia. *Ann Neurol* 56:540–547, 2004.
3. Takakusaki K, Tomita N, Yano M: Substrates for normal gait and pathophysiology of gait disturbances with respect to the basal ganglia dysfunction. *J Neurol* 255(Suppl 4):19–29, 2008.
4. Mena-Segovia J, Bolam JP, Magill PJ: Pedunculopontine nucleus and basal ganglia: distant relatives or part of the same family? *Trends Neurosci* 27:585–588, 2004.
5. Jahn K, Zwergal A: Imaging supraspinal locomotor control in balance disorders. *Restor Neurol Neurosci* 28:5–114, 2010.
6. Herrero MT, Barcia C, Navarro JM: Functional anatomy of thalamus and basal ganglia. *Childs Nerv Syst* 18:386–404, 2002.
7. de Weijer AD, Mandl RC, Sommer IE, et al: Human fronto-tectal and fronto-striatal-tectal pathways activate differently during anti-saccades. *Front Hum Neurosci* 4:41, 2010.
8. Hikosaka O: Basal ganglia mechanisms of reward-oriented eye movement. *Ann N Y Acad Sci* 1104:229–249, 2007.
9. Groenewegen HJ, Trimble M: The ventral striatum as an interface between the limbic and motor systems. *CNS Spectr* 12:887–892, 2007.
10. Balleine BW, O'Doherty JP: Human and rodent homologies in action control: corticostriatal determinants of goal-directed and habitual action. *Neuropsychopharmacology* 35:48–69, 2010.
11. Ding L, Gold JI: Caudate encodes multiple computations for perceptual decisions. *J Neurosci* 30:15747–15759, 2010.
12. Lau B, Glimcher PW: Value representations in the primate striatum during matching behavior. *Neuron* 58(3):451–463, 2008.
13. Watanabe M, Munoz DP: Presetting basal ganglia for volitional actions. *J Neurosci* 30:10144–10157, 2010.
14. DeLong M, Wichmann T: Changing views of basal ganglia circuits and circuit disorders. *Clin EEG Neurosci* 41:61–67, 2010.
15. Samejima K, Doya K: Multiple representations of belief states and action values in corticobasal ganglia loops. *Ann N Y Acad Sci* 1104:213–228, 2007.

16. Lehéricy S, Bardinet E, Tremblay L, et al: Motor control in basal ganglia circuits using fMRI and brain atlas approaches. *Cereb Cortex* 16(2):149–161, 2006.
17. Xue G, Ghahremani DG, Poldrack RA: Neural substrates for reversing stimulus-outcome and stimulus-response associations. *J Neurosci.* 28(44):11196–11204, 2008.
18. Draganski B, Kherif F, Klöppel S, et al: Evidence for segregated and integrative connectivity patterns in the human basal ganglia. *J Neurosci* 28:7143–7152, 2008.
19. Haber SN, Calzavara R: The cortico-basal ganglia integrative network: the role of the thalamus. *Brain Res Bull* 78:69–74, 2009.
20. Narumoto J, Matsushima N, Oka S, et al: Neurobehavioral changes associated with bilateral caudate nucleus infarctions. *Psychiatry Clin Neurosci* 59:109–110, 2005.
21. Richfield EK, Twyman R, Berent S: Neurological syndrome following bilateral damage to the head of the caudate nuclei. *Ann Neurol* 22(6):768–771, 1987.
22. Passarotti AM, Sweeney JA, Pavuluri MN: Neural correlates of incidental and directed facial emotion processing in adolescents and adults. *Soc Cogn Affect Neurosci* 4(4):387–398, 2009.
23. Badre D, Poldrack RA, Paré-Blagoev EJ: Dissociable controlled retrieval and generalized selection mechanisms in ventrolateral prefrontal cortex. *Neuron* 47(6):907–918, 2005.
24. Kringelbach M: The human orbitofrontal cortex: linking reward to hedonic experience. *Nat Rev Neurosci* 6(9):691–702, 2005.
25. Sesack SR, Grace AA: Cortico-basal ganglia reward network: microcircuitry. *Neuropsychopharmacology* 35:27–47, 2010.
26. Smith KS, Tindell AJ, Aldridge JW, et al: Ventral pallidum roles in reward and motivation. *Behav Brain Res* 196(2):155–167, 2009.
27. Korchounov A, Schipper HI, Preobrazhenskaya IS, et al: Differences in age at onset and familial aggregation between clinical types of idiopathic Parkinson's disease. *Mov Disord* 19:1059–1064, 2004.
28. Kang GA, Bronstein JM, Masterman DL, et al: Clinical characteristics in early Parkinson's disease in a central California population-based study. *Mov Disord* 20:1133–1142, 2005.
29. Priano L, Albani G, Brioschi A, et al: Nocturnal anomalous movement reduction and sleep microstructure analysis in parkinsonian

patients during 1-night transdermal apomorphine treatment. *Neurol Sci* 24:207–208, 2003.

30. Pope PA, Praamstra P, Wing AM: Force and time control in the production of rhythmic movement sequences in Parkinson's disease. *Eur J Neurosci* 23:1643–1650, 2006.

31. Marques A, Dujardin K, Boucart M, et al: REM sleep behaviour disorder and visuoperceptive dysfunction: a disorder of the ventral visual stream? *J Neurol* 257:383–391, 2010.

32. Uitti RJ, Baba Y, Wszolek ZK, Putzke DJ: Defining the Parkinson's disease phenotype: initial symptoms and baseline characteristics in a clinical cohort. *Parkinsonism Relat Disord* 11:139–145, 2005.

33. Reijnders JS, Ehrt U, Lousberg R, et al: The association between motor subtypes and psychopathology in Parkinson's disease. *Parkinsonism Relat Disord* 15:379–382, 2009.

34. Ceravolo R, Rossi C, Kiferle L, Bonuccelli U: Nonmotor symptoms in Parkinson's disease: the dark side of the moon. *Future Neurology* 5:851–871, 2010.

35. Jahan I, Hauser RA, Sullivan KL, et al: Sleep disorders in Parkinson's disease. *Neuropsychiatr Dis Treat* 5:535–540, 2009.

36. Clarimón J, Pagonabarraga J, Paisán-Ruíz C, et al: Tremor dominant parkinsonism: clinical description and LRRK2 mutation screening. *Mov Disord* 23:518–523, 2008.

37. Gubellini P, Salin P, Kerkerian-Le Goff L, Baunez C: Deep brain stimulation in neurological diseases and experimental models: from molecule to complex behavior. *Prog Neurobiol* 89:79–123, 2009.

38. Mounsey RB, Teismann P: Mitochondrial dysfunction in Parkinson's disease: pathogenesis and neuroprotection. *Parkinsons Dis* 2011:617472, 2010.

39. Vatalaro M: Fly model of Parkinson's offers hope of simpler, faster research. *NIH Record* L11:3, 2000.

40. de Lau LM, Breteler MM: Epidemiology of Parkinson's disease. *Lancet Neurol* 5:525–535, 2006.

41. Fahn S: Parkinson's disease: 10 years of progress, 1997–2007. *Mov Disord* 25(Suppl 1):S2–14, 2010.

42. Volkmann J: Deep brain stimulation for the treatment of Parkinson's disease. *J Clin Neurophysiol* 21:6–17, 2004.

43. Karimi M, Golchin N, Tabbal SD, et al: Subthalamic nucleus stimulation-induced regional blood flow responses correlate with improvement of motor signs in Parkinson disease. *Brain* 131:2710–2719, 2008.

44. Thevathasan W, Gregory R: Deep brain stimulation for movement disorders. *Pract Neurol* 10:16–26, 2010.

45. Pahwa R, Lyons KE, Wilkinson SB, et al: Long-term evaluation of deep brain stimulation of the thalamus. *J Neurosurg* 104:506–512, 2006.

46. Schupbach WM, Chastan N, Welter ML, et al: Stimulation of the subthalamic nucleus in Parkinson's disease: a 5 year follow up. *J Neurol Neurosurg Psychiatry* 76:1640–1644, 2005.

47. Alam M, Schwabe K, Krauss JK: The pedunculopontine nucleus area: critical evaluation of interspecies differences relevant for its use as a target for deep brain stimulation. *Brain* 134:11–23, 2011.

48. Weaver FM, Follett K, Stern M, et al: CSP 468 Study Group. Bilateral deep brain stimulation vs best medical therapy for patients with advanced Parkinson disease: a randomized controlled trial. *JAMA* 301:63–73, 2009.

49. Arenas E: Towards stem cell replacement therapies for Parkinson's disease. *Biochem Biophys Res Commun* 396:152–156, 2010.

50. Kwakkel G, deGoede CJT, van Wegen E: Impact of physical therapy for Parkinson's disease: a critical review of the literature. *Parkinsonism Relat Disord* 13:S478–S487, 2007.

51. Rao AK: Enabling functional independence in Parkinson's disease: update on occupational therapy intervention. *Mov Disord* 25(Suppl 1):S146–S151, 2010.

52. Dibble LE, Hale TF, Marcus RL, et al: High-intensity resistance training amplifies muscle hypertrophy and functional gains in persons with Parkinson's disease. *Mov Disord* 21:1444–1452, 2006.

53. Zesiewicz TA, Sullivan KL, Gooch CL: Red flags to spot the parkinsonian variant of multiple system atrophy. *Nat Clin Pract Neurol* 4:596–597, 2008.

54. Poewe W, Wenning G: The differential diagnosis of Parkinson's disease. *Eur J Neurol* 9(Suppl 3):23–30, 2002.

55. Bensimon G, Ludolph A, Agid Y, et al, NNIPPS Study Group: Riluzole treatment, survival and diagnostic criteria in Parkinson plus disorders: the NNIPPS study. *Brain* 132:156–171, 2009.

56. Zaccai J, McCracken C, Brayne C: A systematic review of prevalence and incidence studies of dementia with Lewy bodies. *Age Ageing* 34:561–566, 2005.

57. Schrag A, Wenning GK, Quinn N, Ben-Shlomo Y: Survival in multiple system atrophy. *Mov Disord* 23:294–296, 2008.

58. Dujardin K, Defebvre L, Krystkowiak P, et al: Executive function differences in multiple system atrophy and Parkinson's disease. *Parkinsonism Relat Disord* 9:205–211, 2003.

59. Caroff SN, Hurford I, Lybrand J, Campbell EC: Movement disorders induced by antipsychotic drugs: implications of the CATIE schizophrenia trial. *Neurol Clin* 29:127–148, 2011.

60. Gavett BE, Stern RA, McKee AC: Chronic traumatic encephalopathy: a potential late effect of sport-related concussive and subconcussive head trauma. *Clin Sports Med* 30:179–188, 2011.

61. Hurelbrink CB, Lewis SJ, Barker RA: The use of the Actiwatch-Neurologica system to objectively assess the involuntary movements and sleep-wake activity in patients with mild-moderate Huntington's disease. *J Neurol* 252:642–647, 2005.

62. Roos RA: Huntington's disease: a clinical review. *Orphanet J Rare Dis* 5:40, 2010.

63. Adler CH: Strategies for controlling dystonia: overview of therapies that may alleviate symptoms. *Postgrad Med* 108:151–152, 155–156, 159–160, 2000.

64. Elia AE, Lalli S, Albanese A: Differential diagnosis of dystonia. *Eur J Neurol* 17(Suppl 1):1–8, 2010.

65. Adler CH, Crews D, Hentz JG, et al: Abnormal co-contraction in yips-affected but not unaffected golfers: evidence for focal dystonia. *Neurology* 64:1813–1814, 2005.

66. Altenmüller E, Jabusch HC: Focal dystonia in musicians: phenomenology, pathophysiology, triggering factors, and treatment. *Med Probl Perform Art* 25:3–9, 2010.

67. Byl NN: The neural consequences of repetition. *Neurol Rep* 24:60–70, 2000.

68. Lenz FA, Byl NN: Reorganization in the cutaneous core of the human thalamic principal somatic sensory nucleus (ventral caudal) in patients with dystonia. *J Neurophysiol* 82:3204–3212, 1999.

69. McKenzie AL, Nagarajan SS, Roberts TP, et al: Somatosensory representation of the digits and clinical performance in patients with focal hand dystonia. *Am J Phys Med Rehabil* 82:737–749, 2003.

70. Leckman JF, Bloch MH, Smith ME, et al: Neurobiological substrates of Tourette's disorder. *J Child Adolesc Psychopharmacol* 20:237–247, 2010.

71. Krageloh-Mann I, Helber A, Mader I, et al: Bilateral lesions of thalamus and basal ganglia: origin and outcome. *Dev Med Child Neurol* 44:477–484, 2002.

72. Doya K: Complementary roles of basal ganglia and cerebellum in learning and motor control. *Curr Opin Neurobiol* 10:732–739, 2000.

73. Steele CJ, Penhune VB: Specific increases within global decreases: a functional magnetic resonance imaging investigation of five days of motor sequence learning. *J Neurosci* 30:8332–8341, 2010.

74. Xu D, Liu T, Ashe K, Bushara KO: Role of the olivo-cerebellar system in timing. *J Neurosci* 26:5990–5995, 2006.

75. Schoch B, Dimitrova A, Gizewski ER, Timmann D: Functional localization in the human cerebellum based on voxelwise statistical analysis: a study of 90 patients. *Neuroimage* 30:36–51, 2006.

76. Vilis T, Hore J: Effects of changes in mechanical state of limb on cerebellar intention tremor. *J Neurophysiol* 40:1214–1224, 1977.

77. Morton SM, Tseng YW, Zackowski KM, et al: Longitudinal tracking of gait and balance impairments in cerebellar disease. *Mov Disord* 25:1944–1952, 2010.

78. Agrawal Y, Carey JP, Della Santina CC, et al: Disorders of balance and vestibular function in US adults: data from the National Health and Nutrition Examination Survey, 2001–2004. *Arch Intern Med* 169:938–944, 2009.

79. Nashner LM, Black FO, Wall C 3rd: Adaptation to altered support and visual conditions during stance: patients with vestibular deficits. *J Neurosci* 2:536–544, 1982.

80. Cordo PJ, Nashner LM: Properties of postural adjustments associated with rapid arm movements. *J Neurophysiol* 47:287–302, 1982.

81. Burleigh AL, Horak FB, Malouin F: Modification of postural responses and step initiation: evidence for goal directed postural interactions. *J Physiol* 76:2892–2902, 1994.

82. Hesse S, Reiter F, Jahnke M, et al. Asymmetry of gait initiation in hemiparetic stroke subjects. *Arch Phys Med Rehabil* 78(7):719–724, 1997.

83. Gantchev N, Viallet F, Aurenty R, Massion J: Impairment of posturo-kinetic coordination during initiation of forward oriented step in parkinsonian patients. *Electroencephalogr Clin Neurophysiol* 101:110–120, 1996.

84. Yogev-Seligmann G, Hausdorff JM, Giladi N: The role of executive function and attention in gait. *Mov Disord* 23:329–342, 2008.

85. Goodale MA, Westwood DA, Milner AD: Two distinct modes of control for object-directed action. *Prog Brain Res* 144:131–144, 2004.

86. Jeannerod M: *In The neural and behavioral organization of goal-directed movements*, Oxford, 1990, Clarendon Press.

87. Castiello U: The neuroscience of grasping: nature reviews. *Neuroscience* 6:726–736, 2005.

88. von Hofsten C: Development of manual actions from a perceptual perspective. In Forssberg H, Hirschfeld H, editors: *Movement disorders in children*, Basel, Switzerland, 1992, S. Karger, pp 113–123.

89. Bradley NS: What are the principles of motor development? In Forssberg H, Hirschfeld H, editors: *Movement disorders in children*, Basel, Switzerland, 1992, S. Karger, pp 41–49.

90. Freund HJ: Somatosensory and motor disturbances in patients with parietal lobe lesions. *Adv Neurol* 93:179–193, 2003.

91. Kendall FP, McCreary EK, Provance P, et al: *In Muscles: testing and function with posture and pain*, Baltimore, 2005, Lippincott Williams & Wilkins.

92. Hislop HJ, Montogomery J: *In Daniels and Worthingham's muscle testing: techniques of manual examination*, ed 7, Philadelphia, 2002, WB Saunders.

93. Tinetti M: Performance oriented assessment of mobility problems in elderly patients. *J Am Geriatr Soc* 40:479, 1986.

94. Shumway-Cook A, Horak FB: Assessing the influence of sensory interaction on balance. *Phys Ther* 66:1548–1550, 1986.

95. Duncan P, Weiner DK, Chandler J, Studenski S: Functional reach: a new clinical measure of balance. *J Gerontol* 45:192–197, 1990.

# 12 Peripheral Nervous System

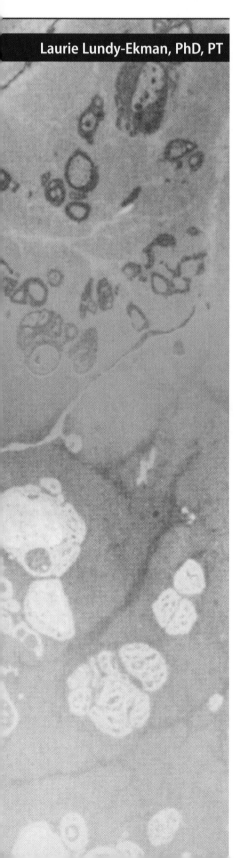

Laurie Lundy-Ekman, PhD, PT

## Chapter Outline

I was a 32-year-old woman working a 40-hour week as a chef's assistant. I first noticed pain in my wrist and hand while working. After work, my hand would be numb and have tingling sensations. As the problem progressed, it became difficult to grip a knife or cleaver.

When I first went to the doctor, the problem was diagnosed as tendonitis, and I was advised to use my other hand more. I kept working, and the condition worsened; on returning to the doctor, I received pain medication and a wrist brace. When these did not help, I was referred to an orthopedic specialist. Nerve conduction studies were performed by a physical therapist. The condition was diagnosed as carpal tunnel syndrome. I went to a physical therapist two times a week for heat treatments and exercises for about 3 months. I was told I could no longer continue my line of work. I ended up with a full cast for 6 weeks to prevent me from using my left arm and hand.

The pain in my wrist and hand continued to be intense, much worse at night. I could only sleep with my arm propped up on a pillow above my head. I ended therapy after having two cortisone shots into my wrist, which did not have any effect.

Today if I garden or use my left hand too long typing or playing tennis, I will have pain and know I need to lighten up.

—*Genevieve Kelly*

**Carpal tunnel syndrome is caused by pressure on the median nerve at the wrist, where the carpal bones and a ligament form a tunnel surrounding the tendons of flexor muscles and the median nerve. The compression leads to pain, numbness, and tingling, in the parts of the hand supplied by the median nerve: skin of the palmar surfaces of the lateral 3 ½ digits and the adjacent palm. Weakness and atrophy may affect the abductor pollicis brevis, opponens pollicis, first and second lumbricals, and half of the flexor pollicis brevis.**

The peripheral nervous system includes all neural structures distal to the spinal nerves. Thus, axons of sensory, motor, and autonomic neurons, along with specialized sensory endings and entire postganglionic autonomic neurons, form the peripheral nervous system. Examples of peripheral nerves include the median, ulnar, and tibial nerves. Although cranial nerves are also peripheral nerves, cranial nerves will be covered in Chapters 14 and 15, because their function can best be understood in the context of brainstem function. In this textbook, all nervous system structures enclosed by bone are considered parts of the central nervous system; nerve roots, dorsal root ganglia, and spinal nerves therefore are within the spinal region (Figure 12-1). Distal to the spinal nerve, the groups of axons split into posterior and anterior rami. Axons in the *posterior rami* innervate the paravertebral muscles, posterior parts of the vertebrae, and overlying cutaneous areas. Axons in the *anterior rami* innervate the skeletal, muscular, and cutaneous areas of the limbs and the anterior and lateral trunk.

Classifying nerve roots, dorsal root ganglia, and spinal nerves as spinal and the remaining axons as peripheral allows the clinical difference between spinal and peripheral lesions to be easily distinguished: sensory, autonomic, and motor deficits in spinal region lesions show a myotomal and/or dermatomal distribution; sensory, autonomic, and motor deficits in peripheral lesions show a peripheral nerve distribution (see Figures 6-5 and 6-6). Signs of peripheral neuron lesions include paresis or paralysis, sensory loss, abnormal sensations, muscle atrophy, and reduced or absent deep tendon reflexes.

### ◎ Clinical Pearl

Peripheral nerve lesions produce signs and symptoms in a peripheral nerve distribution. Spinal region lesions produce signs and symptoms in a myotomal and/or dermatomal distribution.

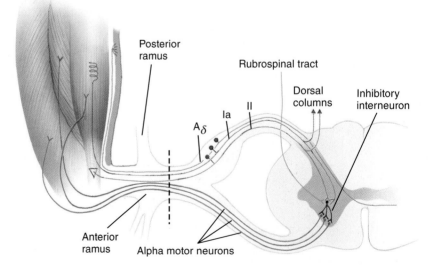

**Fig. 12-1** The vertical dotted line indicates the division between the peripheral and the central nervous systems. Neural structures in the periphery include muscle spindle receptors *(blue spiral in muscle)*, the Golgi tendon organ *(blue triangle in the tendon)*, motor endings in muscle *(red V's)*, and axons. The posterior rami innervate structures along the posterior midline of the body and the anterior rami supply structures in the lateral and anterior body.

## PERIPHERAL NERVES

Peripheral nerves consist of parallel bundles of axons surrounded by three connective tissue sheaths: endoneurium, perineurium, and epineurium. *Endoneurium* separates individual axons, *perineurium* surrounds bundles of axons called *fascicles,* and *epineurium* encloses the entire nerve trunk (Figure 12-2). An outer layer of connective tissue, the *mesoneurium,* surrounds the epineurium. Connective tissues protect the axons and glia and support mechanical changes in length that nerves undergo during movements.

Peripheral nerves receive blood supply via arterial branches that enter the nerve trunk. Within the nerve, axons are

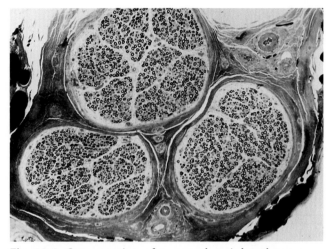

**Fig. 12-2 Cross-section of a normal peripheral nerve, showing three fascicles.** Within each fascicle are many darkly stained myelin sheaths, appearing as small oval structures enclosing the axons, which appear white. Endoneurium surrounds each axon. Perineurium surrounds each fascicle. External epineurium surrounds the three fascicles. Internal epineurium and blood vessels fill the areas between fascicles. *(From Richardson EP Jr, DeGirolami U: Pathology of the peripheral nerve, Philadelphia, 1995, WB Saunders, p 3.)*

electrically insulated from each other by endoneurium and by a myelin sheath. The myelin sheath is provided by Schwann cells, which may partially surround a group of small-diameter axons or may completely envelop a section of a single large axon. The small-diameter axons that share Schwann cells are called *unmyelinated* (although *partially myelinated* would be a more accurate term), and the large-diameter axons that are fully wrapped by individual Schwann cells are designated *myelinated.*

Peripheral nerves supply viscera or somatic structures. The visceral supply, via splanchnic nerves, is discussed in Chapter 9.

Somatic peripheral nerves are usually mixed, consisting of sensory, autonomic, and motor axons. Cutaneous branches supply the skin and subcutaneous tissues; muscular branches supply muscle, tendons, and joints. Cutaneous branches are not purely sensory because they deliver the sympathetic efferent axons to sweat glands and arterioles. Muscular branches are not purely motor because they contain sensory axons from proprioceptive structures.

Peripheral axons are classified into groups according to their speed of conduction and their diameter (Table 12-1). Two classification systems for peripheral axons are in common use. The letter classification system (A, B, C) applies to both afferent and efferent axons; the Roman numeral system applies only to afferent axons.

### Nerve Plexuses

The junctions of anterior rami form four nerve plexuses:
- Cervical plexus
- Brachial plexus
- Lumbar plexus
- Sacral plexus

Please refer to the appendices at the end of this chapter for innervation in the upper and lower extremities.

The cervical plexus arises from anterior rami of C1-C4 and lies deep to the sternocleidomastoid muscle (Figure 12-3, *A*). The cervical plexus provides cutaneous sensory information from the posterior scalp to the clavicle and innervates the anterior neck muscles and the diaphragm. The phrenic nerve, whose

| TABLE 12-1 | PERIPHERAL AXONS | | | | | |
|---|---|---|---|---|---|---|
| | Conduction | Axon | **EFFERENT AXONS** | | **AFFERENT AXONS** | |
| Axon | Speed, m/sec | Diameter, μm | Group | Innervates | Group | Innervates |
| Large myelinated | 70–130 | 12–20 | Aα | Extrafusal muscle fibers | Ia, Ib, II | Spindles, Golgi tendon organs, touch and pressure receptors |
| Medium myelinated | 12–45 | 3–6 | Aγ | Intrafusal muscle fibers | | |
| Small myelinated | 12–30 | 2–10 | | | Aδ | Pain, temperature, visceral receptors |
| | 3–15 | 1–5 | B | Presynaptic autonomic | | |
| Unmyelinated | 0.2–2.0 | 0.4–1.2 | C | Postsynaptic autonomic | C | Pain, temperature, visceral receptors |

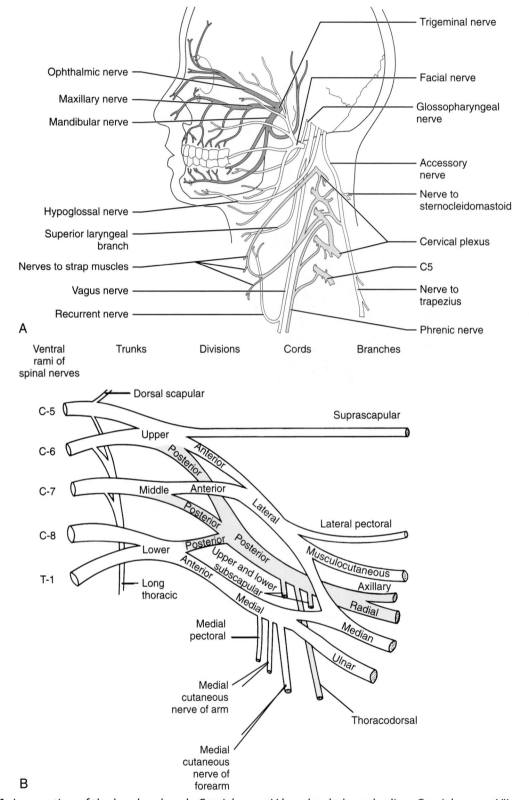

**Fig. 12-3  A,** Innervation of the head and neck. Cranial nerve V has the darkest shading. Cranial nerves VII and IX-XI are not shaded.  The cervical plexus is moderately shaded. **B,** The brachial plexus. *(From Jenkins DB: Hollinshead's functional anatomy of the limbs and back, ed 9, Philadelphia, 2009, WB Saunders.)*

cell bodies are in the cervical spinal cord (C3-C5), is the most important single branch from the cervical plexus because the phrenic nerve is the only motor supply and the main sensory nerve for the diaphragm.

The brachial plexus is formed by anterior rami of C5-T1 (Figure 12-3, *B*). The plexus emerges between the anterior and middle scalene muscles, passes deep to the clavicle, and enters the axilla. In the distal axilla, axons from the plexus become the radial, axillary, ulnar, median, and musculocutaneous nerves. The entire upper limb is innervated by brachial plexus branches (see Appendix 12-1 for additional illustrations of the nerves of the upper limb).

The lumbar plexus is formed by anterior rami of L1-L4 (Figure 12-4, *A*); the plexus forms in the psoas major muscle.

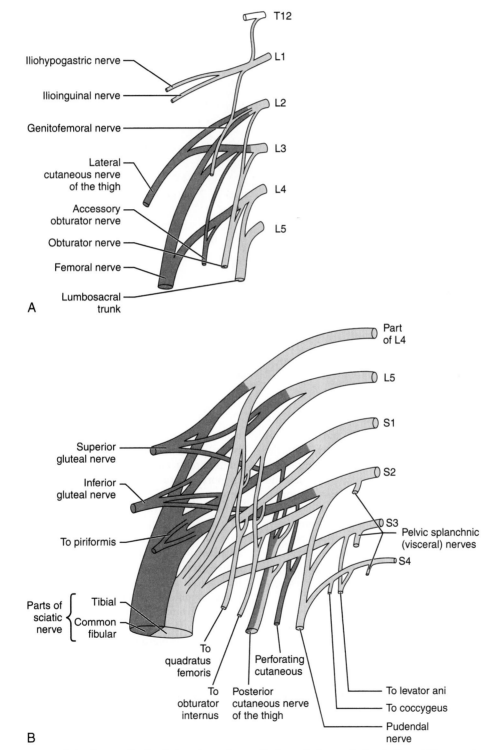

**Fig. 12-4 Innervation of the lower limb. A,** Lumbar plexus. **B,** Sacral plexus. In both **A** and **B** posterior parts have darker shading. **C,** Lumbosacral plexus. The sacral plexus has darker shading. *(From Jenkins DB: Hollinshead's functional anatomy of the limbs and back, ed 9, Philadelphia, 2009, WB Saunders.)*

*Continued*

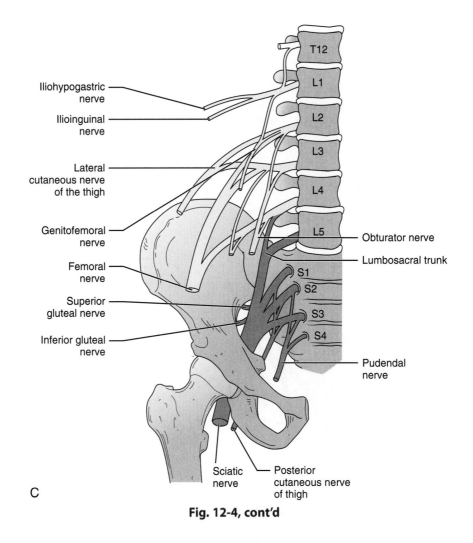

C

**Fig. 12-4, cont'd**

Branches of the lumbar plexus innervate skin and muscles of the anterior and medial thigh. A cutaneous branch from the plexus, the saphenous nerve, continues into the leg to innervate the medial leg and foot. Branches of the cervical, brachial, and lumbar plexuses provide sympathetic innervation via connections with the sympathetic chain. The sacral plexus innervates the posterior thigh and most of the leg and foot (Figure 12-4, *B* and *C*). Unlike the other plexuses, which contain sympathetic axons in addition to somatosensory and somatic motor axons, the sacral plexus contains parasympathetic axons in addition to the somatic axons. See Appendix 12-2 for additional illustrations of the nerves of the lower limb.

## Movement Is Essential for Nerve Health

Movement optimizes the health of nerves by promoting the flow of blood throughout the nerves and the flow of axoplasm through the axons. Normally, fascicles glide within the nerve and nerves glide relative to other structures. Adequate blood flow is necessary to supply nutrition and oxygen and to remove waste from neural tissues. Axoplasm thickens and becomes more resistant to flow when stationary. Movement causes axoplasm to thin and flow more easily, facilitating retrograde and anterograde transport. Retrograde axoplasmic transport moves

chemicals from the axons and surrounding structures to the cell body, providing information for the genetic machinery to adjust production of ion channels, transmitters, vesicles, and support structures. Anterograde axoplasmic transport delivers new structural and signaling components to their proper locations in the neuron.

Connective tissues support the changes in length that nerves undergo during movements. For example, with the shoulder abducted to 90 degrees, the median nerve is approximately 10 cm longer when the elbow and wrist are extended than when the elbow and wrist are flexed.[1] This increase in nerve length without injury is made possible by axons wrinkling within the endoneurium when the nerve is not stretched (Figure 12-5), by connective tissue, and by fascicular plexuses. The fascicular plexuses are connections that spread tensile load among fascicles, preventing excessive loading on a single fascicle.

As a nerve is stretched, first the viscoelastic tubes formed by endoneurium, perineurium, and external epineurium stretch, axons unfold, and fascicles glide relative to each other. As stretching continues, the entire nerve slides relative to surrounding structures. As stretching continues and exceeds the capacity of these mechanisms, tensile stress develops in the neural tissues. As the nerve is shortened, the processes reverse:

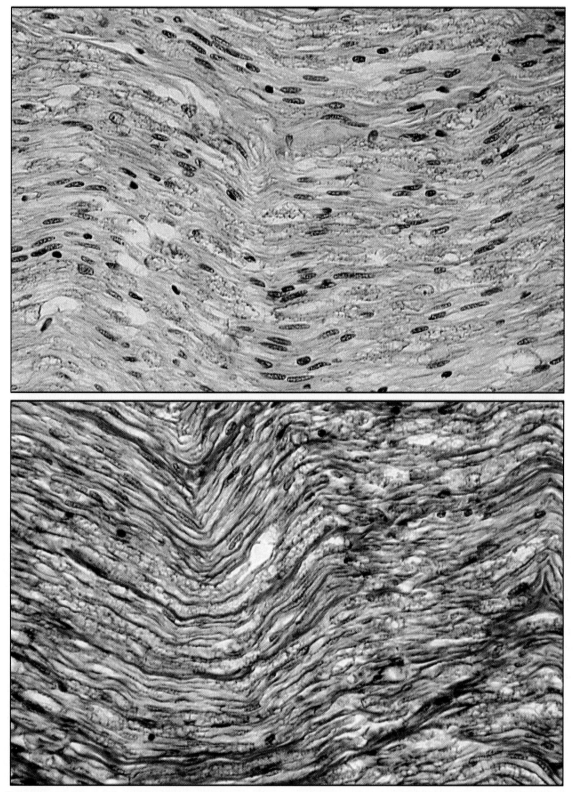

**Fig. 12-5** Normal folding of axons when a nerve is in the shortened position. Longitudinal section of femoral nerve, magnified ×100. Myelin is stained red *(top)* and connective tissue is blue *(bottom)*. *(From Warner JJ: Atlas of neuroanatomy, Maryland Heights, Mo, 2001, Butterworth-Heinemann.)*

tensile stress is relieved first, then the nerve slides relative to surrounding structures, the viscoelastic tubes recoil, and the axons fold. The nerve may also fold, as the median nerve does at the flexed elbow. See Topp and Boyd (2006)[2] and Rempel and Diao (2004)[3] for discussion of the mechanisms that permit nerves to lengthen and shorten without injury to axons or their supporting structures.

## NEUROMUSCULAR JUNCTION

Motor axons synapse with muscle fibers at neuromuscular junctions. This nerve-muscle synapse requires only depolarization of the motor axon, releasing acetylcholine (ACh), which diffuses across the synaptic cleft and binds with receptors to elicit depolarization of the muscle membrane. Unlike with neuron–neuron synapses, no summation of action potentials is required to depolarize the postsynaptic membrane. No inhibition is possible because only one branch of an axon synapses with a muscle fiber, and the action of the neurotransmitter is always excitatory. In a normal motor unit, every depolarization of the motor axon releases sufficient ACh to initiate action potentials in the innervated muscle fibers. Even when a lower motor neuron is inactive (no action potentials are occurring), it spontaneously releases minute amounts of ACh. Binding of the small quantity of ACh to receptors on the muscle membrane causes miniature end-plate potentials. These potentials, although not sufficient to initiate the process of muscle contraction, are believed to supply factors necessary to maintain muscle health. Without miniature end-plate potentials, muscles atrophy.

## DYSFUNCTION OF PERIPHERAL NERVES

Signs of peripheral nerve damage include sensory, autonomic, and motor changes. All signs present in a peripheral nerve distribution.

### Sensory Changes

Sensory changes include decreased or lost sensation and/or abnormal sensations: hyperalgesia, dysesthesia, paresthesia, and allodynia (see Chapter 8).

### Autonomic Changes

Autonomic signs depend on the pattern of axonal dysfunction. If a single nerve is damaged, autonomic signs usually are observed only if the nerve is completely severed. These signs include lack of sweating and loss of sympathetic control of smooth muscle fibers in arterial walls. The latter may contribute to edema in an affected limb. If many nerves are involved, autonomic problems may include impotence and difficulty regulating blood pressure, heart rate, sweating, and bowel and bladder functions.

### Motor Changes

Motor signs of peripheral nerve damage include paresis (weakness) or paralysis. If muscle is denervated, electromyography (EMG) recordings show no activity for about 1 week following injury. Muscle atrophy progresses rapidly. Then muscle fibers begin to develop generalized sensitivity to ACh along the entire muscle membrane, and fibrillation ensues. Fibrillation is spontaneous contraction of individual muscle fibers. Fibrillation is observable only with needle EMG. Unlike fasciculation, fibrillation cannot be observed on the skin surface. Fibrillation is not diagnostic of any specific lesion.

### Denervation: Trophic Changes

When nerve supply is interrupted, trophic changes begin in the denervated tissues. Muscles atrophy, skin becomes shiny, nails become brittle, and subcutaneous tissues thicken. Ulceration of cutaneous and subcutaneous tissues, poor healing of wounds and infections, and neurogenic joint damage are common, secondary to blood supply changes, loss of sensation, and lack of movement.

## CLASSIFICATION OF NEUROPATHIES

Peripheral neuropathy can involve a single nerve (mononeuropathy), several nerves (multiple mononeuropathy), or many nerves (polyneuropathy). Mononeuropathy is focal dysfunction, and multiple mononeuropathy is multifocal. Multiple mononeuropathy presents as asymmetric involvement of individual nerves. Polyneuropathy is a generalized disorder that typically presents distally and symmetrically. Dysfunction can be due to damage to the axon, myelin sheath, or both. Table 12-2 summarizes the types, pathology, and prognosis of peripheral neuropathies.

### Traumatic Injury to a Peripheral Nerve: Mononeuropathy

Various types of trauma, including repetitive stimuli, prolonged compression, or wounds, may injure peripheral nerves. Depending on the severity of damage, traumatic injuries to peripheral nerves are classified into three categories:
* Traumatic myelinopathy
* Traumatic axonopathy
* Severance

### Traumatic Myelinopathy

*Traumatic myelinopathy* is loss of myelin limited to the site of injury. Peripheral myelinopathies interfere with the function of large-diameter axons, producing motor, discriminative touch, proprioceptive, and phasic stretch reflex deficits, and cause neuropathic pain. Unless the injury is unusually severe, autonomic function is intact and the axons are not damaged (if axons are damaged, the lesion is called an *axonopathy;* see later). Recovery from traumatic myelinopathy tends to be complete because remyelination can occur rapidly, before irreversible damage occurs in the target tissues.

Focal compression of a peripheral nerve causes traumatic myelinopathy. Repeated mechanical stimuli, including excessive pressure, stretch, vibration, and/or friction may cause focal compression. The following sequence of events produces traumatic myelinopathy (Figure 12-6):

**TABLE 12-2   PERIPHERAL NEUROPATHIES**

| Neuropathy | Usual Cause | Pathology | Typical Recovery |
|---|---|---|---|
| **MONONEUROPATHY** | | | |
| Traumatic myelinopathy | Trauma | Demyelination | Complete and rapid, by remyelination |
| Traumatic axonopathy | Trauma | Axonal damage | Slow, by regrowth of axons, but good recovery because Schwann cell and connective tissue sheaths intact |
| Traumatic severance | Trauma | Axon and myelin degeneration | Slow, with poor results, owing to inappropriate reinnervation and traumatic neuroma |
| **MULTIPLE MONONEUROPATHY** | Complication of diabetes or blood vessel inflammation | Ischemia of neuron | Slow, by regrowth of axons, usually good recovery |
| **POLYNEUROPATHY** | Complication of diabetes or autoimmune disorder (e.g., Guillain-Barré syndrome) or genetic (hereditary motor and sensory neuropathy) | Metabolic or inflammatory | Diabetic neuropathy may be stable, progressive, or may improve with better blood sugar control; Guillain-Barré syndrome usually improves gradually; hereditary motor and sensory neuropathy is very slowly progressive |

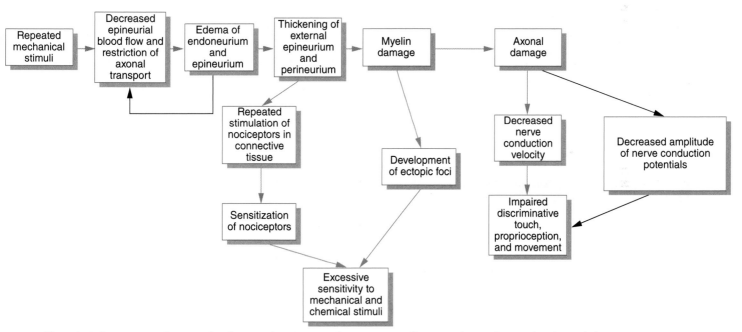

**Fig. 12-6** Sequence of events leading to the signs and symptoms of traumatic myelinopathy. Axonal damage occurs only in unusually severe cases. *(Modified from Nee RJ and Butler D: Management of peripheral neuropathic pain: integrating neurobiology, neurodynamics, and clinical evidence. Physical Therapy in Sport 7:36–49, 2006.)*

1. Nerve compression decreases axonal transport[4] and epineurial blood flow.
2. Decreased blood flow causes edema of the endoneurium and epineurium.
3. Edema further restricts blood and axoplasmic flow, interfering with axon function despite the axons being physically intact.
4. The external epineurium and perineurium thicken, causing myelin damage, leading to decreased nerve conduction velocity and the development of ectopic foci. Signals from the myelin-deficient part of the nerve alter gene activity in the cell body, stimulating the production of excessive numbers of mechanosensitive and chemosensitive ion channels, that are subsequently inserted into the myelin-deficient membrane, producing ectopic foci.[5] Axons that previously conveyed only action potentials can now repeatedly generate action potentials.[5]
5. Decreased nerve conduction velocity results in impaired discriminative touch, proprioception, and movements. Mechanical or chemical stimulation of ectopic foci generates neuropathic pain in the peripheral nerve distribution.[5]

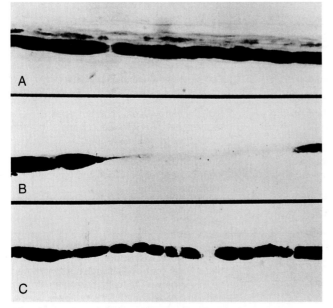

**Fig. 12-7 Nerve fiber with myelin stained to appear black. A,** Normal myelin. **B,** Segmental demyelination severe enough to cause secondary axonal degeneration. **C,** Remyelination, with abnormally short distance between nodes of Ranvier. *(From Richardson EP Jr, DeGirolami U: Pathology of the peripheral nerve, Philadelphia, 1995, WB Saunders, p 18.)*

Nerve entrapment, the mechanical constriction of a nerve within an anatomic canal, often causes traumatic myelinopathy. Entrapment is most common in the following nerves: median (carpal tunnel), ulnar (ulnar groove), radial (spiral groove), and peroneal (fibular head). Prolonged pressure from casts, crutches, or sustained positions (e.g., sitting with knees crossed) may compress nerves. Compression temporarily interferes with blood supply or, in the case of prolonged compression, may cause local demyelination. Local demyelination slows or prevents nerve conduction at the demyelinated site (Figure 12-7).

Carpal tunnel syndrome is a common compression injury of the median nerve in the space between the carpal bones and the flexor retinaculum (Pathology 12-1). Initially, pain and numbness are noted at night. Later, these symptoms persist throughout the day, and sensation is decreased or lost in the lateral 3½ digits and the adjacent palm of the hand. On the dorsum of the hand, the distal halves of the same digits are involved. Paresis and atrophy of the thumb intrinsic muscles may follow (Figure 12-8). Pain from carpal tunnel syndrome may radiate into the forearm and occasionally to the shoulder.[6]

Carpal tunnel syndrome is more prevalent in people whose occupations require working in a cold environment or the gripping of vibrating tools than in the general population. For mild cases, often 1 month of rest, splinting, and anti-inflammatory medication (to reduce trauma and edema), followed by exercises designed to promote gliding of the tendons in the carpal tunnel (to improve blood flow and axonal transport), constitute sufficient intervention. For more severe cases, changing to a different occupation and surgical release by severing the transverse carpal ligament may be necessary.[7]

## PATHOLOGY 12-1    CARPAL TUNNEL SYNDROME

| | |
|---|---|
| Pathology | Compression of median nerve in carpal tunnel |
| Etiology | Gripping vibrating tools, working in cold environment; associated with genetic factors and endocrine and rheumatic diseases[6] |
| Speed of onset | Chronic |
| Signs and symptoms | |
| Consciousness | Normal |
| Communication and memory | Normal |
| Sensory | Numbness, tingling, burning sensation in median nerve distribution. Symptoms may be evoked by compressing the median nerve or by stretching the nerve (neural tension test) |
| Autonomic | If unusually severe, lack of sweating in median nerve distribution |
| Motor | Paresis and atrophy of thenar muscles |
| Region affected | Peripheral |
| Demographics | Most common in people over 30 years of age; women more often affected than men |
| Prevalence | 3%–6% of adults[7] |
| Incidence | 2%[8] |
| Prognosis | Variable. Surgically treated group had slightly better outcome than groups treated with NSAIDs (nonsteroidal anti-inflammatory drugs) and hand therapy (ligament stretching, tendon gliding, splint use, ultrasound)[9] |

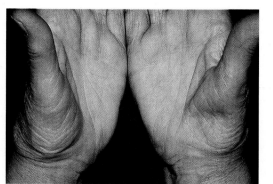

**Fig. 12-8** Carpal tunnel syndrome in the right hand. The thenar eminence has atrophied as a result of compression of the median nerve. *(From Parsons M, Johnson M: Diagnosis in color neurology, St Louis, 2001, Mosby.)*

## Traumatic Axonopathy

*Traumatic axonopathy* disrupts axons, and wallerian degeneration occurs distal to the lesion. Axonopathies affect all sizes of axons, so reflexes, somatosensation, and motor function are markedly reduced or absent. Muscle atrophy ensues. Because the myelin and connective tissues remain intact, regenerating axons are able to reinnervate appropriate targets. Axon regrowth typically proceeds at a rate of 1 mm/day. Recovery from axonopathies is generally good because the connective tissue and myelin sheaths provide guidance and support for axonal sprouts. Traumatic axonopathies usually arise from crushing of the nerve secondary to dislocations or closed fractures.

## Severance

*Severance* occurs when nerves are physically divided by excessive stretch or laceration. The axons and connective tissue are completely interrupted, causing immediate loss of sensation and/or muscle paralysis in the area supplied. Wallerian degeneration begins distal to the lesion 3 to 5 days later. Then axons in the proximal stumps begin to sprout. If proximal and distal nerve stumps are apposed, and scarring does not interfere, some sprouts enter the distal stump and are guided to their target tissue in the periphery. However, in a mixed peripheral nerve, lack of guidance from connective tissue and Schwann cells may allow the axon sprouts to reach inappropriate end-organs, resulting in poor recovery. For example, a motor axon may innervate a Golgi tendon organ; although the lower motor neuron could fire, the tendon organ would not respond, so the connection would be nonfunctional. If the stumps are displaced, or if scar tissue intervenes between the stumps, sprouts may grow into a tangled mass of nerve fibers, forming a traumatic *neuroma* (tumor of axons and Schwann cells). Nerve conduction distal to the injury may never return because of poor regeneration.

## Multiple Mononeuropathy

Involvement of two or more nerves in different parts of the body occurs most commonly when diabetes or vasculitis cause ischemia of the nerves. Vasculitis, the inflammation of blood

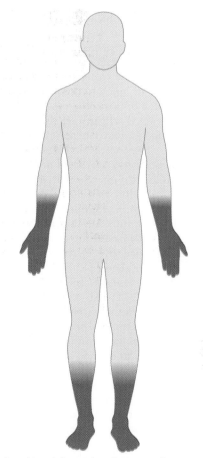

**Fig. 12-9** Stocking/glove distribution of sensory impairment in diabetic neuropathy.

vessels, may cause multiple mononeuropathy by restricting blood flow or by weakening vessel walls, resulting in rupture. In multiple mononeuropathy, individual nerves are affected, producing a random, asymmetric presentation of signs. If vasculitis is suspected, urgent referral should be made for an electrodiagnostic evaluation.[10]

## Polyneuropathy

Symmetric involvement of sensory, motor, and autonomic fibers, often progressing from distal to proximal, is the hallmark of polyneuropathy. Symptoms typically begin in the feet and then appear in the hands—areas of the body supplied by the longest axons. The distal pattern of symptoms is called a stocking/glove distribution (Figure 12-9). Degeneration of the distal part of long axons may occur because of inadequate axonal transport to keep the distal axons viable. Demyelination is also likely to produce distal symptoms first, because the longer axons have more myelin along their length and thus have a greater chance of being affected by the random destruction of myelin.

In contrast to mononeuropathies, polyneuropathies are not due to trauma or ischemia. The cause can be toxic, metabolic, or autoimmune. The most common causes of polyneuropathies are diabetes, nutritional deficiencies secondary to alcoholism, and autoimmune diseases. A variety of therapeutic drugs, industrial and agricultural toxins, and nutritional disorders (including malnutrition secondary to alcoholism) can cause polyneuropathy. In severe polyneuropathy, trophic changes (poor healing, ulceration of skin, neurogenic joint damage) often occur[11]; these changes probably occur because the person is unaware of injury to the part, owing to lack of sensation. Thus, education regarding monitoring and care of insensitive areas is vital. Therapists are likely to treat people with diabetic (metabolic) and Guillain-Barré (autoimmune) polyneuropathies.

In *diabetic polyneuropathy*, axons and myelin are damaged. Usually sensation is affected most severely, often in a stocking/glove distribution. All sizes of sensory axons are damaged (Figure 12-10), resulting in decreased sensation along with pain, paresthesias, and dysesthesias. Impaired vibration sense is often the first sign. Ankle reflexes are decreased. Loss of autonomic regulation of blood flow increases bone reabsorption, motor neuropathy causes abnormal stresses on joints, and lack of pain sensation often leads to damaged joints in the feet (Charcot foot; Figure 12-11) and to foot ulcers. Later in the disease process, muscle weakness and atrophy also tend to occur distally. Patients typically have difficulty walking on their heels but are able to walk on their toes.[12] All autonomic functions are susceptible to diabetic neuropathy: cardiovascular, gastrointestinal, genitourinary, and sweating dysfunction (lack of sweating distally, excessive compensatory sweating proximally) is common (Pathology 12-2). Unfortunately, physicians fail to diagnose peripheral neuropathy in approximately two thirds of mild to moderate cases and in one third of severe cases.[13]

Proper diabetic foot care, including regular sensory testing with monofilaments (see Chapter 7; Figure 12-12), wearing of appropriate shoes, regular self-inspection of the feet, and proper care of the skin and toenails, may prevent or forestall limb amputations in people with diabetes. The mean annual incidence of amputations in a London hospital has been reported as 18.9 per 10,000 subjects with diabetes.[14]

Balance and strength training reduces the risk of falls in people with diabetic neuropathy.[15] Gait and balance improve with exercise.[16] Owing to the risk of exercise-induced hypoglycemia or hyperglycemia, self-monitoring of blood glucose should be performed before, during, and after moderate to intense physical activity.[17] Glycemic control can limit the progression of diabetic neuropathy.[18] Painful diabetic neuropathy can be treated with pregabalin.[19]

Although the incidence of peripheral polyneuropathy is particularly high in people with diabetes, older people without diabetes also develop peripheral polyneuropathy. Among people over 60 years of age with polyneuropathy, no cause can be identified in 10% to 18%.[23]

The polyneuropathy in *Guillain-Barré syndrome* is characterized by more severe effects on the motor than the sensory system (see Pathology 2-1). Contrary to the pattern in most polyneuropathies, paresis may be worse proximally. Onset is rapid, with progressive paralysis, requiring urgent diagnosis and treatment to prevent respiratory failure. One third of Guillain-Barré patients require a ventilator.[24]

The most common inherited form of peripheral neuropathy is *hereditary motor and sensory neuropathy* (HMSN), also known as *Charcot-Marie-Tooth disease*. This disease generally causes paresis of muscles distal to the knee, with resulting foot drop,

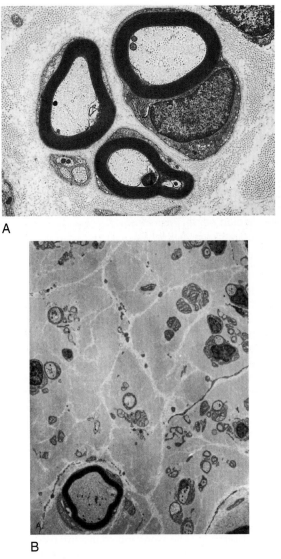

A

B

**Fig. 12-10  Sural nerve biopsies.** The sural nerve is often used for biopsies because it is a purely sensory nerve, thus the removal of a small section does not cause motor loss. **A,** Cross-section of normal nerve, with three myelinated axons (surrounded by darkly stained rings of myelin) and a small group of unmyelinated axons to the left of the bottom myelinated axon. **B,** Cross-section of a nerve with damage by diabetic neuropathy. All sizes of axons have been lost, only one myelinated fiber is present, and many axons have been replaced by collagen. *(From Richardson EP Jr, DeGirolami U: Pathology of the peripheral nerve, Philadelphia, 1995, WB Saunders, pp 5, 80.)*

a steppage gait, frequently tripping, and muscle atrophy (Figure 12-13). As the disease slowly progresses, muscle atrophy and paresis affect the hands. Despite the involvement of sensory neurons, significant numbness is unusual. Instead, ability to sense heat, cold, and painful stimuli is decreased. Neuropathic pain, a frequent complaint, probably is related to the loss of Aδ neurons.[25] Onset typically occurs in adolescence or in young adulthood, but this varies with the specific type of HMSN.

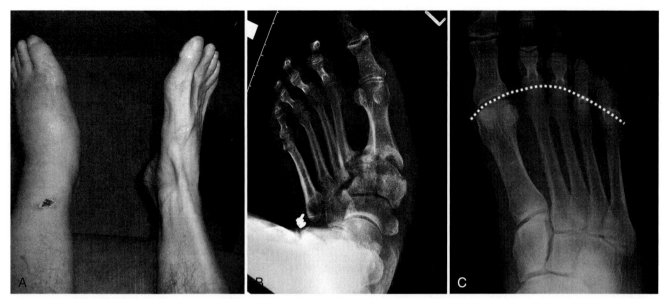

**Fig. 12-11 Charcot foot secondary to neuropathy.** Charcot foot comprises pathologic fracture, joint dislocation, and, if left untreated, disabling joint deformity. **A,** Appearance of Charcot foot on left side; compare with normal foot on right side. **B,** X-ray of Charcot foot on left, showing a shortened first metatarsal, a gap between the base of the first and second metatarsals, and midfoot swelling. **C,** Normal foot x-ray for comparison. (*A from Rogers LC, Bevilacqua NJ: The diagnosis of Charcot foot. Clin Podiatr Med Surg 25:43–51, 2008, Figure 1, p 44;* **B** *from Dreher T: Reconstruction of multiplanar deformity of the hindfoot and midfoot with internal fixation techniques. Foot Ankle Clin 14:489–531, 2009, Figure 22, p 324, panel A;* **C** *from Banerjee R, Nickisch F, Easley ME, et al: Foot injuries. In Browner BD, Levine, AM, editors: Skeletal Trauma, ed 4, Philadelphia, 2009, WB Saunders, Figure 61-82.)*

| PATHOLOGY 12-2 | DIABETIC POLYNEUROPATHY |
|---|---|
| Pathology | Demyelination and axon damage; abnormalities of ion channels impair nerve conduction[20] |
| Etiology | Metabolic |
| Speed of onset | Chronic |
| Signs and symptoms | Distal more involved than proximal |
| Consciousness | Normal |
| Communication and memory | Normal |
| Sensory | Numbness, pain, paresthesias (tingling, pins and needles), dysesthesias (burning, aching) |
| Autonomic | Orthostatic hypotension; impaired sweating; bowel, bladder, digestive, genital, pupil, and lacrimal dysfunction |
| Motor | Balance and coordination problems (secondary to sensory deficits); weakness |
| Cranial nerves | Usually normal; occasionally cranial nerve III is involved, producing drooping of upper eyelid and paresis of four muscles that move the eye to look up, down, and medially |
| Region affected | Peripheral |
| Demographics | Affects all ages; no gender predominance |
| Incidence | 72 per 100,000 population per year[21] |
| Lifetime prevalence | Approximately 8% of people in the United States have diabetes, and of those with diabetes, 60%–70% have diabetic neuropathy[22] |
| Prognosis | Stable or progressive; occasionally better control of blood sugar levels leads to improvement |

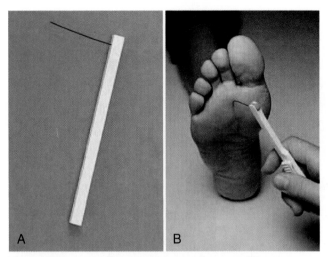

**Fig. 12-12 Monofilament testing. A,** Monofilament.
**B,** The tip of the filament is placed on the patient's skin,
and sufficient pressure is applied to bend the filament.
*(From Seidel HM, Ball  JW, Dains JE, et al. Mosby's Guide to Physical
Examination, ed 7. St. Louis, 2011, Mosby.)*

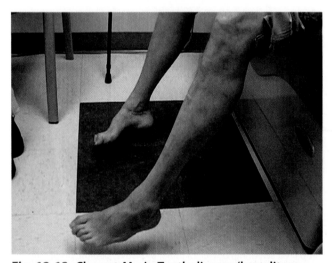

**Fig. 12-13 Charcot-Marie-Tooth disease (hereditary
motor and sensory neuropathy).** Foot deformities
include high arches and hammertoe deformity.
Hammertoe is flexion of the proximal interphalangeal
joint. *(From Pascuzzi RM: Peripheral neuropathy. Med Clin North Am
93:317–42, 2009.)*

Various types of HMSN are caused by different genetic mutations, which affect the production of different proteins essential
to the structure and function of peripheral axons or myelin
sheaths. The pattern of inheritance may be autosomal dominant, autosomal recessive, or X-linked (abnormal gene on the
X chromosome). Rarely HMSN results from a spontaneous
(nonhereditary) gene mutation. Prevalence is 1 per 1214
people.[26] Therapy involves strengthening, stretching, conditioning, and joint, muscle, and skin protection.

## DYSFUNCTIONS OF THE NEUROMUSCULAR JUNCTION

Two disorders that affect the neuromuscular junction have
similar effects. In myasthenia gravis, an autoimmune disease
that damages ACh receptors at the neuromuscular junction,
repeated use of a muscle leads to increasing weakness. In bot-
ulism, ingesting the botulinum toxin from improperly stored
foods causes interference with the release of ACh from the
motor axon. This produces acute, progressive weakness, with
loss of stretch reflexes. Sensation remains intact. Botulinum
toxin (Botox) is used therapeutically in people with spasticity
or dystonia, to weaken overactive muscles. Botox is injected
directly into overactive muscles and interferes with the release
of ACh at the neuromuscular junction and thus reduces
muscle contraction. Botox does not affect muscle contracture.
Botox injection frequently improves function by improving
the person's ability to control antagonistic and synergistic
muscles.

## MYOPATHY

Myopathies are disorders intrinsic to muscle. An example is
muscular dystrophy; random muscle fibers degenerate, leaving
motor units with fewer muscle fibers than normal. Activating
a muscle that lacks a significant number of muscle fibers produces less force than is produced by a healthy motor unit.
Because the nervous system is not affected by myopathy, sensation and autonomic function remain intact. Coordination,
muscle tone, and reflexes are unaffected until muscle atrophy
becomes so severe that muscle activity cannot be elicited.

## ELECTRODIAGNOSTIC STUDIES

Dysfunction of peripheral nerves and the muscles they innervate can be evaluated by electrodiagnostic studies. Recording of
electrical activity from nerves and muscles by nerve conduction
study (NCS) and EMG studies (see Chapters 7 and 11) reveals
the location of pathology and is often diagnostic. Nerve conduction studies can be used to differentiate the following:
- Processes that are primarily demyelinating (myelinopathy)
  and those that primarily damage axons (axonopathy).
  Myelinopathies produce marked slowing of velocity. Axonopathies produce decreases in the amplitude of nerve conduction potentials and may produce slowing of conduction
  velocity.
- Upper motor neuron and lower motor neuron paresis.
  Upper motor neuron lesions have no effect on peripheral
  nerve conduction, so NCS is normal. Lower motor neuron
  lesions produce abnormal NCS.
- Mononeuropathy and polyneuropathy
- Local conduction block and wallerian degeneration. Local
  conduction block interferes with nerve conduction only at
  one site, whereas wallerian degeneration affects the entire
  axon distal to the lesion.

Electromyography differentiates between nerve and muscle
disorders, thus distinguishing neuropathy from myopathy (see
Chapter 11).

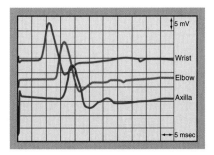

| | Latency (ms) | Amplitude (mV) | Distance (mm) | Velocity (m/s) |
|---|---|---|---|---|
| Recorded values: | | | | |
| Stimulated at wrist | 8.0 (distal) | 13.0 | | |
| Stimulated at elbow | 12.8 | 13.2 | 240 | 49.6 |
| Stimulated at axilla | 15.2 | 11.5 | 145 | 62.1 |
| Normal values for median nerve | Distal latency <4.2 | >5.0 | | >50 |

A

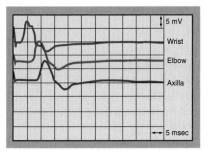

| | Latency (ms) | Amplitude (mV) | Distance (mm) | Velocity (m/s) |
|---|---|---|---|---|
| Recorded values: | | | | |
| Stimulated at wrist | 3.0 (distal) | 8.0 | | |
| Stimulated at elbow | 6.7 | 7.5 | 205 | 55.9 |
| Stimulated at axilla | 8.8 | 7.8 | 150 | 69.2 |
| Normal values for ulnar nerve | Distal latency <3.4 | >5.0 | | >49.5 |

B

**Fig. 12-14  Motor nerve conduction study. A,** Severe demyelination of the median nerve at the wrist. This is indicated by the 8.0 distal latency and the slow forearm conduction velocity, combined with normal amplitude of the recorded potential. **B,** Normal, ipsilateral ulnar nerve conduction study (NCS) in the same person. *(Courtesy Robert A. Sellin, PT.)*

The effect of myelinopathy on nerve conduction is to slow or stop conduction across the site of damage, with normal conduction in the axon segments proximal and distal to the injury (Figure 12-14). In axonopathy, axons lose their ability to conduct action potentials across the damaged site at the time of injury. Thus, the amplitude of the evoked potential is decreased (Figure 12-15). Nerve conduction velocity in the section of nerve distal to the injury gradually decreases over several days, eventually ceasing as a result of wallerian degeneration distal to the lesion. When a nerve is completely severed, nerve conduction may never return distal to the injury.

Generalized neuropathies (i.e., polyneuropathies) are characterized by slowed nerve conduction throughout the affected nerves and by decreased amplitude, particularly with increased distance between stimulation and recording sites. In myopathy, nerve conduction is normal, but the amplitude of the potential recorded from muscle is decreased.

## CLINICAL TESTING

Richardson (2002)[27] identified three clinical signs that detect peripheral neuropathy in outpatients 50 years of age and older.

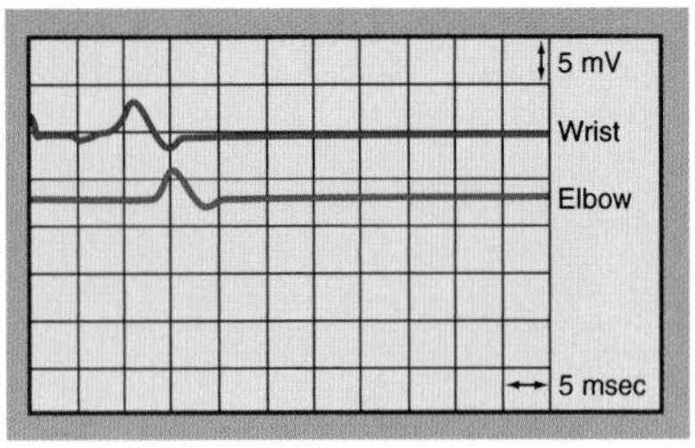

| | Latency (ms) | Amplitude (mV) | Distance (mm) | Velocity (m/s) |
|---|---|---|---|---|
| Recorded values: | | | | |
| Stimulated at wrist | 9.2 | 3.3 | | |
| Stimulated at elbow | 13.2 | 3.2 | 230 | 57.5 |
| Normal values for median nerve | Distal latency <4.2 | >5.0 | | >50 |

**Fig. 12-15** Median motor nerve conduction study, showing severely prolonged distal latency and a marked decrease in amplitude compared with normal. Conduction velocity between the wrist and the elbow is normal. *(Courtesy Robert A. Sellin, PT.)*

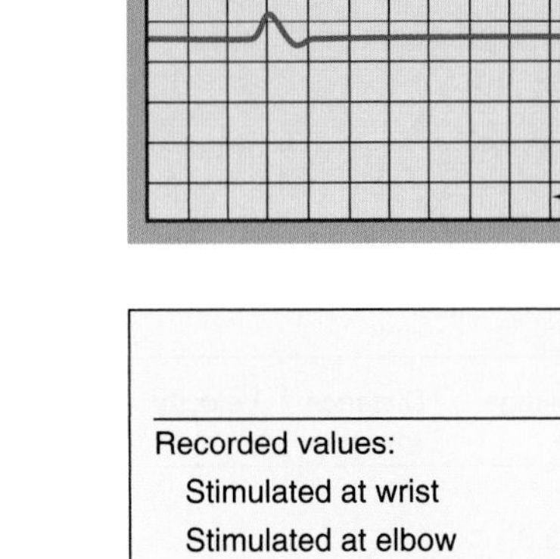

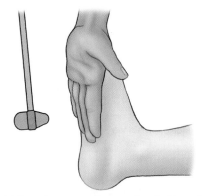

**Fig. 12-16 The plantar strike method of testing the ankle jerk reflex.** The patient is supine with the knees extended. The examiner places the dorsum of the hand against the sole of the patient's foot, passively dorsiflexes the foot, then strikes his or her own fingers with the reflex hammer.

The presence of two or three of these signs correlates highly with electrodiagnostic evidence of peripheral neuropathy. The three signs include absence of ankle jerk reflex despite facilitation, impaired vibration, and impaired position sense of the great toe. The ankle jerk was tested two ways: by striking the tendon, and by striking the plantar surface of the foot, as shown in Figure 12-16. Facilitation techniques for the ankle jerk reflex included having the patient gently plantarflex the foot, close the eyes tightly, or pull against the resistance of their own clasped hands just before the reflex hammer strike. For vibration testing, a 128 Hz tuning fork was struck; it was then placed until the patient reported that the vibration was gone. Sites tested, in order, included the clavicle, just proximal to the nail

bed of the index finger of the dominant upper limb, just proximal to the nail bed of each of the great toes, and at the medial malleolus. Position sense was tested on the dominant great toe. The examiner grasped the medial and lateral surfaces and flexed and extended the great toe. The patient's eyes were open for a few trials, then the patient closed the eyes and ten 1 second movements of approximately 1 cm were administered smoothly. Results indicating peripheral neuropathy included absence of the ankle jerk reflex despite facilitation, decreased vibration sense at the great toe (vibration perceived for less than 8 seconds), and decreased position sense at the toe (correct perception less than 8 times in 10 trials).

## EVALUATION AND INTERVENTION

### Evaluation

As the severity of peripheral neuropathy increases, so do reports of pins and needles sensation.[12] Sensory, autonomic, and motor functions are evaluated as indicated in their respective chapters (see Chapters 7, 9, and 11). Signs of peripheral nervous system damage result from hypoactivity or hyperactivity of neurons. For example, neuronal hypoactivity, a decrease or loss of neuronal activity, may produce loss of proprioception. An example of neuronal hyperactivity is light touch eliciting a painful sensation.

Table 12-3 lists the signs and symptoms of mononeuropathy. In polyneuropathy, the same characteristics are found but in a symmetric distribution, sometimes with additional autonomic signs including postural hypotension, bowel or bladder incontinence, and inability to have a sexual erection.

Clinically, making the distinction between peripheral neuropathy and central nervous system dysfunction is vital. Table 12-4 indicates factors that differentiate peripheral from central nervous system lesions.

**TABLE 12-3**   SIGNS AND SYMPTOMS OF MONONEUROPATHY

|  | Neuronal Hypoactivity | Neuronal Hyperactivity |
|---|---|---|
| Sensory | Decrease or lack of sensation (touch, pressure, proprioception, or pain) | Pain, dysesthesia, allodynia, hyperesthesia |
| Autonomic | Flushing of skin, edema, lack of sweating | Vasoconstriction: cold skin, pallor, cyanosis (dark blue color of skin); excessive sweating; perpetuation of pain in early stage complex regional pain syndrome (see Chapter 9) |
| Motor | Paresis, paralysis, hypotonia, muscle atrophy | Spasms, muscle fasciculations and/or fibrillations |
| Reflexes | Decreased or absent | Normal |

**TABLE 12-4**   DISTINGUISHING PERIPHERAL FROM CENTRAL NERVOUS SYSTEM DYSFUNCTION

|  | Peripheral Nervous System | Central Nervous System |
|---|---|---|
| Distribution of signs and symptoms | Peripheral nerve pattern | Dermatomal or myotomal pattern |
| Nerve conduction study | Slowed or blocked conduction; decreased amplitude of recorded potentials | Normal |
| Muscle tone | If lower motor neuron involvement, hypotonia | If upper motor neuron involvement, hypertonia |
| Muscle atrophy | Rapid muscle atrophy indicates denervation | Muscle atrophy progresses slowly |
| Phasic stretch reflexes | Reduced or absent | Hyperactive or normal |
| Paraspinal sensation and/or paraspinal muscles | Normal | Involved |

## Interventions for Peripheral Neuropathy

Results of sensory, manual muscle, and, if indicated, electrodiagnostic testing guide treatment decisions. Education is necessary to prevent complications from damage due to lack of sensation, disuse, or overuse. The person with peripheral neuropathy that affects sensation should be taught to visually inspect the involved areas daily, using mirrors if necessary, and to monitor for wounds and for reddening of the skin that persists longer than a few minutes. If the feet are involved, proper foot care should be taught. Interventions for edema include elevation of the limb, compression bandaging with an elastic wrap, and electrical stimulation.

Endurance exercise following a peripheral nerve crush injury has been demonstrated to enhance both sensory and motor recovery; resistance training or a combination of resistance and endurance training may delay functional recovery.[28] Exercises should emphasize gradual strengthening and the functional use of individual muscles and muscle groups. Orthoses (braces) are frequently used to stabilize weight-bearing joints, thus preventing sprains and strains, and to prevent dropping of the forefoot during gait in cases of paresis or paralysis of the tibialis anterior muscle. Orthoses are also used to prevent deformities that can result from paresis, paralysis, and lack of sensation. Use of electrical stimulation to prevent atrophy of denervated muscles by evoking muscle contractions may be beneficial.[29]

## SUMMARY

Somatic peripheral nerves convey signals between sensory receptors and the central nervous system, and between the central nervous system and skeletal muscles and autonomic effectors. Somatic peripheral nerves consist of axons, connective tissue, and sensory endings. Peripheral nerve lesions produce signs and symptoms in a peripheral nerve distribution. In contrast, spinal region lesions produce signs and symptoms in a myotomal and/or dermatomal distribution. When peripheral nerves are stretched, axons unwrinkle, connective tissue tubes extend, fascicles glide relative to each other, fascicular plexuses share the loading, and the entire nerve slides relative to surrounding tissues. Normal stretching and shortening of nerves facilitates blood and axoplasm flow, contributing to the health of peripheral nerves.

Mononeuropathy results when excessive mechanical stimuli damage peripheral nerves by compromising blood flow and axonal transport, causing edema and eventual thickening of certain connective tissues, leading to myelin damage, development of ectopic foci, and decreased nerve conduction velocity. Polyneuropathy is symmetric damage to peripheral nerves. Examples include diabetic polyneuropathy, Guillain-Barré syndrome, and hereditary motor and sensory neuropathy (HMSN). Electrodiagnostic studies are useful for evaluating neuropathy and may be used to distinguish neuropathy from myopathy.

## CLINICAL NOTES

### Case 1

R.V. is a 35-year-old man who was brought to the emergency room by a friend 2 days ago. At admission to the hospital, R.V. complained of aching, burning pain in his thighs, and a feeling of weakness that began 2 days before admission. He has no history of trauma. His current condition is as follows:

- He is unable to communicate, so sensation and cognitive functions cannot be tested.
- He is subject to abnormal variations in blood pressure and heart rate.
- He is completely paralyzed. His breathing is maintained by a respirator.
- Nerve conduction velocity is markedly slowed bilaterally in the tested nerves—the median and tibial nerves. Amplitude of recorded potentials is normal.

#### Question

What is the location of the lesion(s) and the probable etiology?

### Case 2

A 16-year-old woman was injured 2 days ago when a load of lumber fell from a shelf, pinning her left forearm. The following signs and symptoms are noted on her left side:

- She does not feel pinprick, touch, temperature differences, or vibration on the medial hand, little finger, and medial half of the ring finger.
- Sweating is absent in the same distribution as the sensory loss.
- Radial wrist extension and flexion and finger extension are normal strength on manual muscle tests.
- She is unable to flex the middle and distal phalanges of the fourth and fifth digits, abduct or adduct her fingers, or adduct the hand.

#### Questions

1. What is the location of the lesion(s)?
2. How could the probable rate of recovery be predicted?

### Case 3

A 7-year-old boy has progressive proximal muscle weakness. Clinical examination and electrodiagnostic tests reveal the following:

- Sensation and coordination are within normal limits.
- He falls twice when walking 100 feet.
- He has difficulty coming to standing and climbing stairs.
- Lumbar lordosis is increased.
- Manual muscle tests indicate that shoulder girdle and hip muscles are approximately 50% of normal strength, knee and elbow muscles are about 75% of normal strength, and distal muscles have near-normal strength.
- Velocity of nerve conduction is normal.
- Electromyographic potentials recorded from hip girdle muscles are of small amplitude.

#### Question

What is the location of the lesion(s) and the probable etiology?

### Case 4

A 22-year-old man sprained his ankle last week and during the physical therapy history mentioned that his ankles seem to gradually be getting weaker. He reported difficulty walking on uneven ground and in the dark. Examination revealed the following:

- Manual muscle tests bilaterally normal for muscles of the hips and knees. Unable to walk on heels; ankle dorsiflexion 4–/5 bilaterally. Unable to rise on toes. All foot intrinsic muscles weak. Upper limb normal strength except 4/5 finger extension and finger abduction
- Observation: hammer toes (flexion contractures affecting the proximal interphalangeal joint of all toes) and high arches both feet
- Pinprick: normal in all tested digits (digits 1, 3, and 5 of both hands and feet). Vibration (128 Hz tuning fork): absent bilaterally at hallux interphalangeal joint and first metatarsal head, present for 4 seconds over medial malleoli. Normal bilaterally at distal interphalangeal joint of the index fingers and at the ulnar styloid process. Proprioception: at toes, unable to detect position or movement direction accurately; ankles, 75% accuracy regarding position, able to detect direction of passive movements greater than 5 degrees accurately; knee and upper limb proprioception normal
- Steppage gait (high stepping to clear mild drop foot)
- Phasic stretch reflexes cannot be elicited with Achilles tendon tap, quadriceps tendon tap, or brachioradialis tendon tap. Trace phasic stretch reflexes can be elicited with biceps tendon tap.

#### Questions

1. What is the location of the lesion(s)?
2. What is the probable diagnosis? What is the next step for the patient?

## REVIEW QUESTIONS

1. What mechanisms allow peripheral nerves to lengthen and shorten without injury?
2. What signs are produced by complete severance of a peripheral nerve?
3. List the trophic changes that occur in denervated tissues.
4. Give an example of a myelinopathy. What part of the nerve is damaged in a myelinopathy? Describe the sequence of events that produces a compression mononeuropathy.
5. Describe an axonopathy.
6. Why is the prognosis for a severed nerve poor?
7. What is multiple mononeuropathy?
8. What are the most common causes of polyneuropathy?
9. Why do the signs and symptoms of polyneuropathy usually appear distally first?
10. How can myelinopathy be distinguished from axonopathy?
11. How can neuropathy be distinguished from myopathy?
12. Classify each of the following signs as resulting from neuronal hyperactivity or hypoactivity: absent reflexes, muscle spasms, lack of sweating, paralysis, muscle fasciculations, and cyanosis of the skin.
13. Sensory loss in a dermatomal pattern, normal NCS, muscle hypertonia, and slowly progressive muscle atrophy that includes the paraspinal muscles are indicative of lesions in what region of the nervous system?
14. What are the signs and symptoms of diabetic polyneuropathy?

## References

1. Dilley A, Lynn B, Greening J, DeLeon N: Quantitative in vivo studies of median nerve sliding in response to wrist, elbow, shoulder and neck movements. *Clin Biomech (Bristol, Avon)* 18:899–907, 2003.
2. Topp KS, Boyd BS: Structure and biomechanics of peripheral nerves: nerve responses to physical stresses and implications for physical therapist practice. *Phys Ther* 86:92–109, 2006.
3. Rempel DM, Diao E: Entrapment neuropathies: pathophysiology and pathogenesis. *J Electromyogr Kinesiol* 14:71–75, 2004.
4. Foti C, Romita P, Vestita M: Unusual presentation of carpal tunnel syndrome with cutaneous signs: a case report and review of the literature. *Immunopharmacol Immunotoxicol* 2011 February 14. [Epub ahead of print]
5. Devor M: Ectopic discharge in Abeta afferents as a source of neuropathic pain. *Exp Brain Res* 196:115–128, 2009.
6. Conolly WB, McKessar JH: Carpal tunnel syndrome—can it be a work related condition? *Aust Fam Physician* 38:684–686, 2009.
7. Leblanc KE, Cestia W: Carpal tunnel syndrome. *Am Fam Physician* 83:952–958, 2011.
8. Shi Q, MacDermid JC: Is surgical intervention more effective than non-surgical treatment for carpal tunnel syndrome? A systematic review. *J Orthop Surg Res* 6:17,1–9, 2011.
9. Jarvik JG, Comstock BA, Kliot M, et al: Surgery versus non-surgical therapy for carpal tunnel syndrome: a randomised parallel-group trial. *Lancet* 374:1074–1081, 2009.
10. England JD, Asbury AK: Peripheral neuropathy. *Lancet* 363:2151–2161, 2004.
11. Vanderhoff BT, Carroll W: Neurology. In RE Rakel: *Textbook of family medicine*, ed 7, Philadelphia, 2007, Elsevier.
12. Costa LA, Maraschin JF, Xavier de Castro JH, et al: A simplified protocol to screen for distal polyneuropathy in type 2 diabetic patients. *Diabetes Res Clin Pract* 73:292–297, 2006.
13. Herman WH, Kennedy L: Underdiagnosis of peripheral neuropathy in type 2 diabetes. *Diabetes Care* 28:1480–1481, 2005.
14. Valabhji J, Gibbs RG, Bloomfield L, et al: Matching the numerator with an appropriate denominator to demonstrate low amputation incidence associated with a London hospital multidisciplinary diabetic foot clinic. *Diabet Med* 27:1304–1307, 2010.
15. Morrison S, Colberg SR, Mariano M, et al: Balance training reduces falls risk in older individuals with type 2 diabetes. *Diabetes Care* 33:748–750, 2010.
16. Allet L, Armand S, de Bie RA, et al: The gait and balance of patients with diabetes can be improved: a randomised controlled trial. *Diabetologia* 53:458–466, 2010.
17. Riddell M, Perkins BA: Exercise and glucose metabolism in persons with diabetes mellitus: perspectives on the role for continuous glucose monitoring. *J Diabetes Sci Technol* 3:914–923, 2009.
18. Habib AA, Brannagan TH 3rd: Therapeutic strategies for diabetic neuropathy. *Curr Neurol Neurosci Rep* 10:92–100, 2010.
19. Freeman R, Durso-Decruz E, Emir B: Efficacy, safety, and tolerability of pregabalin treatment for painful diabetic peripheral neuropathy: findings from seven randomized, controlled trials across a range of doses. *Diabetes Care* 31:1448–1454, 2008.
20. Tomlinson DR, Gardiner NJ: Diabetic neuropathies: components of etiology. *J Periph Nerv Syst* 13:112–121, 2008.
21. Dieleman JP, Kerklaan J, Huygen FJ, et al: Incidence rates and treatment of neuropathic pain conditions in the general population. *Pain* 137:681–688, 2008.
22. Centers for Disease Control and Prevention: *National diabetes fact sheet: national estimates and general information on diabetes and prediabetes in the United States, 2011*, Atlanta, Ga, 2011, U.S. Department of Health and Human Services.
23. Erdmann PG, Teunissen LL, van Genderen FR, et al: Functioning of patients with chronic idiopathic axonal polyneuropathy (CIAP). *J Neurol* 254:1204–1211, 2007.
24. Pascuzzi RM: Peripheral neuropathy. *Med Clin North Am* 93:317–342, 2009.
25. Pazzaglia C, Vollono C, Ferraro D, et al: Mechanisms of neuropathic pain in patients with Charcot-Marie-Tooth 1 A: a laser-evoked potential study. *Pain* 149:379–385, 2010.
26. Braathen GJ, Sand JC, Lobato A, et al: Genetic epidemiology of Charcot-Marie-Tooth in the general population. *Eur J Neurol* 18:39–48, 2011.
27. Richardson JK: The clinical identification of peripheral neuropathy among older persons. *Arch Phys Med Rehabil* 83:1553–1558, 2002.
28. Ilha J, Araujo RT, Malysz T, et al: Endurance and resistance exercise training programs elicit specific effects on sciatic nerve regeneration after experimental traumatic lesion in rats. *Neurorehabil Neural Repair* 22:355–366, 2008.
29. Salmons S, Jarvis JC: Functional electrical stimulation of denervated muscles: an experimental evaluation. *Artif Organs* 32:597–603, 2008.

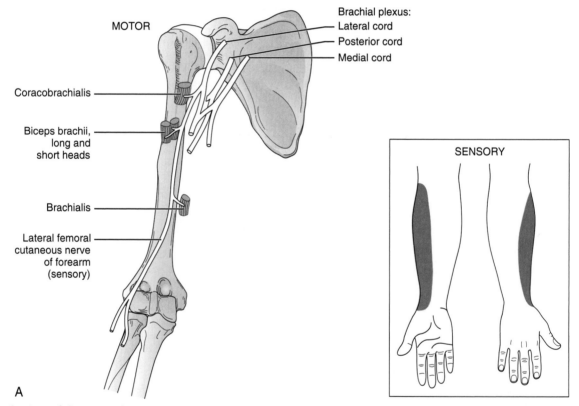

**A,** Distribution of the musculocutaneous nerve. *(From Jenkins DB: Hollinshead's functional anatomy of the limbs and back, ed 9, Philadelphia, 2009, WB Saunders.)*

# MEDIAN NERVE

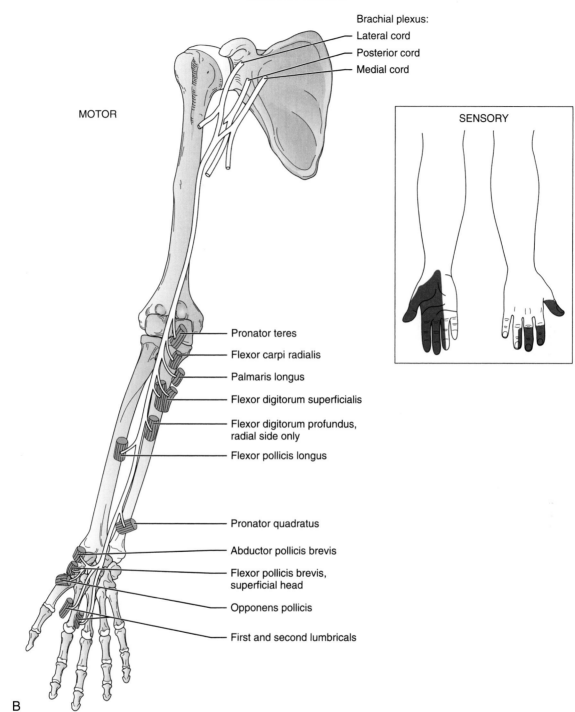

**Brachial plexus:**
Lateral cord
Posterior cord
Medial cord

MOTOR

SENSORY

Pronator teres

Flexor carpi radialis

Palmaris longus

Flexor digitorum superficialis

Flexor digitorum profundus,
radial side only

Flexor pollicis longus

Pronator quadratus

Abductor pollicis brevis

Flexor pollicis brevis,
superficial head

Opponens pollicis

First and second lumbricals

B

**B,** Distribution of the median nerve. *(From Jenkins DB: Hollinshead's functional anatomy of the limbs and back, ed 9, Philadelphia, 2009, WB Saunders.)*

# ULNAR NERVE

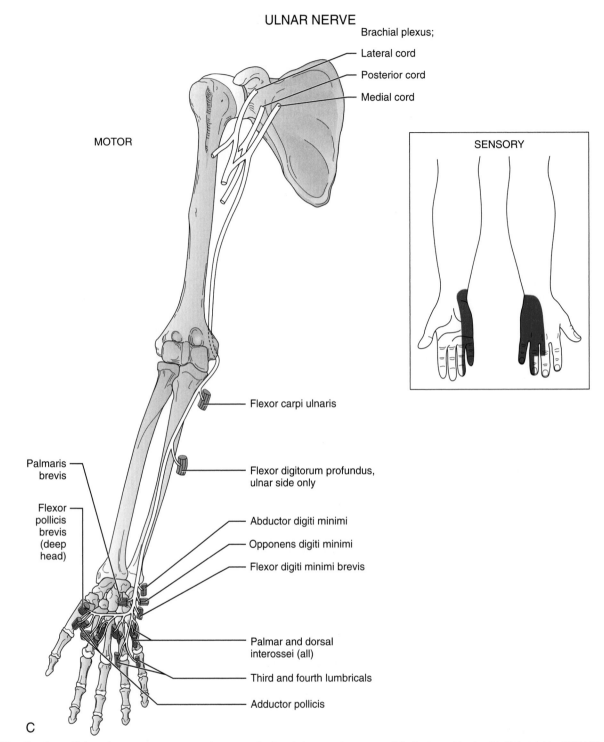

**C,** Distribution of the ulnar nerve. *(From Jenkins DB: Hollinshead's functional anatomy of the limbs and back, ed 9, Philadelphia, 2009, WB Saunders.)*

## RADIAL/AXILLARY NERVES

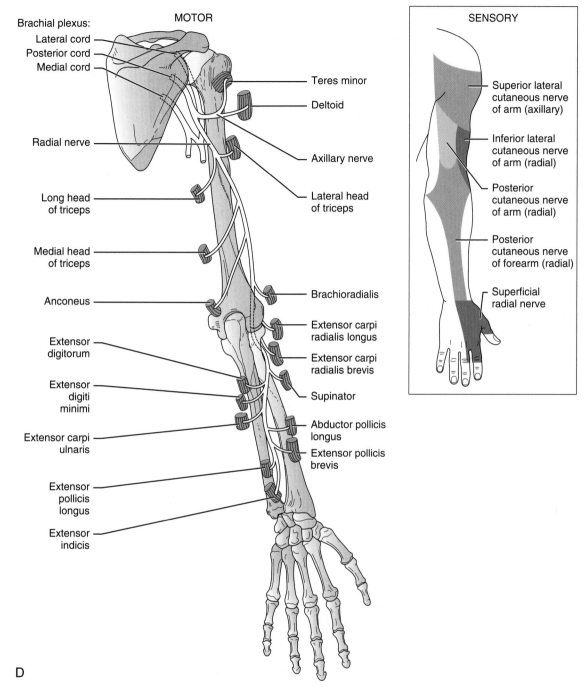

MOTOR

Brachial plexus:
Lateral cord
Posterior cord
Medial cord

Radial nerve

Long head
of triceps

Medial head
of triceps

Anconeus

Extensor
digitorum

Extensor
digiti
minimi

Extensor carpi
ulnaris

Extensor
pollicis
longus

Extensor
indicis

Teres minor

Deltoid

Axillary nerve

Lateral head
of triceps

Brachioradialis

Extensor carpi
radialis longus

Extensor carpi
radialis brevis

Supinator

Abductor pollicis
longus

Extensor pollicis
brevis

SENSORY

Superior lateral
cutaneous nerve
of arm (axillary)

Inferior lateral
cutaneous nerve
of arm (radial)

Posterior
cutaneous nerve
of arm (radial)

Posterior
cutaneous nerve
of forearm (radial)

Superficial
radial nerve

D

**D,** Distribution of the radial and axillary nerves. *(From Jenkins DB: Hollinshead's functional anatomy of the limbs and back, ed 9, Philadelphia, 2009, WB Saunders.)*

# Distribution of Nerves in the Lower Limbs

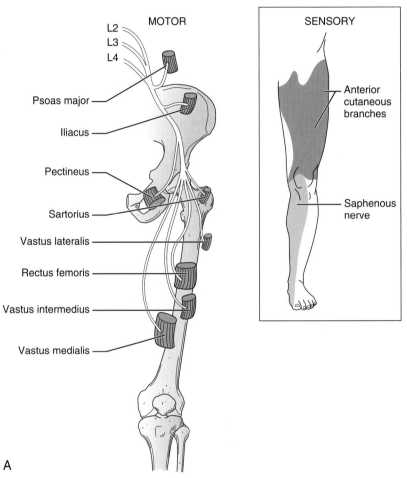

**A,** Distribution of the femoral nerve. *(From Jenkins DB: Hollinshead's functional anatomy of the limbs and back, ed 9, Philadelphia, 2009, WB Saunders.)*

## COMMON FIBULAR NERVE

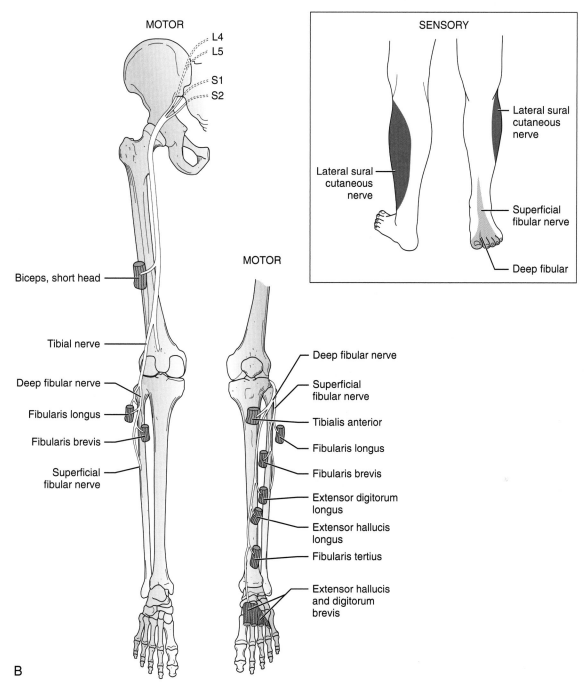

**B,** Distribution of the common fibular nerve. *(From Jenkins DB: Hollinshead's functional anatomy of the limbs and back, ed 9, Philadelphia, 2009, WB Saunders.)*

## OBTURATOR NERVE

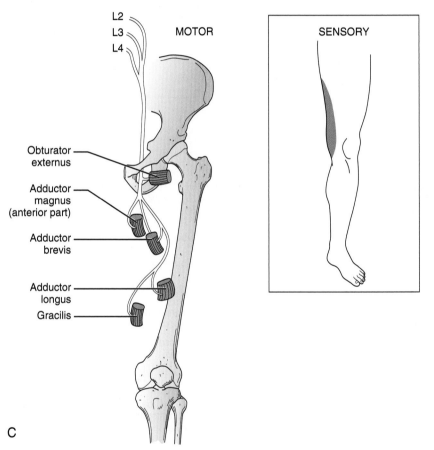

**C,** Distribution of the obturator nerve. *(From Jenkins DB: Hollinshead's functional anatomy of the limbs and back, ed 9, Philadelphia, 2009, WB Saunders.)*

# TIBIAL NERVE

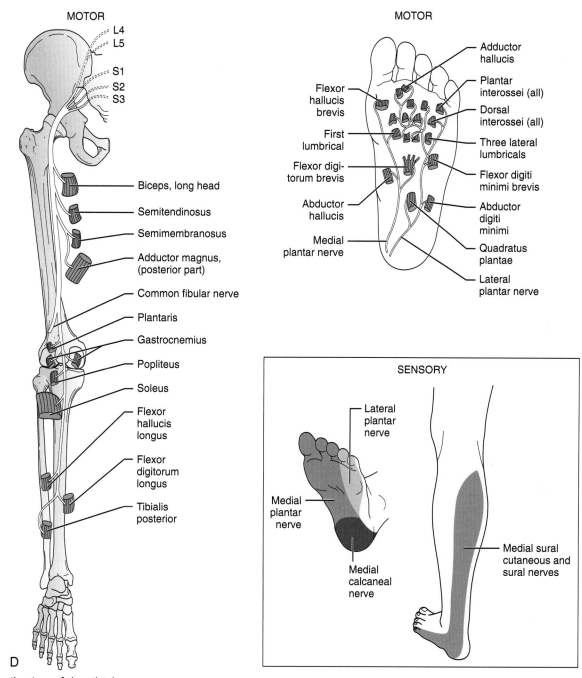

MOTOR

L4
L5

S1
S2
S3

- Biceps, long head
- Semitendinosus
- Semimembranosus
- Adductor magnus, (posterior part)
- Common fibular nerve
- Plantaris
- Gastrocnemius
- Popliteus
- Soleus
- Flexor hallucis longus
- Flexor digitorum longus
- Tibialis posterior

MOTOR

- Adductor hallucis
- Plantar interossei (all)
- Dorsal interossei (all)
- Three lateral lumbricals
- Flexor digiti minimi brevis
- Abductor digiti minimi
- Quadratus plantae
- Lateral plantar nerve

Flexor hallucis brevis
First lumbrical
Flexor digitorum brevis
Abductor hallucis
Medial plantar nerve

SENSORY

Lateral plantar nerve
Medial plantar nerve
Medial calcaneal nerve
Medial sural cutaneous and sural nerves

D

**D,** Distribution of the tibial nerve. *(From Jenkins DB: Hollinshead's functional anatomy of the limbs and back, ed 9, Philadelphia, 2009, WB Saunders.)*

# 13 Spinal Region

**Laurie Lundy-Ekman, PhD, PT**

Five years ago, I had an accident. I recall the doctor saying afterwards: "You have a spinal cord injury, a thoracic 7 lesion, but you can manage yourself in the future."

The last part was most important, since I have two children. What the doctor didn't tell me was how to achieve independence and how to return to a normal life. I am a physical therapist, and my specialty was in treating the neurologic problems of children. I am a pioneer in this field in the Netherlands, and for the past 25 years I have worked with handicapped children in their daily situations.

I left the rehabilitation center after 9 months of therapy and training. It could have been earlier, but my home was not ready for my return. Some things needed to be adapted and made accessible to me from my wheelchair. I have a car that my work paid to have adapted for hand control. I can organize all the daily things in life for me and my children. We are a good team.

Now, I had to work for a new life for myself. Because of my profession and my specialty, I was able to return to my job after only about 6 months. Part of my job involved my own physical therapy practice, and the other part was working as an instructor/senior tutor for children with cerebral palsy. Due to my injury, I sold my physical therapy practice and began teaching, from my wheelchair, at a physical therapy school. In this surrounding, nobody noticed the wheelchair; I was just myself.

Now it has been 5 years, and sometimes I think to myself: "What is different?" I can do all the things I want and enjoy. I cannot walk, and sometimes I have a lot of pain. Once I spilled hot tea on my stomach and burned myself quite severely without realizing it until later. Because I lack sensation in my abdomen and legs, I did not become aware of the burn until I saw blisters on my skin. But I am happy in my wheelchair and I am happy with my son (18) and my daughter (16). The doctor was right. It is a hard and long way to come, but it is possible.

Last year, while visiting the United States, I learned how to catheterize my bladder while remaining sitting in my wheelchair. This was very important to my independence. Now I can go anywhere and not need special equipment. This year I went to the United States for my work and was driving a car on the interstate. I thought to myself, "It really is true; you can do almost anything if you have friends and your own desires." When I use the terms *impairment, disability,* and *handicap,* I can say that I am not handicapped.

I use no medications. I can deal with the spasticity very well, since for 25 years in my profession I worked with spasticity in other people. I control the spasticity by using slow stretch, correct foot and leg positioning, prolonged positions, and making sure to empty my bladder on schedule. My professional knowledge helped me a lot, but on the other hand I am now a patient and sometimes need the guidance of professionals.

—*Tineke Dirks*

## ANATOMY OF THE SPINAL REGION

The spinal region includes all neural structures contained within the vertebrae: spinal cord, dorsal and ventral roots, spinal nerves, and meninges (Figure 13-1). Lateral enlargements of the cord at the cervical and lumbosacral levels accommodate the neurons for upper and lower limb innervation. The spinal cord is continuous with the medulla and ends at the L1-L2 intervertebral space in adults (Figure 13-2). Table 13-1 lists the correspondence between spinal cord segments and vertebrae in adults.

Inferior to the end of the spinal cord is the *filum terminale,* a bundle of connective tissue and glia that connects the end of the cord to the coccyx. Because the spinal cord is not present below the L1 vertebral level, long roots are required for axons from the termination of the cord to exit the lumbosacral vertebral column. These long roots form the cauda equina within the lower vertebral canal (Figure 13-3).

**TABLE 13-1   ANATOMIC RELATIONSHIP BETWEEN SPINAL CORD SEGMENTS AND VERTEBRAE IN ADULTS**

| Spinal Cord Segment | Vertebral Bodies | Bony Spinous Process |
| --- | --- | --- |
| C8 | C6-7 | C6 |
| T1 | C7-T1 | T3 |
| T12 | T10-11 | T8 |
| L5 | T12-L1 | T10 |
| S | L1-2 | T12, L1 |

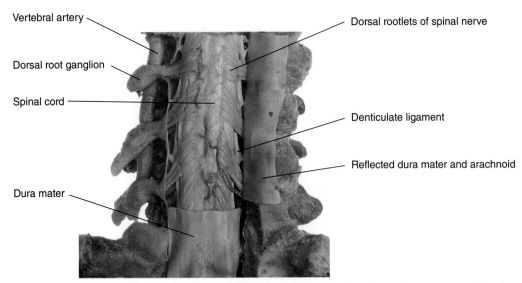

**Fig. 13-1 Posterior view of part of cervical spinal region.** The vertebral arches have been removed and part of the dura and arachnoid have been reflected. *(With permission from Abrahams PH, Marks SC, Hutchings R: McMinn's color atlas of human anatomy, ed 6, Philadelphia, 2008, Mosby.)*

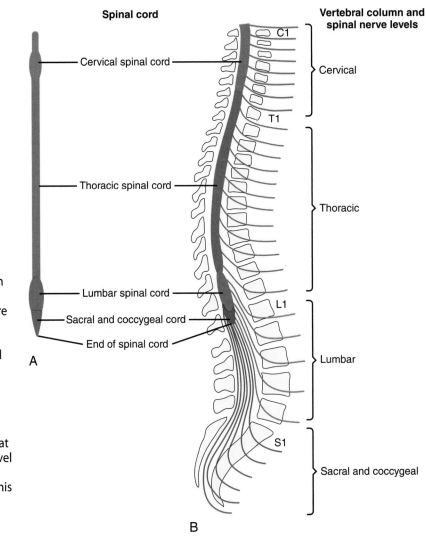

**Fig. 13-2 Relationship of spinal cord segments to the vertebral column. A,** An anterior view of the spinal cord. **B,** Spinal cord segment levels (neurologic levels) are indicated on the left. Vertebral levels and spinal nerves are indicated on the right. Spinal nerves are named for the vertebral level where they exit the vertebral canal. The spinal cord ends at the L2 vertebral level. Because the spinal cord is significantly shorter than the vertebral column, only at C1 and C2 are the spinal cord segment levels and vertebral levels at the same level. The L2-S5 nerve roots travel downward below the end of the spinal cord before exiting the vertebral canal. This collection of nerve roots inferior to the spinal cord within the bony canal is the cauda equina.

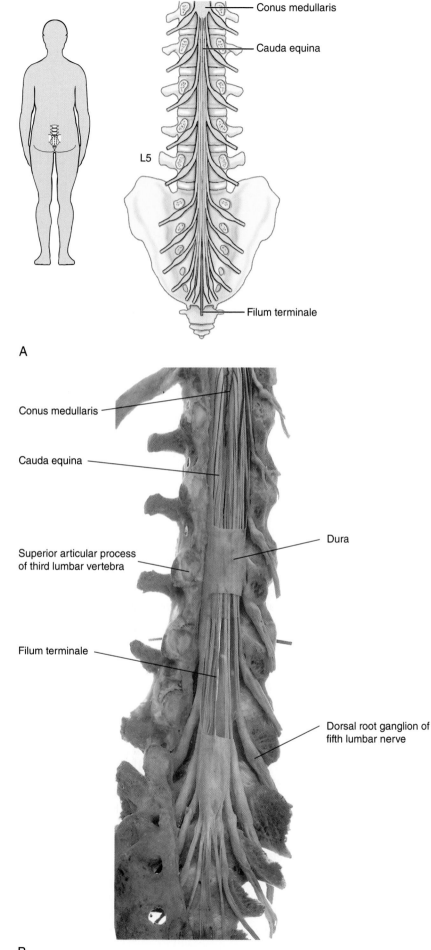

Conus medullaris

Cauda equina

L5

Filum terminale

A

Conus medullaris

Cauda equina

Superior articular process
of third lumbar vertebra

Filum terminale

Dura

Dorsal root ganglion of
fifth lumbar nerve

B

**Fig. 13-3 Cauda equina. A,** Dorsal
view of the cauda equina in relationship
to the vertebral column. Note the end
of the spinal cord (conus medullaris)
at the L1-L2 intervertebral space.
**B,** Vertebral arches and part of the dura
and arachnoid have been removed to
reveal the cauda equina. *(B with permission
from Abrahams PH, Marks SC, Hutchings R: McMinn's
color atlas of human anatomy, ed 6, Philadelphia,
2008, Mosby.)*

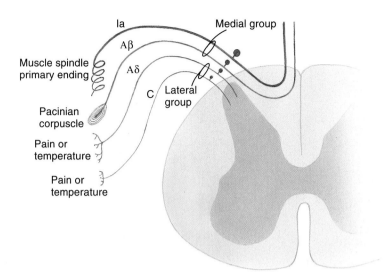

**Fig. 13-4** In the dorsal root entry zone, axons conveying information from touch and proprioceptive receptors enter the cord medially, and axons carrying information about tissue damage or threat to tissue and temperature enter the cord laterally.

Vertical grooves mark the external spinal cord. The anterior cord has a deep median fissure, and the posterior cord has a shallow median sulcus. The anterior cord also has two anterolateral sulci, where nerve rootlets emerge from the cord. The posterior cord has two posterolateral sulci, where nerve rootlets enter the cord.

## Ventral and Dorsal Roots

Axons sending information to the periphery (motor) leave the anterolateral cord in small groups called *rootlets*. Ventral rootlets from a single segment coalesce to form a *ventral root*. The *dorsal root* contains sensory axons that bring information into the spinal cord and enters the posterolateral spinal cord via rootlets. Unlike the ventral roots, each dorsal root has a *dorsal root ganglion* located outside the spinal cord. The dorsal root ganglion contains the cell bodies of sensory neurons. Where sensory axons enter the spinal cord, the large-diameter fibers, transmitting proprioceptive and touch information, are located medially, and the small-diameter fibers, transmitting pain and temperature information, are located laterally (Figure 13-4).

The dorsal and ventral roots join briefly to form a *spinal nerve*. The spinal nerve is a mixed nerve because it contains both sensory and motor axons. Spinal nerves are located in the intervertebral foramen.

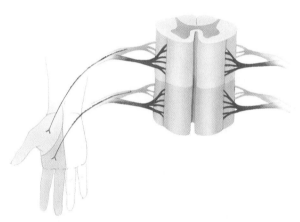

**Fig. 13-5 Two segments of the spinal cord.** Axons traveling through the rootlets, roots, and spinal nerves connect a spinal segment with a specific part of the body. The axons shown are sensory axons, conveying information from the C6 and C7 dermatomes through the dorsal root into the C6 and C7 spinal cord segments.

> ### ◎ Clinical Pearl
>
> The ventral root contains motor axons. The dorsal root contains sensory neurons. The somas of sensory neurons are found in the dorsal root ganglion. The spinal nerve consists of all sensory and motor axons connected with a single segment of the cord.

## Segments of the Spinal Cord

A striking and significant feature of the spinal cord is *segmental organization*. Each segment of the cord is connected to a specific region of the body by axons traveling through a pair of

spinal nerves. The connections of nerve rootlets to the exterior of the cord indicate the segments (Figure 13-5). Segments are identified by the same designation as their corresponding spinal nerves. For example, the term *L4 spinal segment* refers to the section of the cord whose spinal nerve traverses the L4 intervertebral foramen. However, within the cord, distinct segments are not evident because the cord consists of continuous vertical columns extending from the brain to the cord termination.

## Spinal Nerves and Rami

*Spinal nerves* are unique in that they carry all of the motor and sensory axons of a single spinal segment. In the cervical region, spinal nerves are found above the corresponding vertebra, except for the eighth spinal nerve, which emerges between the

**Spinal nerve innervation of skeletal muscles**

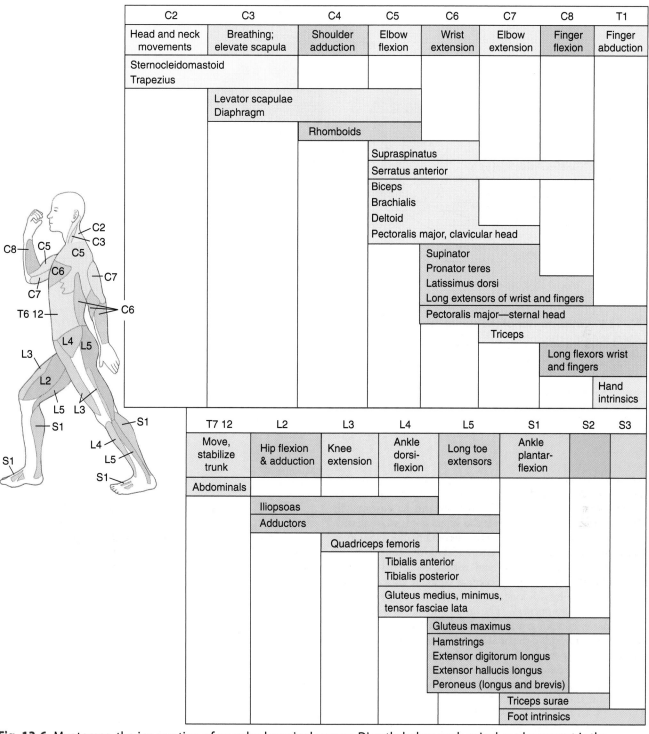

| C2 | C3 | C4 | C5 | C6 | C7 | C8 | T1 |
|---|---|---|---|---|---|---|---|
| Head and neck movements | Breathing; elevate scapula | Shoulder adduction | Elbow flexion | Wrist extension | Elbow extension | Finger flexion | Finger abduction |

Sternocleidomastoid
Trapezius

Levator scapulae
Diaphragm

Rhomboids

Supraspinatus

Serratus anterior

Biceps
Brachialis
Deltoid
Pectoralis major, clavicular head

Supinator
Pronator teres
Latissimus dorsi
Long extensors of wrist and fingers

Pectoralis major—sternal head

Triceps

Long flexors wrist and fingers

Hand intrinsics

| T7 12 | L2 | L3 | L4 | L5 | S1 | S2 | S3 |
|---|---|---|---|---|---|---|---|
| Move, stabilize trunk | Hip flexion & adduction | Knee extension | Ankle dorsi-flexion | Long toe extensors | Ankle plantar-flexion | | |

Abdominals

Iliopsoas

Adductors

Quadriceps femoris

Tibialis anterior
Tibialis posterior

Gluteus medius, minimus, tensor fasciae lata

Gluteus maximus

Hamstrings
Extensor digitorum longus
Extensor hallucis longus
Peroneus (longus and brevis)

Triceps surae

Foot intrinsics

**Fig. 13-6** Myotomes, the innervation of muscles by spinal nerves. Directly below each spinal cord segment is the movement associated with that segment.

C7 and T1 vertebrae. In the remainder of the cord, spinal nerves lie below the corresponding vertebra. Spinal nerve innervation of muscles in the upper and lower limbs is summarized in Figure 13-6.

After a brief transit through the intervertebral foramen, the spinal nerve splits into two rami; this division marks the end of the spinal region and the beginning of the peripheral nervous system. The dorsal rami innervate the paravertebral muscles, posterior parts of the vertebrae, and overlying cutaneous areas. The ventral rami innervate the skeletal, muscular, and cutaneous areas of the limbs and of the anterior and lateral trunk. Both rami are mixed nerves.

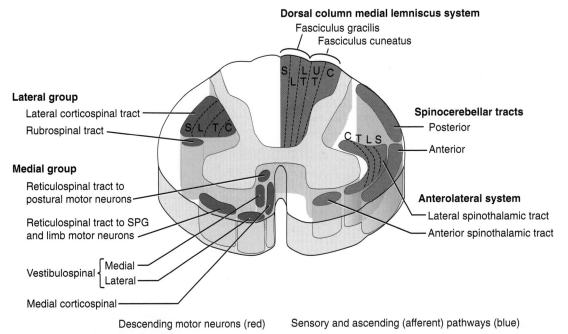

**Fig. 13-7  White matter of the spinal cord.** The sensory tracts are indicated in blue, and the motor tracts in red. The letters indicate the somatotopic organization of the tracts: C cervical, T thoracic, LT lower thoracic, UT upper thoracic, L lumbar, and S sacral. SPG, stepping pattern generator.

---

> ⊚ *Clinical Pearl*
>
> A segment of the spinal cord is connected to a specific region of the body by a pair of spinal nerves.

## Internal Structure of the Spinal Cord

The internal structure of the spinal cord can be observed in horizontal sections. Throughout the spinal cord, white matter surrounds gray matter. White matter contains the axons that connect various levels of the cord and link the cord with the brain. Axons that begin and end within the spinal cord are called *propriospinal*. The propriospinal axons are adjacent to the gray matter. Cells with long axons connecting the spinal cord with the brain are *tract cells*. The dorsal and lateral columns of white matter contain axons of tract cells, transmitting sensory information upward to the brain. The lateral and anterior white matter contains axons of upper motor neurons, conveying information descending from the brain to interneurons and lower motor neurons. Specific tracts have been discussed in Chapters 6 and 10. Tracts in the spinal cord are illustrated in Figure 13-7.

The central part of the cord is marked by a distinctive H-shaped pattern of gray matter (Figure 13-8). Lateral sections of spinal gray matter are divided into three regions called *horns*:
• Dorsal horn
• Lateral horn
• Ventral horn

The *dorsal horn* is primarily sensory, containing endings and collaterals of first-order sensory neurons, interneurons, and dendrites and somas of tract cells. For example, the somas of second-order neurons in the spinothalamic pathway are in the dorsal horn. The *lateral horn* (present only at T1-L2 spinal

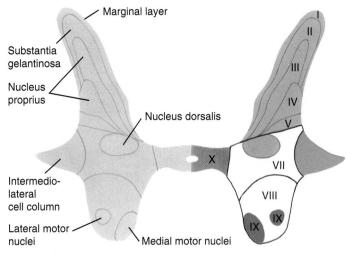

**Fig. 13-8  Gray matter of lower thoracic spinal cord.** Named regions are indicated on the left, and Rexed's laminae are indicated on the right. Lamina VI is present in the segments of the spinal cord that innervate the limbs and is not present between T4 and L2. The correspondence between Rexed's laminae and the named areas is inconsistent. For example, some authors include laminae III to VI in the nucleus proprius.

segments) contains the cell bodies of preganglionic sympathetic neurons. A region analogous to the lateral horn in the S2-S4 spinal segments includes the preganglionic parasympathetic cell bodies. Preganglionic autonomic neurons are efferent neurons. Both sympathetic and parasympathetic preganglionic neurons exit the cord via the ventral root. The *ventral horn* primarily consists of cell bodies of lower motor neurons whose axons exit the spinal cord via the ventral root.

> ### ◎ *Clinical Pearl*
>
> The dorsal horn processes sensory information, the lateral horn processes autonomic information, and the ventral horn processes motor information. Much of the gray matter is composed of spinal interneurons, cells with their somas in the gray matter that act upon other cells within the cord. Spinal interneurons include cells that remain entirely within the gray matter and cells whose axons travel in white matter to different levels of the cord.

### Rexed's Laminae

Spinal gray matter has been classified into 10 histologic regions called *Rexed's laminae;* these regions are illustrated in Figure 13-8. In the dorsal horn, laminae I through VI are numbered from dorsal to ventral. Lamina VII includes the intermediolateral horn and part of the ventral horn. In the ventral horn, locations of laminae VII through IX vary, depending on the level of the cord. Lamina X is the central region of gray matter.

Laminae I and II, called the *marginal layer* and the *substantia gelatinosa*, respectively, process information about noxious stimuli. Laminae III and IV, together known as the *nucleus proprius*, process proprioceptive and two-point discrimination information.* Lamina V cells process information about noxious stimuli and information from the viscera. Lamina VI cells process proprioceptive information. Lamina VII includes the nucleus dorsalis, or Clarke's column, extending from T1-L3 and the intermediolateral horn. The nucleus dorsalis receives proprioceptive information, and its axons relay unconscious proprioceptive information to the cerebellum. The intermediolateral horn contains somas of autonomic efferents. Lamina VIII cells connect with the contralateral cord and the brain. Lamina IX contains cell bodies of lower motor neurons, whose axons travel through a ventral root, a spinal nerve, and then a peripheral nerve to innervate skeletal muscles. Lamina X consists of axons crossing to the opposite side of the cord.

> ### ◎ *Clinical Pearl*
>
> Rexed's laminae consist of 10 histologic and functionally specific regions in the spinal cord gray matter.

### Meninges

The meninges, layers of connective tissue surrounding the spinal cord, are continuous with the meninges surrounding the brain. The pia mater closely adheres to the spinal cord surface, the arachnoid is separated from the pia by cerebrospinal fluid in the subarachnoid space, and the dura is the tough, outer layer. Between the arachnoid and the dura is the subdural space, and the epidural space separates the dura from the vertebrae.

---

*The correspondence between Rexed's laminae and some of the named spinal cord areas is controversial. For example, some authors include laminae III through VI in the nucleus proprius.

## MOVEMENTS OF THE SPINAL CORD AND ROOTS WITHIN THE VERTEBRAL COLUMN

Static and dynamic deformations of the vertebral column and movements of the limbs are directly transmitted to spinal cord, nerve roots, and spinal nerves via the meninges. Because the meninges surrounding the spinal cord are anchored to the skull and to the vertebrae, flexion of the vertebral column stretches the spinal cord and the spinal nerves. The nervous system connective tissue is continuous, so stretching the sciatic and tibial nerves by flexion of the hip joint, extension of the knee, and dorsiflexion of the ankle generates tension in the lumbosacral trunk and the spinal cord.[1] Hip flexion produces anterior movement of the cauda equina,[2] stretching the lumbosacral roots.

You can demonstrate the continuity of neural connective tissue by comparing your ability to fully extend your knee in different sitting postures. First, sit upright with your thighs fully supported and extend one knee while your foot is plantarflexed. Second, flex your lumbar and thoracic spine, place your hands behind your head and flex your neck, dorsiflex your foot, and then extend your knee. Decreased knee extension in the slumped position is probably the result of tension in the neural structures, created by stretch of the meninges and peripheral nerve connective tissue.[3] Flexion of any part of the vertebral column can produce longitudinal stretch of the entire spinal cord and nerve roots. The length of the cord increases by as much as 10% when a person flexes the spine. However, magnetic resonance imaging (MRI) studies indicate that the cauda equina moves very little—a maximum of 4 mm (0.16 of an inch)—when people move from a neutral spine to a flexed spine.[4] Extension of the spine reduces the stretch of central nervous system (CNS) structures.

Nerve roots and spinal nerves are protected from excessive mechanical loads by:
- Occupying 23% to 50% of available space within the intervertebral foramina[5]
- Cushioning by fat
- Dural sleeves surrounding the nerve roots within the intervertebral foramen
- Ligaments that maintain the spinal nerve within the intervertebral space and relieve traction on the spinal nerve[6,7]

Although physiologic motions do not significantly change the vertebral canal space in people with normal vertebral canals, extending and/or lateral bending of the neck increases the intervertebral foramen pressure at all cervical levels.[8] Therefore, neck extension and lateral bending increase cervical nerve root signs and symptoms.

## FUNCTIONS OF THE SPINAL CORD

Segments of the spinal cord exchange information with other spinal cord segments, with peripheral nerves, and with the brain. Tracts convey this information, yet spinal cord functions are far more complex than a simple conduit. Only for one type of information does the spinal cord serve as a simple conduit: axons carrying touch and proprioceptive information enter the dorsal column and project to the medulla without synapsing. All other tracts conveying information in the spinal cord

**TABLE 13-2**   ORIGINS AND FUNCTIONS OF TRACTS OF THE SPINAL CORD

| Tract | Origin | Function |
|---|---|---|
| Dorsal column/medial lemniscus | Peripheral receptors; first-order neuron synapses in medulla | Conveys information about discriminative touch and conscious proprioception |
| Spinothalamic | Dorsal horn of spinal cord | Conveys discriminative information about pain and temperature |
| Spinolimbic, spinomesencephalic, spinoreticular | Dorsal horn of spinal cord | Nonlocalized perception of pain; arousal, reflexive, motivational, and analgesic responses to nociception |
| Spinocerebellar | High-fidelity paths originate in peripheral receptors; first-order neurons synapse in nucleus dorsalis or medulla | Conveys unconscious proprioceptive information |
|  | Internal feedback tracts originate in the dorsal horn of the spinal cord | Conveys information about activity in upper motor neuron pathways and spinal interneurons |
| Lateral corticospinal | Supplementary motor, premotor, and primary motor cerebral cortex | Contralateral fractionation of movement, particularly of hand movements |
| Medial corticospinal | Supplementary motor, premotor, and primary motor cerebral cortex | Control of neck, shoulder, and trunk muscles |
| Rubrospinal | Red nucleus of midbrain | Facilitates contralateral upper limb extensors |
| Reticulospinal | Reticular formation in medulla and pons | Facilitates postural muscles and gross limb movements |
| Medial vestibulospinal | Vestibular nuclei in medulla and pons | Adjusts activity in neck and upper back muscles |
| Lateral vestibulospinal | Vestibular nuclei in medulla and pons | Ipsilaterally facilitates lower motor neurons to extensors; inhibits lower motor neurons to flexors |
| Ceruleospinal | Locus coeruleus in brainstem | Enhances the activity of interneurons and lower motor neurons in spinal cord |
| Raphespinal | Raphe nucleus in brainstem | Same as ceruleospinal |

synapse in the cord, and thus their information is subject to processing and modification within the cord.

For example, after one hammers a thumb, pain signals can be modified by rubbing the thumb and/or by activity of the descending pain inhibition pathways (see Chapter 7). Pain information is modified within the spinal cord by signals from large-diameter sensory afferents and by signals in the descending tracts, both of which decrease the frequency of signals in slow pain pathways. Similarly, information conveyed by an upper motor neuron axon in a descending tract to a lower motor neuron is only one of many influences on that lower motor neuron (see Chapter 10). The origins and functions of the tracts in the spinal cord are listed in Table 13-2.

## Classification of Spinal Interneurons

In most textbooks, spinal interneurons are considered only in the context of reflexes. To study interneurons, experimenters have often disconnected the spinal cord from the brain, stimulated only one type of afferent neuron, and then recorded from interneurons. These experiments led to the concept of reflexes as an invariant coupling of input and output, with discrete spinal circuits dedicated to each reflex. Voluntary movement was considered to be entirely separate from reflexes. Although reductionism may be required to simplify the system

for experiments, interneurons do not normally function with isolated inputs. Subsequent research has demonstrated the following:

- Natural stimuli simultaneously excite a variety of receptor types. For example, flexing a joint stimulates muscle spindles, Golgi tendon organs, joint stretch and pressure receptors, and cutaneous stretch and pressure receptors.
- Afferent and descending information converges on the same spinal interneurons.
- Reflexes and voluntary control act together to produce goal-oriented movements. Reflexes are not hardwired but depend on the environmental context and the task.

By integrating volleys of peripheral, ascending, and descending inputs, spinal circuitry provides the following:
- Modulation of sensory information
- Coordination of movement patterns
- Autonomic regulation

In this text, interneurons are categorized by function.* Modulation of sensory information was covered in Chapter 7

---

*Historical Note: Until recently, spinal interneurons were categorized according to the earliest discovery of associated afferents. Thus, interneurons activated by type Ia spindle afferents are often called type Ia inhibitory interneurons, despite subsequent findings that these interneurons are also strongly influenced by other afferents and by descending tracts.

and will not be considered here. The other mechanisms will be discussed individually for simplicity; however, recall that none of these mechanisms acts in isolation.

## SPINAL CORD MOTOR COORDINATION

Interneuronal circuits integrate activity from all sources and then adjust the output of lower motor neurons. Thus interneurons coordinate activity in all muscles when a limb moves.

What determines whether a single alpha motor neuron will fire? The summation of activity at 20,000 to 50,000 synapses determines whether an alpha motor neuron will fire. These synapses provide information from the following:

- Ia, Ib, and II afferents
- Interneurons
- Descending upper motor neurons, including medial, lateral, and nonspecific tracts

In normal movement, motor activity elicited by descending commands can be modified by afferent input. The contribution of interneurons to this modification is illustrated in Figure 13-9.

Alternatively, descending commands can modify the motor activity elicited by afferent input. *Jendrassik's maneuver* provides a demonstration of the effects of descending influences on alpha motor neurons. The maneuver consists of voluntary contraction of certain muscles during reflex testing of other muscles. For example, subjects hook their flexed fingers together and then pull isometrically against their own resistance; this activity facilitates the quadriceps deep tendon reflex by producing a generalized increase in spinal interneuron activity. In Jendrassik's maneuver, signals from upper motor neurons contribute to increasing the general level of excitation in the cord.

The following pattern-generating, reflexive, and inhibitory circuits are examples of connections that use interneuron activity to shape motor output.

### Stepping Pattern Generators

Stepping pattern generators are adaptable neural networks that produce rhythmic output (see Chapter 10). Stepping pattern generators (SPGs) contribute to stepping by activating lower motor neurons, eliciting alternating flexion and extension at the hips and knees. In humans, SPGs are normally activated when the person voluntarily sends signals from the brain to the SPGs in the spinal cord to initiate walking. SPG neurons are activated in sequence (Figure 13-10, *A*). At specific times in the sequence, signals from branches of SPG neurons activate lower motor neurons innervating flexor muscles. At other times in the sequence, lower motor neurons to extensor muscles are activated. Thus spinal SPG activity elicits repetitive, rhythmic, alternating flexion and extension movements of the hips and knees. Each of the lower limbs has a dedicated SPG. Reciprocal movements of the lower limbs during walking are coordinated by signals conveyed in the anterior commissure of the spinal cord.[9]

Processing of proprioceptive information in the SPG produces a biomechanical snapshot at a specific time. When a person is walking or running, information from all of the activated proprioceptors is processed to create a proprioceptive image of time and space. The SPG computes the exact position

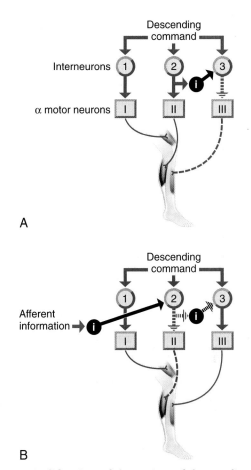

A

B

**Fig. 13-9 Modification of the action of descending commands by afferent information.** At the bottom of both **A** and **B** are three muscles in the lower limb. Solid lines indicate active axons. Dotted lines indicate inactive axons. **A,** Descending commands stimulate all three interneurons (1, 2, and 3). A collateral of interneuron 2 excites an interneuron *(black)* that inhibits interneuron 3. As a result, alpha motor neurons I and II fire, and III is silent. **B,** Afferent input excites an interneuron *(black)* that inhibits interneuron 2. As a result, alpha motor neurons I and III fire, and II is silent. *(Modified by permission from McCrea DA: Can sense be made of spinal interneuron circuits? In Cordo P, Harnad S, editors: Movement control, Cambridge, 1994, Cambridge University Press, pp 31-41.)*

of the limb, the status of muscle contractions, and the relationship of the limb to the environment. The somatosensory information affecting SPG function is shown in Figure 13-10, *B.* Thus SPGs interpret somatosensory input within the context of a task and the environment, then predict and program the appropriate actions.[10] For example, proprioceptive input from the stretched iliopsoas at the end of stance phase triggers initiation of the swing phase.[11]

SPG output is adapted to the task, the environment, and the stage of the walking cycle. Walking requires different SPG output than running. If you step off a sidewalk onto sand, your SPGs alter their output to adapt your stepping movements to the changed environment. The effect of somatosensation on

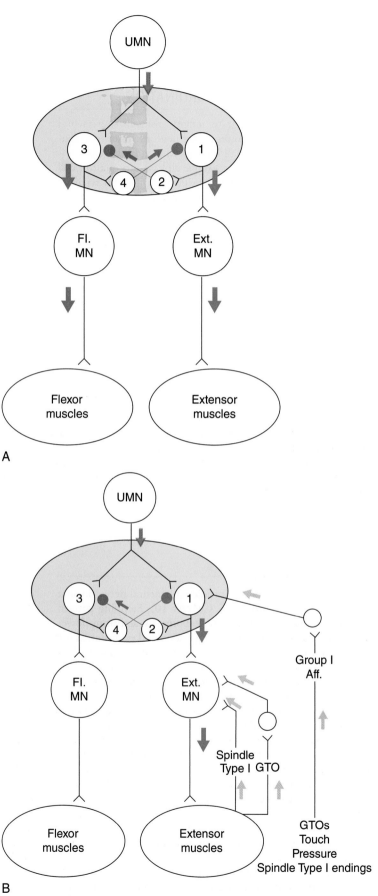

**Fig. 13-10  A simplified conceptual model of a stepping pattern generator. A,** Only the motor pathways are shown. The stepping pattern generator (SPG) is represented by neurons within the large oval. Firing of the upper motor neuron (UMN) initiates cycles of activity in the SPG. SPG neuron 1 activates extensor motor neurons that signal extensor muscles to contract. Collaterals from neuron 1 synapse with an inhibitory interneuon (neuron 2), inhibiting neuron 3. When the interneuron fatigues, neuron 3 begins firing, activating flexor motor neurons that signal flexor muscles to contract. Collaterals from neuron 3 synapse with an inhibitory interneuron (neuron 4) inhibiting neuron 1. When this interneuron fatigues, neuron 1 resumes firing. **B,** Sensory pathways have been added to the right side of the illustration. Neural activity during stance phase is indicated by the arrows. Sensory information from muscle spindle type I endings and from Golgi tendon organs (GTOs) feeds back to the extensor motor neurons. The pathway from the GTO to the extensor motor neuron pool involves an interneuron (IN). Group I afferents convey information from muscle spindle type I endings, Golgi tendon organs, and touch and pressure receptors to adjust activity in the SPG. During stance phase, GTO input facilitates the extensor motor neurons. Similar sensory pathways are present on the left (flexor) side but have been omitted to simplify the diagram. *(Developed from models in Rybak IA, Stecina K, Shevtsova NA, and McCrea DA: Modelling spinal circuitry involved in locomotor pattern generation: insights from the effects of afferent stimulation. J Physiol 577(Pt 2):641-58, 2006, and Quevedo J, Fedirchuk B, Gosgnach S, McCrea DA: Group I disynaptic excitation of cat hindlimb flexor and bifunctional motoneurones during fictive locomotion. J Physiol 525 (Pt 2):549-64, 2000.)*

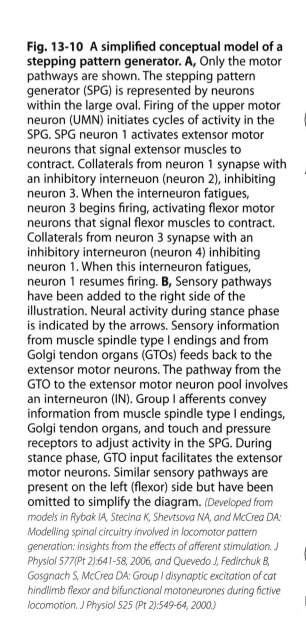

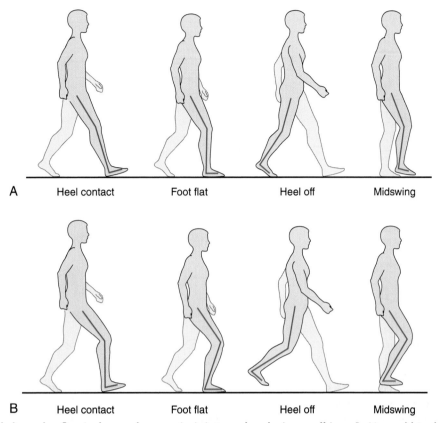

**Fig. 13-11** **The withdrawal reflex induces changes in joint angles during walking. A,** Normal hip, knee, and ankle joint angles at four points during the gait cycle. **B,** Joint angle changes induced by electrically stimulating the mid-medial sole of the foot. Maximal increases in joint angles occurred when stimulation occurred during the swing phase. During swing, the response to electrical stimulation increased the average maximal hip flexion by 9 degrees, knee flexion by 20 degrees, and dorsiflexion by 4 degrees. *(Created from data in Spaich EG, Arendt-Nielsen L, Andersen OK: Modulation of lower limb withdrawal reflexes during gait: a topographical study. J Neurophysiol 91(1):258-66, 2004.)*

SPG activity depends on the stage of the step cycle. For example, during the flexor phase of walking, input from flexor muscle GTOs facilitates lower motor neurons to flexor muscles, and during the extensor phase, the same input inhibits lower motor neurons to flexor muscles.[12] Another example is the modification of the withdrawal reflex elicited during gait (Figure 13-11).

When a person is walking, electrical stimulation to a single point on the foot produces different responses depending on the phase of the gait cycle. If the stimulus occurs at the onset of the swing phase, tibialis anterior activity increases. If the stimulus occurs at the end of the swing phase, tibialis anterior activity decreases and antagonist muscle activity increases.[13] This response reversal adapts the ongoing activity of SPGs to the task and environment. At the start of the swing phase, dorsiflexion is required to clear the foot. However, at the end of the swing phase, increasing tibialis anterior contraction would prevent appropriate positioning of the foot for weight bearing. Plantarflexion during late swing would result in faster whole foot contact with the ground.[13]

Human SPGs are normally activated when a person initiates walking by sending signals from the brain to the spinal cord. After spinal cord injury, SPGs can be activated by artificial stimulation. When the spinal cord is completely severed, the brain cannot communicate with the cord below the level of the lesion. Therefore, a complete thoracic lesion causes paralysis of voluntary movements of the lower limbs. However, a lumbar spinal cord isolated from the brain is still capable of generating near-normal reciprocal lower limb movements similar to walking. Patients with complete spinal cord injuries can experience stepping-like movements of the lower limbs following nonpatterned electrical stimulation of the posterior lumbar spinal cord. Minassian and associates (2007)[14] electrically stimulated the lumbar spinal cord in people with complete spinal cord lesions, using an electrode on the surface of the dura mater. During stimulation, an electromyogram (EMG, recording of the electrical activity produced by muscle fibers) and lower limb joint movement were recorded. The electrical stimulation elicited rhythmic step-like EMG activity and flexion-extension movements of the lower limbs (Figure 13-12). However, without additional neural control, the alternating flexion/extension elicited by SPG activity is inadequate to produce walking. Postural control, cortical control of dorsiflexion,[15] and afferent information to adapt movements to the environment and the task are also essential for normal human walking.

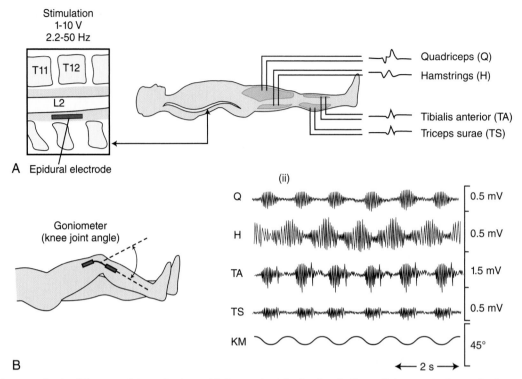

**Fig. 13-12 In a patient with complete spinal cord injury, electrical stimulation of the posterior spinal roots elicits stepping-like movements. A,** A stimulating electrode has been implanted inside the T11 and T12 vertebrae, outside the dura at the L2-L4 spinal cord levels. The patient is supine during electrical stimulation. **B,** Epidural electrical stimulation at a rate of 31 Hz produces rhythmic electromyographic (EMG) activity in the quadriceps (Q), hamstrings (H), tibialis anterior (TA), and triceps surae (TS). EMG activity produces alternating knee flexion and extension. *KM,* Knee movement.
*(Modified with permission from Minassian K, Jilge B, Rattay F, et al: Stepping-like movements in humans with complete spinal cord injury induced by epidural stimulation of the lumbar cord: electromyographic study of compound muscle action potentials. Spinal Cord 42:401-16, 2004.)*

Sensory input strongly influences the output of stepping pattern generators in people with spinal cord lesions. When subjects with minimal or no sensory or voluntary motor function below the level of the injury are manually assisted in walking on a treadmill, their lower motor neuron output is modulated by sensory input. Despite the lack of upper motor neuron input to lower motor neurons, information about hip joint position, cutaneous stimulation, and contralateral limb position contributes to patterns of lower motor neuron activity.[14] Sensory input from bilateral alternate leg movements amplifies induced stepping-type activity of the lower limbs in people with complete spinal cord injuries, indicating that the spinal cord is able to coordinate lower limb walking movements despite being deprived of information from the brain.[14]

### Reflexes

Except for the monosynaptic phasic stretch reflex, spinal reflexes involve interneurons. Phasic and tonic stretch reflexes, reciprocal inhibition, and withdrawal reflexes were introduced as spinal region reflexes in Chapter 10. In this chapter, the focus is on the capacity of interneuronal circuits to generate complex movements. This is demonstrated by the *withdrawal reflex.* Afferent information from skin, muscles, and/or joints can elicit a variety of withdrawal movements. Each withdrawal

movement is specific for most effectively removing the stimulated area away from the provocation. For example, if one steps on a tack, the involved lower limb flexes to remove the foot from the stimulus. However, if a bee stings the inside of one's calf, the lower limb abducts. The specificity of the movement pattern is referred to as *local sign,* indicating that the response depends on the site of stimulation. Because the muscles removing the part from the stimulation usually are not innervated by the same cord segment that received the afferent input, information is relayed to other cord segments by collaterals of the primary afferent and by interneurons. In an intact nervous system, the stimulation must be quite strong to evoke a powerful withdrawal reflex. If one is standing when one lower limb is abruptly withdrawn, another interneuronal circuit quickly adjusts the muscle activity in the stance limb to prevent falling; this is the *crossed extension reflex.* Withdrawal and associated crossed extension reflexes are illustrated in Figure 13-13.

### Inhibitory Circuits

Interneurons in inhibitory circuits also contribute to spinal cord motor coordination. Inhibitory interneurons provide the following:
* Reciprocal inhibition
* Recurrent inhibition

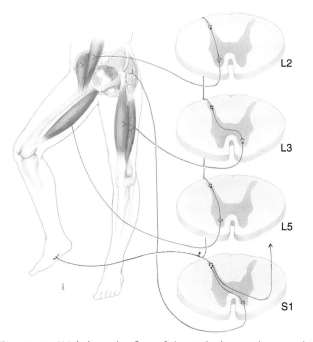

**Fig. 13-13** Withdrawal reflex of the right leg and crossed extension reflex in the left leg. Interaction of several spinal cord segments is required to produce the coordinated muscle action.

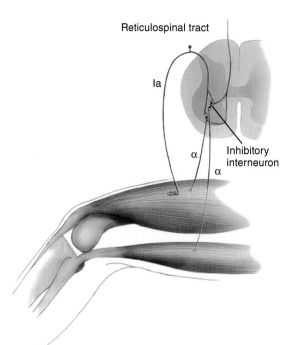

**Fig. 13-14 Reciprocal inhibition.** For simplicity, only the reticulospinal input to an alpha motor neuron activating fibers in the quadriceps and to a reciprocal inhibition interneuron inhibiting an alpha motor neuron to fibers in the semitendinosus muscle are shown.

## Reciprocal Inhibition

*Reciprocal inhibition* decreases activity in an antagonist when an agonist is active, allowing the agonist to act unopposed. When agonists are voluntarily recruited, reciprocal inhibition interneurons prevent unwanted activity in the antagonists (Figure 13-14). Thus, reciprocal inhibition separates muscles into agonists and antagonists. For efficient motor control, collaterals of upper motor neurons activate reciprocal inhibitory interneurons simultaneously with excitation of selected lower motor neurons.

Type Ia, cutaneous, and joint afferents, other interneurons, and corticospinal, rubrospinal, and vestibulospinal tracts provide input to reciprocal inhibition interneurons.[16] Reciprocal inhibition occurs with afferent input, as well as during voluntary movement. For example, during a quadriceps stretch reflex, reciprocal inhibition interneurons inhibit the hamstrings. Occasionally, reciprocal inhibition is suppressed to allow cocontraction of antagonists. This occurs in people with intact nervous systems when they are anxious, anticipate unpredictable movement disturbances, or are learning new movements.

## Recurrent Inhibition

*Recurrent inhibition* has effects opposite to those of reciprocal inhibition: inhibition of agonists and synergists, with disinhibition of antagonists (Figure 13-15). *Renshaw cells,* interneurons that produce recurrent inhibition, are stimulated by a recurrent collateral branch from the alpha motor neuron. A recurrent collateral branch is a side branch of an axon that turns back toward its own cell body. Renshaw cells inhibit the

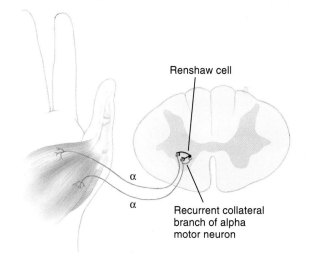

**Fig. 13-15 Recurrent inhibition.** The recurrent collateral branch of the alpha motor neuron stimulates the Renshaw cell. The Renshaw cell inhibits agonists and synergists and facilitates antagonists. For simplicity, the antagonist facilitation is not shown.

same alpha motor neuron that gives rise to the collateral and also inhibit alpha motor neurons of synergists. Renshaw cells focus motor activity, thus isolating desired motor activity from gross activation.[16] Loss of descending influence on Renshaw cell activity may cause difficulty in achieving fine motor control.

## SPINAL CONTROL OF PELVIC ORGAN FUNCTION

The sacral spinal cord contains centers for the control of urination, bowel function, and sexual function. In a normal infant, when the bladder is empty, sympathetic efferents from T11-L2 levels inhibit contraction of the bladder wall and maintain contraction of the internal sphincter (Figure 13-16, *A*). When the bladder fills, proprioceptors sense stretching of the bladder wall, impulses regarding fullness of the bladder are transmitted to the reflex center in the sacral cord, and efferent impulses initiate voiding. Parasympathetic impulses stimulate bladder wall contraction and open the internal sphincter; somatic efferents (S2-S4) cease firing to allow opening of the external sphincter (Figure 13-16, *B*). Thus, *reflexive bladder function*, which is normal in infants, requires the following:

- Afferents
- T11-L2 and S2-S4 cord levels
- Somatic, sympathetic, and parasympathetic efferents

Even when voluntary control of voiding is achieved, bladder filling remains primarily an involuntary process, controlled by sympathetic signals that induce relaxation of the bladder wall and contraction of the internal sphincter. For voluntary control of voiding, three central nervous system urination centers are essential. These centers are located in the frontal cortex, pons, and sacral spinal cord. When the bladder is filling, the frontal cortex urination center inhibits the pontine urination center, to prevent the pons from signaling the sacral urination center to empty the bladder. If the bladder is full but circumstances are not appropriate for urination, the frontal lobe urination center signals corticospinal neurons to lower motor neurons that control pelvic floor muscle contraction. Contraction of the levator ani compresses the bladder neck, thus assisting the external sphincter in preventing urination.

When the bladder is full and conditions are appropriate, the frontal cortex initiates voiding by disinhibition of the pontine urination center. The pontine urination center then signals "GO" to the sacral spinal cord urination center, which sends

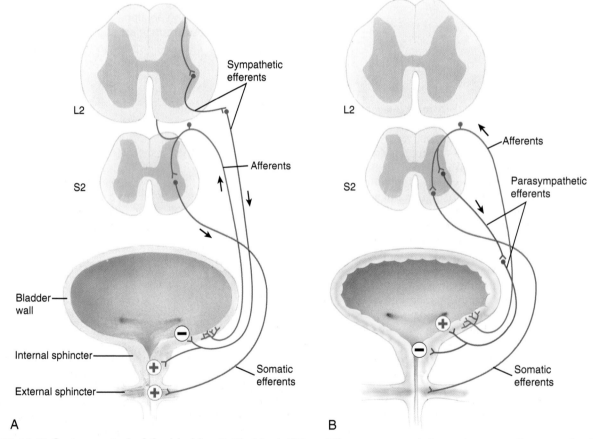

**Fig. 13-16 Reflexive control of the bladder. A,** Bladder is filling. Afferents convey information regarding stretch of the bladder wall to the spinal cord. Signals in sympathetic efferents maintain relaxation of the bladder wall and constriction of the internal sphincter. Somatic efferent signals elicit contraction of the external sphincter. **B,** When the bladder is full, reflexive voiding is initiated by signals in the parasympathetic efferents, producing contraction of the bladder wall and relaxation of the internal sphincter. Decreased somatic efferent activity allows relaxation of the external sphincter. Plus signs indicate facilitation, minus signs indicate inhibition.

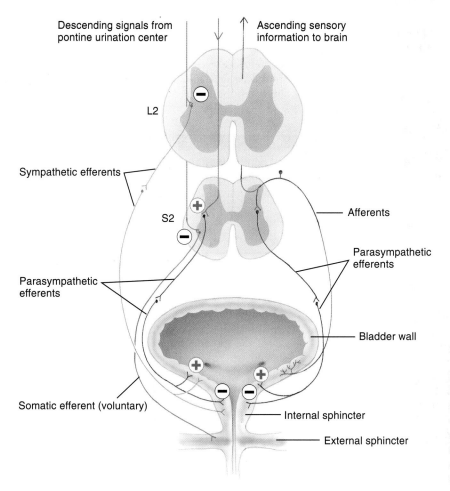

Descending signals from pontine urination center

Ascending sensory information to brain

L2

Sympathetic efferents

S2

Afferents

Parasympathetic efferents

Parasympathetic efferents

Bladder wall

Somatic efferent (voluntary)

Internal sphincter

External sphincter

**Fig. 13-17 Neural control of the bladder.** Efferents and descending signals from the brain are indicated on the left side of the illustration. Ascending sensory neurons, afferents, and a reflexive connection between afferents and parasympathetic efferents are shown on the right side.

signals via parasympathetic neurons to stimulate contraction of the bladder wall and relax the internal sphincter (Figure 13-17). Simultaneously, signals from the pontine center to the spinal cord inhibit alpha motor neurons that elicit contraction of the external sphincter and pelvic floor muscles; together, these actions empty the bladder. See Box 13-1, which summarizes neural control of the bladder.

Bowel control is similar to bladder control. The signal to empty the bowels is stimulation of stretch receptors in the wall of the rectum. Afferent fibers transmit the information to the lumbar and sacral cord, the information is conveyed to the brain, and, if appropriate, the efferent signal is sent to relax the sphincters.

The lower spinal cord is also vital for sexual function. Erection of the penis or clitoris is controlled by parasympathetic fibers from S2-S4 spinal cord levels, and ejaculation is elicited by sympathetic nerves originating in L1-L2 and the pudendal nerve with cell bodies in S2-S4.

### ◎ Clinical Pearl

Reflexive functions of the bladder, bowels, and male sexual organ require intact afferents, lumbar and sacral cord segments, and somatic and autonomic efferents. Voluntary control of these functions requires intact neural pathways between the organ and the cerebral cortex.

### BOX 13-1 NEURAL CONTROL OF THE BLADDER

**To Allow Bladder Filling**
- *Frontal cortex* inhibits the pontine urination center, to prevent bladder wall from contracting until voiding is socially appropriate.
- From sacral spinal cord urination center:
  - *Sympathetic signals* relax the bladder wall and constrict internal sphincter.
  - *Somatic signals* constrict external sphincter.
- If the urge to void is powerful but circumstances are inappropriate, *corticospinal signals* to lower motor neurons elicit *contraction* of pelvic floor muscles to reinforce the contraction of the external sphincter.

**To Empty the Bladder**
- *Frontal cortex* releases the pontine urination center from inhibition.
- *Pontine urination center* provides the "GO" signal to the sacral spinal cord for emptying the bladder; signals from the pons facilitate sacral spinal cord parasympathetic activity and inhibit sympathetic activity.
- From sacral spinal cord urination center: parasympathetic signals elicit contraction of the bladder wall and relax the internal sphincter.

## EFFECTS OF SEGMENTAL AND TRACT LESIONS IN THE SPINAL REGION

A lesion in the spinal region may interfere with the following:
- Segmental function
- Vertical tract function
- Both segmental and vertical tract function

### Segmental Function

Segmental function is the function of a spinal cord segment. Segmental lesions interfere with neural function only at the level of the lesion. For example, complete severance of the C5 dorsal root (roots are considered within the spinal region, although not in the spinal cord) would prevent sensory information from the C5 dermatome, myotome, and sclerotome from reaching the spinal cord.

### Vertical Tract Function

Vertical tracts convey ascending and descending information. Lesions that interrupt the vertical tracts result in loss of function below the level of the lesion. A complete lesion prevents sensory information from below the lesion from ascending to higher levels of the central nervous system and prevents descending signals from reaching levels of the spinal cord below the lesion.

### Segmental and Vertical Tract Function

Spinal region lesions may cause both segmental and tract signs. A lesion at the C5 level on the right that involves the right dorsal quadrant would prevent discriminative touch and conscious proprioception from the right side of the body below C5 from reaching the brain (tract signs), and sensory information from the C5 dermatome, myotome, and sclerotome would be lost (segmental signs).

### Signs of Segmental Dysfunction

A focal lesion involving a single level of the spinal cord, the dorsal or ventral roots, or a spinal nerve results in segmental signs due to interruption of pathways. At the level of the lesion, sensory, motor, and/or reflexive changes occur. In Figure 13-18, the effects of a C5 spinal nerve lesion are contrasted with the effects of a C5 hemisection of the spinal cord. Autonomic signs are difficult to detect with a lesion at a single level because of the overlapping distribution of autonomic fibers from adjacent cord segments.

A lesion of the dorsal root, spinal nerve, or dorsal horn interferes with sensory function in a spinal segment, causing abnormal sensations or loss of sensation in a dermatomal distribution. For example, a dorsal root can be avulsed (forcibly detached) from the cervical spinal cord by extreme traction on the upper limb. If avulsion occurs at C5, the spinal cord is deprived of sensory information from the C5 dermatome, myotome (proprioceptive and muscle pain information), and sclerotome innervated by that dorsal root.

A lesion of the ventral horn, ventral root, or spinal nerve interferes with lower motor neuron function. Signs of lower motor neuron dysfunction include flaccid weakness, atrophy,

fibrillation, and fasciculation. If lower motor neuron signs occur in a myotomal pattern (see Chapter 10), the lesion is in the spinal region. A myotome includes paraspinal muscles, so signs of paraspinal involvement help differentiate spinal region from peripheral nerve lesions. Reflexes are absent if motor or sensory fibers contributing to the reflex circuit are damaged.

> ◎ **Clinical Pearl**
>
> Segmental signs include abnormal or lost sensation in a dermatomal distribution and/or lower motor neuron signs in a myotomal distribution.

### Signs of Vertical Tract Dysfunction

Lesions interrupting the vertical tracts result in loss of communication to and/or from the spinal levels below the lesion. Therefore, all signs of damage to the vertical tracts occur below the level of the lesion. Ascending tract (sensory information) signs are ipsilateral if the dorsal column is interrupted and contralateral if the spinothalamic tracts are involved, because the dorsal columns remain ipsilateral throughout the cord, while the spinothalamic tracts cross the midline within a few levels of where the information enters the cord. Autonomic signs may include problems with regulation of blood pressure, sweating, and bladder and bowel control.

Descending tract (upper motor neuron) signs include paralysis, spasticity, and muscle hypertonia; if the lateral corticospinal tract is interrupted, Babinski's sign (see Chapter 10) is present. Deep tendon reflex testing (biceps, triceps, patellar, and tendo calcaneus [see Chapter 7]) may help to distinguish between upper motor neuron and lower motor neuron involvement: hyperreflexia indicates upper motor neuron, and hyporeflexia or areflexia may indicate lower motor neuron involvement. However, hyporeflexia or areflexia may also occur with damage to type Ia afferents.

An incomplete bilateral lesion at the C5 level limited to the dorsal columns would prevent ascending conscious proprioceptive and discriminative touch information from reaching the brain. Thus a person with a spinal cord tumor that damaged the dorsal columns at C5 would not be aware of the location of light touch or passive joint movement below the C5 level but would be able to distinguish among sharp and dull stimuli, locations of pinprick, and different temperatures. Information in the descending pathways would also be intact, although coordination would be somewhat impaired because of the lack of conscious proprioceptive information.

### Differentiating Spinal Region From Peripheral Region Lesions

Peripheral region lesions produce deficits in the distribution of a peripheral nerve. Peripheral nerve lesions cause:
- Altered or lost sensation in a peripheral nerve distribution
- Decrease or loss of muscle power in a peripheral nerve distribution
- No vertical tract signs

Spinal region segmental signs occur when nerve roots and/or spinal nerves are compromised. Segmental signs include:

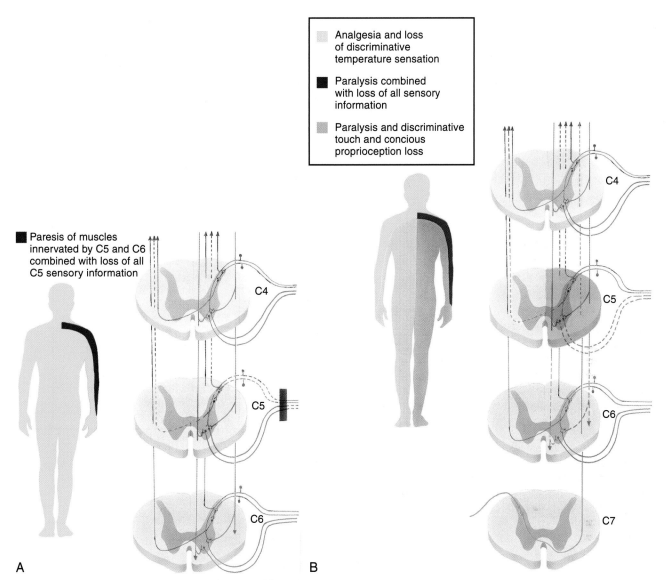

**Fig. 13-18 Spinal region lesions: segmental signs versus vertical tract signs.** Dotted lines indicate neural pathways that have been interrupted and do not convey information. **A,** The lesion interrupts all axons in the left C5 spinal nerve. This produces loss of sensation from the C5 dermatome and weakness of the biceps and brachioradialis, partially innervated by the C5 spinal nerve. The biceps and brachioradialis are not paralyzed because C6 also supplies these muscles. Thus the losses are limited to only part of the left arm. The entire remainder of the nervous system functions normally. **B,** In contrast, the hemisection of the cord at C5 produces the following conditions below the C5 level: paralysis on the left side, loss of discriminative touch and conscious proprioceptive information from the left side, and analgesia and loss of discriminative temperature sensation from the right side. In addition, segmental losses are the same as in lesion **A.**

- Altered or lost sensation in a dermatome
- Decreased or lost muscle power in a myotome
- Decreased or lost phasic stretch reflex
  Spinal region vertical tract signs include:
- Altered or lost sensation below the level of the lesion
- Altered or lost descending control of blood pressure, pelvic viscera, and thermoregulation
- Upper motor neuron signs including: decrease or loss of muscle power, spasticity, muscle hypertonia, and if the lateral corticospinal tract is involved, positive Babinski's sign and clonus

## SPINAL REGION SYNDROMES

Syndromes are collections of signs and symptoms that do not indicate a specific cause. The following syndromes usually result from tumors or trauma (Figure 13-19):

- Anterior cord syndrome (Figure 13-19, *A*) interrupts ascending spinothalamic tracts and descending motor tracts and damages the somas of lower motor neurons. Thus anterior cord syndrome interferes with pain and temperature sensation and with motor control. Because tracts that convey proprioception and discriminative touch

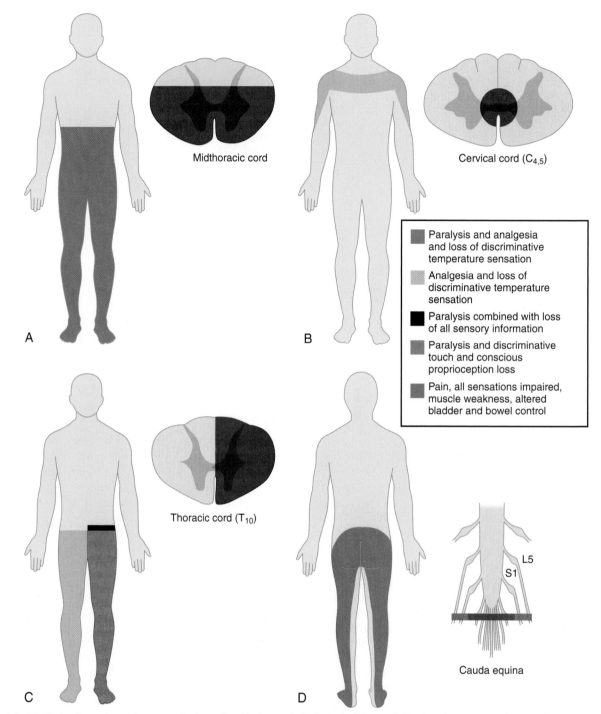

**Fig. 13-19** **Spinal cord syndromes. A,** Anterior. **B,** Central. **C,** Brown-Séquard. **D,** Cauda equina. The cauda equina syndrome shown affects nerve roots L5 through S5, causing paralysis of the foot and toe dorsiflexors and plantarflexors and the bladder and anal sphincters.

information are located in the posterior cord, these functions are spared.

- Central cord syndrome (Figure 13-19, *B*) usually occurs at the cervical level. If the lesion is small, loss of pain and temperature information occurs at the level of the lesion because spinothalamic fibers crossing the midline are interrupted. Larger lesions additionally impair upper limb motor

function due to the medial location of upper limb fibers in the lateral corticospinal tracts.

- Brown-Séquard syndrome (Figure 13-19, *C*) results from a hemisection of the cord. Segmental losses are ipsilateral and include loss of lower motor neurons and all sensations. Below the level of the lesion, voluntary motor control, conscious proprioception, and discriminative touch are lost

| **PATHOLOGY 13-1** | CAUDA EQUINA SYNDROME |
|---|---|
| Pathology | Compression and/or irritation of nerve roots below the L2 vertebral level |
| Etiology | Decreased space in the vertebral canal below L2. Common causes include herniated disk (may be secondary to narrowing of the vertebral canal and/or long history of heavier than normal loading of the lumbar spine due to work and/or recreation), vertebral fracture, and tumor. 90% of lumbar disk herniations occur at L4-L5 or L5-S1. |
| Speed of onset | Usually acute (develops in less than 24 hours); rarely subacute or chronic |
| Signs and symptoms | |
| Consciousness | Normal |
| Communication and memory | Normal |
| Sensory | Low back pain and sciatica aggravated by Valsalva maneuver and by sitting; relieved by lying down. Decreased sensation: extent of decreased sensation depends on the level of the cauda equina affected. The "saddle area" (part of the body that would be in contact with the saddle on a horse; innervated by S2-S5) is usually affected. |
| Autonomic | Retention or incontinence of urine and/or stool. Impotence |
| Motor | Paresis or paralysis; distribution depends on the nerve roots affected |
| Reflexes | Impairment of nerve roots causes decrease or loss of reflexes |
| Region affected | Spinal region lumbosacral nerve roots; the lesion does not directly affect the spinal cord |
| Demographics | Rare |
| Incidence | Cauda equina syndrome: 1–3 per 100,000 population[17]<br>Operated disk cases: between 2% and 3%[18] |
| Prevalence | In people with low back pain: 4 per 10,000 population[17] |
| Prognosis | Markedly improves with surgical decompression. Without surgery, greater chance of persistent problems with bladder function, severe motor deficits, pain, and sexual dysfunction.[19] Outcomes correlate with presurgical neurologic deficits.[20] |
| Red flag | Low back pain and/or sciatica combined with bladder or bowel retention or incontinence requires emergency medical referral because cauda equina syndrome may progress to paraplegia and/or to permanent problems with bladder and/or bowel control. |

ipsilaterally; pain and temperature sensation is lost contralaterally. This syndrome is also illustrated and explained in Figure 13-18, *B*.

- Cauda equina syndrome (Figure 13-19, *D*) indicates damage to the lumbar and/or sacral spinal roots, causing sensory impairment and flaccid paresis or paralysis of lower limb muscles, bladder, and bowels. Muscle hypertonia and hyperreflexia do not occur because the upper motor neurons are intact (Pathology 13-1).
- *Tethered cord syndrome* (not illustrated). During development, the vertebral column grows longer than the spinal cord (see Chapter 5). Infrequently, the spinal cord becomes attached to surrounding structures during early development. Scar tissue, a fatty mass (lipoma), or abnormal development can lead to tethering of the spinal cord. As the vertebral column elongates, the tethered spinal cord becomes stretched. Stretch injury damages the spinal cord and/or cauda equina. Consequences of a tethered spinal cord include low back and lower limb pain, difficulty walking, excessive lordosis, scoliosis, problems with bowel and/or bladder control, and foot deformities. Lower motor neuron signs (weakness, flaccidity) occur if the anterior cauda equina is stretched. Upper motor neuron signs (abnormal reflexes, paresis, and changes in skeletal muscles) occur if

the spinal cord is excessively stretched. Often, abnormal signs on the lower back indicate a tethered cord: an unusually located dimple, a tuft of hair, a hemangioma (tangle of blood vessels), or the bulge of a fatty mass. Tethered cord is often associated with myelomeningocele at the L4, L5, or S1 level. In severe cases, surgery may be indicated to untether the cord. Tethered cord occurs most often in children, and sometimes in teenagers during a growth spurt.

> **◉ Clinical Pearl**
>
> Syndromes are collections of signs and symptoms that occur together. Spinal cord syndromes indicate the location of a lesion but do not signify cause. Thus, an anterior cord syndrome could be caused by trauma, loss of blood supply, or other pathology.

## EFFECTS OF SPINAL REGION DYSFUNCTION ON PELVIC ORGAN FUNCTION

Control of bladder, bowel, and sexual function depends on the level of cord damage. Lesions above the sacral level of the cord produce signs similar to upper motor neuron lesions. Lesions

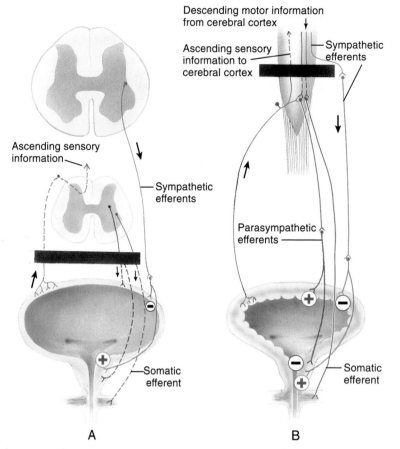

**Fig. 13-20  Bladder dysfunction after spinal region injury.** Dotted lines indicate neural pathways that have been interrupted and do not convey information. **A,** Flaccid bladder due to a complete lesion of the cauda equina. All neural connections with the bladder are severed, except the sympathetic efferents. A complete lesion of spinal cord levels S2 to S4 would also produce a flaccid bladder, owing to interruption of the reflexive bladder emptying circuit. **B,** Hypertonic bladder caused by a complete lesion above the S2 level. Communication between the brain and the sacral level parasympathetic neurons controlling the bladder are interrupted, preventing voluntary control. The reflexive connections between the bladder and spinal cord are intact, so reflexive emptying of the bladder can occur.

in the S2-S4 spinal cord levels, the afferents, and/or the parasympathetic efferents produce signs similar to lower motor neuron lesions.

Complete lesions that damage any part of the reflexive bladder emptying circuit, that is, levels S2-S4—or afferents or parasympathetic efferents—produce a flaccid, paralyzed bladder (Figure 13-20, *A*). The flaccid, paralyzed bladder overfills with urine, and when the bladder cannot stretch any further, urine dribbles out.

In contrast, complete lesions above the sacral cord interrupt descending axons that normally control bladder function but do not interrupt sacral level reflexive control of the bladder. This results in a hypertonic, hyperreflexive bladder with reduced bladder capacity (Figure 13-20, *B*). Because the reflex circuit for bladder emptying is intact, reflexive emptying may occur automatically whenever the bladder is stretched, or, if the sphincter is also hypertonic, flow of urine is functionally obstructed, and the reflexive contraction of the bladder wall may force urine back into the kidneys causing kidney damage.

Bowel control and sexual organ function are similarly affected by spinal cord lesions because the parasympathetic reflexive connections for these organs are also located at levels S2-S4. The person with a spinal cord lesion above the sacral cord is unaware of rectal stretch and has no voluntary control of sphincters, yet rectal stretch can elicit reflexive emptying of the lower bowel because the reflexive lower bowel emptying circuit is intact. If the bowel emptying reflex circuit is interrupted by a lesion of S2-S4 or the parasympathetic connections with S2-S4, the parasympathetic influence on peristalsis and reflex emptying of the bowels is lost.

Reflexive sexual erection can occur if the sacral cord is intact. In some men with complete spinal lesions above the lumbar level in whom the lumbosacral cord is intact, ejaculation can be elicited reflexively because sympathetic axons from the L1 and L2 levels and somatic nerves from the S2-S4 levels control ejaculation. Fertile women with spinal cord lesions can conceive and often have a normal pregnancy, but they frequently require cesarean delivery.

## TRAUMATIC SPINAL CORD INJURY

Traumatic injuries to the spinal cord usually are caused by motor vehicle accidents, sports injuries, falls, or penetrating wounds. The first three types of injuries typically do not sever the cord. Instead, damage is due to crush, hemorrhage, edema, and infarction. Penetrating wounds, by a knife or a bullet, directly sever neurons in the cord.

Immediately after a traumatic injury to the spinal cord, cord functions below the lesion are depressed or lost. This condition, known as *spinal shock,* is due to interruption of descending tracts that supply tonic facilitation to the spinal cord neurons. During spinal shock, the following may occur:

- Somatic reflexes, including stretch reflexes, withdrawal reflexes, and crossed extension reflexes, are lost.
- Autonomic reflexes, including smooth muscle tone and reflexive emptying of the bladder and bowels, are lost or impaired.

- Autonomic regulation of blood pressure is impaired, resulting in hypotension.
- Control of sweating and piloerection is lost.

Several weeks after the injury, most people experience some recovery of function in the cord, leading to return of reflex activity below the lesion. In some people, spinal neurons become excessively excitable, resulting in stretch reflex hyperreflexia (see Chapter 10). Hyperreflexia develops as neuroplasticity produces new synapses in the reflex pathway.[21]

Damage to the cervical cord results in *tetraplegia* (quadriplegia) with impairment of arm, trunk, lower limb, and pelvic organ function. People with lesions above the C4 level cannot breathe independently, because the phrenic nerve (C3-C5) innervates the diaphragm, and thoracic nerves innervate the intercostal and abdominal muscles. *Paraplegia* results from damage to the cord below the cervical level, sparing arm function. Function of the trunk, lower limbs, and pelvic organs in paraplegia depends on the level of the lesion. Table 13-3 lists the motor capabilities and sensations mediated by each spinal cord level.

### Abnormal Interneuron Activity in Chronic Spinal Cord Injury

Chronic spinal cord injury is the period after recovery from spinal shock when the neurologic deficit is stable, neither progressing nor improving (Pathology 13-2). This period can last for decades.

| **PATHOLOGY 13-2** | **CHRONIC SPINAL CORD INJURY** |
|---|---|
| Pathology | Crush, severance, hemorrhage, edema, and/or infarction |
| Etiology | Trauma |
| Speed of onset | Acute |
| Signs and symptoms | |
| Consciousness | Normal |
| Communication and memory | Normal |
| Sensory | Depends on what part of the spinal cord is damaged. In a complete spinal cord lesion, all sensation is lost below the level of the lesion. |
| Autonomic | Depends on what part of the spinal cord is damaged. In a complete spinal cord lesion, all descending autonomic regulation is lost below the level of the lesion, including voluntary bladder and bowel control; if the lesion is above T6, autonomic dysreflexia, poor thermoregulation, and orthostatic hypotension may occur. |
| Motor | Depends on what part of the spinal cord is damaged. In a complete spinal cord lesion, all voluntary motor control below the level of the lesion is lost. |
| Region affected | Spinal region |
| Demographics | 4:1 ratio of males to females[23] |
| Incidence | 1.9 per 100,000 population per year[24] |
| Lifetime prevalence | 0.7 per 1000 population[23] |
| Prognosis | Currently, no functional regeneration of neurons in the central nervous system occurs in humans. Neurologic recovery, if it occurs, is rapid initially (hours to weeks) as the edema and hemorrhage resolve. People with incomplete spinal cord injury have much better recovery of function than people with complete spinal cord injury. Once the lesion is stable (no more bleeding, infarction, edema), the neurologic deficit does not change. People with spinal cord injury may live a normal life span. |

**TABLE 13-3** FUNCTIONAL ABILITIES ASSOCIATED WITH COMPLETE SPINAL CORD LESIONS AT VARIOUS LEVELS

| Level of Lesion | Motor Capability* | Intact Sensation | Mobility | ADLs/Transfers | Limitations |
|---|---|---|---|---|---|
| C1-C3 | Facial muscles, upper trapezius, sternocleidomastoid | Neck and head (cranial nerves from face; C2: posterior head, upper neck; C3: lower neck) | Breath/chin controlled power wheelchair (WC) | Dependent in all activities of daily living (ADLs)/transfers | Ventilator dependent |
| C4 | Diaphragm | Upper shoulder | Breath/chin controlled power WC | Dependent in all ADLs/transfers | No upper limb movement |
| C5 | Elbow flexors | Lateral upper arm | Hand controlled power WC; able to use manual WC with rim projections but requires excessive time and energy | Able to perform some ADLs with adaptive equipment if an assistant sets up required items. Dependent in transfers | Unable to extend elbow or move hand |
| C6 | Wrist extensors | Lateral forearm and lateral hand | Manual WC with rim projections; drive using hand controls | Independent ADLs except lower limb dressing. Transfers independent except toilet | Unable to extend elbow or move hand |
| C7 | Elbow extensors | Middle finger | WC on level surfaces | Independent except floor/WC transfers | Unable to move fingers and thumb |
| C8 | Finger flexors | Medial hand | Up/down 2–4 inch curbs in WC | Independent living | Some intrinsic hand muscle function; difficulty with fine motor tasks |
| T1 | Finger abductors | Medial forearm | | | No lower abdominals |
| T2-T6 | | T2: medial upper arm; T3-T6: torso | WC up/down 6 inch curbs | | No lower abdominals |
| T7-T12 | Abdominals, lateral spine flexion | T7-T12: torso (T10: level of umbilicus) | Sit-to-stand and walk with orthoses indoors | | No hip flexors |
| L1 | — | Anterior upper thigh | | | |
| L2 | Hip flexors | Anterior thigh, below L1 | Community walking with orthoses | | No quadriceps |
| L3 | Knee extensors | Anterior knee | | | No gluteus maximus |
| L4 | Ankle dorsiflexors | Medial leg | | | |
| L5 | Long toe extensors | Lateral leg, dorsum of foot | | | |
| S1 | Ankle plantarflexors | Posterior calf and lateral foot | | | No bowel/bladder voluntary control |
| S2 | — | Posterior thigh | | | |
| S3 | — | Ring surrounding S4-S5 | | | |
| S4-S5 | Voluntary anal contraction | Ring surrounding anus | | | |

*Each additional level adds functions to the capabilities of the higher levels. Muscles listed may be only partially innervated at the level indicated. Thus the quadriceps usually has some voluntary activity if the L3 level is intact; however, the action is weak unless the L4 level is also intact. ADLs (activities of daily living) include eating, bathing, dressing, grooming, work, homemaking, and leisure.

In chronic spinal cord injury, two abnormalities in interneuron activity occur below the level of the lesion:
- Inhibitory interneuron response to type Ia afferent activity is diminished.
- Transmission from cutaneous afferents to lower motor neurons is facilitated.

The first change correlates with hyperreflexia, and the second change occurs because of the loss of descending inhibition. Upper motor neurons normally inhibit interneurons that produce the withdrawal reflex. Without this inhibition, an exaggerated withdrawal reflex occurs in response to normally innocuous stimuli in some people with spinal cord injury.[22] For example, light touch on the thigh may trigger a withdrawal reflex of the entire lower limb. Additional changes secondary to spinal cord injury include loss of lower motor neurons and changes in mechanical properties of muscle fibers: atrophy of muscle fibers, fibrosis, and alteration of contractile properties toward tonic muscle characteristics.

## Classification of Spinal Cord Injuries

Spinal cord injuries are classified according to two criteria[25]:
- Whether the injury is complete or incomplete
- The neurologic level of injury

A *complete injury* is defined as lack of sensory and motor function in the lowest sacral segment. An *incomplete injury* is defined as preservation of sensory and/or motor function in the lowest sacral segment.

The *neurologic level* is the most caudal level with normal sensory and motor function bilaterally. However, motor function may be impaired at a level different from sensory function, and the losses may be asymmetric. In these cases, up to four different neurologic segments may be described in a single patient: right sensory, left sensory, right motor, and left motor.

## Determination of Neurologic Levels

The American Spinal Injury Association (ASIA) has developed a standardized assessment for evaluating neurologic level in spinal cord injury. The ASIA classification form is presented in Figure 13-21. Key sensory points (28 bilateral points) are tested with a safety pin to determine the person's ability to distinguish sharp from dull, and with light touches with cotton to determine the ability to localize light touch. In addition, testing of deep pressure and of position sense in the index fingers and great toes is recommended. Key muscles are tested on the right and left sides of the body. Scoring criteria for each test are listed on the form.

## Autonomic Dysfunction in Spinal Cord Injury

During spinal shock, neural control of the pelvic organs is depressed. Therefore, the bladder and bowel walls are atonic, allowing overfilling of these viscera, and overflow leaking occurs (see Figure 13-19, *A*). Overfilling and overflow leaking can be avoided by establishing a regular bladder and bowel emptying routine. After recovery from spinal shock, a complete lesion above the sacral level usually allows some reflexive functioning of the pelvic organs, but voluntary control is not possible, and the person is deprived of conscious awareness of the state of the pelvic organs.

Complete lesions at higher levels of the spinal cord cause more serious abnormalities of autonomic regulation because more segments of the cord are free from descending sympathetic control. Loss of descending sympathetic control due to lesions above T6 results in three dysfunctions:
- Autonomic dysreflexia
- Poor thermoregulation (body temperature regulation)
- Orthostatic hypotension

### Autonomic Dysreflexia

*Autonomic dysreflexia* (also called *mass reflex*) is excessive activity of the sympathetic nervous system elicited by noxious stimuli below the lesion. Often the precipitating stimulus is overstretching of the bladder or rectum. Collaterals from tract neurons conveying signals regarding noxious input facilitate sympathetic neurons. Normally this facilitation is balanced by inhibitory signals from the brain. Lesions above the T6 level prevent most of the spinal cord from receiving signals from the brain that inhibit sympathetic activity. The excessive sympathetic response is characterized by an abrupt increase in blood pressure and a pounding headache. In addition, flushing of the skin and profuse sweating occur above the level of the lesion. The sudden spike in blood pressure may be life threatening. Figure 13-22 compares the normal response to visceral distention or pain with autonomic dysreflexia.

### Poor Thermoregulation

*Poor thermoregulation* may interfere with the ability to maintain homeostasis. Normally, body temperature regulation is achieved by descending sympathetic innervation. In spinal cord injury, reflexive sweating below the lesion may be intact; however, interruption of sympathetic pathways prevents thermoregulatory sweating (response to increased ambient temperature) below the level of injury. To compensate, excessive sweating may occur above the level of the lesion. People with complete lesions above the T6 level should avoid exposure to high ambient temperatures because of the risk of heat stroke. Signs of heat stroke include high body temperature, rapid pulse, and dry, flushed skin. These signs indicate a medical emergency because untreated heat stroke can cause permanent brain damage or convulsions and death. In cold weather, hypothermia is a risk because the person with a complete lesion above T6 has lost descending control of blood vessels and the ability to shiver below the lesion. Signs of hypothermia include irritability, mental confusion, hallucinations, lethargy, clumsiness, slow respiration, and slowing of the heartbeat.

### Orthostatic Hypotension

*Orthostatic hypotension* is a 20 mm Hg or greater fall in systolic blood pressure or a 10 mm Hg or greater fall in diastolic blood pressure on assuming an upright position. In people with spinal cord injury, this is caused by loss of sympathetic vasoconstriction combined with loss of muscle-pumping action for blood return. Figure 13-23 summarizes the autonomic dysfunctions associated with various levels of spinal cord injury.

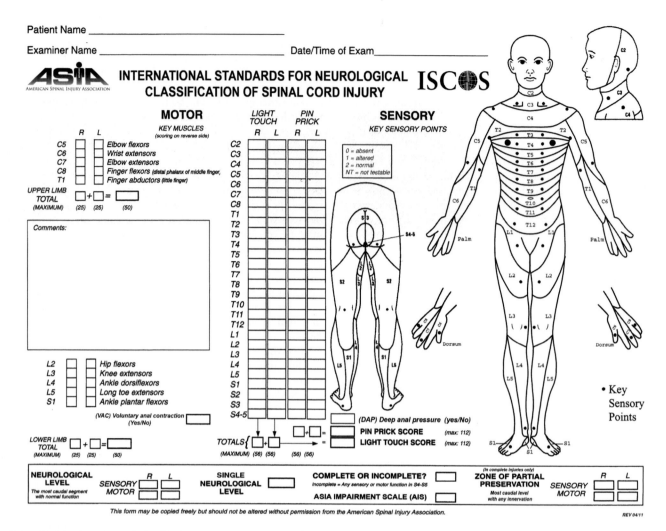

**Fig. 13-21** **American Spinal Injury Association classification of spinal cord injury.** Motor scores are recorded on the left half of the form. The scoring criteria are listed in the large box. The two columns, headed by the letters *R* (*right*) and *L* (*left*), are used to record the scores of the listed muscles. To the left of the columns is a list of segments of the spinal cord. Sensory scores are recorded on the right half of the form. Scoring criteria are in the small box. Areas of impaired or absent sensation can be indicated on the dermatome diagrams. At the bottom of the motor and sensory sections are small boxes for totaling motor and sensory scores. The neurologic level is recorded at the bottom of the form, according to the criteria listed there. *(From American Spinal Injury Association. Reference Manual of the International Standards for Neurological Classification of Spinal Cord Injury, Chicago, IL, 2006, American Spinal Injury Association.)*

## Prognosis and Treatment in Spinal Cord Injury

Unlike axons in the peripheral nervous system, severed axons in the adult spinal cord fail to functionally regenerate. Barriers to regeneration include inhibitory molecules on oligodendrocytes, impenetrable glial scars, and decreased rate of growth (compared with embryonic neurons) in mature neurons.[26–28] However, some of the functional losses after spinal cord injury are not due to the original trauma but instead are due to secondary changes; these include bleeding, edema, ischemia, pain, and inflammation.

People with incomplete paraplegia have the highest rate of recovery during the first 3 months post injury, with relatively small gains after 3 months. The contrast between functional recovery in complete versus incomplete paraplegia at 1 year post

injury is striking. Table 13-4 summarizes the ambulation prognosis for people with paraplegia.

Typical complications after spinal cord injury include urinary tract infection, spasticity, chills and fever, decubiti, autonomic dysreflexia, contractures, heterotropic ossification, and pneumonia. Upright posture can provide some protection against urinary tract infection and pneumonia; mobility can help avoid contractures and decubiti. Currently, strengthening and range-of-motion exercises, mobility and activities of daily living training, adaptive equipment, and environmental modifications are commonly used in spinal cord injury rehabilitation.

A recent study of 64 people with incomplete spinal cord injury longer than 1 year post injury compared four body weight supported training methods for improving gait:

| TABLE 13-4 PERCENTAGE OF PEOPLE WITH DIFFERING ASIA* SCORES ABLE TO WALK AT TIME OF DISCHARGE FROM HOSPITAL | |
| --- | --- |
| ASIA Impairment Scale Score at Admission | Able to Walk at Time of Discharge |
| A: complete—no motor or sensory function is preserved in the sacral segments S4-S5 | 6% |
| B: incomplete—sensory but not motor function is preserved below the neurologic level and includes the sacral segments S4-S5 | 23% |
| C: incomplete—motor function is preserved below the neurologic level, and more than half of key muscles below the neurologic level have a muscle grade less than 3 | 50% |
| D: incomplete—motor function is preserved below the neurologic level, and at least half of key muscles below the neurologic level have a muscle grade of 3 or more | 89% |

*ASIA Impairment Scale from the American Spinal Injury Association (2006). Data on walking ability at discharge from Morganti et al. (2005).

treadmill with manual assistance, treadmill with electrical stimulation, treadmill with robotic assistance, and overground training with electrical stimulation. Body weight support used a lift and an overhead harness. Gait speed improved in all groups, with no differences in gait speed among the groups. The overground training group improved significantly more than the other groups in distance walked. The authors suggested that overground training may have been superior because subjects learned to maximize their remaining upper motor neuron control of the spinal cord circuitry, but the treadmill training groups relied on afferent stimulation provided by the moving treadmill.[29]

## SPECIFIC DISORDERS AFFECTING SPINAL REGION FUNCTION

Other disorders in addition to traumatic spinal cord injury interfere with spinal region function. These include meningomyelocele, spastic cerebral palsy, lesions of dorsal and ventral nerve roots, multiple sclerosis, and lesions that cause compression in the spinal cord.

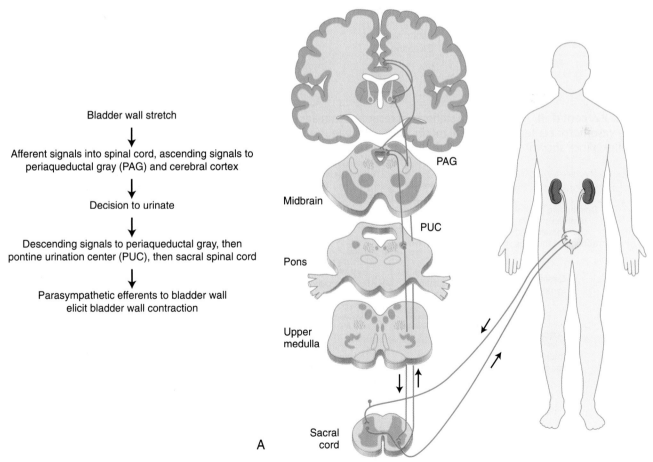

Bladder wall stretch

↓

Afferent signals into spinal cord, ascending signals to periaqueductal gray (PAG) and cerebral cortex

↓

Decision to urinate

↓

Descending signals to periaqueductal gray, then pontine urination center (PUC), then sacral spinal cord

↓

Parasympathetic efferents to bladder wall elicit bladder wall contraction

**Fig. 13-22** **Normal response to bladder distention versus autonomic dysreflexia. A,** Normal response to bladder distention.

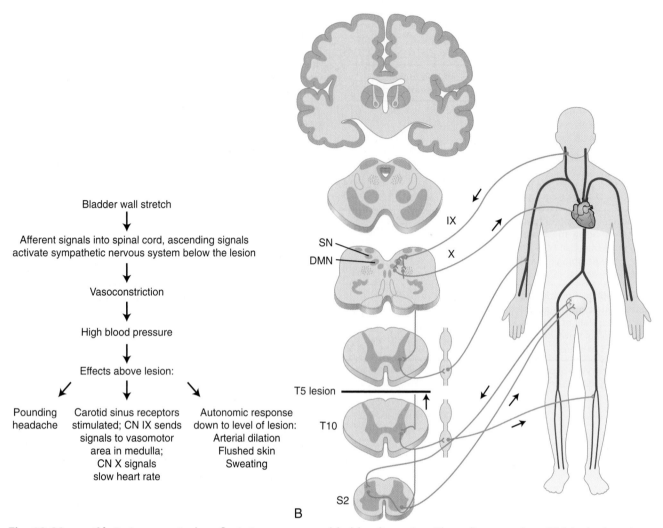

Bladder wall stretch

↓

Afferent signals into spinal cord, ascending signals
activate sympathetic nervous system below the lesion

↓

Vasoconstriction

↓

High blood pressure

↓

Effects above lesion:

↙    ↓    ↘

Pounding
headache

Carotid sinus receptors
stimulated; CN IX sends
signals to vasomotor
area in medulla;
CN X signals
slow heart rate

Autonomic response
down to level of lesion:
Arterial dilation
Flushed skin
Sweating

B

**Fig. 13-22, cont'd   B,** Autonomic dysreflexia in response to bladder distention. The solitary nucleus (SN) is the location of the vasomotor center. DMN, dorsal motor nucleus of vagus nerve (efferents to heart). Other causes of autonomic dysreflexia (not shown) include bowel distention and visceral pain.

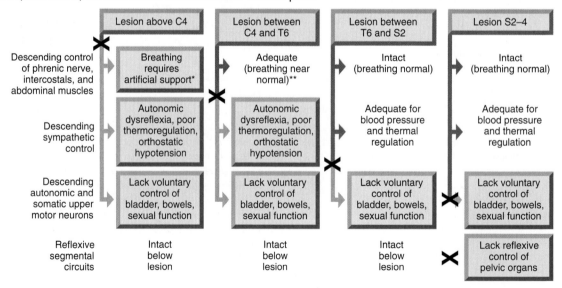

| | Lesion above C4 | Lesion between C4 and T6 | Lesion between T6 and S2 | Lesion S2–4 |
|---|---|---|---|---|
| Descending control of phrenic nerve, intercostals, and abdominal muscles | Breathing requires artificial support* | Adequate (breathing near normal)** | Intact (breathing normal) | Intact (breathing normal) |
| Descending sympathetic control | Autonomic dysreflexia, poor thermoregulation, orthostatic hypotension | Autonomic dysreflexia, poor thermoregulation, orthostatic hypotension | Adequate for blood pressure and thermal regulation | Adequate for blood pressure and thermal regulation |
| Descending autonomic and somatic upper motor neurons | Lack voluntary control of bladder, bowels, sexual function | Lack voluntary control of bladder, bowels, sexual function | Lack voluntary control of bladder, bowels, sexual function | Lack voluntary control of bladder, bowels, sexual function |
| Reflexive segmental circuits | Intact below lesion | Intact below lesion | Intact below lesion | Lack reflexive control of pelvic organs |

\* Ventilator or phrenic nerve stimulator dependent; may learn to breathe using glossopharyngeal technique for short periods.
\*\* Abdominal muscles and lower intercostal muscles do not receive descending control.

**Fig. 13-23** Autonomic dysfunctions associated with various levels of spinal cord injury.

## Meningomyelocele

Outcomes of meningomyelocele, a developmental defect arising from failure of the inferior neuropore to close (see Chapter 5), are roughly equivalent to those of spinal cord injury in later life. If the lesion is in the lower lumbar spinal cord, anterior thigh muscles may be functional and sensation intact in the overlying skin, with the remainder of the lower limbs nonmoving and insensitive to sensory stimulation, and with no voluntary or reflexive control of the pelvic organs. If the lesion is below S1, skeletal muscle control is intact throughout the body (except the bladder external sphinter and the anal sphincter), and dermatomes are intact above the S2 level; however, reflexive and voluntary control of the bladder and bowel is absent because the sacral cord contains the connections for these reflexes.

## Spastic Cerebral Palsy

Cerebral palsy is a motor disorder that develops in utero or during infancy. Spastic cerebral palsy is characterized by excessive muscle contraction and phasic stretch hyperreflexia. The hyperreflexia resulting from overexcitation of local reflex circuits can be inhibited by surgically cutting selected dorsal rootlets, thus decreasing sensory input to the reflex circuit. Thus, to alleviate lower limb hyperreflexia in children with spastic cerebral palsy, selected dorsal rootlets sometimes are surgically severed *(dorsal rhizotomy)*. Dorsal rhizotomy reduces hyperreflexia by interrupting the afferent limb of the stretch reflex. Each rootlet is electrically stimulated, and only rootlets that contribute to abnormal muscle activity are cut. Dorsal rhizotomy typically is performed at the L2-L5 level. Goals of surgery are to improve motor function and to make bathing, positioning, and dressing easier. Dorsal rhizotomy combined with physical therapy improves: lower limb spasticity and range of motion; range of motion during walking in children able to walk; the level of ambulation in children unable to independently ambulate before surgery; and upper limb function. Adverse events, although uncommon, include back pain, spinal deformity, transient urinary retention, and temporary dysesthesia.[30] Careful evaluation of the child's potential for improved function is vital before surgery is performed.

## Lesions of Dorsal and Ventral Nerve Roots

A lesion of a nerve root is termed *radiculopathy;* however, this term also is often used clinically to refer to damage to a spinal nerve. Mechanical irritation or infection of a dorsal root produces pain in the innervated dermatome and in the muscles innervated by the spinal cord segment. Mechanical irritation can be produced by a herniated intervertebral disk, a tumor, or a dislocated fracture. However, herniated vertebral disks do not always cause symptoms; between 60% and 90% of people with herniated disks are asymptomatic.[31] When a dorsal root is irritated, coughing or sneezing often aggravates the pain.

Other conditions affecting the spinal nerve roots include infection, avulsion, and severance. Avulsion or complete severance of the dorsal root causes loss of sensation in the dermatome. Avulsion or complete severance of a ventral root deprives the muscles in its myotome of motor innervation, resulting in muscle atrophy and fibrillation.

Traumatic avulsion of the C5 and C6 motor nerve roots causes *Erb's paralysis.* This paralysis is the result of forceful separation of the head and shoulder. Birth trauma, produced by traction pulling the head away from the shoulder, and motorcycle accidents in which a person lands on a shoulder often cause Erb's paralysis. Shoulder abduction, external rotation, and elbow flexion are lost, producing the characteristic "waiter's tip" position of the upper limb. Biceps and brachioradialis stretch reflexes are lost.

*Klumpke's paralysis,* due to avulsion of the motor roots of C8 and T1, results in paralysis and atrophy of the hand intrinsic muscles and the long flexors and extensors of the fingers. The precipitating injury is traction on the abducted arm.

## Lesions of Dorsal Root Ganglia

Dorsal root ganglia (DRG), located within the intervertebral foramina, are more sensitive to mechanical damage than are proximal or distal axons of primary nociceptive afferents. DRG compression induces alterations in the production of neuropeptides, receptors (including *N*-methyl-D-aspartate [NMDA] receptors), and ion channels in primary nociceptive afferents. DRG develop ectopic foci that generate action potentials in response to mechanical stimulation.[32] Normally action potentials are generated only at the axon hillock (tract and interneurons) or near the receptor (sensory neurons). DRG-generated action potentials are perceived as pain in the distribution of the peripheral axon, resulting in severe hyperalgesia. An example is *sciatica*—pain radiating from the low back and down the lower limb along the path of the sciatic nerve. Sciatica is a symptom typically caused by compression of dorsal roots and/or dorsal root ganglia by a herniated disk, spinal stenosis, spondylolisthesis (anterior slipping of one vertebra relative to another), or piriformis syndrome. In piriformis syndrome, the muscle compresses the sciatic nerve. If DRG compression causes sciatica, the pain may be incapacitating. If nerve roots or peripheral axons are compressed, the pain is less intense. Sciatica may be accompanied by numbness, weakness, and/or tingling sensations.

A common infection of the somas in the dorsal root is varicella zoster, also called *herpes zoster* or *shingles* (see Chapter 7).

## Multiple Sclerosis

*Multiple sclerosis* is characterized by random, multifocal demyelination limited to the central nervous system (see Chapter 2). Signs and symptoms of multiple sclerosis are exceptionally variable because the demyelination can occur in a wide variety of locations, and the extent of the lesions varies. Sensory complaints may include numbness, paresthesias, and *Lhermitte's sign.* Lhermitte's sign is the radiation of a sensation similar to electric shock down the back or limbs, elicited by neck flexion. Frequently, multiple sclerosis of the spinal cord produces asymmetric weakness caused by plaques interfering with the descending motor tracts and ataxia of the lower limbs due to interruption of conduction in the dorsal columns.

## Transverse Myelitis

*Transverse myelitis* is a rare immune disorder that damages a limited part of the spinal cord. The resulting inflammation spreads across the width of the spinal cord (transversely), producing spinal segment losses and blocking signals traveling up and down the spinal cord. Signs and symptoms are bilateral. Segmental effects include myotomal weakness and dermatomal sensory loss. Damage to vertical tracts produces upper motor neuron signs, loss of somatosensation, and bladder, bowel, and sexual dysfunction, depending on the location of the lesion. Typically, transverse myelitis begins with acute back pain and a band-like area of tightness surrounding the chest or abdomen around affected spinal segments. Within hours to a few days, weakness, tingling, and numbness affect the feet; then the signs and symptoms move upward. Transverse myelitis progressively worsens following onset, for up to 3 weeks. Most of the recovery occurs within 3 months of onset, although improvement may continue for longer than a year. Causes include multiple sclerosis and multisystemic disease, or the condition may be idiopathic. The incidence is 0.13 to 0.8 per 100,000.[33] Recovery usually begins within 6 months. Good recovery occurs in about one third of cases; another one third have moderate permanent disability, and one third have severe disabilities.[34]

## Compression in the Spinal Region

Pressure in the spinal region or restriction of blood flow due to compression can cause any of the following symptoms: pain (usually constant), sensory changes, weakness, paralysis, hypertonia, ataxia, and impaired bladder and/or bowel function. The clinical presentation depends on the location of the lesion. Gradual onset, progressive worsening, no history of trauma, and the combination of segmental and vertical tract signs indicate the possibility of a spinal region tumor, cervical spondylosis, or syringomyelia.

## Spinal Region Tumors

Tumors outside the dura mater or in the subarachnoid space may compress the spinal cord, nerve roots, and spinal nerve, or their blood supply. Tumors can also occur within the spinal cord, resulting in pressure on the neurons and vascular supply from within the cord. Pain, aggravated by coughing or sneezing, is the most common initial symptom. Tumors can produce segmental and/or vertical tract signs, depending on their location.

## Vertebral Canal Stenosis

Stenosis is narrowing of the vertebral canal (Figure 13-24) that results in compression of neural and vascular structures. Stenosis is usually a degenerative disorder caused by bone growth,

facet hypertrophy, bulging disks, and hypertrophy of the ligamentum flavum. Figure 13-25 shows spinal cord compression in a patient with multilevel cervical spinal stenosis.

### Cervical Stenosis

Signs and symptoms vary, depending upon whether the lesion affects the intervertebral foramina or the central canal and how many cervical vertebral levels are involved. Narrowing of the intervertebral foramina compresses spinal nerves, resulting in a dermatomal distribution of abnormal sensations (tingling, prickling, burning, and/or electrical sensations), pain, and numbness, along with myotomal (lower motor neuron) distribution of weakness and atrophy in the upper limb.

Narrowing of the central canal compresses the spinal cord, causing cervical spondylotic myelopathy (myelo = spinal cord). The injury interferes with segmental and vertical tract function. Although the location of the lesion is in the spinal cord, the effects on segmental function (somatosensory abnormalities and lower motor neuron dysfunction) are the same as when the spinal nerve is compressed because the lesion compromises the proximal axons of the somatosensory neurons and the lower motor neuron cell bodies. In addition, compression of the vertical tracts affects both the upper and lower limbs.

Some cervical spondylotic myelopathy cases may cause only axial neck pain and/or scapular pain.[35] More severe cases involve the vertical tracts.

Compression of the somatosensory vertical tracts causes:
- abnormal sensations (tingling, prickling, burning, electrical) and
- numbness in the upper and lower limbs.

Compression of vertical tracts conveying proprioceptive and motor information causes:
- abnormal gait,
- incoordination, and
- upper motor neuron (UMN) signs.

Abnormal gait is often the first sign of cervical myelopathy, caused by damage to the spinocerebellar and UMN tracts. Additional UMN signs in the lower limb may include paresis, hyperreflexia of the stretch reflex, Babinski's sign, clonus, and spasticity. Later, as the stenosis progresses, upper limb coordination and fine motor control are impaired by damage to the spinocerebellar tracts and corticospinal tracts. Neural control of the bladder and bowels may be compromised.

The incidence of cervical spondylotic myelopathy is 2 cases per 100,000 people per year, with a prevalence of 0.4 per 1000 people.[36] Recent research indicates that people with moderate to severe cervical spondylotic myelopathy benefit from surgery, and that those with minimal neurologic signs and larger space within the spinal canal can be managed with a soft collar,

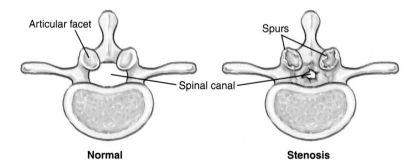

**Fig. 13-24 Spinal stenosis.** Narrowing of the spinal canal and intervertebral foramina compresses the spinal cord and/or spinal nerve roots.

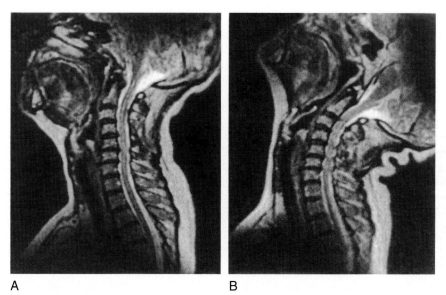

A                                         B

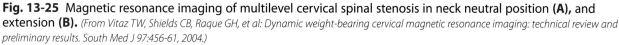

**Fig. 13-25** Magnetic resonance imaging of multilevel cervical spinal stenosis in neck neutral position **(A)**, and extension **(B)**. *(From Vitaz TW, Shields CB, Raque GH, et al: Dynamic weight-bearing cervical magnetic resonance imaging: technical review and preliminary results. South Med J 97:456-61, 2004.)*

nonsteroidal anti-inflammatory drugs, and avoidance of activities that have a high risk of neck trauma.[35]

*Lumbar stenosis* produces lower limb and lower back pain that may be aggravated by walking and improves with rest. If stenosis is severe, compression of spinal nerve roots and/or the cauda equina causes additional signs and symptoms. In severe stenosis, paresis, clumsiness, falling, foot drop during gait, numbness, tingling, and/or a heavy, tired feeling in the lower limbs may occur. Flexing the lumbar spine often relieves these signs and symptoms.

## Syringomyelia

*Syringomyelia* is a rare, progressive disorder that most frequently occurs in people 35 to 45 years of age. A syrinx, or a fluid-filled cavity, develops in the spinal cord, almost always in the cervical region. Syringomyelia usually is congenital but may occur secondary to trauma or tumor. Accumulation of cerebrospinal fluid in the syrinx causes increased pressure inside the spinal cord, expanding the cavity and compressing adjacent nerve fibers. Segmental signs occur in the upper limbs: loss of sensitivity to pain and temperature stimuli, due to interruption of axons crossing the midline in the anterior white commissure; paresis; and muscle atrophy. Sensory loss is often distributed like a cape draped over the shoulders (see Figure 13-19, *B*). Upper motor neuron signs in the lower limbs include paresis, muscle hypertonia, spasticity, and loss of bowel and bladder control.

## RED FLAGS FOR THE SPINAL REGION

Signs and symptoms that indicate a spinal cord lesion include the following:
- Bilateral alteration or loss of somatosensation
- Incoordination, caused by inadequate somatosensory information to the cerebellum. Confirm that the ataxia is

somatosensory and is not cerebellar or vestibular by findings of impaired proprioception, vibration, and two-point discrimination.
- Upper motor neuron signs: decreased muscle power, spasticity, muscle hypertonia, Babinski's sign, and clonus

Signs and symptoms that indicate a possible cauda equina lesion include:
- Difficulty with urination/defecation
- Decreased or lost sensation in the saddle area
- Low back pain
- Unilateral or bilateral sciatica
- Lower limb paresis and sensory deficits
- Decreased or lost lower limb reflexes

In cauda equina syndrome, no upper motor neuron signs occur because the lesion is inferior to the end of the spinal cord; thus, only nerve roots are affected. Sudden onset of cauda equina syndrome is a medical emergency requiring immediate referral.

Signs and symptoms that indicate intermittent claudication, a vascular disorder that must be differentiated from sciatica, include the following:
- Pain in the buttock, posterior lower limb, and/or foot while walking or exercising that disappears after a brief rest
- Decreased pulse in the lower limb
- Cyanosis (bluish color of the skin due to deoxygenated hemoglobin in blood vessels near the surface of the skin)

## SUMMARY

Lesions of the spinal cord produce segmental and/or vertical tract signs. Segmental signs include the following:
- Sensory changes: impaired sensations, paresthesias, and dysesthesias, in a dermatomal distribution
- Lower motor neuron signs (paresis or paralysis, atrophy, cramps) in a myotomal distribution

- If dorsal nerve roots are involved, increasing intra-abdominal pressure by straining, sneezing, or coughing may produce sharp, radiating pain.
  Common vertical tract signs include the following:
- Sensory changes: decreased or lost sensation below the level of the lesion

- Autonomic signs: decreased or lost voluntary control of pelvic organs, autonomic dysreflexia, poor thermoregulation, and/or orthostatic hypotension
- Upper motor neuron lesion signs: muscle hypertonia, paresis, spasticity, Babinski's sign

## CLINICAL NOTES

### Case 1

P.E. is a 17-year-old woman. She fractured the C7 vertebra in a diving accident 2 months ago. The fracture is stable. Current findings are as follows:
- Sensation is intact (pinprick, temperature, conscious proprioception, and discriminative touch) in her head, neck, and lateral upper limbs.
- She has no sensation in the medial upper limbs, the trunk below the sternal angle, and the lower limbs.
- All head and shoulder movements are normal strength except shoulder extension.
- Elbow flexion and radial wrist extensors are normal strength.
- The remaining upper limb, trunk, and lower limb muscles have no trace of voluntary movement.
- Babinski's sign is present bilaterally.

Without adaptive equipment, P.E. is unable to care for herself. Using adaptive equipment, she is able to eat, dress, and groom independently. She uses a wheelchair. She cannot voluntarily control her bladder or bowels.

#### Questions
1. Is the lesion in the dorsal or ventral root or in the spinal cord?
2. What neurologic level is the lesion? Note: The neurologic level in a spinal cord injury is the most caudal level with normal sensory and motor function bilaterally. Refer to Table 13-4 to determine the neurologic level. Is the lesion complete or incomplete?

### Case 2

B.D. is a 16-year-old adolescent. He sustained a spinal cord injury 2 months ago in a fall from a bicycle. Current findings are as follows:
- Pinprick and temperature sensation are impaired, as indicated in Figure 13-26. All other sensations are fully intact.
- Manual muscle test scores are also indicated in Figure 13-26.
- Babinski's sign is present bilaterally.
- He is independent in all activities. He is able to walk 30 meters using an ankle-foot orthosis on his left leg and a cane.

#### Questions
1. What level is the cord lesion? Is the lesion complete, or does the pattern indicate a spinal cord syndrome?
2. Why is this patient independent, while the patient in Case 1 requires adaptive equipment, a wheelchair, and maximal assistance on stairs?

### Case 3

V.K. is a 30-year-old man. He plays recreational sports 4 days a week and is a highly competitive soccer player. Two years ago, he experienced temporary weakness in his left lower leg, which gradually resolved without consultation or treatment. His primary complaint now is inability to control his right foot. He first noticed poor kicking skills 3 weeks ago. Sensation and motor control are normal except in the right lower limb. The following deficits are observed in the right lower limb:
- Discriminative touch, vibration sense, and position sense are impaired throughout.
- Pain and temperature sensations are intact.
- Movement is ataxic. Gait deficits: dragging of toes on the ground during the swing phase of walking (foot drop), poor placement of the foot on the ground, weight bearing on the right lower limb only half the time spent weight bearing on the left lower limb
- Gluteals, hamstrings, and all muscles originating below the knee are weak, less than half the strength of the homologous muscles on the left. The same muscles are hypertonic. Reflex testing reveals gastrocnemius hyper-reflexia and Babinski's sign on the left.

## CLINICAL NOTES—cont'd

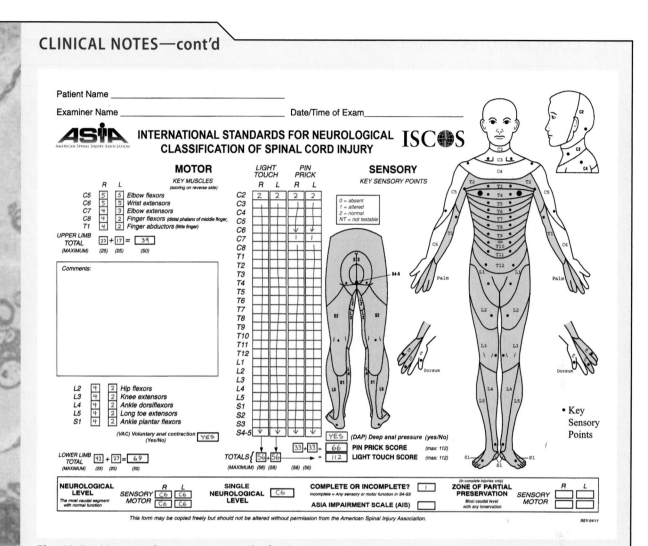

**Fig. 13-26** Motor and sensory test results for Case 2. *(Form courtesy of American Spinal Injury Association. Reference Manual of the International Standards for Neurological Classification of Spinal Cord Injury. Chicago, IL, 2006, American Spinal Injury Association.)*

### Questions

1. Why are pain and temperature sensations intact bilaterally?
2. Where is the lesion?
3. What is the probable etiology?

## Case 4

E.V. is a 62-year-old woman. She reports constant burning pain radiating down the back of her left leg into her foot. When she coughs or sneezes, sharp, stabbing pains become excruciating. The pain began as a backache 3 months ago. Pain intensity has been consistently increasing. Following are the results of testing:

- Sensation is intact in the right lower limb.
- Sensory testing results for the left lower limb are shown in Table 13-5.
- Strength in all limbs is within normal limits.
- Ankle deep tendon reflex is absent on the left side.

### Questions

1. Where is the lesion?
2. What is the probable etiology?
3. Why is discriminative touch more affected than pain and temperature sensations?

*Continued*

## CLINICAL NOTES—cont'd

**TABLE 13-5    SENSORY TESTING RESULTS FOR LEFT LOWER LIMB FOR CASE 4\***

| Spinal Level | Discriminative Touch | Joint Kinesthesia | Pinprick | Warm | Cold |
|---|---|---|---|---|---|
| L4 | 2 | Knee 2 | 2 | 2 | 2 |
| L5 | 2 | Ankle 1 | 2 | 2 | 2 |
| S1 | 0 | Ankle 1 | 0 | 0 | 0 |
| S2 | 0 | — | 1 | 1 | 1 |
| S3 | 0 | — | 1 | 1 | 1 |
| S4 | 2 | — | 2 | 2 | 2 |
| S5 | 2 | — | 2 | 2 | 2 |

*Scoring: 2, intact; 1, impaired; 0, absent.

### Case 5

A 48-year-old woman has a 5 year history of intermittent low back pain. She is otherwise healthy. Yesterday she had abrupt onset of severe pain in the perineal and sacral region and intermittent shooting pain down the back of her right lower limb, exacerbated by sitting and by coughing. Two hours later, she developed increased urinary frequency and a sensation of being unable to fully empty her bladder. Defecation frequency also increased.

- Somatosensation: decreased light touch and pinprick in perineal and sacral region. Somatosensation intact throughout rest of body. With the patient in the supine position, shooting pain is elicited in the posterior right leg when the therapist lifts the patient's leg to 30 degrees of hip flexion with the knee straight. The same maneuver flexing the left hip to 70 degrees does not elicit pain. Normally, this test, the straight leg raise, does not elicit pain with hip flexion to 70 degrees.
- Autonomic: increased frequency of urination and defecation; abnormal sensation of inability to completely empty bladder
- Motor: weak contraction of anal sphincter. MMT (manual muscle test) grade is 5 throughout both lower limbs.

#### Questions

1. Where is the lesion?
2. What is the probable etiology?
3. After the examination, what is the next step with this patient?

## REVIEW QUESTIONS

1. What is a spinal nerve?
2. What is the difference between a ventral root and a ventral primary ramus?
3. What is a spinal segment?
4. What is the function of the dorsal horn?
5. Which of Rexed's laminae is also known as the substantia gelatinosa?
6. Are reflexes and voluntary motor control entirely separate systems?
7. What is the function of reciprocal inhibition?
8. What aspects of walking are controlled by stepping pattern generators in the spinal cord? Why are stepping pattern generators by themselves inadequate to control walking?
9. How is voluntary voiding of urine controlled?
10. What are the differences in signs between segmental and vertical tract lesions?
11. List the four adult-onset spinal region syndromes, and draw spinal cord cross-sections that illustrate the location of the lesion in each syndrome.
12. Why are cord functions below the lesion depressed or lost immediately after a spinal cord injury?
13. Why do some people with spinal cord injuries have exaggerated withdrawal reflexes?
14. What is an incomplete spinal cord injury? Give two examples of syndromes that may result from incomplete spinal cord injury.
15. List the three conditions that arise when the spinal cord below the T6 level is deprived of descending sympathetic innervation.

# References

1. Shacklock M: *Clinical neurodynamics*, Oxford, 2005, Elsevier.
2. Ranger MR, Irwin GJ, Bunbury KM, et al: Changing body position alters the location of the spinal cord within the vertebral canal: a magnetic resonance imaging study. *Br J Anaesth* 101:804–809, 2008.
3. Laessoe U, Voigt M: Modification of stretch tolerance in a stooping position. *Scand J Med Sci Sports* 14:239–244, 2004.
4. Fettes PD, Leslie K, McNabb S, et al: Effect of spinal flexion on the conus medullaris: a case series using magnetic resonance imaging. *Anaesthesia* 61:521–523, 2006.
5. Morganti B, Scivoletto G, Ditunno P, et al: Walking index for spinal cord injury (WISCI): criterion validation. *Spinal Cord* 43:27–33, 2005.
6. Kraan GA, Hoogland PV, Wuisman PI: Extraforaminal ligament attachments of the thoracic spinal nerves in humans. *Eur Spine J* 18:490–498, 2009.
7. Kraan GA, Smit TH, Hoogland PV, et al: Lumbar extraforaminal ligaments act as a traction relief and prevent spinal nerve compression. *Clin Biomech (Bristol, Avon)* 25:10–15, 2010.
8. Nuckley DJ, Konodi MA, Raynak GC, et al: Neural space integrity of the lower cervical spine: effect of normal range of motion. *Spine* 27:587–595, 2002.
9. Fawcett JP, Georgiou J, Ruston J, et al: Nck adaptor proteins control the organization of neuronal circuits important for walking. *Proc Natl Acad Sci U S A* 104:20973–20978, 2007.
10. Edgerton VR, Roy RR: Activity-dependent plasticity of spinal locomotion: implications for sensory processing. *Exerc Sport Sci Rev* 37:171–178, 2009.
11. Norton JA, Mushahwar VK: Afferent inputs to mid- and lower-lumbar spinal segments are necessary for stepping in spinal cats. *Ann N Y Acad Sci* 1198:10–20, 2010.
12. McCrea DA, Rybak IA: Organization of mammalian locomotor rhythm and pattern generation. *Brain Res Rev* 57:134–146, 2008.
13. Duysens J, Bastiaanse CM, Smits-Engelsman BC, Dietz V: Gait acts as a gate for reflexes from the foot. *Can J Physiol Pharmacol* 82:715–722, 2004.
14. Minassian K, Persy I, Rattay F, et al: Human lumbar cord circuitries can be activated by extrinsic tonic input to generate locomotor-like activity. *Hum Mov Sci* 26:275–295, 2007.
15. Barthélemy D, Willerslev-Olsen M, Lundell H, et al: Impaired transmission in the corticospinal tract and gait disability in spinal cord injured persons. *J Neurophysiol* 104:1167–1176, 2010.
16. Mukherjee A, Chakravarty A: Spasticity mechanisms—for the clinician. *Front Neurol* 1:149, 2010.
17. Ma B, Wu H, Jia LS, et al: Cauda equina syndrome: a review of clinical progress. *Chin Med J (Engl)* 122:1214–1222, 2009.
18. Fraser S, Roberts L, Murphy E: Cauda equina syndrome: a literature review of its definition and clinical presentation. *Arch Phys Med Rehabil* 90:1964–1968, 2009.
19. Olivero WC, Wang H, Hanigan WC, et al: Cauda equina syndrome (CES) from lumbar disc herniations. *J Spinal Disord Tech* 22:202–206, 2009.
20. Gitelman A, Hishmeh S, Morelli BN, et al: Cauda equina syndrome: a comprehensive review. *Am J Orthop* 37:556–562, 2008.
21. Lynskey JV, Belanger A, Jung R: Activity-dependent plasticity in spinal cord injury. *J Rehabil Res Dev* 45:229–240, 2008.
22. Andersen OK, Finnerup NB, Spaich EG, et al: Expansion of nociceptive withdrawal reflex receptive fields in spinal cord injured humans. *Clin Neurophysiol* 115:2798–2810, 2004.
23. DeVivo MJ, Chen Y: Trends in new injuries, prevalent cases, and aging with spinal cord injury. *Arch Phys Med Rehabil* 92:332–338, 2011; Med Clin North Am 17:877–893, 1999.
24. Divanoglou A, Levi R: Incidence of traumatic spinal cord injury in Thessaloniki, Greece and Stockholm, Sweden: a prospective population-based study. *Spinal Cord* 47:796–801, 2009.
25. American Spinal Injury Association: *Reference Manual of the International Standards for Neurological Classification of Spinal Cord Injury*, Chicago, IL, 2006, American Spinal Injury Association.
26. Fitch MT, Silver J: CNS injury, glial scars, and inflammation: inhibitory extracellular matrices and regeneration failure. *Exp Neurol* 209:294–301, 2008.
27. Raiker SJ, Lee H, Baldwin KT, et al: Oligodendrocyte-myelin glycoprotein and Nogo negatively regulate activity-dependent synaptic plasticity. *J Neurosci* 30:12432–12445, 2010.
28. Sun F, He Z: Neuronal intrinsic barriers for axon regeneration in the adult CNS. *Curr Opin Neurobiol* 20:510–518, 2010.
29. Field-Fote EC, Roach KE: Influence of a locomotor training approach on walking speed and distance in people with chronic spinal cord injury: a randomized clinical trial. *Phys Ther* 91:48–60, 2011.
30. Steinbok P: Selective dorsal rhizotomy for spastic cerebral palsy: a review. *Childs Nerv Syst* 23:981–990, 2007.
31. Manchikanti L, Glaser SE, Wolfer L, et al: Systematic review of lumbar discography as a diagnostic test for chronic low back pain. *Pain Physician* 12:541–559, 2009.
32. Devor M: Ectopic discharge in Abeta afferents as a source of neuropathic pain. *Exp Brain Res* 196:115–128, 2009.
33. Frohman EM, Wingerchuk DM: Clinical practice: transverse myelitis. *N Engl J Med* 363:564–572, 2010.
34. Kaplin AI, Krishnan C, Deshpande DM, et al: Diagnosis and management of acute myelopathies. *The Neurologist* 11:2–18, 2005.
35. Klineberg E: Cervical spondylotic myelopathy: a review of the evidence. *Orthop Clin North Am* 41:193–202, 2010.
36. MacDonald BK, Cockerel OC, Sander JW, Shorvon SD: The incidence and lifetime prevalence of neurological disorders in a prospective community-based study in the UK. *Brain* 123:665–676, 2000.

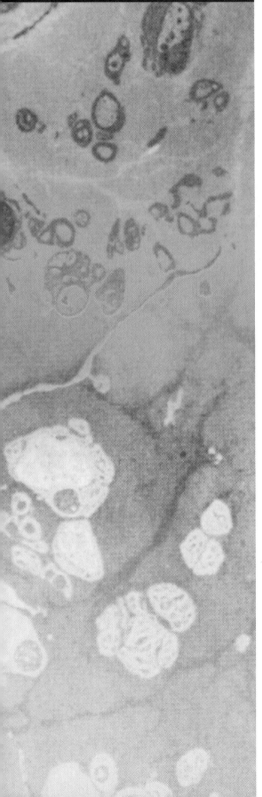

# 14

# Cranial Nerves

Laurie Lundy-Ekman, PhD, PT

I'm 25 years old. A few years ago, I swam in very cold water on a Saturday. The next day, the right side of my tongue and mouth had a coated feeling, and by that evening my lips were twitching ever so slightly. Monday, my right eyelids were occasionally twitching uncontrollably. Tuesday morning I had only 25% to 50% control over my right eyelid and facial muscles; I could get only three quarters of a smile. Wednesday morning I had 0% to 5% control of the right facial muscles. I couldn't close my right eye. I felt like I had Novocain in the right side of my face, except that I had sensation in the affected area. It was scary. The physician performed a nerve conduction velocity test, eye blink reflex tests, and needle electromyography to determine the status of the nerve. The disorder was diagnosed as Bell's palsy.

—*Darren Larson*

Bell's palsy affects the axons of cranial nerve VII, the facial nerve. Cranial nerve VII innervates the muscles of the face, including the orbicularis oculi that closes the eye, the taste receptors of the anterior tongue, skin around the ear, and the lacrimal gland that produces tears. As Darren describes, people with Bell's palsy often have a feeling of numbness on the affected side despite having intact pinprick and touch sensation. The facial skin is innervated by a different cranial nerve, number V, the trigeminal nerve. Absence of proprioceptive feedback from paretic/paralyzed muscles causes the feeling of numbness. Inability to close the eye and lack of tears create a high risk of injury to the cornea; to prevent eye injury, the person wears an eye patch, and to prevent drying of the cornea, he or she uses lubricating drops and ointments. Inability to contract muscles that move the lips causes drooping of the corner of the mouth and drooling, and difficulty with eating and speaking. In Bell's palsy, the ipsilateral facial paralysis may be psychologically devastating because the face is disfigured and the social consequences are distressing. In rare cases, people with severe unilateral facial paralysis become homebound because they are unwilling to be seen in public.

Cranial nerves exchange information between the peripheral and central nervous systems. Twelve pairs of these nerves emanate from the surface of the brain and innervate structures of the head and neck. Cranial nerve X (the vagus) innervates thoracic and abdominal viscera, in addition to structures in the head and neck. Axons and receptors of the cranial nerves outside the skull are part of the peripheral nervous system and are myelinated by Schwann cells. Two cranial nerves, the olfactory and optic nerves, are entirely within the skull and have no peripheral component. The olfactory and optic nerves are myelinated by oligodendroglia and therefore can be affected by diseases that affect oligodendroglia, including multiple sclerosis.

Similar to peripheral nerves connected to the spinal cord, cranial nerves serve sensory, motor, and autonomic functions. Cell bodies of sensory neurons in cranial nerves are usually located in ganglia outside the brainstem (the exception is neurons that convey proprioceptive information from the face, which have cell bodies inside the brainstem). This location is similar to the dorsal root ganglion location of peripheral somatosensory neurons that connect to the spinal cord. Cranial nerve motor cell bodies are located in nuclei inside the brainstem, similar to the location of spinal cord motor neuron cell bodies inside the spinal cord.

Cranial nerves differ from spinal nerves in specialization. Some cranial nerves are only motor, others are only sensory, and some are both sensory and motor. Cranial nerve fibers that innervate muscles of the head and neck are lower motor neurons. As in the spinal cord, these motor neurons are influenced by input from upper motor neurons and sensory afferent fibers. Several cranial nerves have unique functions not shared by any other nerves, such as conveying visual, auditory, or vestibular information.

Cranial nerves have four functions:
- Supply motor innervation to muscles of the face, eyes, tongue, jaw, and two neck muscles (sternocleidomastoid and trapezius)
- Transmit somatosensory information from the skin and muscles of the face and the temporomandibular joint

- Transmit special sensory information related to visual, auditory, vestibular, gustatory, olfactory, and visceral sensations
- Provide parasympathetic regulation of pupil size, curvature of the lens of the eye, heart rate, blood pressure, breathing, and digestion

Cranial nerve connections are illustrated in Figure 14-1. All cranial nerve connections to the brain are visible on the inferior brain except cranial nerve IV, which emerges from the posterior

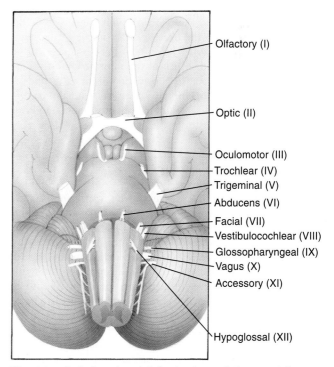

**Fig. 14-1 Inferior view of the brain and the cranial nerves.** The brainstem connection of the trochlear nerve is located posteriorly, inferior to the colliculi.

**TABLE 14-1    CRANIAL NERVES**

| Number | Name | Related Function | Connection to Brain |
|---|---|---|---|
| I | Olfactory | Smell | Inferior frontal lobe |
| II | Optic | Vision | Diencephalon |
| III | Oculomotor | Moves eye up, down, medially; raises upper eyelid; constricts pupil; adjusts the shape of the lens of the eye | Midbrain (anterior) |
| IV | Trochlear | Moves eye medially and down | Midbrain (posterior) |
| V | Trigeminal | Facial sensation, chewing, sensation from temporomandibular joint | Pons (lateral) |
| VI | Abducens | Abducts eye | Between pons and medulla |
| VII | Facial | Facial expression, closes eye, tears, salivation, taste | Between pons and medulla |
| VIII | Vestibulocochlear | Sensation of head position relative to gravity and head movement; hearing | Between pons and medulla |
| IX | Glossopharyngeal | Swallowing, salivation, taste | Medulla |
| X | Vagus | Regulates viscera, swallowing, speech, taste | Medulla |
| XI | Accessory | Elevates shoulders, turns head | Spinal cord and medulla |
| XII | Hypoglossal | Moves tongue | Medulla |

midbrain. Cranial nerve names, primary functions, and connections to the brain are listed in Table 14-1.

# CRANIAL NERVE I: OLFACTORY

The *olfactory nerve* is sensory, conducting information from nasal chemoreceptors to the olfactory bulb. Signals from the olfactory bulb travel in the olfactory tract to the medial temporal lobe of the cerebrum. The sense of smell is dependent on olfactory nerve function. Much of the information attributed to taste is olfactory because information from taste buds is limited to chemoreceptors for salty, sweet, sour, umami (savory flavor, found in fish, cured meat, shellfish, mushrooms, and ripe tomatoes), and bitter tastes.

# CRANIAL NERVE II: OPTIC

The *optic nerve* is sensory, transmitting visual information from the retina to the *lateral geniculate body* of the thalamus and to nuclei in the midbrain (Figure 14-2). The retina is the inner layer of the posterior eye, formed by photosensitive cells. Light striking the retina is converted to neural signals by photosensitive cells. Axons from neurons in the retina travel in the optic nerve, through the optic chiasm, and in the optic tract before synapsing in the lateral geniculate body. The lateral geniculate body is a relay along a pathway to the primary visual cortex. This pathway projects to areas involved in analysis and conscious awareness of visual information. The central processing of visual signals will be discussed in Chapter 16.

Visual signals sent to the midbrain are involved in reflexive responses of the pupil, awareness of light and dark, and orienting of the head and eyes. Reflexes involving cranial nerves are listed in Table 14-2.

# CRANIAL NERVES III, IV, AND VI: OCULOMOTOR, TROCHLEAR, AND ABDUCENS

The *oculomotor, trochlear,* and *abducens nerves* are primarily motor, containing motor neuron axons innervating the six extraocular muscles that move the eye (Figure 14-3) and control reflexive constriction of the pupil.

## Control of Eye Movement

The extraocular muscles include four straight (rectus) muscles and two oblique muscles. The rectus muscles attach to the anterior half of the eyeball. The lateral rectus moves the pupil laterally, and the medial rectus moves the pupil medially; thus, these muscles form a pair, controlling horizontal eye movement. With the eyes looking straightforward, the actions of the superior and inferior rectus are primarily elevation and depression of the pupil, respectively. The two oblique muscles attach to the posterior half of the eyeball (see Figure 14-3, *B*). If the pupil is abducted, the obliques primarily rotate the eye around the axis of the pupil. When the pupil is adducted, the superior oblique muscle depresses the pupil, and the inferior oblique muscle elevates it (see Figure 14-3, *C*). The cranial nerve supply to the extraocular muscles is shown in Figure 14-4.

Cranial nerve III, the oculomotor nerve, controls contraction of the superior, inferior, and medial rectus, the inferior oblique, and the levator palpebrae superioris muscles. These muscles move the pupil upward, downward, and medially; rotate the eye around the axis of the pupil; and assist in elevating

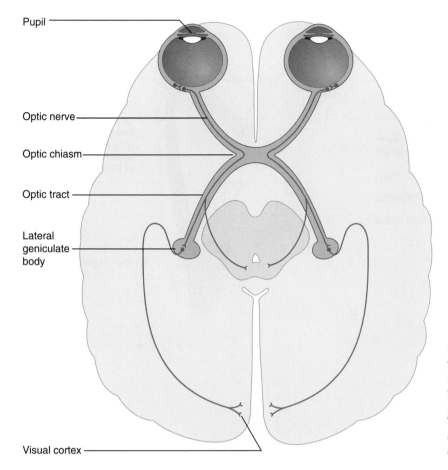

Pupil

Optic nerve

Optic chiasm

Optic tract

Lateral geniculate body

Visual cortex

**Fig. 14-2 The optic nerve projects from the retina to the midbrain and to the lateral geniculate.** Reflex connections in the midbrain control constriction of the pupil and reflexive eye movements. Visual information relayed by the lateral geniculate to the visual cortex provides conscious vision.

| TABLE 14-2 | CRANIAL NERVE REFLEXES | | |
|---|---|---|---|
| **Reflex** | **Description of Reflex** | **Afferent Neurons** | **Efferent Neurons** |
| Pupillary | Pupil of eye constricts when light is shined into eye | Optic | Oculomotor |
| Consensual | Pupil of eye constricts when light is shined into other eye | Optic | Oculomotor |
| Accommodation | Lens of eye adjusts to focus light on the retina, pupil constricts, and pupils move medially when viewing an object at close range | Optic | Oculomotor |
| Masseter | When masseter is tapped with a reflex hammer, the muscle contracts | Trigeminal | Trigeminal |
| Corneal (blink) | When the cornea is touched, the eyelids close | Trigeminal | Facial |
| Gag | Touching of pharynx elicits contraction of pharyngeal muscles | Glossopharyngeal | Vagus |
| Swallowing | Food touching entrance of pharynx elicits movement of the soft palate and contraction of pharyngeal muscles | Glossopharyngeal | Vagus |

the upper eyelid. The upper eyelid is also elevated by the sympathetically innervated superior tarsal muscle (see Figure 9-8). Oculomotor motor neuron cell bodies are located in the oculomotor nucleus.

Cranial nerve IV, the trochlear nerve, controls the superior oblique muscle, which rotates the eye or, if the pupil is adducted, depresses the pupil. The trochlear nerve cell bodies are located in the trochlear nucleus in the midbrain, and this nerve is the only cranial nerve to emerge from the dorsal brainstem, below the inferior colliculus.

Cranial nerve VI, the abducens nerve, controls the lateral rectus muscle, which moves the pupil laterally. The abducens nerve cell bodies are located in the abducens nucleus in the pontine tegmentum.

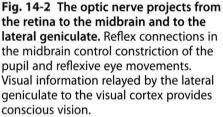

**Clinical Pearl**

Cranial nerves III, IV, and VI (oculomotor, trochlear, and abducens) control eye and upper eyelid movements. Their nuclei are in the midbrain and pons.

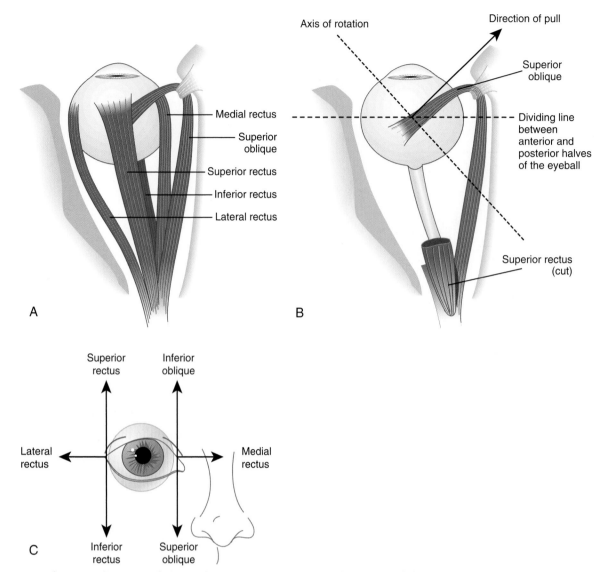

**Fig. 14-3 Left eye and extraocular muscles. A,** Superior view. **B,** The action of the superior oblique muscle. When the eye is directed straightforward or is abducted, contraction of the superior oblique muscle rotates the eye around the axis of the pupil. When the eye is adducted, contraction of the superior oblique muscle moves the pupil downward *(not shown).* **C,** Movements of the right eye by the extraocular muscles. The lateral rectus abducts the eye, and the medial rectus adducts the eye. When the eye is adducted, the superior oblique moves the eye downward and the inferior oblique moves the eye upward. These actions of the oblique muscles occur because of the angle of muscle pull, and because the obliques attach to the posterior half of the eyeball (see part **B** for attachment of the superior oblique).

## Coordination of Eye Movements

Coordination of the two eyes is maintained via synergistic action of the eye muscles. For example, to look toward the right, the abducens nerve activates the lateral rectus to move the right pupil laterally, and the oculomotor nerve activates the medial rectus to move the left pupil medially. This coordination requires connections among the cranial nerve nuclei that control eye movements. Signals conveyed by a brainstem tract, the *medial longitudinal fasciculus,* coordinate head and eye movements by providing bilateral connections among vestibular, oculomotor, and spinal accessory nerve nuclei in the brainstem

(Figure 14-5). The medial longitudinal fasciculus is discussed further in Chapter 15.

> ### ◎ *Clinical Pearl*
> Eye and head movements are coordinated by signals in the medial longitudinal fasciculus.

## Parasympathetic Fibers of Cranial Nerve III

In addition to motor neurons that control voluntary eye movements, cranial nerve III has parasympathetic neurons that elicit

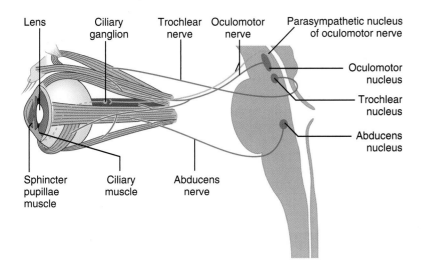

| Cranial Nerve | Muscle | Movement |
|---|---|---|
| III: oculomotor | Levator palpebrae superioris | Lifts eyelid |
| | Superior rectus | Pupil up |
| | Medial rectus | Pupil medial |
| | Inferior rectus | Pupil down |
| | Inferior oblique | If eye adducted, pupil up; if eye abducted, rotates eye |
| | Pupillary sphincter | Constricts pupil |
| | Ciliary | Increases curvature of lens of eye |
| IV: trochlear | Superior oblique | If eye adducted, pupil down and in; if eye abducted, rotates eye |
| VI: abducens | Lateral rectus | Pupil lateral |

**Fig. 14-4 The innervation of extraocular and intraocular eye muscles.** The red nuclei and axons are motor; the orange nuclei and axons are autonomic. *CN*, Cranial nerve.

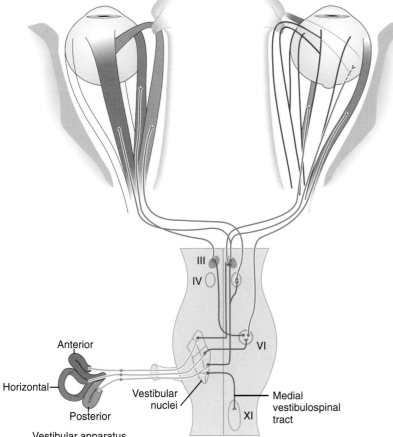

**Fig. 14-5** Axons in the medial longitudinal fasciculus (color coded green) connect the oculomotor, trochlear, abducens, vestibular, and accessory nerve nuclei. Signals conveyed in this tract coordinate head and eye movements.

reflexive constriction of the pupil and contraction of the muscles controlling the lens of the eye. When the pupillary sphincter constricts, the amount of light reaching the retina is decreased. When looking at objects closer than 20 cm, the ciliary muscle contracts, increasing the curvature of the lens. This action, called *accommodation,* increases refraction of light rays so that the focal point will be maintained on the retina. The parasympathetic cell bodies are located in the parasympathetic nucleus of the oculomotor nerve (also called the *Edinger-Westphal nucleus*). The preganglionic parasympathetic fibers synapse with postganglionic fibers behind the eyeball in the ciliary ganglion. The parasympathetic connections innervate the intrinsic muscles of the eye: the pupillary sphincter and the ciliary muscle.

## Pupillary, Consensual, and Accommodation Reflexes

The pupillary, consensual, and accommodation reflexes involve the optic and oculomotor nerves (Figures 14-6 and 14-7). The pupillary and consensual reflexes are elicited by the same stimulus: shining a bright light into one eye. The pupillary reflex is pupil constriction in the eye directly stimulated by bright light. Consensual reflex is constriction of the pupil in the other eye.

The optic nerve is the afferent (i.e., sensory) limb of these reflexes, and the oculomotor nerve provides the efferent (i.e.,

motor) limb. Pathways for the pupillary and consensual reflexes consist of neurons that sequentially connect the following:
- The retina to the pretectal nucleus in the midbrain
- The pretectal nucleus to the parasympathetic nuclei of the oculomotor nerve
- The parasympathetic nuclei of the oculomotor nerve to the ciliary ganglion
- The ciliary ganglion to the pupillary sphincter

> **◎ Clinical Pearl**
>
> The size of the pupil and the shape of the lens of the eye are reflexively controlled by afferents in the optic nerve (CN II) and by parasympathetic efferents in the oculomotor nerve (CN III).

The accommodation reflex consists of adjustments to view a near object: the pupils constrict, the eyes converge (adduct), and the lens becomes more convex. This reflex requires activation of the visual cortex and an area in the frontal lobe of the cerebral cortex—the frontal eye field. The circuitry is shown in Figure 14-7. Table 14-3 summarizes the autonomic innervation of the eye and eyelid.

**Fig. 14-6 Eye reflexes.** Both pupillary and consensual reflexes are responses to bright light shined into one eye. Light shined into the left eye elicits reflexive constriction of both pupils. The optic nerve conveys information from the retina to the pretectal area. Interneurons from the pretectal area synapse in the parasympathetic nucleus of the oculomotor nerve. Efferents travel in the oculomotor nerve and then in the ciliary nerve. **A,** The pupillary reflex is produced by ipsilateral neural connections. **B,** The consensual reflex, constriction of the opposite pupil, is elicited by the neuron connecting the left pretectal area with the right parasympathetic nucleus of the oculomotor nerve.

A

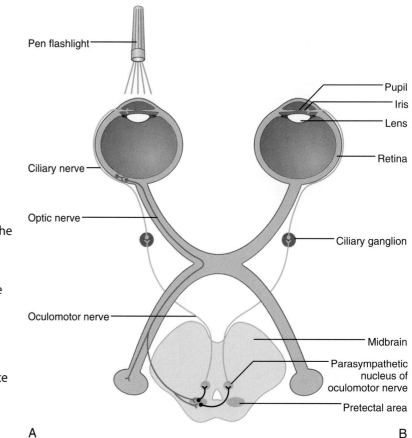

Pen flashlight

Pupil
Iris
Lens
Retina

Ciliary nerve

Optic nerve

Ciliary ganglion

Oculomotor nerve

Midbrain
Parasympathetic nucleus of oculomotor nerve
Pretectal area

B

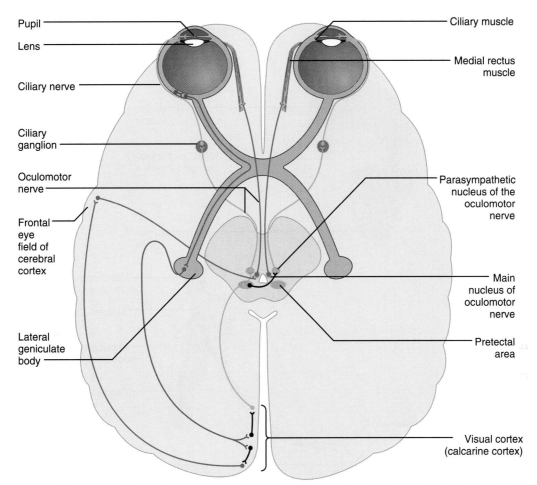

**Fig. 14-7 Accommodation is a change in curvature of the lens, contraction of the pupil, and position of the eyes in response to viewing a near object.** The afferent limb is the retinogeniculocalcarine pathway. The efferent limb to control the curvature of the lens and to contract the pupil is from the visual cortex to nuclei in the midbrain, then via parasympathetic neurons to the ciliary muscle. The efferent limb to move the pupils toward the midline is from the visual cortex to the frontal eye fields, then to the main oculomotor nucleus, then the oculomotor nerve, which controls contraction of the medial rectus muscles.

| TABLE 14-3 | AUTONOMIC INNERVATION OF THE EYE AND EYELID | | |
|---|---|---|---|
| | **Affects** | **Smooth Muscle** | **Action** |
| Parasympathetic (cranial nerve [CN] III, oculomotor) | Lens | Ciliary muscle | Accommodation for near vision. Provides focus for near vision by decreasing tension of fibers that hold the lens in place. This increases the natural curvature of the lens |
| | Iris | Sphincter pupillae | Constricts pupil |
| Sympathetic (cell bodies of three-neuron path located in: Lateral hypothalamus T1 spinal segment Superior cervical ganglion) (see Figure 9-8) | Upper eyelid | Superior tarsal muscle | Assists levator palpebrae superioris (a skeletal muscle innervated by CN III) in raising upper eyelid. If sympathetic innervation is lost, ptosis results |
| | Iris | Dilator muscle | Dilates the pupil |

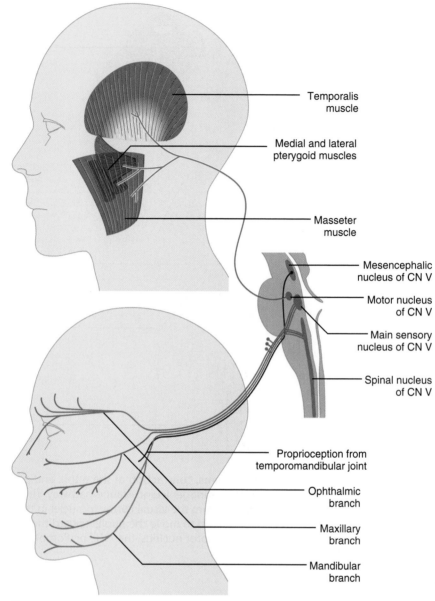

A

**Fig. 14-8 Trigeminal nerve. A,** Distribution to skin of the face, temporomandibular joint, and muscles of mastication.

## CRANIAL NERVE V: TRIGEMINAL

The *trigeminal nerve* is a mixed nerve containing both sensory and motor fibers. Sensory fibers transmit information from the face and the temporomandibular joint. Motor fibers innervate the muscles of mastication. The trigeminal nerve is named for its three branches: ophthalmic, maxillary, and mandibular (Figure 14-8, *A*). All three branches convey somatosensory signals; the *mandibular branch* also contains motor neuron axons to the muscles used in chewing. Pathways carrying information from the trigeminal nerve are illustrated in Figure 14-8, *B*.

Cell bodies of the neurons carrying sensory information for *discriminative touch* are found in the trigeminal ganglion. The

central axons synapse in the *main sensory nucleus* in the pons. Second-order neurons cross the midline and project to the ventral posteromedial nucleus of the thalamus. Third-order neurons then project to the somatosensory cortex, where discriminative touch signals are consciously recognized.

*Proprioceptive information* from the muscles of mastication is transmitted ipsilaterally by axons of cranial nerve V to the *mesencephalic nucleus* in the midbrain. The primary sensory neuron cell bodies are found inside the brainstem, in the mesencephalic nucleus rather than in the trigeminal ganglion. This location for sensory cell bodies is atypical because the usual location of primary neuron cell bodies is cranial nerve or dorsal root ganglia outside the brainstem or spinal cord. Central branches of mesencephalic tract neurons

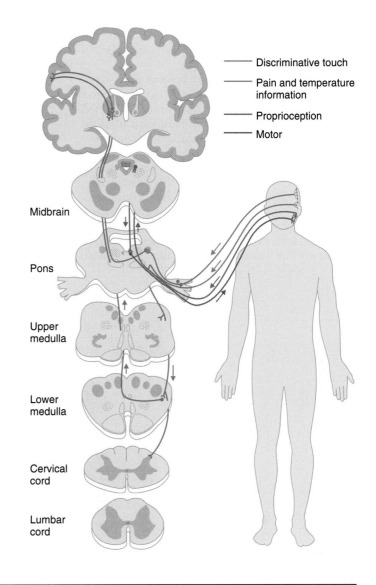

Midbrain

Pons

Upper
medulla

Lower
medulla

Cervical
cord

Lumbar
cord

— Discriminative touch
— Pain and temperature
   information
— Proprioception
— Motor

B

| Sensation | Primary Neuron Cell Body | First Synapse | Second Synapse | Termination |
|---|---|---|---|---|
| Discriminative touch | Trigeminal ganglion | Main sensory nucleus | Ventral posteromedial nucleus of thalamus | Somatosensory cortex |
| Proprioception | Mesencephalic nucleus | Reticular formation | Unknown | Unknown |
| Fast pain | Trigeminal ganglion | Spinal trigeminal nucleus | Ventral posteromedial nucleus of thalamus | Somatosensory cortex |
| Slow pain | Trigeminal ganglion | Reticular formation | Reticular formation and intralaminar nuclei | Limbic system and throughout cortex |

**Fig. 14-8, cont'd B,** Pathways conveying somatosensory information from the face and motor signals to the muscles involved in chewing.

project to the reticular formation. Pathways from the reticular formation to conscious awareness are not known. Collaterals of proprioceptive fibers project to the trigeminal motor nucleus (reflex connections) and to the cerebellum (motor coordination).

The cell bodies of nociceptive (Aδ and C) fibers are in the trigeminal ganglion. The central axons of Aδ neurons enter the pons, then descend as the spinal tract of the trigeminal nerve into the cervical spinal cord. These neurons synapse

with second-order neurons in the *spinal trigeminal nucleus.* Axons of second-order neurons transmitting fast pain information cross the midline and ascend in the trigeminal lemniscus to the ventral posteromedial nucleus of the thalamus. Third-order neurons arise in the ventral posteromedial nucleus and project to the somatosensory cortex. Slow pain information travels in the *trigeminoreticulolimbic pathway.* C fibers from the trigeminal nerve synapse in the reticular formation. Projection neurons end in the intralaminar nuclei.

Projections from the intralaminar nuclei are similar to the spinolimbic pathways, with projections to many areas of cortex.

Reflex actions are also mediated by the trigeminal nerve. Ophthalmic fibers of the trigeminal nerve provide the afferent limb of the *corneal (blink) reflex*. When the cornea is touched, information is relayed to the spinal trigeminal nucleus via the trigeminal nerve. From the spinal trigeminal nucleus, interneurons convey information bilaterally to the facial nerve (VII) nuclei. The facial nerve then reflexively activates muscles to close eyelids of both eyes. Another reflex, the *masseter reflex*, relies entirely on trigeminal nerve connections. When a light downward tap is delivered to the chin, a monosynaptic stretch reflex closing the jaw occurs. Afferent information from the muscle spindles and efferent signals to the muscles travel in the trigeminal nerve. The synapse is in the motor trigeminal nucleus.

> ### ◎ *Clinical Pearl*
>
> Somatosensory information from the face and the anterior ear is conveyed by the trigeminal nerve (CN V) and is distributed to the three trigeminal nuclei: mesencephalic (proprioceptive), main sensory (discriminative touch), and spinal (fast pain and temperature). Slow pain information projects to the reticular formation. CN V also innervates the muscles of mastication and supplies the afferent and efferent limbs of the masseter reflex, and the afferents for the corneal reflex.

## CRANIAL NERVE VII: FACIAL

The *facial nerve* (Figure 14-9) is a mixed nerve containing both sensory and motor fibers. Sensory fibers transmit touch, pain, and pressure information from the tongue, pharynx, and skin

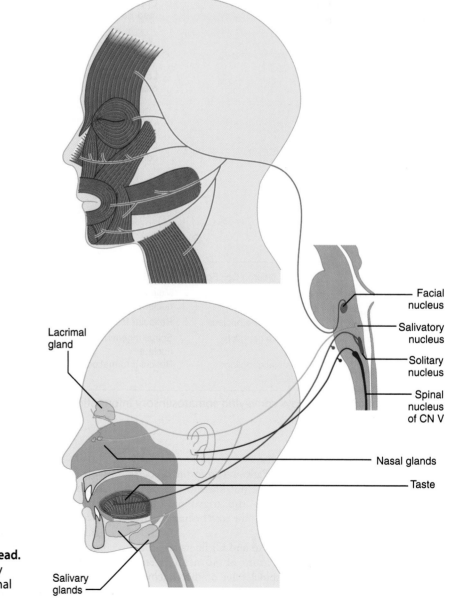

**Fig. 14-9 Facial nerve, supplying innervation to the muscles of facial expression and most glands in the head.** The facial nerve also transmits sensory information from skin near the ear canal and from the tongue and pharynx.

Lacrimal gland

Facial nucleus

Salivatory nucleus

Solitary nucleus

Spinal nucleus of CN V

Nasal glands

Taste

Salivary glands

near the ear canal to the trigeminal spinal nucleus, and information from the chemoreceptors located in the taste buds of the anterior tongue to the solitary nucleus.

Motor innervation by the facial nerve includes the muscles that close the eyes, move the lips, and produce facial expressions. The facial nerve provides the efferent limb of the corneal reflex. The trigeminal nerve provides afferent information from the cornea, and the facial nerve activates eyelid closure. Cell bodies for the motor fibers are in the motor nucleus of the facial nerve. The facial nerve also innervates salivary, nasal, and lacrimal (tear-producing) glands. Cell bodies for the preganglionic parasympathetic neurons that innervate the glands are located in the superior salivary nucleus of the medulla.

> ### ◎ *Clinical Pearl*
>
> The facial nerve (CN VII) innervates the muscles of facial expression and most glands in the head; it also conveys sensory information from the posterior ear canal and taste from the anterior tongue. CN VII carries efferent signals for the corneal (blink) reflex. Signals to and from CN VII are processed in nuclei located in the pons, medulla, and upper spinal cord.

## CRANIAL NERVE VIII: VESTIBULOCOCHLEAR

Cranial nerve VIII, the *vestibulocochlear nerve,* is a sensory nerve with two distinct branches. The vestibular branch transmits information related to head position and head movement. The cochlear branch transmits information related to hearing. Peripheral receptors for these functions are located in the inner ear, in a structure called the *labyrinth.* The labyrinth consists of the vestibular apparatus and the cochlea (Figure 14-10). The vestibular apparatus and the functions of the vestibular system are discussed in Chapter 15. The cochlear nerve and the structures essential for processing auditory information are discussed in subsequent sections.

### Cochlea

The *cochlea* is a snail shell–shaped organ formed by a spiraling, fluid-filled tube (Figure 14-11, *A*). A basilar membrane extends almost the full length of the cochlea, dividing the cochlea into

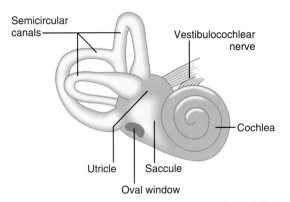

**Fig. 14-10** The vestibulocochlear nerve and the labyrinth of the inner ear.

upper and lower chambers. The basilar membrane consists of fibers oriented across the width of the cochlea. The upper chamber (scala vestibuli) is further divided by a membrane that separates the *cochlear duct* from the remainder of the upper chamber. Within the cochlear duct, resting on the basilar membrane, is the *organ of Corti,* the organ of hearing. The organ of Corti is composed of receptor cells (hair cells), supporting cells, a tectorial membrane, and the terminals of the cochlear branch of cranial nerve VIII (Figure 14-11, *B*). The tops of the hairs that project from hair cells are embedded in the overlying tectorial membrane.

### Converting Sound to Neural Signals

Sound is converted to neural signals by a sequence of mechanical actions. The tympanic membrane (eardrum), small bones called *ossicles,* and a membrane at the opening of the upper chamber of the cochlea are connected in series. When sound waves enter the external ear, the vibration of the tympanic membrane moves the ossicles. The ossicles in turn vibrate the membrane at the opening of the upper chamber, moving the fluid contained in the upper chamber. This moves the fluid inside the cochlea, vibrating the basilar membrane and its attached hair cells. Because the tips of the hair cells are embedded in the tectorial membrane, movement of the hair cells bends the hairs. This bending results in excitation of the hair cell and stimulation of the cochlear nerve endings (Figure 14-12). Neural signals travel in the cochlear nerve to the cochlear nuclei, located at the junction of the medulla and the pons.

The shape of the basilar membrane is important in coding the frequency of sounds. Because the basilar membrane is narrowest near the middle ear and widest at the free end, the fibers at the free end of the basilar membrane are longer than the fibers at the attached end. The longer fibers vibrate at a lower frequency than the shorter fibers. A low-frequency (low-pitched) sound will cause the longer fibers at the free end to vibrate more than fibers at the attached end of the membrane. When the free end of the basilar membrane vibrates, the resulting neural signals are eventually perceived as low-pitch sounds.

> ### ◎ *Clinical Pearl*
>
> The organ of Corti converts mechanical energy from sound into neural signals conveyed by the cochlear branch of CN VIII. The vestibular branch of CN VIII provides information regarding head position relative to gravity and head movement. The nuclei of cranial nerve VIII (vestibulocochlear) are located in the pons and the medulla.

### Auditory Function Within the Central Nervous System

Auditory information
- Orients the head and eyes toward sounds
- Increases the activity level throughout the central nervous system
- Provides conscious awareness and recognition of sounds

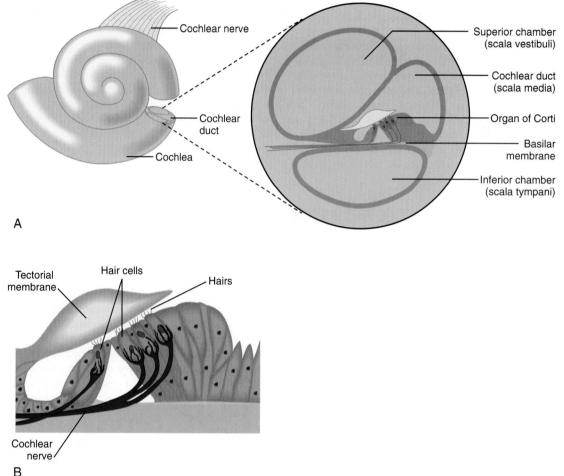

**Fig. 14-11 A,** Cochlea with a small section cut away and enlarged to show the fluid-filled spaces inside and the organ of Corti. **B,** Organ of Corti.

For auditory information to be used for any of these functions, signals are first processed by the cochlear nuclei. From the cochlear nuclei, auditory information is transmitted to three structures (Figure 14-13):

- Reticular formation
- Inferior colliculus (directly and via the superior olive)
- Medial geniculate body

The reticular formation connections account for the activating effect of sounds on the entire central nervous system. For example, loud sounds can rouse a person from sleep. The inferior colliculus integrates auditory information from both ears to detect the location of sounds. When the location information is conveyed to the superior colliculus, neural activity in the superior colliculus elicits movement of the eyes and face toward the sound. The *medial geniculate body* serves as a thalamic relay station for auditory information to the primary auditory cortex, where sounds reach conscious awareness. The routing of auditory information is illustrated in Figure 14-14.

Three cortical areas are dedicated to processing auditory information. The primary auditory cortex is the site of conscious awareness of the intensity of sounds. An adjacent cortical area, the secondary auditory cortex, compares sounds with memories of other sounds, then categorizes the sounds as language, music, or noise. Comprehension of spoken language occurs in yet another cortical area, called *Wernicke's area*. These cortical areas are discussed further in Chapters 17 and 18.

## CRANIAL NERVE IX: GLOSSOPHARYNGEAL

The *glossopharyngeal nerve* is a mixed nerve containing both sensory and motor fibers. Sensory fibers transmit somatosensation from the soft palate and pharynx and information from taste receptors in the posterior tongue (Figure 14-15). Autonomic afferents from the carotid sinus signal blood pressure in the carotid artery. The motor component innervates a pharyngeal muscle and the parotid salivary gland.

Glossopharyngeal sensory fibers contribute the afferent limb of the gag reflex, which can be activated by touching the pharynx with a cotton-tipped swab. Information is conveyed to the spinal nucleus located in the dorsal medulla, then by interneurons to the nucleus ambiguus located in the lateral medulla. Cranial nerve X (see subsequent section) provides

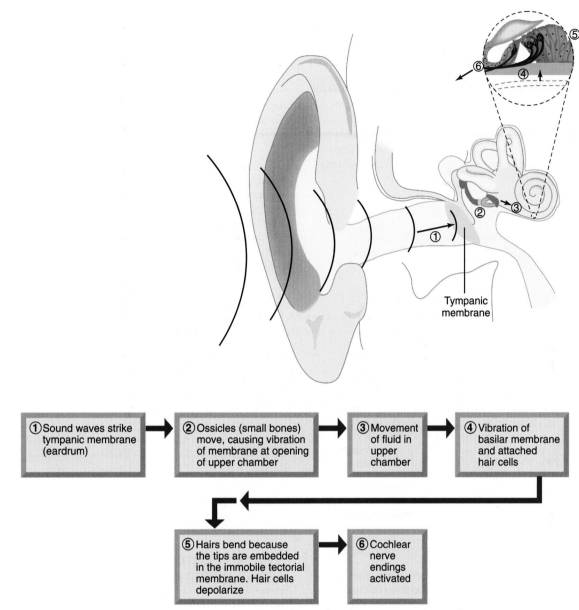

**Fig. 14-12** The conversion of sound waves into neural signals.

① Sound waves strike tympanic membrane (eardrum) → ② Ossicles (small bones) move, causing vibration of membrane at opening of upper chamber → ③ Movement of fluid in upper chamber → ④ Vibration of basilar membrane and attached hair cells

⑤ Hairs bend because the tips are embedded in the immobile tectorial membrane. Hair cells depolarize → ⑥ Cochlear nerve endings activated

the efferent signals, causing the pharyngeal muscles to contract. The swallowing reflex, triggered when the palate is stimulated, uses the same afferent (CN IX) and efferent (CN X) limbs.

> ### ◎ Clinical Pearl
>
> The glossopharyngeal nerve (IX) conveys somatosensory information from the soft palate and the pharynx; this information provides the afferent limb of the gag and swallowing reflexes. Cranial nerve IX also supplies taste information from the posterior tongue, and innervates the carotid sinus, the parotid gland, and one pharyngeal muscle. Information in CN IX is processed in nuclei in the medulla and the upper cervical spinal cord.

## CRANIAL NERVE X: VAGUS

The *vagus nerve* provides afferent and efferent innervation of the larynx, pharynx, and viscera (Figure 14-16). Vagal parasympathetic fibers, both afferent and efferent, are extensively distributed to the larynx, pharynx, trachea, lungs, heart, gastrointestinal tract (except the lower large intestine), pancreas, gallbladder, and liver. These far-reaching connections allow the vagus to decrease heart rate, constrict the bronchi, affect speech production, and increase digestive activity. The motor function of the vagus nerve can be tested by eliciting the gag reflex, as discussed in the previous section.

Cell bodies of the visceral afferent fibers are located in the inferior nucleus of the vagus, outside the brainstem. Cell bodies of the efferent fibers are in the nucleus ambiguus and the dorsal motor nucleus of the vagus, both in the medulla. Figure 14-17 summarizes cranial nerve autonomic innervation. Figure 14-18 summarizes the innervation of the external ear.

> **◎ Clinical Pearl**
>
> The vagus nerve (X) innervates the larynx, pharynx, and thoracic and abdominal viscera. The parasympathetic functions of CN X include decreasing heart rate, constricting the bronchi, and stimulating digestion. CN X supplies the efferent signals for the gag and swallowing reflexes. The nuclei associated with CN X are in the medulla.

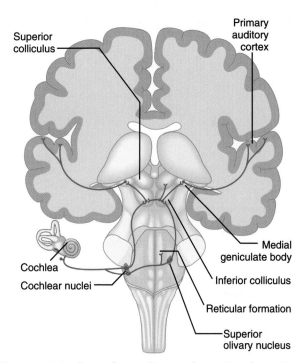

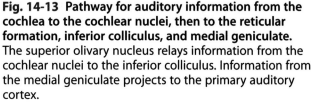

**Fig. 14-13 Pathway for auditory information from the cochlea to the cochlear nuclei, then to the reticular formation, inferior colliculus, and medial geniculate.** The superior olivary nucleus relays information from the cochlear nuclei to the inferior colliculus. Information from the medial geniculate projects to the primary auditory cortex.

## CRANIAL NERVE XI: ACCESSORY

The *accessory nerve* is motor, providing innervation to the trapezius and sternocleidomastoid muscles. The accessory nerve (Figure 14-19) originates in the spinal accessory nucleus in the upper cervical cord, travels upward through the foramen magnum, and then leaves the skull through the jugular foramen. The cell bodies are in the ventral horn at levels C1 to C4.

## CRANIAL NERVE XII: HYPOGLOSSAL

The *hypoglossal nerve* is motor, providing innervation to intrinsic and extrinsic muscles of the ipsilateral tongue (Figure 14-20). Cell bodies are located in the hypoglossal nucleus of the medulla. The activity of the hypoglossal nerve is controlled by both voluntary and reflexive neural circuits.

## CRANIAL NERVES INVOLVED IN SWALLOWING AND SPEAKING

### Swallowing

Swallowing involves three stages: *oral, pharyngeal/laryngeal,* and *esophageal.* Table 14-4 describes the participation of the cranial nerves at each stage.

### Speaking

Speaking requires cortical control, which will be discussed in Chapter 17. At the cranial nerve level, sounds generated by the larynx (CN X) are articulated by the soft palate (CN X), lips (CN VII), jaws (CN V), and tongue (CN XII).

## SYSTEMS CONTROLLING CRANIAL NERVE LOWER MOTOR NEURONS

Cranial nerves III through VII and IX through XII contain lower motor neurons. The activity of motor neurons in cranial nerves is controlled via descending inputs from voluntary and limbic structures of the brainstem and cerebrum, and also via local reflex mechanisms.

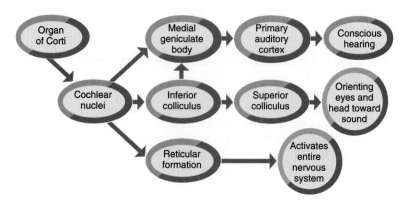

**Fig. 14-14** Flow of signals from the hearing apparatus (organ of Corti) to the outcomes of hearing: conscious hearing, orientation toward sound, and increased general arousal level.

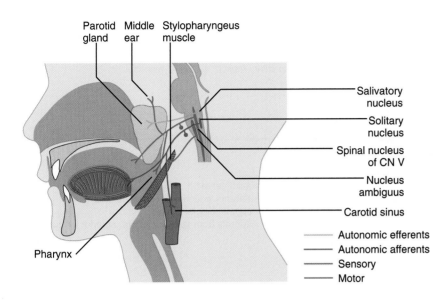

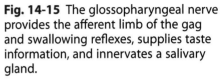

**Fig. 14-15** The glossopharyngeal nerve provides the afferent limb of the gag and swallowing reflexes, supplies taste information, and innervates a salivary gland.

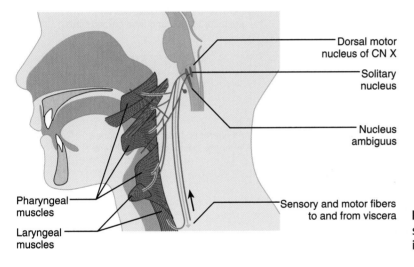

**Fig. 14-16** The vagus nerve regulates viscera, swallowing, and speech and supplies taste information. *CN,* Cranial nerve.

| TABLE 14-4 | PHASES OF SWALLOWING | |
| --- | --- | --- |
| **Stage** | **Description** | **Cranial Nerve** |
| Oral | Food in mouth, lips close | VII |
| | Jaw, cheek, and tongue movements manipulate food | V, VII, XII |
| | Tongue moves food to pharynx entrance | XII |
| | Larynx closes | X |
| | Swallow reflex triggered | IX |
| Pharyngeal/laryngeal | Food moves into pharynx | IX |
| | Soft palate rises to block food from nasal cavity | X |
| | Epiglottis covers trachea to prevent food from entering lungs | X |
| | Peristalsis moves food to entrance of esophagus, sphincter opens, food moves into esophagus | X |
| Esophageal | Peristalsis moves food into stomach | X |

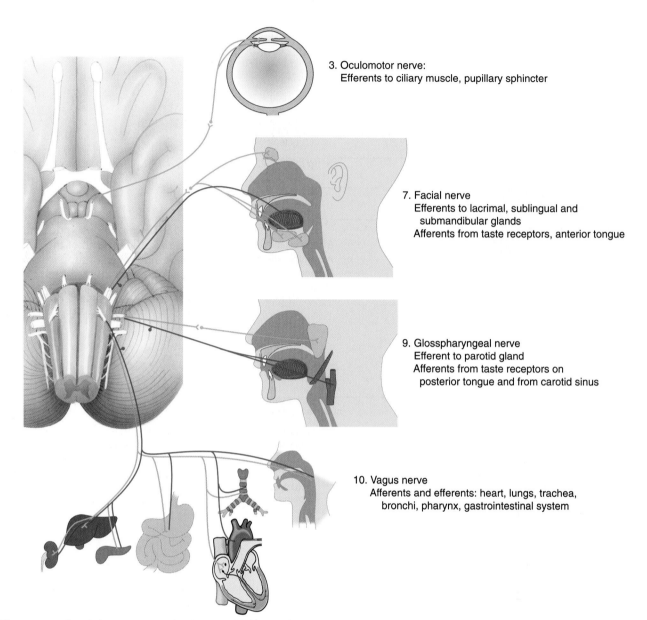

3. Oculomotor nerve:
   Efferents to ciliary muscle, pupillary sphincter

7. Facial nerve
   Efferents to lacrimal, sublingual and
      submandibular glands
   Afferents from taste receptors, anterior tongue

9. Glossopharyngeal nerve
   Efferent to parotid gland
   Afferents from taste receptors on
      posterior tongue and from carotid sinus

10. Vagus nerve
   Afferents and efferents: heart, lungs, trachea,
      bronchi, pharynx, gastrointestinal system

**Fig. 14-17  Cranial nerve autonomic innervation.** Only cranial nerves III, VII, IX, and X contain autonomic fibers. In this figure, green indicates afferent axons and orange indicates efferent axons.

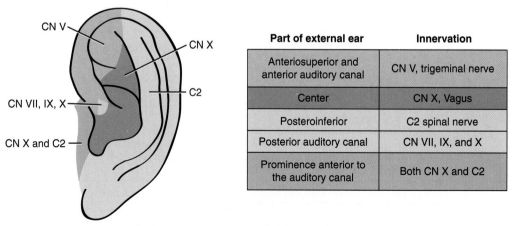

| Part of external ear | Innervation |
| --- | --- |
| Anteriosuperior and anterior auditory canal | CN V, trigeminal nerve |
| Center | CN X, Vagus |
| Posteroinferior | C2 spinal nerve |
| Posterior auditory canal | CN VII, IX, and X |
| Prominence anterior to the auditory canal | Both CN X and C2 |

**Fig. 14-18** Innervation of the external ear.

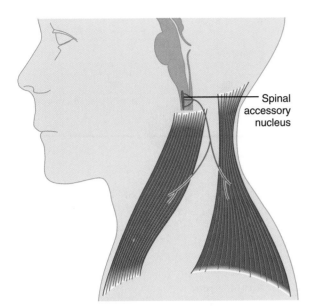

**Fig. 14-19** The accessory nerve innervates the sternocleidomastoid and trapezius muscles.

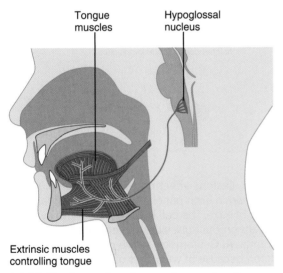

**Fig. 14-20** The hypoglossal nerve innervates the muscles of the tongue.

## Descending Control of Motor Cranial Nerves

Similar to motor neurons in the spinal cord, cranial nerve efferents receive descending regulation by the corticobrainstem tracts and the limbic system. Thus, their activity can be affected by voluntary, emotional, or, as mentioned previously for individual nerves, reflexive pathways. Descending limbic pathways are separate from corticobrainstem tracts.[1]

An example of the dissociation of limbic and voluntary controlled movements is the facial nerve activity that produces a spontaneous smile—a result of limbic innervation and an expression of true emotion—versus an insincere smile—produced voluntarily and usually can be detected. Facial expressions associated with powerful emotions are difficult to suppress voluntarily, but the same expressions may be difficult to produce intentionally.

Similarly, eye movements can be voluntarily controlled, or the eyes may be automatically drawn toward or may avoid disturbing sights. Speaking is mainly voluntary but can occur automatically in highly emotional contexts. In some instances in which brain damage interferes with voluntary speech, the ability of the limbic system to produce emotionally charged words, such as profanity, may be preserved. Extreme emotions, by activating limbic pathways that influence motor activity, can interfere with the ability to eat and speak.

## DISORDERS AFFECTING CRANIAL NERVE FUNCTION

### Olfactory Nerve

Lesions of the olfactory nerve can result in an inability to smell. However, smoking or excessive nasal mucus may also interfere with the function of the olfactory nerve.

### Optic Nerve

Complete interruption of the optic nerve results in ipsilateral blindness and loss of the pupillary light reflex. The pupillary light reflex is pupil constriction in response to a light shining into the eye. Loss of the pupillary light reflex may also occur with a lesion of cranial nerve III, because the oculomotor nerve is the efferent limb of the reflex. Lesions at other sites in the visual pathway can also cause blindness (see Chapter 16). The optic nerve is entirely myelinated by oligodendroglia and is frequently involved in multiple sclerosis.

### Oculomotor Nerve

A complete lesion of the oculomotor nerve causes the following deficits (Figure 14-21):
- Ptosis (drooping of the eyelid), which occurs because the voluntary muscle fibers that elevate the eyelid are paralyzed. The autonomic muscle fibers may be able to keep the eyelid partially elevated.
- The ipsilateral eye looks outward and down because the actions of the lateral rectus and the superior oblique muscles are unopposed.
- *Diplopia* (double vision), which is caused by the difference in position of the eyes. Because the eyes do not look in the same direction, light rays from objects do not fall on corresponding areas of both retinas, producing double vision.
- Deficits in moving the ipsilateral eye medially, downward, and upward
- Loss of pupillary reflex and consensual response to light
- Loss of constriction of the pupil in response to focusing on a near object

The signs of an oculomotor nerve lesion are illustrated in Figure 14-22, *A.* The eye movement deficits seen in an oculomotor nerve lesion must be differentiated from the asymmetric eye movements that occur with upper motor neuron lesions or medial longitudinal fasciculus lesions. The reflexes that produce pupillary constriction will be spared in upper motor neuron or medial longitudinal fasciculus lesions. Either of these disorders

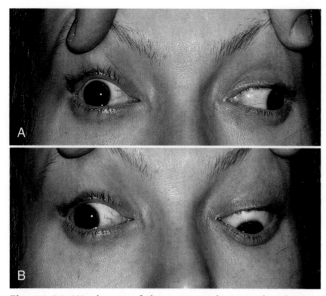

**Fig. 14-21 Weakness of the extraocular muscles due to a lesion involving the right oculomotor nerve (cranial nerve III). A,** With the eyelids held open, on lateral gaze to the left, the right eye does not adduct. The unopposed pull of the lateral rectus (due to paresis of the medial rectus) abducts the right eye. The pupil is dilated and unresponsive to light. **B,** On looking downward, the vessels in the white part of the right eye show that the right eye is rotated clockwise by the intact superior oblique. *(From Parsons M, Johnson M:* Neurology: diagnosis in color, *St Louis, 2001, Mosby.)*

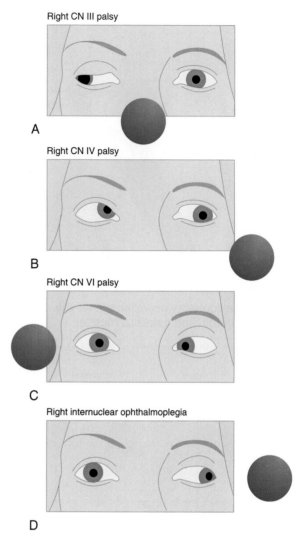

**Fig. 14-22 Lesions affecting eye movements.** The ball is positioned in each panel to illustrate an impaired direction of gaze. The ball is distant from the eyes. All lesions are on the right side. Movements of the left eye are normal. **A,** Oculomotor nerve palsy. The right eye is abducted because of weakness of the medial rectus, the right eyelid droops, and the pupil is dilated. **B,** Trochlear nerve palsy. The right eye adducts but is elevated owing to weakness of the superior oblique muscle. **C,** Abducens nerve palsy. The right eye does not abduct because the lateral rectus muscle is weak. **D,** Internuclear ophthalmoplegia. The lesion affects the right medial longitudinal fasciculus, interrupting signals from the abducens nucleus to the oculomotor nucleus. The right eye does not adduct on voluntary gaze. However, the right eye does adduct during convergence eye movements (not illustrated) because different neural connections are involved in convergence eye movements.

will be accompanied by more extensive brainstem or cerebral signs and symptoms (see Chapter 15).

## Trochlear Nerve

A lesion of the trochlear nerve prevents activation of the superior oblique muscle, so the ipsilateral eye cannot look downward and inward (Figure 14-22, *B*). People with lesions of the trochlear nerve complain of double vision, difficulty reading, and visual problems when descending stairs. Other possible causes of eye movement asymmetry must be ruled out, as was discussed for the oculomotor nerve.

## Trigeminal Nerve

Complete severance of a branch of the trigeminal nerve results in anesthesia of the area supplied by the ophthalmic, maxillary, or mandibular branch. If the ophthalmic division is affected, the afferent limb of the blink reflex will be interrupted, preventing blinking in response to touch stimulation of the cornea. If the mandibular branch is completely severed, the jaw will deviate toward the involved side when the mouth is opened, and the masseter reflex will be lost.

| **PATHOLOGY 14-1** | TRIGEMINAL NEURALGIA (TIC DOULOUREUX) |
|---|---|
| Pathology | Demyelination, ectopic foci, sensitization |
| Etiology | Most frequently caused by compression of the nerve branch by a blood vessel |
| Speed of onset | Abrupt |
| Signs and symptoms | |
| Consciousness | Normal |
| Communication and memory | Normal |
| Sensory | Normal except for sharp, severe pains that last less than 2 minutes, usually only in one branch of the trigeminal nerve distribution and typically triggered by chewing, talking, brushing the teeth, or shaving |
| Autonomic | Normal |
| Motor | Normal |
| Region affected | Peripheral part of cranial nerve V; may also involve spinal nucleus of cranial nerve V |
| Demographics | Women are 1.5 times more likely than men to have trigeminal neuralgia; mean age at onset is 55 years |
| Incidence | 12.6 cases per 100,000 population per year[2] |
| Prognosis | Variable; may resolve spontaneously after a few bouts, may recur, or may require medication or surgery to decompress the nerve |

## Trigeminal Neuralgia

*Trigeminal neuralgia* (also known as *tic douloureux*) is a dysfunction of the trigeminal nerve that produces severe, sharp, stabbing pain in the distribution of one or more branches of the trigeminal nerve (Pathology 14-1). Pain is triggered by stimuli that normally are not noxious, such as eating, talking, or touching the face. The pain begins and ends abruptly, lasts less than 2 minutes, and is not associated with sensory loss.

In most cases, pressure of a blood vessel on the nerve causes local demyelination and ectopic foci that sensitize the trigeminal nerve root and the trigeminal nerve nucleus.[3,4] Four percent of people with trigeminal neuralgia have multiple sclerosis plaques affecting the trigeminal nerve root.[3] Rarely viral neuritis or tumors cause trigeminal neuralgia. Trigeminal neuralgia can be often be treated effectively by drugs or surgery.[5] The differential diagnosis includes trauma, temporomandibular disorders, and postherpetic neuralgia. The first division of the trigeminal nerve is rarely affected,[5] and patients with first division symptoms should be referred to a specialist.

## Abducens Nerve

A complete lesion of the abducens nerve will cause the pupil to look inward, because paralysis of the lateral rectus muscle leaves the pull of the medial rectus muscle unopposed. A person with this lesion will be unable to voluntarily abduct the pupil and will have double vision (Figure 14-22, *C*). Other causes of asymmetric eye movements must be ruled out, as was discussed regarding the oculomotor nerve.

## Medial Longitudinal Fasciculus

A lesion affecting the medial longitudinal fasciculus produces *internuclear ophthalmoplegia* (INO) by interrupting signals from the abducens nucleus to the oculomotor nucleus. Normally, when a person voluntarily moves his or her eyes in a horizontal direction, an area in the frontal lobe sends signals via an area in the pons to the abducens nucleus. In turn, the abducens nucleus sends signals to the ipsilateral lateral rectus muscle and to the contralateral oculomotor nucleus. The oculomotor nucleus sends signals to the medial rectus muscle via the oculomotor nerve. Therefore, when the connection between the abducens nucleus and the oculomotor nucleus is interrupted, the eye contralateral to the lesion moves normally, but the pupil ipsilateral to the lesion cannot adduct past the midline when the fellow pupil moves laterally (Figure 14-22, *D,* and Figure 14-23).

## Facial Nerve

A lesion of the facial nerve causes paralysis or paresis of the ipsilateral muscles of facial expression. This causes one side of the face to droop and prevents the person from being able to completely close the ipsilateral eye. Unilateral facial palsy can result from a lesion of the cranial nerve VII nucleus or from a lesion of the axons of cranial nerve VII. If the lesion involves the axons, the disorder is called *Bell's palsy* (Figure 14-24 and Pathology 14-2). Table 14-5 lists criteria for distinguishing an upper motor neuron lesion from a facial nerve lesion. Bell's palsy is a diagnosis of exclusion, remaining after other causes of facial paralysis have been ruled out. Other causes of facial nerve paralysis include trauma, Lyme disease (a bacterial infection transmitted by ticks), multiple sclerosis, cyst in the middle ear, tumor, and Ramsay-Hunt syndrome (see next section). Thirty-two percent of people with unilateral facial nerve paresis have an identifiable cause and thus do not have Bell's palsy.[6]

Both facial and vestibulocochlear nerves are affected in *Ramsay-Hunt syndrome*. The syndrome, caused by varicella zoster (shingles) infection, usually consists of acute facial

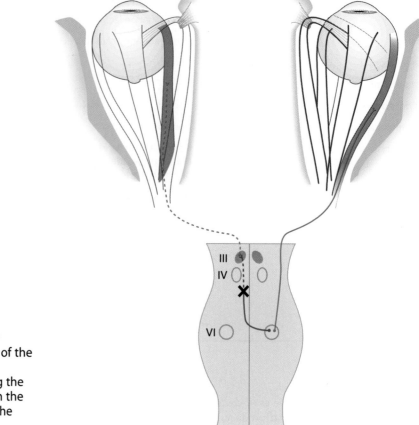

**Fig. 14-23  Mechanism of internuclear ophthalmoplegia.** The indicated lesion of the medial longitudinal fasciculus prevents abducens nucleus signals from reaching the contralateral oculomotor nucleus. When the person attempts to voluntarily look to the right, the left pupil does not adduct.

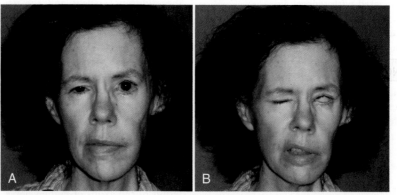

**Fig. 14-24  Bell's palsy, paralysis of the muscles innervated by the facial nerve affecting the left side of the face. A** The vertical space between the eyelids is wider on the left side, and the left side of the mouth droops. **B** The patient is attempting to close her eyes. Note deviation of the mouth toward the unaffected side and inability to close the left eyelid. Upward movement of the left eye is a normal movement when closing the eyes that normally is obscured by closing of the eyelid. *(From Friedman NJ:* Massachusetts Eye & Ear Infirmary illustrated manual of ophthalmology, *ed 3, Philadelphia, 2009, Saunders.)*

paralysis accompanied by ear pain and blisters on the external ear. In some cases, blisters in the mouth and problems with balance, gaze stability, vertigo, hearing, and rarely *tinnitus* (the perception of ringing, hissing, or buzzing sounds in the absence of external sounds) may also occur. Facial muscle control recovers fully in mild to moderate cases but remains impaired 6 months post onset in severe cases. When early treatment with corticosteroids and antiviral drugs is provided, motor and vestibular recovery is good, but hearing tends not to recover.[10]

| **PATHOLOGY 14-2**  BELL'S PALSY | |
|---|---|
| Pathology | Paralysis of the muscles innervated by the facial nerve (cranial nerve VII) on one side of the face, including the orbicularis oculi and frontalis muscles |
| Etiology | Viral infection or immune disorder causing swelling of facial nerve within the temporal bone, resulting in compression and ischemia of the nerve |
| Speed of onset | Acute |
| Signs and symptoms | |
|    Consciousness | Normal |
|    Communication and memory | Normal |
|    Sensory | Facial somatosensation is normal, although people may report feeling numbness; the numbness is caused by lack of proprioceptive feedback from the paretic/paralyzed muscles. Pinprick and light touch sensation are normal (facial skin is innervated by cranial nerve [CN] V). In some cases, hearing is louder in the affected ear owing to loss of CN VII signals to the stapedius muscle, which damps movements of one of the ossicles in the inner ear. In some cases, pain in or posterior to the ear occurs, often before the development of paresis/paralysis. Somatosensation may be impaired in the posterior external ear canal. |
|    Autonomic | In severe cases, salivation and production of tears may be affected. Loss of taste sensation from anterior two thirds of the tongue |
|    Motor | Paresis or paralysis of entire half of face, including frontalis and orbicularis oculi muscles. In severe cases, the ipsilateral eye cannot be closed, and the eyelids must be taped or sutured closed or the eye covered by an eye patch. Paralysis is complete in 45% of cases.[7] |
| Region affected | Peripheral part of CN VII |
| Demographics | Men and women affected equally; usually affects older adults |
| Incidence | 20 to 25 cases per 100,000 population per year[7] |
| Prognosis | Eighty percent recover neural control of facial muscles within 2 months; recovery depends on severity of damage, which can be assessed by nerve conduction velocity and electromyography; paresis typically is followed by complete recovery; outcome after complete paralysis varies from complete recovery to permanent paralysis. In some cases, abnormal reinnervation of facial muscle causes synkinesis—involuntary movements that accompany voluntary movements; an example is the eye closing whenever the person smiles. Synkinesis is treated with cognitive strategies and, if severe, with botulinum toxin. Early corticosteroid treatment to reduce inflammation of CN VII reduces the incidence of poor outcomes and the incidence of synkinesis.[8] |

**TABLE 14-5**  DISTINGUISH AMONG UPPER MOTOR NEURON LESIONS AND FACIAL NERVE LESIONS

| Patient Response | Facial Nerve Lesion | UPPER MOTOR NEURON (UMN) LESION | |
|---|---|---|---|
| | | Voluntary UMNs | Limbic UMNs |
| When asked to "Close your eyes" | One eye does not close | Both eyes close completely | Both eyes close completely |
| When asked to "Smile" | Weakness affecting one side of mouth | Weakness affecting one side of mouth | More symmetric smile than in response to absurd situation |
| Response to "What if a horse walked in here?" | Same amount of weakness affecting one side of mouth as in response to "smile" | More symmetric smile than when requested to smile | More weakness than in response when requested to "smile" |

Location of lesion: Facial nerve lesion affects the facial nerve nucleus in pons or axons of facial nerve; voluntary UMN lesion affects the corticobrainstem neurons from contralateral hemisphere; limbic UMN lesion affects the cingulate neurons.[9]

## Vestibulocochlear Nerve and Disorders of the Auditory System

Deafness usually results from disorders affecting peripheral structures of the auditory system: the cochlea, the organ of Corti within the cochlea, or the cochlear branch of the vestibulocochlear nerve. Loss of hearing in one ear interferes with the ability to locate sounds, because normally the timing of input from each ear is compared to locate sounds in space. Deafness due to peripheral disorders may be classified as either conductive or sensorineural deafness.

*Conductive deafness* occurs when transmission of vibrations is prevented in the outer or middle ear. Common causes of conductive deafness are excessive wax in the outer ear canal and otitis media (inflammation in the middle ear). In otitis media, movement of the ossicles is restricted by thick fluid in the middle ear.

*Sensorineural deafness,* due to damage to receptor cells or the cochlear nerve, is less common than conductive deafness. The usual causes include acoustic trauma (prolonged exposure to loud noises), ototoxic drugs, Ménière's disease (see discussion of vestibular disorders in Chapter 16), and acoustic neuroma. Ototoxic drugs have a poisoning effect on auditory structures, damaging cranial nerve VIII and/or the hearing and vestibular organs. An acoustic neuroma is a benign tumor of myelin cells surrounding cranial nerve VIII within the cranium. An acoustic neuroma causes slow, progressive, unilateral loss of hearing. Tinnitus and problems with balance occur frequently. As the acoustic neuroma grows, additional cranial nerves are compressed, producing facial palsy (cranial nerve VII) and decreased sensation from the face (cranial nerve V). Very large tumors may interfere with the functions of cranial nerves VI through XII. Acoustic tumors are usually removed surgically.

Tinnitus in the form of infrequent, mild, high-pitched sounds lasting for seconds to minutes is normal, particularly in quiet environments. Tinnitus may be caused by medications (most often aspirin), stimulation of receptors in the ear, or central sensitization following deafferentation. Contraction of muscles (in the eustachian tube, middle ear, palate, or pharynx) or turbulence in vascular structures near the ear can stimulate receptors in the ear, producing tinnitus. Central tinnitus is caused by sensitization of the auditory cerebral cortex, similar to phantom limb pain.[11] The auditory illusion can cause significant psychological distress and can interfere with sleep. Treatment, including masking sounds provided by a hearing aid, medication, habituation techniques, and transcranial magnetic stimulation of the central auditory system, may be effective.[12]

Disorders within the central nervous system rarely cause deafness because auditory information projects bilaterally in the brainstem and the cerebrum. Thus, small lesions in the brainstem typically do not interfere with the ability to hear. In the cerebral cortex, each primary auditory cortex receives auditory information from both ears, so that hearing remains fairly normal when one primary auditory cortex is damaged. If the primary auditory cortex is destroyed on one side, the only loss is the ability to consciously identify the location of sounds, because conscious location of sound is accomplished by comparing the time lag between auditory information reaching the cortex on one side versus the time required for auditory information to reach the opposite cortex.

A complete lesion of the cochlear branch of cranial nerve VIII causes unilateral deafness. Vestibular dysfunctions are discussed in Chapter 16.

### Glossopharyngeal Nerve

A complete lesion of cranial nerve IX interrupts the afferent limb of both the gag reflex and the swallowing reflex (cranial nerve X provides the efferent limb for both reflexes). Salivation is also decreased.

### Vagus Nerve

A complete lesion of the vagus nerve results in difficulty speaking and swallowing, poor digestion due to decreased digestive enzymes and decreased peristalsis, asymmetric elevation of the palate, and hoarseness.

### Accessory Nerve

A complete lesion of the accessory nerve paralyzes the ipsilateral sternocleidomastoid and trapezius muscles. Upper motor neuron lesions, in contrast, cause paresis rather than paralysis because cortical innervation is bilateral, and the muscles become hypertonic rather than hypotonic.

### Hypoglossal Nerve

A complete lesion of the hypoglossal nerve causes atrophy of the ipsilateral tongue. When a person with this lesion is asked to stick out the tongue, the tongue protrudes ipsilaterally rather than in the midline. Problems with tongue control result in difficulty speaking and swallowing.

### Dysphagia

Difficulty swallowing is *dysphagia.* Frequent choking, lack of awareness of food in one side of the mouth, or food coming out of the nose may indicate dysfunction of cranial nerve V, VII, IX, X, or XII. Upper motor neuron lesions may also cause swallowing dysfunctions.

### Dysarthria

Poor control of speech muscles is *dysarthria.* In dysarthria, only vocal speech, that is, motor production of sounds is affected. People with dysarthria can understand spoken language and can write and read. Lower motor neuron involvement of cranial nerve V, VII, X, or XII can cause dysarthria. Dysarthria can also result from upper motor neuron lesions or muscle dysfunction.

## OBSERVING AND TESTING CRANIAL NERVES

Table 14-6 lists observations of cranial nerve function. In addition to observation, standard tests are used to assess cranial nerve function. Table 14-7 lists the cranial nerve tests and the effects of lesions of individual cranial nerves.

**TABLE 14-6    OBSERVING CRANIAL NERVES**

| Nerve | Observation |
|---|---|
| II, III (optic, oculomotor) | Asymmetric pupils |
| III (oculomotor) | Drooping upper eyelid (ptosis) |
| III, IV, VI (oculomotor, trochlear, abducens) | Abnormal eye position |
| VII (facial) | Drooping or asymmetry of facial muscles |
| V, VII, X, XII (trigeminal, facial, vagus, hypoglossal) | Difficulty with articulating words |

**TABLE 14-7** CRANIAL NERVE TESTS

| Nerve | Test | Normal Response | Cranial Nerve Lesion | Differentiate From |
|---|---|---|---|---|
| Olfactory | Patient closes eyes, closes one nostril, then smells coffee or cloves. | Patient identifies substance. | Lack of ability to smell; however, mucus or smoking may interfere with the ability to smell. | |
| Optic | Patient and examiner are about two feet apart. With patient's left eye covered, patient looks into examiner's eye. Examiner covers his or her own right eye. Examiner tells patient, "Keep looking into my eye. I'm testing what you can see at the edges of your vision. Say 'now' when you see my finger." Examiner positions finger about one foot from patient's ear. Examiner moves the finger slowly toward the visual center until patient reports seeing the finger. Then test patient's right eye. | Patient reports seeing finger. | If optic nerve is completely interrupted, patient is ipsilaterally blind. | Lesions at other sites in the visual pathway also interfere with vision (see Chapter 16). |
| | Dim room lights if necessary. Shine light into one of the patient's eyes. Observe pupil (pupillary reflex). | Both pupils constrict (cranial nerve III provides the reflex efferent limb). The ipsilateral constriction is the direct reflex, and the contralateral constriction is the consensual reflex. | Response is slow or absent. | Lesion in the pretectal area or parasympathetic nuclei of the oculomotor nerve. Other brainstem signs (see Chapter 15) will accompany either of these lesions. |
| Oculomotor | Ask patient to look straight ahead. Examine the height of the space between upper and lower eyelids and the position of eyelids relative to the iris and pupil. Then ask the patient to look upward without moving the head. | The position of the eyelids is symmetric, and the upper eyelid covers the upper iris, superior to the pupil. The upper eyelid retracts with upward gaze. | The height of the space between the eyelids is asymmetric, and the drooping eyelid (ptosis) does not retract with upward gaze. This finding indicates an oculomotor nerve lesion. Additional signs of oculomotor nerve lesion include dilated pupil, lateral and downward deviation of the eye when attempting to look forward, and diplopia. | The height of the space between the eyelids is asymmetric, yet the drooping eyelid retracts with upward gaze. This finding indicates a lesion involving the sympathetic innervation of the head. Additional signs of such a lesion include absence of sweating, redness of one side of the face, and constriction of the pupil (Horner's syndrome). |
| | Observe position of patient's eyes with patient looking forward. | Both eyes appear to look in the same direction; no nystagmus (involuntary back-and-forth movements of the eyes). | Ipsilateral eye looks outward and down (pulled by unopposed lateral rectus and superior oblique). Patient reports double vision. | |
| | Observe size of pupil in room light. | Moderate size | Dilated pupil | Extremely small pupil: sympathetic dysfunction (Horner's syndrome—see Chapter 9). |
| | Patient's eyes follow examiner's finger, moving eyes up, down, and in (testing superior, medial, and inferior rectus muscles). | Eyes move symmetrically and smoothly. | Deficits in adduction, depression, or elevation of the eye | Asymmetric eye movements; due to upper motor neuron or medial longitudinal fasciculus lesion |

*Continued*

**TABLE 14-7    CRANIAL NERVE TESTS—cont'd**

| Nerve | Test | Normal Response | Cranial Nerve Lesion | Differentiate From |
|---|---|---|---|---|
| | Patient's eye follows examiner's finger to about 50 degrees adduction, then up (testing inferior oblique muscle). | Eye follows finger movement. | Unable to adduct and elevate eye | Asymmetric eye movements; due to upper motor neuron or medial longitudinal fasciculus lesion |
| | Dim the room lights, then shine light into patient's eye (pupillary reflex and consensual response to light). | Constriction of pupils (requires cranial nerve II for afferent limb of reflex). | Pupil unchanged | Lesion in the pretectal area or parasympathetic nuclei of the oculomotor nerve. Other brainstem signs (see Chapter 15) will accompany either of these lesions. |
| | Patient looks at examiner's finger, then examiner's nose. Observe pupillary response to near and far objects. | Near object: constriction Far object: dilation | Pupil unchanged | |
| | Convergence is adduction of the eyes. Ask patient to look at the tip of a pen as it is slowly moved from about 2 feet away toward the patient's nose. | Both eyes are directed toward the pen tip until the pen is within 10 cm (4 inches) of the nose. | Only one eye moves toward the midline; the other eye moves outward. | Asymmetric eye movements due to upper motor neuron lesion |
| Trochlear | Patient's eye follows examiner's finger to about 50 degrees adduction, then down (testing superior oblique muscle). | Eye moves in, then down. | Deficit in looking inferomedially. Patient reports double vision and difficulty reading, descending stairs. | Asymmetric eye movements; due to upper motor neuron or medial longitudinal fasciculus lesion |
| Trigeminal | With patient's eyes closed, use light touch and pin to assess facial sensation in three areas: forehead, cheek, chin. | Distinguishes between sharp and dull and can localize stimulus | Anesthesia in affected area; or patient reports severe pain in trigeminal branch distribution (trigeminal neuralgia, a severe neuropathic pain). | |
| | Touch outer cornea with a wisp of cotton (corneal reflex). | Both eyes blink (requires efferent limb via cranial nerve VII). | Eye does not close (because response is bilateral, can stimulate other eye to determine whether absence of reflex is due to problem with afferent or efferent limb). | |
| | Manual muscle test: jaw opening and closing strength | Jaw opens strongly and symmetrically. Jaw closes strongly. Palpate the masseter muscles while patient clenches the teeth, then relaxes. | Unilateral damage: jaw deviates toward weak side. | |
| | Tap downward on patient's chin with reflex hammer. | Masseter contracts, elevating chin. | Lost or decreased reflex | Hyperreflexia; due to upper motor neuron lesion |
| Abducens | Observe position of eyes with patient looking forward. | Both eyes appear to look in same direction; no nystagmus | One eye looks inward (pulled by unopposed medial rectus); patient reports double vision. | |
| | Patient follows examiner's finger to look laterally. | Eye moves laterally. | Deficit of abduction | Asymmetric eye movements; due to descending motor neuron or medial longitudinal fasciculus lesion |

**TABLE 14-7**　CRANIAL NERVE TESTS—cont'd

| Nerve | Test | Normal Response | Cranial Nerve Lesion | Differentiate From |
|---|---|---|---|---|
| Facial | Facial movements: raise eyebrows, close eyes, smile, puff cheeks | Able to perform requested movements | Paralysis or paresis, with upper and lower face equally involved: cranial nerve VII nucleus or Bell's palsy. Bell's palsy affects axons of facial nerve, preventing patient from completely closing ipsilateral eye. | Corticobrainstem lesion interfering with signals to cranial nerve VII spares the frontalis and orbicularis oculi muscles and causes paresis of the lower face. |
| Vestibulocochlear Cochlear branch (see Chapter 16 for vestibular function tests) | Examiner rubs fingers together near patient's ear; performance can be compared with examiner's own hearing. | Patient reports hearing the stimulus equally in each ear. | Difference in acuity of patient's ears or in patient's and examiner's ability to hear should be investigated further. | |
| | Rinne test: Hold vibrating tuning fork on mastoid bone; when patient no longer hears it, move tuning fork into the air about 1 inch from ear canal. | Patient hears through air after cannot hear through bone. | Patient hears through air after cannot hear through bone, but volume is reduced for both air and bone conduction (sensorineural hearing loss). | Hearing longer through bone indicates conduction loss; due to auditory canal or middle ear lesion. |
| | Weber test: Hold vibrating tuning fork on the top of the patient's head; ask the patient where the sound appears to be coming from. | Sound is coming from the midline. | Sound is louder in one ear than in the other. In sensorineural loss, sound is louder in the unaffected ear because neural function is impaired in the affected ear. | In unilateral conductive hearing loss, sound is louder in the affected ear because bone conduction is normal and the conductive loss dulls the ambient noise in the room. |
| Glossopharyngeal | Touch soft palate with cotton swab (gag reflex). | Gagging and symmetric elevation of soft palate; requires cranial nerve X efferents | Lack of gag reflex, or asymmetric elevation of soft palate | |
| Vagus | Patient opens mouth and says "ah." Examiner observes soft palate. | Elevation of soft palate | Asymmetric elevation of soft palate; hoarseness | |
| Accessory | Manual muscle test: sternocleidomastoid and upper trapezius | Normal strength | Paralysis or paresis | Upper motor neuron lesion: paresis with hypertonia; bilateral cortical innervation prevents complete paralysis. |
| Hypoglossal | Patient protrudes tongue. | Tongue protrudes in midline. | Protruded tongue deviates to the side of the lesion, and ipsilateral tongue atrophies. | |
| | Patient pushes tongue into cheek. On outside of cheek, examiner pushes against the tongue. | Tongue able to resist moderate force. | Force of tongue easily overcome by examiner's pressure. | |

## SUMMARY

The cranial nerves innervate the head, neck, and viscera. Cranial nerves I and II are part of the central nervous system and convey olfactory and visual information. Cranial nerves III through XII continue into the periphery. Cranial nerves III, IV, and VI innervate eye muscles. Cranial nerve V conveys somatosensory information from the face and mouth and motor signals to the muscles of mastication. Cranial nerve VII innervates muscles of facial expression, salivary glands, and taste receptors. Cranial nerve VIII conveys auditory and vestibular information. The last four cranial nerves innervate the mouth, neck, and viscera. Cranial nerve IX carries information from the tongue and larynx. Cranial nerve X is motor to the palate, pharynx, larynx, heart, and glands, and afferent for visceral sensations. Cranial nerve XI is motor to the sternocleidomastoid and trapezius muscles. Cranial nerve XII is motor to the tongue. Because these nerves are frequently damaged by trauma or disease, knowing their functions and the disorders that affect the cranial nerves is essential for clinical practice.

## CLINICAL NOTES

### Case 1

R.F. is a 62-year-old man who was involved in a car accident 5 days ago. He sustained fractures of the skull, both femurs, and the right tibia. He complains of double vision.
- Consciousness, cognition, language, memory, and somatosensation are normal.
- All autonomic functions, including pupillary and accommodation reflexes, are normal.
- Motor function is normal except for an inability to look downward and inward with the right eye. All other eye movements, including the ability to look medially and laterally with the right eye, are normal. When asked, he says he has been having trouble reading since the accident.

#### Question

What is the most likely location of the lesion?

### Case 2

A.K., a 46-year-old engineer, is complaining of double vision. She cannot read or drive unless she closes one eye. Results of the cranial nerve examination:
- Olfaction, vision, facial sensation, control of the muscles of facial expression, mastication, hearing, equilibrium, gag and swallowing reflexes, and contraction of the sternocleidomastoid, trapezius, and tongue muscles are normal. Pupillary responses and movements of the left eye are normal.
- When A.K. is instructed to look straight ahead, her right eye looks outward and down.
- A.K. cannot look in, down, or up with her right eye.
- A.K. can open the right eyelid only halfway.
- No pupillary reflex or consensual response occurs when a flashlight is shined into her right eye, nor does the pupil constrict when she focuses on an object 6 inches from her right eye.

#### Questions

1. Is this an upper motor neuron lesion? Why or why not?
2. Where is the lesion?

### Case 3

M.R., a 56-year-old electrician, awoke with an inability to move the left side of his face. His neurologic examination was normal, including facial sensation and control of the muscles of mastication and the tongue, except for the following:
- Drooping of the left side of the face
- Complete lack of movement of the muscles of facial expression on the left. Examples include M.R.'s inability to voluntarily smile, pucker his lips, or raise his eyebrow on the left side. Emotional facial expressions were also absent; when he smiled with the right side of his lips, the left half of his lips did not move.
- Inability to close his left eye

#### Question

What is the most likely location of the lesion?

## CLINICAL NOTES—cont'd

### Case 4

P.F., a 52-year-old accountant, was referred to physical therapy for Bell's palsy. She had right facial paralysis, pain on the right side of the face, and increased loudness of sound in the right ear. The onset of paralysis was gradual, progressively worsening for 3 weeks. The pain began after the paralysis. At the time of referral, she was 5 months post onset. The neurologic examination was normal, except for the following:

- Inability to feel touch or pinprick in the mandibular division of the right CN V (chin and lower mandible region)
- No contraction of the right masseter and temporalis muscles when asked to clench teeth
- Complete paralysis of muscles of facial expression on the right; inability to close the right eye

### Question

What is the most likely location of the lesion?

## REVIEW QUESTIONS

1. How are the eyes voluntarily moved to follow an examiner's finger to the right and then look up? Include both muscle and cranial nerve activity in the answer.
2. Which cranial nerve provides efferents for the pupillary reflex?
3. Which cranial nerve provides efferents to the tongue muscles?
4. Which cranial nerve provides afferents for the gag reflex?
5. Which cranial nerve provides control of the muscles of facial expression?
6. Which cranial nerve provides somatosensation from the face?
7. Diagram the accommodation reflex.
8. What is the function of the organ of Corti?
9. Why is there a difference between an authentic smile and a false smile?
10. Which cranial nerves are required for swallowing?
11. Lesions of what structures could cause double vision?

## References

1. Holstege G: The emotional motor system and micturition control. *Neurourol Urodyn* 29:42–48, 2010.
2. Koopman JS, Dieleman JP, Huygen FJ, et al: Incidence of facial pain in the general population. *Pain* 147:122–127, 2009.
3. Becker M, Kohler R, Vargas MI, et al: Pathology of the trigeminal nerve. *Neuroimaging Clin N Am* 18:283–307, 2008.
4. Obermann M: Treatment options in trigeminal neuralgia. *Ther Adv Neurol Disord* 3:107–115, 2010.
5. Zakrzewska JM: Assessment and treatment of trigeminal neuralgia. *Br J Hosp Med (Lond)* 71:490–494, 2010.
6. Ljøstad U, Økstad S, Topstad T, et al: Acute peripheral facial palsy in adults. *J Neurol* 252:672–676, 2005.
7. Halperin JJ: Bell's palsy. In Squire L, et al: *The encyclopedia of neuroscience*, London, 2009, Elsevier, pp 155–160.
8. Salinas RA, Alvarez G, Daly F, et al: Corticosteroids for Bell's palsy (idiopathic facial paralysis). *Cochrane Database Syst Rev* (3): CD001942, 2010.
9. Menon V, Uddin LQ: Saliency, switching, attention and control: a network model of insula function. *Brain Struct Funct* 214:655–667, 2010.
10. Boemo RL, Navarrete ML, García-Arumí AM, et al: Ramsay-Hunt syndrome: our experience. *Acta Otorrinolaringol Esp* 61:418–421, 2010.
11. De Ridder D, Elgoyhen AB, Romo R, et al: Phantom percepts: tinnitus and pain as persisting aversive memory networks. *Proc Natl Acad Sci U S A* 108:8075–8080, 2011.
12. Lustig LR, Schindler J: Chapter 8, Ear, nose, & throat disorders. In McPhee SJ, Papadakis MA, Rabow MW, editors: *Current medical diagnosis and treatment 2011*, ed 50, New York, 2011, McGraw-Hill Medical.

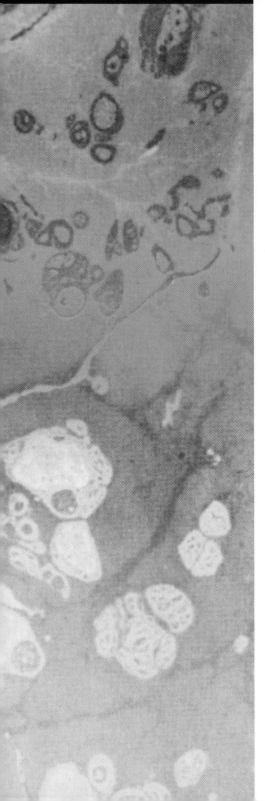

# 15

# Brainstem Region

Laurie Lundy-Ekman, PhD, PT

The brainstem is superior to the spinal cord and inferior to the cerebrum, with the cerebellum appended posteriorly (Figure 15-1, *A*). From inferior to superior, the parts of the brainstem are the medulla, pons, and midbrain (Figure 15-1, *B*). The connection of cranial nerves with the brainstem follows a 2-4-4 rule: two CNs (III and IV), connect with the midbrain; four CNs (V through VIII) connect with the pons; and the remaining four CNs (IX through XII) connect with the medulla (Figure 15-1, *C*).

## ANATOMY OF THE BRAINSTEM

### Vertical Tracts in the Brainstem

Sensory, autonomic, and motor vertical tracts travel through the brainstem, just as in the spinal cord. The sensory tracts conveying information from the spinal cord to the brain, and the motor tracts conveying signals from the cortex to the brainstem and spinal cord, have been discussed in Chapters 6, 9 and 10. Some of these tracts continue through the brainstem without alteration. For these tracts, the brainstem acts as a conduit. Other vertical tracts leave the brainstem or synapse in brainstem nuclei. One tract, the trigeminal lemniscus, ascends to the thalamus from the main sensory nucleus and the spinal nucleus of the trigeminal nerve. The trigeminal lemniscus conveys fast pain, temperature, and tactile information from the face. Modifications of the vertical tracts in the brainstem are summarized in Table 15-1 and illustrated in Figure 15-2.

Upper motor neuron tracts that originate in the brainstem and project to the spinal cord are the rubrospinal, reticulospinal, vestibulospinal, ceruleospinal, and raphespinal. The origins and functions of these tracts are discussed in Chapter 10.

### Longitudinal Sections of the Brainstem

The brainstem is divided longitudinally into two sections: the basilar section and the tegmentum. Throughout the brainstem, the basilar section is located anteriorly and contains predominantly motor system structures:
- Descending axons from the cerebral cortex: corticospinal, corticobrainstem, corticopontine, and corticoreticular tracts
- Motor nuclei: substantia nigra, pontine nuclei, and inferior olive
- Pontocerebellar axons
  The tegmentum, located posteriorly, includes the following:
- The reticular formation, which adjusts the general level of activity throughout the nervous system
- Sensory nuclei and ascending sensory tracts
- Cranial nerve nuclei (discussed later in this chapter)
- The medial longitudinal fasciculus, a tract that coordinates eye and head movements

In addition to basilar and tegmentum sections, the midbrain has a longitudinal section, posterior to the tegmentum, called the *tectum*. The tectum includes structures involved in reflexive control of intrinsic and extrinsic eye muscles and in movements of the head:
- Pretectal area
- Superior and inferior colliculi

The preceding structures are discussed in the context of their location in the medulla, pons, or midbrain. Because the reticular formation extends vertically throughout the brainstem, it is discussed next.

---

### ◎ *Clinical Pearl*

The longitudinal sections of the brainstem are the basilar, the tegmentum, and, in the midbrain, the tectum. The basilar section is primarily motor. The tegmentum is involved in adjusting the general level of neural activity, integrating sensory information, and cranial nerve functions. The tectum regulates eye reflexes and reflexive head movements.

---

### TABLE 15-1   VERTICAL TRACTS IN THE BRAINSTEM

| | Vertical Tract | Modification of Tract in Brainstem |
|---|---|---|
| Sensory (ascending) tracts | Spinothalamic | Not modified (tract passes through brainstem without alteration) |
| | Dorsal column | Axons synapse in nucleus gracilis or cuneatus; second-order neurons cross midline to form medial lemniscus |
| | Spinocerebellar | Axons leave brainstem via inferior and superior cerebellar peduncles to enter the cerebellum |
| | Trigeminal lemniscus | Second-order neuron cell bodies are in the main sensory nucleus and the spinal nucleus of the trigeminal nerve and cross the midline |
| Autonomic (descending) tracts | Sympathetic | Not modified (tract passes through brainstem without alteration) |
| | Parasympathetic | Axons synapse with brainstem parasympathetic nuclei or continue through brainstem and cord to the sacral level of the spinal cord |
| Motor (descending) tracts | Corticospinal | Not modified (tract passes through brainstem without alteration) |
| | Corticobrainstem | Axons synapse with cranial nerve nuclei in brainstem |
| | Corticopontine | Axons synapse with nuclei in pons |
| | Corticoreticular | Axons synapse within reticular formation |

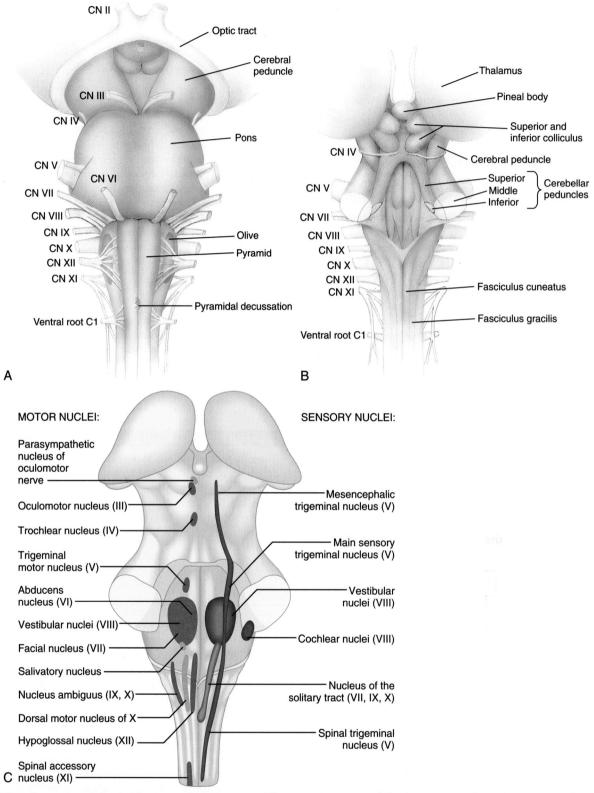

**Fig. 15-1  Anatomy of the brainstem.  A,** Anterior and **B,** posterior views of the brainstem.  **C,** Posterior view of cranial nerve nuclei inside the brainstem. On the left side, motor nuclei are indicated in red, and autonomic efferent nuclei in bright orange. On the right side, sensory nuclei are indicated in blue, and the autonomic nucleus that receives afferent information is green.

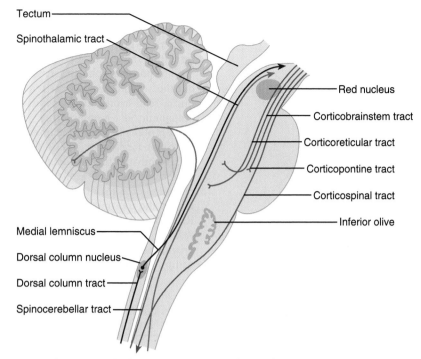

Tectum

Spinothalamic tract

Red nucleus

Corticobrainstem tract

Corticoreticular tract

Corticopontine tract

Corticospinal tract

Inferior olive

Medial lemniscus

Dorsal column nucleus

Dorsal column tract

Spinocerebellar tract

**Fig. 15-2** Vertical tracts in the brainstem. For simplicity, the autonomic tracts are omitted.

## RETICULAR FORMATION

The reticular formation is a complex neural network that includes the reticular nuclei, their connections, and ascending and descending reticular pathways (Figure 15-3). The reticular formation:

- Integrates sensory and cortical information
- Regulates somatic motor activity, autonomic function, and consciousness
- Modulates nociceptive/pain information

## RETICULAR NUCLEI AND THEIR NEUROTRANSMITTERS

Reticular nuclei regulate neural activity throughout the central nervous system. Neurons in each nucleus produce a different neurotransmitter. The transmitters released by the reticular nuclei are all slow acting or neuromodulating, although the same transmitter may be fast acting in other neural subsystems. For example, acetylcholine (ACh) released from a reticular nucleus is slow acting, and ACh released in the peripheral nervous system is fast acting.[1] Slow-acting neurotransmitters alter the release of fast-acting neurotransmitters or the response of receptors to fast-acting neurotransmitters. The slow action is achieved by indirect opening of ion channels or by activating a cascade of intracellular events (see Chapter 3). These slow-acting or neuromodulating neurotransmitters markedly influence activity in other parts of the brainstem and in the cerebrum and cerebellum. Several also influence neural activity in the spinal cord.

Although the reticular nuclei are confined to small regions in the brainstem, their axons project to widespread areas of the

brain and, in some cases, to the spinal cord. The major reticular nuclei are:

- Ventral tegmental area
- Pedunculopontine nucleus
- Raphe nuclei
- Locus coeruleus and the medial reticular area

### Ventral Tegmental Area: Dopamine

Most neurons that produce dopamine are located in the midbrain. Of the two midbrain areas that produce dopamine, only one, the ventral tegmental area (VTA), is part of the reticular formation. The other dopamine-producing area is the substantia nigra, discussed in Chapter 11 as part of the basal ganglia circuit that supplies dopamine to the caudate and putamen. The VTA provides dopamine to cerebral areas important in motivation and in decision making (Figure 15-4, *A*). Activation of the VTA affects the ventral striatum, producing feelings of pleasure and reward.[2] The powerful effect of VTA activity is demonstrated in addiction to amphetamines and cocaine. Both drugs activate the VTA dopamine system. Morphine is habit forming because it inhibits inhibitory inputs to the VTA, thus increasing dopamine release. Excessive VTA activity has been hypothesized to explain certain aspects of schizophrenia, because drugs that block a particular type of dopamine receptor ($D_2$) have antipsychotic effects.[3] Schizophrenia is a disorder of perception and thought processes characterized by withdrawal from the outside world.

### Pedunculopontine Nucleus: Acetylcholine

The pedunculopontine nucleus (PPN) is located in the caudal midbrain (Figure 15-4, *B*). Ascending axons from the

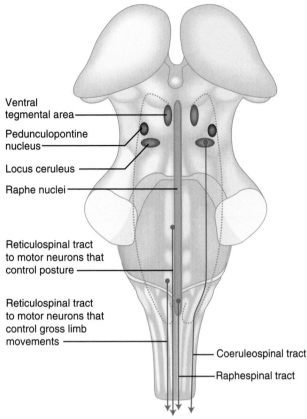

Ventral
tegmental area

Pedunculopontine
nucleus

Locus ceruleus

Raphe nuclei

Reticulospinal tract
to motor neurons that
control posture

Reticulospinal tract
to motor neurons that
control gross limb
movements

Coeruleospinal tract

Raphespinal tract

**Fig. 15-3 Reticular formation: reticular nuclei and tracts.** The dotted lines indicate the extent of the reticular formation. Reticular nuclei include the ventral tegmental area, the pedunculopontine nucleus, the locus coeruleus, and the raphe nuclei. Four upper motor neuron tracts arise in the reticular formation: two reticulospinal tracts, one ceruleospinal tract, and one raphespinal tract *(tracts shown in red)*. Ascending projections of the reticular nuclei are illustrated in Figure 15-5.

pedunculopontine nucleus project to the inferior part of the frontal cerebral cortex and the intralaminar nuclei of the thalamus. The PPN influences movement via connections with the following[4,5]:

• Globus pallidus and subthalamic nucleus
• Limbic system
• Reticular areas that give rise to the reticulospinal tracts

In cats that have a lesion separating the brainstem from the cerebrum, electrical stimulation of the PPN can induce walking despite the lack of cerebral connection with the spinal cord. In people with Parkinson's disease, loss of pedunculopontine neurons explains the dopamine-resistant signs, including difficulty with gait initiation, postural instability, and sleep problems.[5] Deep brain stimulation of the PPN or adjacent regions improves gait and posture in Parkinson's disease.[4]

### Raphe Nuclei: Serotonin

Most cells that produce serotonin are found along the midline of the brainstem, in the raphe nuclei (Figure 15-4, *C*). The

midbrain raphe nuclei project throughout the cerebrum. Serotonin levels have profound effects on mood. The antidepressant fluoxetine (Prozac) prolongs the availability of serotonin by inhibiting the reuptake of serotonin.[6]

The pontine raphe nuclei modulate neural activity throughout the brainstem and in the cerebellum. The medullary raphe nuclei send axons into the spinal cord to modulate sensory, autonomic, and motor activity.[7] Some medullary raphe nuclei are part of the fast-acting neuronal pathway for descending pain inhibition (see Figure 7-12). Ascending pain information stimulates both the periaqueductal gray and the medullary raphe nuclei. In response, axons from the medullary raphe nuclei release serotonin onto interneurons in the dorsal horn that inhibit the transmission of pain information (see Chapter 7). Raphespinal endings in the lateral horn influence the cardiovascular system. Raphespinal endings in the anterior horn provide nonspecific activation of interneurons and lower motor neurons (see Chapter 10).

### Locus Coeruleus and Medial Reticular Zone: Norepinephrine

The locus coeruleus and the medial reticular zone are the sources of most norepinephrine in the central nervous system (Figure 15-4, *D*). Axons from the locus coeruleus project throughout the brain and spinal cord. The locus coeruleus is most active when a person is attentive and is inactive during sleep. Activity of ascending axons from the locus coeruleus provides the ability to direct attention.[8] Descending axons from the locus coeruleus form the ceruleospinal tract, providing nonspecific activation of interneurons and lower motor neurons in the spinal cord. Ceruleospinal endings in the dorsal horn provide direct inhibition of spinothalamic neurons conveying pain information.

The medial reticular zone produces both norepinephrine and epinephrine. It regulates autonomic functions—respiratory, visceral, and cardiovascular—through projections to the hypothalamus, brainstem nuclei, and lateral horn of the spinal cord.

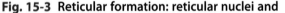

> ◎ **Clinical Pearl**
>
> Arousal levels in the cerebrum are influenced by the raphe nuclei, and attention is directed by the locus coeruleus. Descending axons from the locus coeruleus and the raphe nuclei determine the general level of neuronal activity in the spinal cord.

### Regulation of Consciousness by the Ascending Reticular Activating System

Consciousness is awareness of self and surroundings. The consciousness system governs alertness, sleep, and attention. Brainstem components of the consciousness system are the reticular formation and its *ascending reticular activating system* (ARAS; Figure 15-5). The axons of the ARAS project to cerebral

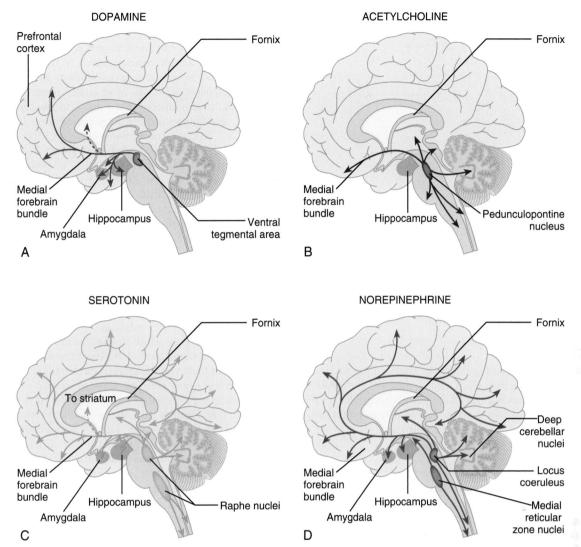

**Fig. 15-4 Slow-acting neurotransmitters are produced in the brainstem by reticular nuclei.** Ascending fibers from the reticular nuclei form the ascending reticular activating system, which regulates activity in the cerebral cortex. Descending fibers adjust activity in the spinal cord. **A,** The ventral tegmental area supplies dopamine to the frontal cortex and limbic areas. **B,** The pedunculopontine nucleus provides acetylcholine to the thalamus, frontal cerebral cortex, brainstem, and cerebellum and inhibits the reticulospinal tract to lower motor neurons that control postural muscles. **C,** The raphe nuclei supply serotonin to the thalamus, midbrain tectum, striatum, amygdala, hippocampus, and cerebellum; throughout the cerebral cortex; and to the spinal cord (raphespinal tract). **D,** The locus coeruleus and medial reticular zone nuclei provide norepinephrine in a wide distribution similar to the pattern of serotonin distribution. The tracts descending from reticular nuclei into the spinal cord are the reticulospinal, raphespinal, and ceruleospinal tracts.

components of the consciousness system: basal forebrain (anterior to the hypothalamus), thalamus, and cerebral cortex.[9] For normal sleep-wake cycles and the ability to direct attention while awake, all brainstem and cerebral components of the consciousness system must be functional.

Sleep, a periodic loss of consciousness, is actively induced by activity of areas within the ascending reticular activating system. The function of sleep is controversial. Current speculation on the role of sleep includes consolidation of memory, particularly memory for motor skills, and adjusting immune activity.[10,11]

## MEDULLA

The medulla is the inferior part of the brainstem, continuous with the spinal cord inferiorly and the pons superiorly (Figure 15-6).

### External Anatomy of the Medulla

Anteriorly, the medulla has two vertical bulges, called *pyramids*. Lateral to the pyramids are two small oval lumps, called *olives* (see Figure 15-1). Cranial nerve XII connects with the medulla

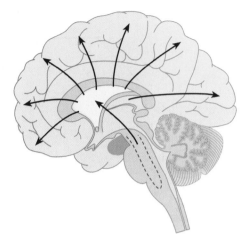

**Fig. 15-5 Ascending reticular activating system (ARAS).** Reticular formation *(indicated by the dotted line)* cells project to midline and intralaminar nuclei of the thalamus, then axons from these thalamic nuclei project throughout the cerebral cortex. When activated, the ARAS produces arousal of the entire cerebral cortex.

between the pyramid and the olive. In a vertical groove lateral to the olive, cranial nerves IX, X, and XI attach to the medulla. The most prominent features of the posterior medulla are the inferior cerebellar peduncle and widening of the central canal to become a larger space, the fourth ventricle.

## Inferior Medulla

The inferior half of the medulla contains a central canal that is continuous with the central canal of the spinal cord. Anteriorly, the pyramids are formed by descending axons of the corticospinal tract. Most lateral corticospinal axons (88%) cross the midline in the pyramidal decussation at the inferior border of the medulla (see Chapter 10). The spinothalamic tracts maintain an anterolateral position, similar to their location in the cord (see Figure 15-6, *B*). Dorsal column tracts synapse in their associated nuclei, the nucleus gracilis and cuneatus. Second-order fibers cross the midline in the decussation of the medial lemniscus, attaining a position posterior to the pyramids before ascending.

In addition to connections between spinal cord and cerebrum, the lower medulla contains cranial nerve structures. The spinal tract and the nucleus of the trigeminal nerve are located anterolateral to the nucleus cuneatus and convey pain and temperature information from the face. The medial longitudinal fasciculus, located near the center of the inferior medulla, coordinates eye and head movements via connections between vestibular nuclei, spinal accessory nucleus, and the nuclei that control eye movements (see Figure 14-5).

> **◎ Clinical Pearl**
>
> The corticospinal and dorsal column/medial lemniscus pathways cross the midline in the caudal medulla. Thus, these tracts connect the spinal cord with the opposite cerebral cortex. Cranial nerve V fibers conveying pain and temperature synapse in the caudal medulla.

## Upper Medulla

In the upper half of the medulla, the central canal widens to form part of the fourth ventricle. Tracts in the upper medulla maintain approximately the same positions as in the caudal medulla (see Figure 15-6, *A*). Most cranial nerve nuclei in the upper medulla are clustered in the dorsal section; from medial to lateral, these nuclei include the hypoglossal nucleus (cranial nerve [CN] XII), the dorsal motor nucleus of the vagus (CN X), the solitary nucleus (visceral afferents from CN VII, IX, and X), and the vestibular nuclei (CN VIII). The solitary nucleus receives visceral and taste afferent information. The nucleus ambiguus is the only cranial nerve nucleus in the medulla that is separate from the dorsally located group. The nucleus ambiguus is located more anteriorly and contributes motor fibers to striated muscles in the pharynx, larynx, and upper esophagus via cranial nerves IX and X. Corticobrainstem tracts provide cortical input to the nucleus ambiguus and the hypoglossal nucleus. The corticobrainstem projections are usually bilateral; however, occasionally, projections to the hypoglossal nucleus are contralateral.

At the junction of the medulla and the pons are the cochlear and vestibular nuclei, which receive auditory and vestibular information via cranial nerve VIII. Auditory information from the cochlea of the inner ear is transmitted to the cochlear nuclei by the cochlear nerve. Head movement and head position relative to gravity are signaled by receptors in the labyrinths of the inner ear (see Chapter 16); the vestibular nerve relays this information to the vestibular nuclei. The medial and lateral vestibulospinal tracts (see Chapter 10) that arise from the vestibular nuclei contribute to the control of postural muscle activity.

Deep to the olive is the inferior olivary nucleus (see Figure 15-6, *A*). Shaped like a wrinkled paper bag, this nucleus receives input from most motor areas of the brain and spinal cord. Axons from the inferior olivary nucleus project to the contralateral cerebellar hemisphere via the olivocerebellar tract. Current theory on the role of the inferior olivary nucleus is that these neurons are important for the perception of time.[12]

The medulla sends many fibers (spinocerebellar, olivocerebellar, vestibulocerebellar, and reticulocerebellar) to the cerebellum via the inferior cerebellar peduncle. Only one fiber tract, the cerebellovestibular tract, sends information from the cerebellum to the medulla.

> **◎ Clinical Pearl**
>
> The upper medulla contains nuclei for cranial nerves VII through X and XII. Most of the cranial nerve nuclei are located dorsally. Vestibular nuclei help regulate head and eye movements and postural activity.

## Functions of the Medulla

Medullary neuronal networks coordinate cardiovascular control, breathing, head movement, and swallowing. These activities are partially executed by cranial nerves with nuclei in the medulla: VII through X and XII. The medullary neuronal networks regulating these functions are normally influenced by cerebral activity. For example, the tonic neck reflexes seen in infants

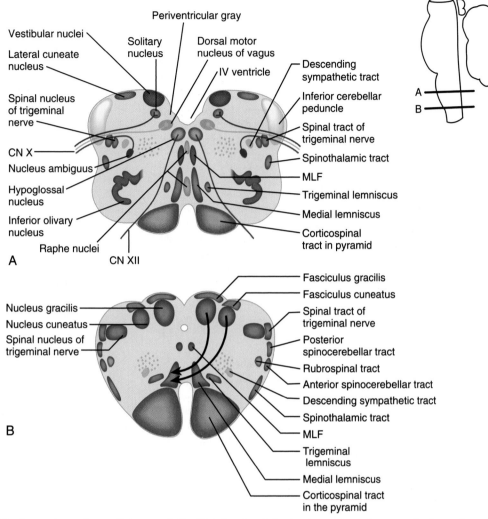

**Fig. 15-6 Horizontal sections of the medulla.** The levels of the horizontal sections are indicated on the lateral view of the brainstem. Nuclei are labeled on the left side of each horizontal section. Tracts are labeled on the right side. *A,* Upper medulla; *B,* inferior medulla; *CN,* cranial nerve; and *MLF,* medial longitudinal fasciculus. Color coding: red, motor; blue, sensory; purple, motor and sensory or bidirectional; green, autonomic afferents; bright orange, autonomic efferents; and orange, modulates motor and nociceptive activity in the spinal cord.

younger than 6 months old require reflex circuits in the medulla (see Chapter 11). As the cerebral cortex matures, information from the cortex modulates the activity of the reflex circuit, modifying the reflexive activity.

---

> ### ◎ *Clinical Pearl*
>
> The medulla contributes to control of eye and head movements, coordinates swallowing, and helps regulate cardiovascular, respiratory, and visceral activity.

---

## PONS

The pons is located between the midbrain and the medulla (Figure 15-7). The posterior pons borders on the fourth ventricle. Most vertical tracts continue unchanged through the pons. Only the corticopontine tracts and some corticobrainstem tracts synapse in the pons. The corticopontine tracts synapse on pontine nuclei; then the postsynaptic axons, called *pontocerebellar fibers,* leave the pons to enter the cerebellum via the middle cerebellar peduncle. The corticobrainstem tracts synapse with neurons in the trigeminal motor nucleus and the facial nucleus.

The basilar (anterior) section of the pons contains descending tracts (corticospinal, corticobrainstem, and corticopontine axons), pontine nuclei, and pontocerebellar axons. The posterior section of the pons, the tegmentum, contains sensory tracts, reticular formation, autonomic pathways, the medial longitudinal fasciculus, and nuclei for cranial nerves V through VII. These cranial nerves are involved in the following:

- Processing sensation from the face (cranial nerve V)
- Controlling lateral movement of the eye (cranial nerve VI)
- Controlling facial and chewing muscles (cranial nerves VII and V, respectively)

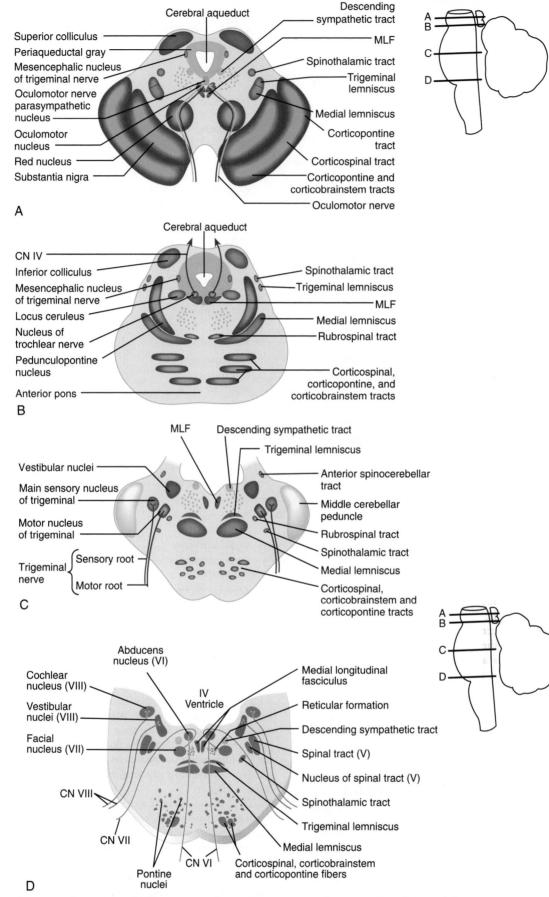

**Fig. 15-7** Horizontal sections of **(A)** upper midbrain, **(B)** junction of pons and midbrain, **(C)** upper pons, and **(D)** lower pons. The levels of the horizontal sections are indicated on the lateral view of the brainstem. Nuclei are labeled on the left side of each horizontal section. Tracts are labeled on the right side. *CN,* Cranial nerve; *MLF,* medial longitudinal fasciculus. Stippled areas are the reticular formation. Color coding: red, motor; blue, sensory; purple, motor and sensory or bidirectional; green, autonomic afferent or, in the case of locus coeruleus, modulates attention and motor and nociceptive activity in the spinal cord; and bright orange, autonomic efferent.

The pons processes motor information from the cerebral cortex and forwards the information to the cerebellum. Pontine cranial nerve nuclei process sensory information from the face (CN V) and control contraction of muscles involved in facial expression (CN VII), lateral movement of the eye (CN VI), and chewing (CN V).

## MIDBRAIN

The uppermost part of the brainstem, the midbrain, connects the diencephalon and the pons. The cerebral aqueduct, a small canal through the midbrain, joins the third and fourth ventricles. The midbrain can be divided into three regions, from anterior to posterior: basis pedunculi, tegmentum, and tectum.

### Basis Pedunculi

Anteriorly, the basis pedunculi is formed by the cerebral peduncles (composed of descending tracts from the cerebral cortex) and an adjacent nucleus, the substantia nigra (see Figure 15-7, *A*). The substantia nigra is one of the nuclei in the basal ganglia circuit (see Chapter 11). The other basal ganglia nuclei are the caudate, putamen, globus pallidus, pedunculopontine nucleus, and subthalamic nucleus.

### Midbrain Tegmentum

The middle region of the midbrain, the tegmentum, contains vertical sensory tracts, the superior cerebellar peduncle, the red nucleus, the pedunculopontine nucleus (see Figure 15-7, *B*), and the nuclei of cranial nerves III and IV. Most vertical tracts occupy similar positions as in the pons, except that the spinothalamic tract and the medial lemniscus are located more laterally in the midbrain. The superior cerebellar peduncle connects the midbrain with the cerebellum, transmitting primarily efferent information from the cerebellum.

The red nucleus is a sphere of gray matter that receives information from the cerebellum and the cerebral cortex and projects to the cerebellum, spinal cord (via rubrospinal tract), and reticular formation. Activity in the rubrospinal tract contributes to control of distal upper limb extension. Pedunculopontine nucleus neurons are part of the basal ganglia circuit and are involved in regulation of muscle tone.[13-15]

Anterior to the cerebral aqueduct are the oculomotor complex (nuclei of cranial nerve III) and the nucleus of the trochlear nerve (cranial nerve IV). The oculomotor complex consists of the oculomotor nucleus, supplying efferent somatic fibers to the extraocular muscles innervated by the oculomotor nerve, and the oculomotor parasympathetic (Edinger-Westphal) nucleus, supplying parasympathetic control of the pupillary sphincter and the ciliary muscle. The oculomotor complex is superior to the trochlear nucleus. The trochlear nerve innervates the superior oblique muscle that moves the eye.

Surrounding the cerebral aqueduct is the periaqueductal gray. Involvement of the periaqueductal gray in pain suppression was discussed in Chapter 7. The periaqueductal gray also coordinates somatic and autonomic reactions to pain, threats,

and emotions. Periaqueductal gray activity elicits the fight-or-flight reaction[16] and vocalization during laughing and crying.[17]

### Midbrain Tectum

The posterior region of the midbrain, the tectum, contains the pretectal area and the colliculi. The pretectal area is involved in the pupillary, consensual, and accommodation reflexes of the eye (see Chapter 14). The inferior colliculi relay auditory information from the cochlear nuclei to the superior colliculus and to the medial geniculate body of the thalamus (see Chapter 14). The superior colliculi are involved in reflexive eye and head movements (see Chapter 16).

## CEREBELLUM

The cerebellum is discussed briefly in this chapter because cerebellar function is entirely dependent on input and output connections with the brainstem. Furthermore, the cerebellum and the brainstem share the tightly confined space of the posterior fossa, bringing them into a close anatomic relationship. The following list summarizes cerebellar functions:
- Coordination of movement, including fine finger movements, limb and head movements, postural control, and eye movements
- Motor planning
- Cognitive functions, including rapid shifts of attention.[18] Axons from the cerebellum synapse with neurons in the reticular formation to achieve their role in directing attention.

In addition to its roles in motor control and motor planning, the cerebellum contributes to voluntary shifting of attention.

## DISORDERS IN THE BRAINSTEM REGION

Evaluating the function of cranial nerves (see Chapter 14) and vertical tracts can be used localize lesions within the brainstem. A single brainstem lesion may cause a mix of ipsilateral and contralateral signs (see Figure 7-5). The mix of ipsilateral and contralateral signs occurs because cranial nerves supply the ipsilateral face and neck, while many of the vertical tracts cross the midline in the brainstem to supply the contralateral body. In addition to vertical tract and cranial nerve damage, lesions in the brainstem may interfere with vital functions and consciousness.

### Vertical Tract Signs

The lateral corticospinal, dorsal column/medial lemniscus, and spinothalamic tracts connect the spinal cord with the contralateral cerebrum. Lesions of the lateral corticospinal and dorsal column tracts in the brainstem usually cause contralateral signs because these tracts cross the midline in the inferior medulla. The only location where a brainstem lesion would cause ipsilateral corticospinal or dorsal column/medial lemniscus signs

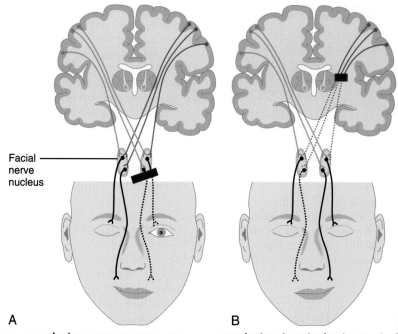

**Fig. 15-8 Lower motor neuron lesion versus upper motor neuron lesion (corticobrainstem) affecting the facial nerve.** In both **A** and **B**, the person has been asked to close the eyes and smile. Dotted lines indicate axons that, subsequent to the lesions, do not convey information. **A**, With a facial nerve lesion, lower motor neurons are interrupted, preventing control of the ipsilateral muscles of facial expression. Therefore the person cannot close the eye or contract the muscles that move the lips on the left. **B**, An upper motor neuron lesion prevents information from the left cortex from reaching the facial nerve nuclei. Because the contralateral cortex controls the muscles of the lower face, the person is unable to generate a smile on the right side. However, because the upper face is innervated bilaterally, the person with this upper motor neuron lesion can close both eyes.

would be the corticospinal tract or dorsal column nuclei in the inferior medulla. The spinothalamic tract crosses the midline in the spinal cord, so any brainstem lesion that damages the spinothalamic tract causes contralateral signs.

## Corticobrainstem Lesions

The corticobrainstem tracts convey motor signals from the cerebral cortex to cranial nerve nuclei in the brainstem. Thus, neurons with axons in the corticobrainstem tract serve as upper motor neurons to the motor neurons in cranial nerves V, VII, IX, X, XI, and XII. Although both upper and lower motor neuron lesions cause paresis or paralysis, upper motor neuron lesions are associated with muscle hypertonia, and lower motor neuron lesions are associated with hyporeflexia and muscle flaccidity. Corticobrainstem projections are bilateral, except to lower motor neurons innervating the muscles of the lower face and sometimes to the hypoglossal nucleus.

## Facial Nerve vs. Corticobrainstem Tract Lesions

A complete lower motor neuron lesion of the facial nerve, cranial nerve VII, prevents commands from reaching all ipsilateral facial muscles. The result is flaccid paralysis of the muscles in the ipsilateral face. A person with a complete facial nerve lesion is completely unable to contract the muscles of facial expression and cannot close the ipsilateral eye. In contrast, unilateral upper motor neuron lesions interrupt voluntary

control of contralateral facial muscles in the lower half of the face. The muscles in the upper half of the face are spared because the right and left cerebral cortices have bilateral projections to lower motor neurons innervating muscles of the forehead and surrounding the eye. Thus, an upper motor neuron lesion that prevents corticobrainstem information from the left cerebral cortex from reaching the facial nerve nuclei causes paresis or paralysis of the right lower face, but cerebral control of muscles of the upper face is relatively unaffected. The difference between a lesion of the facial nerve (lower motor neuron lesion) and a corticobrainstem lesion (upper motor neuron lesion) is illustrated in Figure 15-8. People with upper motor neuron lesions that prevent voluntary control of the contralateral lower face are able to laugh and cry normally because the pathway involved in emotional vocalization is separate from the corticobrainstem tract for the same activity.[19]

### Clinical Pearl

In the brainstem, lesions cause contralateral vertical tract signs unless the lesion affects the corticospinal tracts or dorsal column nuclei in the inferior medulla. Complete lesions of the facial cranial nerve cause ipsilateral paralysis of the facial muscles; lesions of the corticobrainstem axons to the facial nucleus cause paralysis of the contralateral lower face with sparing of control of the upper face.

## Contralateral and Ipsilateral Signs

A lesion in the brainstem often causes a combination of ipsilateral and contralateral signs, analogous to the effect of a spinal cord hemisection causing Brown-Sequard syndrome. For example, a lesion in the lateral medulla produces ipsilateral limb ataxia and ipsilateral loss of pain and temperature sensation from the face, combined with contralateral loss of pain and temperature sensation from the body (Figure 15-9, *A*) Because axons in the inferior cerebellar peduncle and the spinal tract and nucleus of the trigeminal nerve remain ipsilateral, the effects of a lesion affecting these structures are ipsilateral. Because axons in the spinothalamic tract cross the midline in the spinal cord, a lesion that interrupts the spinothalamic tract in the brainstem causes contralateral loss of pain and temperature sensation from the body. Additional examples of brainstem lesions are provided in Figure 15-9.

## Disorders of Vital Functions

Disruption of vital functions secondary to brainstem damage may cause the heart to stop beating, blood pressure to fluctuate, and/or breathing to cease. Areas in the medulla and pons regulate vital functions.

## Four D's of Brainstem Region Dysfunction

Dysphagia, dysarthria, diplopia, and dysmetria are the cardinal signs of brainstem dysfunction. Dysphagia is difficulty in swallowing, dysarthria is difficulty in speaking, diplopia is double vision, and dysmetria is the inability to control the distance of movements. The first three of these disorders are covered in Chapter 14; dysmetria is discussed in Chapter 11.

## Disorders of Consciousness

States of altered consciousness may occur with lesions affecting the brainstem or the cerebrum, because structures in both regions are required for consciousness. Brainstem damage that affects the reticular formation and/or the axons of the ascending reticular activating system interferes with consciousness. Damage to the cerebrum that interferes with hypothalamic/thalamic activating areas or with the function of the entire cerebral cortex may also impair consciousness. States of altered consciousness are defined in Table 15-2.

People in vegetative and minimally conscious states have loss of tissue in subcortical, thalamic, and brainstem regions. In the vegetative state, the loss is greater in the thalamic and subcortical white matter than in the minimally conscious state.[21]

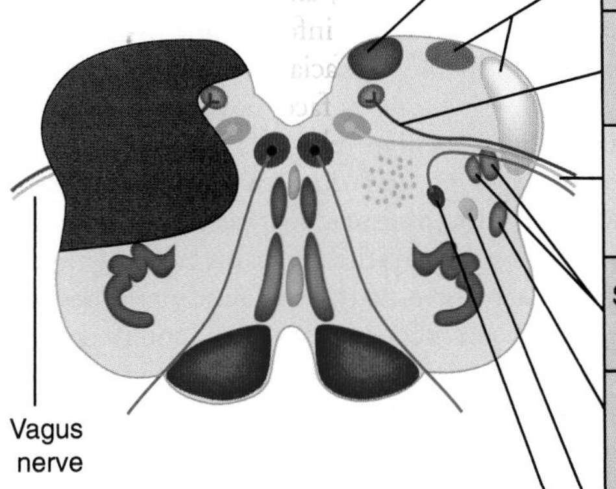

| Structures involved | Function | Lesion causes |
|---|---|---|
| Vestibular nuclei | Control of posture, head position, eye movements | Vertigo, nausea, vomiting, nystagmus, tilted head position, balance problems |
| Lateral cuneate nucleus and inferior cerebellar peduncle | Proprioceptive information into cerebellum | Ataxia |
| Afferents to solitary nucleus | Afferents from pharynx, larynx, GI system, thoracic viscera | Loss of taste from ipsilateral anterior tongue |
| Efferents from dorsal motor nucleus of vagus | Parasympathetic signals to thoracic and abdominal viscera | Problems with digestion and decreased ability to slow heart rate |
| Spinal tract and nucleus of trigeminal nerve | Information regarding tissue damage and temperature from ipsilateral face | Loss of pain and temperature sensation from ipsilateral face |
| Spinothalamic tract | Information regarding tissue damage and temperature from contralateral body | Loss of pain and temperature sensation from contralateral body |
| Descending sympathetic tract | Sympathetic signals from the hypothalamus to the T 1-2 spinal cord | Ispilateral Horner's syndrome |
| Nucleus ambiguus CN IX, X, XI) | Innervate striated muscles in pharynx, larynx, palate | Problems swallowing, speaking, loss of gag reflex, hoarseness |

Vagus nerve

A

**Fig. 15-9 Frequent sites of brainstem stroke.** The charts summarize structures damaged by the lesion and results of the damage. **A,** The most frequent site of brainstem stroke is illustrated: lateral medulla. The stroke affects the posterior inferior cerebellar artery and produces lateral medullary syndrome (also called *Wallenberg's syndrome*).

*Continued*

| Structures involved | Function | Lesion causes |
|---|---|---|
| Cochlear nucleus | Hearing relay | Unilateral deafness |
| Descending sympathetic tract | Sympathetic signals from the hypothalamus to the T1-2 spinal cord | Ispilateral Horner's syndrome |
| Vestibular nuclei | Control of posture, head position, eye movements | Vertigo, nausea, vomiting, nystagmus |
| Spinal tract and nucleus of trigeminal nerve | Information regarding tissue damage and temperature from ipsilateral face | Loss of pain and temperature sensation from ipsilateral face |
| Inferior cerebellar peduncle | Provide proprioceptive information from the body to the cerebellum | Ataxia |
| Salivatory nucleus | Innervate salivary and lacrimal glands | Lack of tears in the eye and decreased salivation |
| Spinothalamic tract | Information regarding tissue damage and temperature from contralateral body | Loss of pain and temperature sensation from contralateral body |
| Facial nucleus | Innervates muscle of face including orbicularis oculi; also innervates stapedius muscle | Ipsilateral paralysis muscles of face, loss of efferent limb of corneal reflex and stapedial reflex (causes sounds to be louder due to loss of stapes bone movement damping) |

Facial nerve

Vestibulo-cochlear nerve

B

**Fig. 15-9, cont'd  B,** The second most frequent site of brainstem stroke is illustrated: lateral inferior pons. The stroke affects the anterior inferior cerebellar artery.

A disconnection syndrome, called *locked-in syndrome,* may mimic the signs of impaired consciousness. In locked-in syndrome, consciousness is intact, but damage to upper motor neurons completely prevents the person from voluntarily moving, or in some cases, the person is able to voluntarily control eye movements and can communicate by coded eye movements. Figure 15-10 shows a section of medulla from a patient with locked-in syndrome.

The integrity of brainstem function can be assessed with auditory evoked potentials. As in somatosensory evoked potentials, a sense organ is stimulated, and the resulting electrical activity is recorded from electrodes on the scalp. For auditory evoked potentials, a brief burst of tone is presented and the brainstem response is recorded. Auditory evoked potentials are most commonly used to assess brainstem function in comatose patients. Auditory evoked potentials can also be used to evaluate whether the cochlea, the cochlear nerve, and auditory nuclei in the brainstem are functioning.

### Tumors in the Brainstem Region

Tumors within the cerebellum or brainstem cause increased intracranial pressure. This pressure may cause headache,

nausea, vomiting, cranial nerve disorders, and/or hydrocephalus. If the tumor is within the cerebellum, ataxia commonly occurs.

Damage caused by a benign tumor may be extensive because the unyielding bone and dura prevent brain tissue from moving away from the pressure. For example, an acoustic neuroma is a benign tumor of the Schwann cells surrounding the vestibulocochlear nerve. If the surrounding bones did not confine the nerve, the acoustic neuroma could enlarge without compromising function. Unfortunately, bony restriction causes the enlarging tumor to compress the vestibulocochlear nerve, resulting in tinnitus and eventual deafness. If the tumor continues to grow, more and more structures are compressed. The trigeminal and facial nerves will be the next structures compressed by the enlarging tumor, causing loss of sensation from the face and paresis of the facial muscles. Next, cerebellar signs, including ipsilateral limb ataxia, intention tremor, and nystagmus (abnormal eye movements), appear as pressure builds on the cerebellum. Eventually, brainstem compression interferes with vertical tracts and nuclear functions. Acoustic neuromas affect approximately 1 in 100,000 adults per year.[22] Acoustic tumors can be surgically removed at any stage of their growth.

| Structures involved | Function | Lesion causes |
|---|---|---|
| Oculomotor nerve parasympathetic nucleus | Innervates pupillary sphincter muscle and the ciliary muscles that adjust the lens for near vision | Dilation of pupil and unable to focus on near objects |
| Trigeminal lemniscus | Discriminative somatosensation from the face | Contralateral loss of sensation from the face |
| Medial lemniscus | Discriminative somatosensation from the face | Contralateral loss of sensation from the body |
| Cerebellothalamic axons | Coordinates movements | Contralateral cerebellar ataxia |
| Oculomotor nucleus | Innervates extraoccular muscles that move eye up, down, and in; partially innvervates levator palpebrae (partially raises upper eyelid) | Unable to move eye up, down, and in; drooping of upper eyelid. Eye abduction and depression by intact lateral rectus (CN VI) and superior oblique (CN IV); double vision |
| Red nucleus | Facilitate LMNs that elicit extension of wrist and fingers | Mild weakness wrist and finger extensors, obscured by ataxia |
| Corticopontine tract | Signals from somato-sensory and motor cerebral cortex to pons; synapses with ponto-cerebellar neurons; information used to coordinate distal limb movements | Contralateral cerebellar ataxia |

C

**Fig. 15-9, cont'd C,** The most frequent site of midbrain stroke: anteromedial midbrain.

| TABLE 15-2 | STATES OF ALTERED CONSCIOUSNESS |
|---|---|
| Coma | Unarousable; no response to strong stimuli including strong pinching of the Achilles tendon |
| Stupor | Arousable only by strong stimuli, including strong pinching of the Achilles tendon |
| Obtunded | Sleeping more than awake; drowsy and confused when awake |
| Vegetative state | Complete loss of consciousness, without alteration of vital functions. Vegetative state is distinguished from coma by the following signs: spontaneous eye opening, regular sleep-wake cycles, and normal respiratory patterns |
| Minimally conscious state | Severely altered consciousness with at least one behavioral sign of consciousness. Signs include following simple commands, gestural or verbal yes/no responses, intelligible speech, and movements or affective behaviors that are not reflexive[20] |
| Syncope (fainting) | Brief loss of consciousness due to a drop in blood pressure* |
| Delirium | Reduced attention, orientation, and perception, associated with confused ideas and agitation |

*Benign syncope results from overactivity of the vagus nerve (vasovagal syncope). Orthostatic hypotension (decreased blood pressure in the upright position) may cause syncope in patients with spinal cord injury and in people who have experienced prolonged bed rest.

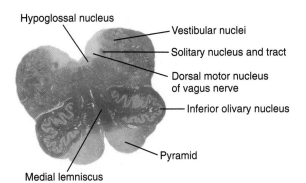

**Fig. 15-10 Section of the medulla, myelin darkly stained, illustrating degeneration of the medullary pyramids.** Destruction of the corticospinal tract, indicated by the pale appearance of the pyramids (normally the tract would be darkly stained), and other descending pathways produced locked-in syndrome.

## Brainstem Region Ischemia

Typically, ischemia in the brainstem region produces an abrupt onset of neurologic symptoms, including dizziness, visual disorders, weakness, incoordination, and somatosensory disorders. Vertebrobasilar artery insufficiency produces transient symptoms of brainstem region ischemia when the neck is extended and rotated.

Strokes that affect the lateral medulla produce Wallenberg's syndrome, also called *posterior inferior cerebellar artery syndrome* (see Figure 1-20). This syndrome consists of ipsilateral limb ataxia, dysarthria, dysphagia, vertigo (sensation of spinning), *pathologic nystagmus* (abnormal involuntary eye movements), ipsilateral Horner's syndrome, ipsilateral impairment of pain and temperature sensation in the face, and contralateral loss of pain and temperature sensation in the body. Ataxia results from damage to the inferior cerebellar peduncle, dysarthria and dysphagia from damage to the nucleus ambiguus, vertigo and nystagmus from damage to the vestibular nuclei (see Chapter 16), Horner's syndrome from damage to the descending sympathetic pathway, and somatosensory disorders from damage to the spinothalamic tract and the spinal nucleus of the trigeminal nerve (see Figure 15-8, *B*).

## SUMMARY

The brainstem contains the origin of most upper motor neurons (excluding corticospinal and corticobrainstem neurons), axons transmitting somatosensory information, and nuclei for cranial nerves III through X and XII and the reticular formation. The reticular formation is essential for modulation of neural activity throughout the central nervous system. A mnemonic for remembering the effects of a brainstem region lesion is the four *D*'s: dysphagia, dysarthria, diplopia, and dysmetria.

## CLINICAL NOTES

### Case 1

P.C. is a 32-year-old man who was found unconscious at home 4 days ago. He regained consciousness today. The therapist's evaluation reveals the following:
- Lack of pain and temperature sensation on the right side of the body
- Lack of somatosensation on the left side of the face
- Ataxia on the left side of the body
- Paralysis of muscles of facial expression on the left side
- Loss of corneal reflex on the left side

The therapist also notes nystagmus, vertigo, nausea, and vomiting when P.C. turns his head.

#### Questions
1. List the structure associated with each loss.
2. Where is the lesion?

### Case 2

L.D., a 78-year-old woman, awoke with an inability to voluntarily move the muscles of facial expression in her right lower face. In the clinic, the following signs are noted:
- Sensation is intact throughout the body and face, and movements of the limbs and trunk are normal.
- Movement of the upper face and the left lower face are normal. She is able to completely close both eyes on request. When she is asked to smile or frown, muscles in the right lower face do not contract. However, when she frowns in response to frustration, muscles in the right lower face contract.
- Test results for all cranial nerves other than cranial nerve VII are normal.

#### Question
Where is the lesion?

### Case 3

M.Z. is 17 years old. He suffered a severe head injury in a car accident 2 months ago. After a month-long hospitalization, M.Z. has been in a long-term care facility for 4 weeks. Notes in his chart indicate that he is in a vegetative state and is not expected to recover. M.Z. is completely immobile except for eye movements. His family believes that he is aware and able to communicate with them via eye movements. When the therapist asks him to blink three times, M.Z. complies. When the therapist asks him to look toward his right, he does. However, M.Z. does not move any other part of his body on request.

#### Questions
1. Is M.Z.'s behavior consistent with a vegetative state?
2. If not, what is the condition?

## CLINICAL NOTES—cont'd

### Case 4

R.V., a 58-year-old man, was in a meeting when suddenly he lost control of the right side of his body, including his face. He slumped in his chair, and the right side of his face appeared to sag, but he did not lose consciousness. R.V. complains of double vision. Clinical findings are as follows:

- Somatosensation is intact.
- Movement and strength on the left side of his body are normal. He is able to sit unassisted in a chair with arm and back support but cannot sit unassisted without support. R.V. is able to voluntarily move his right upper limb at the shoulder and his right lower limb at the hip, but strength is less than half that of the left side. He cannot move any other joints in his limbs on the right.
- All cranial nerves are intact except for the following:
  - He is unable to voluntarily move his right lower face.
  - He cannot move his left eye medially, downward, or upward.
  - He cannot fully open his left eye (left eyelid droops).
  - The left pupil is dilated and does not contract in response to light shined into either eye.

### Questions

1. List the structures associated with the functional losses.
2. Where is the lesion?

## REVIEW QUESTIONS

1. List the vertical tracts that are modified in the brainstem.
2. What are the functions of the reticular formation?
3. List the major reticular nuclei and the slow-acting neurotransmitters produced by these nuclei.
4. Which neurotransmitter produced in the brainstem is important in the cerebral processes of motivation and decision making?
5. How does the pedunculopontine nucleus affect movement?
6. Which medullary nuclei are included in a system that inhibits the transmission of pain information?
7. What is the role of ascending fibers from the locus coeruleus?
8. For each of the following functions, list the cranial nerve nucleus responsible for the function and the part of the brainstem where the nucleus is located (lower medulla, upper medulla, junction of the medulla and pons, pons, junction of the pons and midbrain, midbrain):
   - Control of voluntary muscles in the pharynx and larynx
   - Integration and transmission of pain information from the face
   - Control of tongue muscles
   - Processing of information about sounds
   - Control of muscles of mastication
   - Contraction of the pupillary sphincter and change in curvature of the lens to focus on near objects

9. Which nuclei in the midbrain are included in the basal ganglia circuit?
10. What are the functions of the cerebellum?
11. Why do brainstem lesions above the inferior medulla cause contralateral loss of discriminative touch information from the body?
12. What midbrain region coordinates somatic and autonomic reactions to pain, threats, and emotions?
13. What tracts convey motor signals from the cerebral cortex to cranial nerve motor nuclei?
14. How can a complete lesion of the facial nerve be differentiated from a lesion affecting the corticobrainstem tracts that convey information from the cerebral cortex to the facial nerve nucleus?
15. Would a person with a complete facial nerve lesion on the left side be able to smile involuntarily on the left side of the face? Why or why not?
16. Disorders of consciousness can occur with damage to what brainstem structures?
17. A person who has complete loss of consciousness combined with normal vital functions is in what state of altered consciousness?
18. Why are space-occupying lesions in the brainstem region, including benign tumors, so disruptive of brainstem function?

## References

1. Mena-Segovia J, Sims HM, Magill PJ, et al: Cholinergic brainstem neurons modulate cortical gamma activity during slow oscillations. *J Physiol* 586:2947–2960, 2008.

2. Mark GP, Shabani S, Dobbs LK, et al: Cholinergic modulation of mesolimbic dopamine function and reward. *Physiol Behav* 104:76–81, 2011.

3. Beaulieu J-M, Gainetdinov RR: The physiology, signaling, and pharmacology of dopamine receptors. *Pharmacol Rev* 63:182–217, 2011.

4. Alam M, Schwabe K, Krauss JK: The pedunculopontine nucleus area: critical evaluation of interspecies differences relevant for its use as a target for deep brain stimulation. *Brain* 134:11–23, 2011.

5. Jahn K, Zwergal A: Imaging supraspinal locomotor control in balance disorders. *Restor Neurol Neurosci* 28:5–114, 2010.

6. Haenisch B, Bönisch H: Depression and antidepressants: insights from knockout of dopamine, serotonin or noradrenaline re-uptake transporters. *Pharmacol Ther* 129:352–368, 2011.

7. Hornung JP: The human raphe nuclei and the serotonergic system. *J Chem Neuroanat* 26:331–343, 2003.

8. Carter ME, Yizhar O, Chikahisa S, et al. Tuning arousal with optogenetic modulation of locus coeruleus neurons. *Nat Neurosci* 13:1526–1533, 2010.

9. Reinoso-Suárez F, de Andrés I, Garzón M: Functional anatomy of the sleep-wakefulness cycle: wakefulness. *Adv Anat Embryol Cell Biol* 208:1–128, 2011.

10. Diekelmann S, Born J: The memory function of sleep. *Nat Rev Neurosci* 11:114–126, 2010.

11. Lange T, Born J: The immune recovery function of sleep—tracked by neutrophil counts. *Brain Behav Immun* 25:14–15, 2011.

12. Wu X, Nestrasil I, Ashe J, et al: Inferior olive response to passive tactile and visual stimulation with variable interstimulus intervals. *Cerebellum* 9:598–602, 2010.

13. Karachi C, Grabli D, Bernard FA, et al: Cholinergic mesencephalic neurons are involved in gait and postural disorders in Parkinson disease. *J Clin Invest* 120:2745–2754, 2010.

14. Matsamura M: The pedunculopontine tegmental nucleus and experimental parkinsonism: a review. *J Neurol* 252(Suppl 4): IV/5–12, 2005.

15. Takakusaki K, Tomita N, Yano M: Substrates for normal gait and pathophysiology of gait disturbances with respect to the basal ganglia dysfunction. *J Neurol* 255(Suppl 4):19–29, 2008.

16. Mobbs D, Petrovic V, Marchant JL, et al: When fear is near: threat imminence elicits prefrontal-periaqueductal gray shifts in humans. *Science* 317:1079–1083, 2007.

17. Jurgens U: The neural control of vocalization in mammals: a review. *J Voice* 23:1–10, 2009.

18. Rønning C, Sundet K, Due-Tønnessen B, et al: Persistent cognitive dysfunction secondary to cerebellar injury in patients treated for posterior fossa tumors in childhood. *Pediatr Neurosurg* 41:15–21, 2005.

19. Simonyan K, Horwitz B: Laryngeal motor cortex and control of speech in humans. *Neuroscientist* 17:197–208, 2011.

20. Giacino JT, Kalmar K: Diagnostic and prognostic guidelines for the vegetative and minimally conscious states. *Neuropsychol Rehabil* 15:166–174, 2005.

21. Fernández-Espejo D, Bekinschtein T, Monti MM, et al: Diffusion weighted imaging distinguishes the vegetative state from the minimally conscious state. *Neuroimage* 54:103–112, 2011.

22. Arthurs BJ, Lamoreaux WT, Giddings NA, et al: Gamma knife radiosurgery for vestibular schwannoma: case report and review of the literature. *World J Surg Oncol* 7:100, 2009.

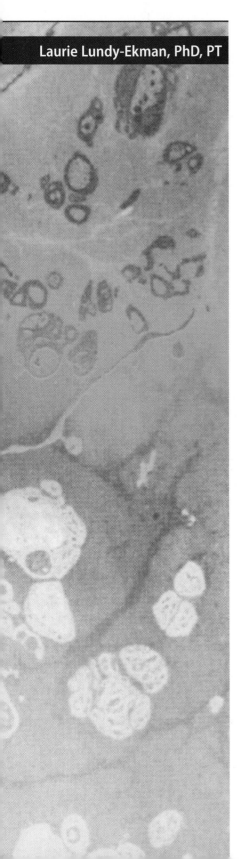

# 16

# Vestibular and Visual Systems

Laurie Lundy-Ekman, PhD, PT

When I was 37 years old, I awoke one morning in my completely dark bedroom. I stood up, took a step, and fell to the floor. Lying on the floor, I decided I had one of two problems: a stroke or a vestibular lesion. I quickly checked my brainstem cranial nerves: except for the vestibular nerve, the other brainstem cranial nerves and my hearing were intact. I concluded I hadn't had a stroke, because a stroke would affect more cranial nerve functions than just one vestibular nerve. When I turned my head, I experienced an intense sensation of spinning, complete disorientation, and nausea. If I didn't move my head, everything was normal. Using the bed to steady myself, and moving my head very slowly, I got up and turned on the light. I found I could use vision to maintain upright, but when I tried walking, my path curved dramatically. I diagnosed myself with vestibular neuritis, a viral infection of the vestibular nerve. A mismatch between signals from the infected vestibular nerve and the intact vestibular nerve caused the illusion of spinning, disorientation and nausea. The mismatched vestibular signals elicited abnormal vestibulospinal tract activity, causing asymmetrical contraction of postural muscles and thus my fall in the dark and, with the light on, my inability to walk in a straight line.

For the next three days, whenever I moved my head, the spinning, disorientation, and disequilibrium were severe. I noticed that I couldn't read street signs when I was walking because the visual world appeared to bounce up and down when I walked. On the fourth day, I felt recovered enough to drive. As I pulled onto the freeway on ramp, I quickly turned my head to check traffic. Immediately I felt as if the car were flipping over. I told myself that if the car were flipping, there would be metallic noises and I would be thrown around inside; instead there was only the convincing illusion of the car flipping. I pulled onto the shoulder of the freeway ramp and called my husband to pick me up and drive the car home. I avoided fast head movements for five more days, continued to feel unsteady while walking for another week, then gradually fully recovered.

*—Laurie Lundy-Ekman*

Vestibular receptors and cranial nerve axons in the periphery, vestibular nuclei in the brainstem, and an area of the cerebral cortex are dedicated to vestibular function. The visual system includes specialized neurons in the retina, cranial nerve afferents that are myelinated by oligodendroglia (and thus part of the central nervous system), a relay nucleus in the thalamus, the visual cortex, and areas of the cerebral cortex and midbrain that direct eye movements. The function of the visual system is partially dependent on the vestibular system because vestibular information contributes to compensatory eye movements that maintain the stability of the visual world when the head moves. (*Note:* The auditory system is covered in Chapter 14, "Cranial Nerves.")

## VESTIBULAR SYSTEM

Vestibular information is essential for postural control and for control of eye movements. The vestibular apparatus, located in the inner ear, contains sensory receptors that respond to the position of the head relative to gravity and to head movements. This information is converted into neural signals conveyed by the vestibular nerve to the vestibular nuclei. The vestibular nuclei are located in the brainstem, at the junction of the pons and medulla. Projections from the vestibular nuclei contribute to:

- Sensory information about head movement and head position relative to gravity
- Gaze stabilization (control of eye movements when the head moves)
- Postural adjustments
- Autonomic function and consciousness

### Vestibular Apparatus

The vestibular apparatus consists of bony and membranous labyrinths and hair cells. The bony labyrinth is a convoluted space within the skull that contains three semicircular canals and two otolithic organs (Figure 16-1). The membranous labyrinth is within the bony labyrinth. The membranous labyrinth is hollow and is filled with a fluid called *endolymph*. Receptors inside the membranous labyrinth are hair cells. Bending of the hairs determines the frequency of signals conveyed by the vestibular nerve (a branch of the vestibulocochlear nerve, cranial nerve VIII).

### Semicircular Canals

Receptors in the semicircular canals detect movement of the head by sensing the motion of endolymph. The semicircular canals are three hollow rings arranged perpendicular to each other. Each semicircular canal opens at both ends into the utricle, one of the otolithic organs. Each semicircular canal has a swelling, called the *ampulla*, containing a crista. The crista consists of supporting cells and sensory hair cells. The hairs are embedded in a gelatinous mass, the *cupula*. When the head is stationary, the hair cells fire at a baseline rate. If the head begins to turn, inertia causes the fluid in the canal to lag behind, resulting in bending of the cupula and the hairs of the hair cells (see Figure 16-1, *B*). Bending of the hairs results in an increase or decrease in the baseline rate of hair cell firing, depending on the direction of bend. The receptors in semicircular canals are sensitive only to rotational acceleration or deceleration (i.e., speeding up or slowing down rotation of the head).

If the head rotates at a constant speed, the effects of friction gradually cause the endolymph to move at the same speed as the head. When rotation is constant, the hair cells fire at a constant rate. As head rotation slows or stops, the endolymph continues moving at a faster rate than the head due to inertia. The continued endolymph movement bends the cupulae in the opposite direction to that during the head rotation. For example, if the head rotates to the right, during acceleration the bending of the hair cells in the cupula will cause the right vestibular nerve to fire more frequently than before head movement. During deceleration, the hair cells will bend in the opposite

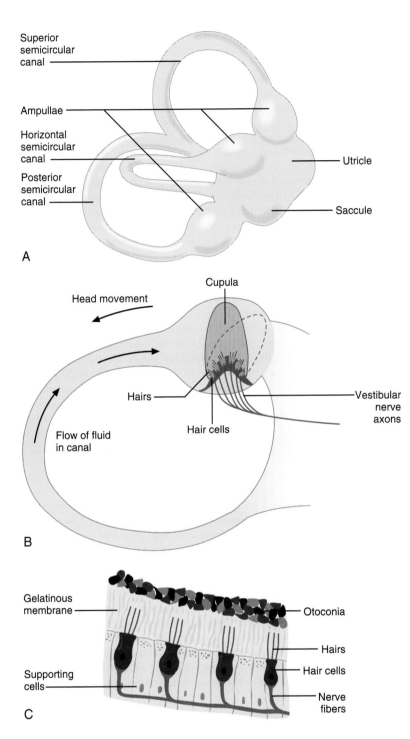

Superior semicircular canal

Ampullae

Horizontal semicircular canal

Posterior semicircular canal

Utricle

Saccule

A

Head movement

Cupula

Hairs

Flow of fluid in canal

Hair cells

Vestibular nerve axons

B

Gelatinous membrane

Supporting cells

Otoconia

Hairs

Hair cells

Nerve fibers

C

**Fig. 16-1 A,** The vestibular apparatus consists of the utricle, saccule, and semicircular canals. The three semicircular canals are at right angles to each other. Each semicircular canal has a swelling, the ampulla, that contains a receptor mechanism, the crista. **B,** A section through a semicircular canal shows the crista inside the ampulla. Flow of fluid in the canal, indicated by the arrow, moves the cupula and in turn bends the hair cells. Bending of the hair cells changes the pattern of firing in the vestibular neurons. **C,** Inside the utricle and the saccule is a receptor called the *macula.* In the macula, hairs projecting from hair cells are embedded in a gelatinous material. Atop the gelatinous material are otoconia: small, heavy, sand-like crystals. When the macula is moved into different positions, the weight of the otoconia bends the hairs, stimulating the hair cells and changing the pattern of vestibular neuron firing.

direction and the right vestibular nerve will fire less frequently than its baseline rate.

Maximum fluid flow in each semicircular canal and thus maximal change in the frequency of signals generated by bending of the hairs embedded in the cupula occur when the head turns on the canal's axis of rotation (Figure 16-2, *A*). Two semicircular canals that have maximal fluid flow during rotation in a single plane form a pair. For example, when the head is flexed 30 degrees, the horizontal canals are parallel to the ground. Rotation of the head in 30 degrees of flexion around

the vertical axis maximizes fluid flow in both horizontal canals. The horizontal canals are classified as a pair because maximal fluid flow occurs during movement in a single plane. When the horizontal canals are parallel to the ground, the anterior and posterior canals are vertical.

The anatomic arrangement of the canals, with the semicircular canals oriented at 90 degree angles to each other, ensures that acceleration or deceleration in a plane of movement that causes maximal fluid flow in a pair of semicircular canals does not stimulate the other semicircular canals. The anterior and

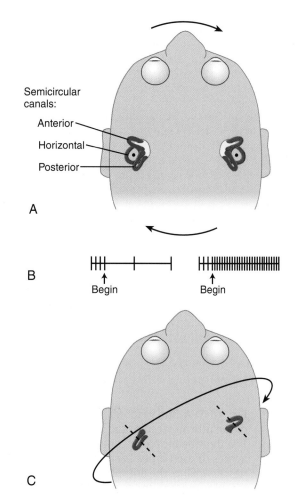

A

B

Begin　　　　Begin

C

**Fig. 16-2 Axis of rotation of the semicircular canals.** The three pairs of canals—horizontal, the right anterior with left posterior, and the left anterior with right posterior—are indicated by colors. **A,** The axes of the horizontal canals are indicated by a dot in the center of each horizontal canal. Rotating the head toward the right as indicated by the arrows causes maximum fluid flow in both horizontal canals. **B,** The graphs indicate vestibular nerve firing. When the head is not moving, the resting discharge rate for both right and left hair cells is about 90 spikes/sec. As the head turns, hair cells on the side away from the direction of turn hyperpolarize, decreasing vestibular nerve signals on the left side. Simultaneously, hair cells toward the direction of the turn depolarize, increasing vestibular nerve signals on the right (side toward the turn). **C,** Only the left posterior and right anterior canals are shown. The axes are indicated by dotted lines. Because their axes are parallel, rotation in one plane *(indicated by the arrow)* simultaneously maximally stimulates both canals in the pair.

degrees to each other, there is no plane of movement in which fluid flow in the anterior canals can be maximized simultaneously. However, the same somersault causes maximal fluid flow in the left posterior canal. Because movement in a single plane maximizes fluid flow in the right anterior and left posterior canals, these canals are classified as a pair (Figure 16-2, *C*). Similarly, the left anterior and right posterior canals are a pair. The influence of the semicircular canals on eye movement is discussed in the section on vestibulo-ocular reflexes.

Each of the canals in a pair produces reciprocal signals, that is, increased signals from one canal occur simultaneously with decreased signals from its partner. These reciprocal signals are essential for normal vestibular function. If the signals from a pair of semicircular canals are not reciprocal, difficulties with control of posture, abnormal eye movements, and nausea may result.

## Otolithic Organs

The two otolithic organs, the *utricle* and the *saccule,* are membranous sacs within the vestibular apparatus. They are not sensitive to rotation but instead respond to head position relative to gravity and to linear acceleration and deceleration. In each of these sacs is a macula, consisting of hair cells enclosed by a gelatinous mass topped by calcium carbonate crystals (see Figure 16-1, *C*). These crystals, called *otoconia,* are more dense than the surrounding fluid and their gelatinous support. Changing the position of the head tilts the macula, and the weight of the otoconia displaces the gelatinous mass, bending the embedded hairs. Bending the hairs stimulates or inhibits the hair cells (depending on the direction of bend), and this determines the frequency of firing of neurons in the vestibular nerve.

The utricular macula is on the floor of the utricle when the head is upright; thus its orientation is horizontal. The utricular macula responds maximally to head tilts that begin with the head in the upright position, as in bending forward to pick up something off the floor. The saccular macula is oriented vertically. The saccular macula responds maximally when the head moves from a laterally flexed position, as in moving from side-lying to standing. In addition to head position, the utricular maculae respond to linear acceleration and deceleration. As the head begins to move forward, the otoconia in the utricular macula fall back, bending the hairs and changing the firing rate of hair cells. The resulting impulses are conveyed via the vestibular nerve into the brainstem, signaling head acceleration.

---

**◎ Clinical Pearl**

Much of the information derived from the semicircular canals is used to stabilize vision, that is, the information keeps the eyes on a target when the head turns. Most of the information provided by the otolithic organs affects the spinal cord, adjusting activity in the lower motor neurons to postural muscles.

---

posterior semicircular canals are oriented vertically at a 45 degree angle to the midline. Turning the head 45 degrees to the left and then doing somersaults causes maximal fluid flow in the right anterior canal. This somersault causes no fluid flow in the left anterior canal because the left anterior canal is moving perpendicular to its axis. Because the anterior canals are 90

Information from the semicircular canals and from otolithic organs is transmitted by the vestibular nerve to the vestibular nuclei in the medulla and pons, and to the flocculonodular lobe of the cerebellum. Cell bodies of the vestibular primary afferents are in the vestibular ganglion, within the internal auditory canal. The peripheral part of the vestibular system consists of the vestibular apparatus and the peripheral part of the vestibular nerve. The central vestibular system is far more extensive.

## Central Vestibular System

The effects of activating the central vestibular system can be demonstrated by rapidly rotating the head. Simply spinning around or by riding a spinning amusement park ride activates the semicircular canal connections, eliciting:

- Altered postural control (leading to leaning or falling)
- Head orientation adjustment
- Eye movement reflexes
- Autonomic changes (nausea, vomiting)
- Changes in consciousness (light-headedness)
- Altered conscious awareness of head orientation and head movement

The central vestibular system comprises four nuclei, six pathways, the vestibulocerebellum, and the vestibular cortex (Figure 16-3). The vestibular nuclei are located bilaterally at the junction of the pons and the medulla, near the fourth ventricle. The nuclei are the lateral (or Deiter's nuclei), medial, inferior (or spinal), and superior vestibular nuclei. The flow of information from vestibular receptors to the consequences of vestibular information is summarized in Figure 16-4. In addition to vestibular information, the vestibular nuclei receive visual, proprioceptive, tactile, and auditory information (Figure 16-5). Thus, the vestibular nuclei integrate information from multiple senses. The six pathways that convey vestibular information to other areas within the central nervous system and their effects are listed in Table 16-1.

**TABLE 16-1 PATHWAYS THAT CONVEY INFORMATION FROM THE VESTIBULAR NUCLEI**

| | |
|---|---|
| Medial longitudinal fasciculus | Bilateral connections with the extraocular nuclei (cranial nerves III, IV and VI) and superior colliculus, influencing eye and head movements |
| Vestibulospinal tracts | Both medial and lateral, to lower motor neurons that influence posture |
| Vestibulocolic pathways | To the nucleus of the spinal accessory nerve (cranial nerve XI), influencing head position |
| Vestibulothalamocortical pathways | Providing conscious awareness of head position and movement and input to the corticospinal tracts |
| Vestibulocerebellar pathways | To the vestibulocerebellum, which controls the magnitude of muscle responses to vestibular information (including the gain of the vestibulo-ocular reflex) |
| Vestibuloreticular pathways | To the reticular formation, influencing the reticulospinal tracts and autonomic centers for nausea and vomiting |

The vestibulocerebellum (see Figure 11-14) is the section of the cerebellum that receives vestibular information and influences postural muscles and eye movements. The vestibulocerebellum adjusts the gain of responses to head movement via connections with the vestibular apparatus, vestibular nuclei, spinal cord, and inferior olive. Thus the magnitude of the reflex responses to changes in position and movement (of the head, body, or external objects) depends on vestibulocerebellar processing of vestibular and visual information. For example, when maintaining visual fixation on a target while turning the head, the eyes move precisely opposite the direction of head movement. The gain of the response (the ratio of head movement to eye movement) is 1. The vestibulocerebellum is vital for adaptation to vestibular disorders and to alterations in the postural and balance systems.

### Vestibular Role in Motor Control

In addition to providing sensory information about head movement and position, the vestibular system has two roles in motor control: gaze stabilization and postural adjustments (see Figure 16-4). Gaze stabilization operates by the vestibulo-ocular reflex, discussed later in this chapter.

Postural adjustments are achieved by reciprocal connections between the vestibular nuclei and the spinal cord, reticular formation, superior colliculus, nucleus of cranial nerve XI, vestibular cerebral cortex, and the cerebellum (Figure 16-5). The *lateral vestibulospinal tract,* which originates in the lateral vestibular nucleus, is the primary tract for vestibular influence on lower motor neurons to postural muscles in the limbs and trunk. The *medial vestibulospinal tract,* via projections to the cervical spinal cord, conveys signals that adjust head position to upright according to information signals from the vestibular apparatus. The vestibular nuclei are linked with areas that affect signals in the corticospinal and reticulospinal tracts. By these connections, the vestibular nuclei strongly influence the posture of the head and body.

## VISUAL SYSTEM

The visual system provides:
- Sight, for the recognition and location of objects
- Eye movement control
- Information used in postural and limb movement control

### Sight: Information Conveyed From Retina to Cortex

The visual pathway begins with cells in the retina that convert light into neural signals. These signals are processed within the retina and are conveyed to the retinal output cells. Retinal output is conveyed by the axons that travel in the optic nerve, optic chiasm, and optic tract, then synapse in the lateral geniculate nucleus of the thalamus. The optic nerve is the bundle of axons passing from the retina to the optic chiasm. The optic nerves merge at the optic chiasm, where some axons cross the midline. The optic tract conveys visual information from the chiasm to the lateral geniculate.

Postsynaptic neurons travel from the lateral geniculate in the geniculocalcarine tract (optic radiations) to the primary visual cortex. As the optic radiations emerge from the lateral

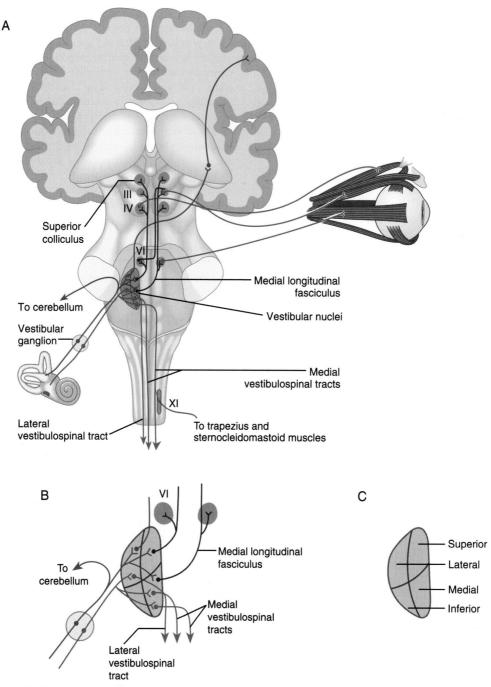

**Fig. 16-3 The vestibular system and the medial longitudinal fasciculus. A,** Direct connections from the vestibular apparatus to the cerebellum are indicated. The four vestibular nuclei are shown only on the left side. The medial longitudinal fasciculus connects the vestibular nuclei with the nuclei that control eye movements, with the superior colliculus, and with the nucleus of cranial nerve XI (accessory nerve). Note the connection between the left abducens nucleus and the right oculomotor nucleus. The medial and lateral vestibulospinal tracts convey vestibular information to the spinal cord, to adjust activity in postural muscles. Indirect connections from vestibular nuclei to the cerebral cortex via the thalamus (ventroposterolateral nucleus) carry information that contributes to conscious awareness of head position. **B,** An enlargement of the left vestibular nuclei and their connections. **C,** The vestibular nuclei.

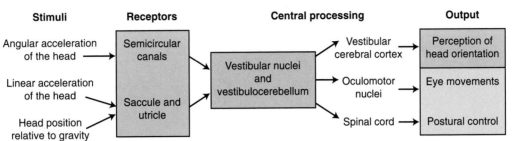

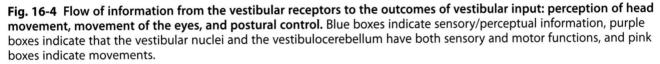

**Fig. 16-4** **Flow of information from the vestibular receptors to the outcomes of vestibular input: perception of head movement, movement of the eyes, and postural control.** Blue boxes indicate sensory/perceptual information, purple boxes indicate that the vestibular nuclei and the vestibulocerebellum have both sensory and motor functions, and pink boxes indicate movements.

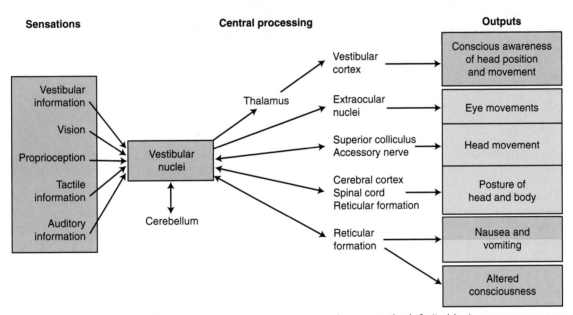

**Fig. 16-5** **Connections of the vestibular nuclei.** Sensory inputs are shown on the left *(in blue)*, motor output on the right *(in pink)*, and perceptual information on the right *(in blue)*. Note the wide variety of sensory information feeding into the vestibular nuclei. The vestibular nuclei integrate all types of sensory information that can be used for orientation—not only information from the vestibular receptors.

geniculate, they travel in the posterior part of the internal capsule. The primary visual cortex is the region of the cortex that receives direct projections of visual information. Thus, to reach conscious awareness, neural signals travel to the visual cortex via the retinogeniculocalcarine pathway (Figure 16-6).

The cortical destination of visual information depends on which half of the retina processes the visual information—the nasal retina, nearest the nose, or the temporal retina, nearest the temporal bone. Information from the nasal half of each retina crosses the midline in the optic chiasm and projects to the contralateral visual cortex. Information from the temporal half of each retina continues ipsilaterally through the optic chiasm and projects to the ipsilateral cortex.

The outcome of the fiber rearrangement in the chiasm is that all visual information from one visual field is delivered to the opposite visual cortex. For example, the right visual field is the part of the environment that people see to the right of their own midline when looking straight ahead. Light from the right visual field strikes the left half of each retina. The left half of the left retina is temporal and projects to the ipsilateral visual cortex. The left half of the right retina is nasal, and its projections cross the midline in the chiasm. Thus, all axons leaving the chiasm in the left optic tract carry information from the right visual field. Axons of the left optic tract synapse in the left lateral geniculate, and then the information is relayed to the left visual cortex via the geniculocalcarine tract. This results in

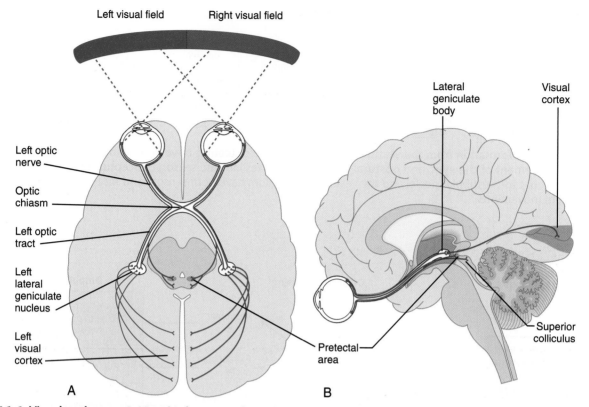

**Fig. 16-6 Visual pathways. A,** Visual information from the right visual field activates neurons in the left half of the retina of both eyes. Axons from the temporal half of the retina project ipsilaterally to the lateral geniculate body, and axons from the nasal half of the retina cross the midline in the optic chiasm to project to the contralateral lateral geniculate body. Thus all visual information from the right visual field projects to the left lateral geniculate, then through the optic radiations to the left visual cortex. Collaterals from axons in the optic tract to the pretectal area and to the superior colliculus are also shown. **B,** Lateral view of the projections from the retina to the superior colliculus, pretectal area, and lateral geniculate/visual cortex.

projection of the right visual field information to the left visual cortex. Similarly, left visual field information is projected to the right visual cortex.

---

**◎ Clinical Pearl**

The retinogeniculocalcarine pathway conveys visual information that reaches conscious awareness. Information from a visual field is conveyed to the contralateral visual cortex.

---

## Processing of Visual Information

Visual information reaching the primary visual cortex stimulates neurons that discriminate the shape, size, or texture of objects. Information conveyed to adjacent cortical areas, called the *secondary visual cortex,* is analyzed for colors and motion. From the secondary visual cortex, the information flows to other areas of the cerebral cortex, where the visual information is used to adjust movements or to visually identify objects (see Chapter 17). The stream of visual information that flows

dorsally is called the *action stream* because this information is used to direct movement, and the stream of visual information that flows ventrally is called the *perception stream* because this information is used to recognize visual objects (Figure 16-7).

Two areas that process nonconscious visual information are discussed in Chapter 14: the superior colliculus and the pretectal area. Projections from the retina to these areas in the brainstem and to the visual cortex are illustrated in Figure 16-6. The conscious and nonconscious pathways transmitting visual information are summarized in Figure 16-7.

## Eye Movement System

Normal eye movements require synthesis of information about:
• Head movements (vestibular information)
• Visual objects (vision)
• Eye movement and position (proprioceptive information)
• Selection of a visual target (brainstem and cortical areas)

Precise control of eye position is vital for vision because the best visual acuity is available only in a small region of the retina (the fovea), and because binocular perception of an object as a

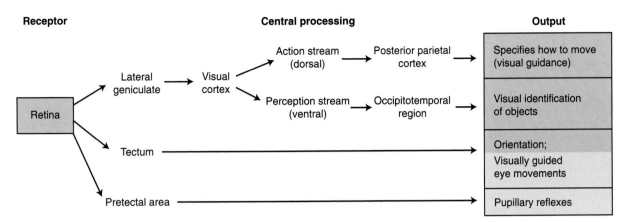

**Fig. 16-7 Flow of visual signals from the retina to the visual cortex, tectum, and pretectal area.** Signals arriving in the visual cortex are analyzed and then sent to other areas of the cerebral cortex, where directions for movement are created and where objects are recognized visually. Signals arriving in the tectum are used for orientation and eye movement control. Signals arriving in the pretectal area produce pupillary reflexes. Blue indicates sensory receptors and perception; pink indicates movement.

single object requires that the image be received by corresponding points on both retinas. The medial longitudinal fasciculus, reflexes, and cerebral centers achieve this exquisite control of eye position. The superior colliculus coordinates reflexive orienting movements of the eyes and head via the medial longitudinal fasciculus.

## Types of Eye Movements

Eye movements have two objectives: keeping the position of the eyes stable during head movements so that the environment does not appear to bounce, and directing the gaze at visual targets. Eye movements are either conjugate or vergence movements. In conjugate movements, both eyes move in the same direction. In vergence movements, the eyes move toward the midline or away from the midline. Vergence movements occur when looking at an object near the eyes or when switching the gaze from a near object to a far object.

**Gaze stabilization** (also called *visual fixation*) during head movements is achieved by:
- The vestibulo-ocular reflex: the action of vestibular information on eye position during fast movements of the head
- The optokinetic reflex: the use of visual information to stabilize images during slow movements of the head
**Direction of gaze** is accomplished by:
- Saccades: fast eye movements to switch gaze from one object to another. The high-speed eye movements bring new objects into central vision, where details of images are seen.
- Smooth pursuits: eye movements that follow a moving object
- Vergence movements: movement of the eyes toward or away from midline to adjust for different distances between the eyes and the visual target

## Vestibulo-ocular Reflexes

Vestibulo-ocular reflexes (VORs) stabilize visual images during head movements. This stabilizing prevents the visual world from appearing to bounce or jump around when the head

moves, especially during walking. Lack of visual image stability can be seen in videotapes when the videographer walks with the camera: the videotaped objects appear to bounce. Even more disconcerting to the viewer are abrupt swings of the video image, causing the visual objects to jump. Although these visual effects can be entertaining in giant-screen movies of airplanes swooping over canyons, in daily life lack of image stability can be disabling because the ability to use vision for orientation is lost.

Normally, when the head turns to the right, signals from the right horizontal semicircular canal increase and signals from the left horizontal semicircular canal decrease. This information is relayed to the vestibular nuclei for coordination of visual stabilization. Information is sent from the vestibular nuclei to the nuclei of cranial nerves III and VI, activating the rectus muscles that move the eyes to the left and inhibiting the rectus muscles that move the eyes to the right (Figures 16-8 and 16-9).

Similarly, vertical VORs can be elicited by flexion of the head and extension of the head. All VORs move the eyes in the direction opposite to the head movement to maintain stability of the visual field and visual fixation on objects. The effect of stimulation of each semicircular canal on extraocular muscles is illustrated in Figure 16-10. Stimulating a pair of semicircular canals induces eye movements in roughly the same plane as the canals.[1]

Sometimes when a person turns the head, the intent is to look in the new direction rather than have the eyes fixate on the previous target. To accomplish this, suppression of the VOR is essential. The flocculus of the cerebellum adjusts the gain of the VOR and can completely suppress the VOR when appropriate.

## Optokinetic Reflex

The optokinetic reflex adjusts eye position during slow head movements. *Optokinetic* means that the reflex is elicited by moving visual stimuli. When a person is walking, the head moves relative to objects in the environment. The optokinetic system allows the eyes to follow large objects in the visual field.

Experimentally, the optokinetic system can be studied by having a person watch a cylinder covered with vertical stripes rotating slowly. A normal response is for the person's eyes to follow a single stripe to the edge of the visual field, and then a saccade moves the eyes to the next stripe. Neurologic control of the optokinetic reflex involves the following structures in sequence: retina, optic nerve, optic chiasm, optic tract, pretectal area (in the midbrain; see Figure 14-6), medial vestibular nucleus, and oculomotor nuclei (Figure 16-11).

The influence of optokinetic stimuli on the perception of movement is illustrated by responses to unexpected movement of nearby large objects. For example, a person stopped at a stoplight may misinterpret the sudden movement of a bus in the adjacent lane as the person's car rolling backward. The person hits the brakes, only to realize the car was not moving. This illusion of motion is called *vection*.

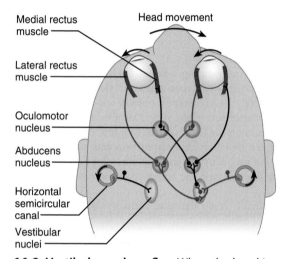

**Fig. 16-8 Vestibulo-ocular reflex.** When the head is turned to the right, inertia causes the fluid in the horizontal semicircular canals to lag behind the head movement. This bends the cupula in the right semicircular canal in a direction that increases firing in the right vestibular nerve. The cupula in the left semicircular canal bends in a direction that decreases the tonic activity in the left vestibular nerve. Neurons whose activity level increases with this movement are indicated in red. Neurons whose activity level decreases are black. For simplicity, the connections of the left vestibular nuclei are not shown. Via connections between the vestibular nuclei and the nuclei of cranial nerves III and VI, both eyes move in the direction opposite to the head turn.

## Direction of Gaze

Saccades, smooth pursuits, and convergence are eye movements that serve to direct gaze toward selected objects. Brainstem centers control horizontal and vertical eye movements. An area in the pons, the paramedian pontine reticular formation (PPRF), controls voluntary horizontal saccades. The abducens nucleus, as the source of the abducens nerve and via connections with the oculomotor nucleus, controls horizontal pursuits and reflexive saccades. The midbrain reticular formation controls vertical eye movements.

Cortical centers influencing eye movements include the frontal, occipital, and temporal eye fields (Figure 16-12). The frontal eye fields provide voluntary control of eye movements when a decision is made to look at a particular object. The occipital and temporal eye fields contribute to the ability to visually pursue moving objects (pursuit eye movements). The dorsolateral prefrontal cortex inhibits reflexive eye movements as appropriate. Another area, in the posterior parietal cortex, provides cortical input for smooth pursuit movements.

The following may influence eye movements:

- Auditory information (via the superior colliculus)
- Vestibulo-ocular reflex
- Visual stimuli
- Sensory information from extraocular muscles
- Limbic system (see Chapters 17 and 18) and voluntary control

Saccades quickly switch vision from one object to another. If a person is reading and someone comes into the room, a saccadic eye movement shifts the reader's gaze from the text to the person. For voluntary saccades, the posterior parietal cortex directs visual attention to the stimulus. The posterior parietal cortex signals the superior colliculus, the brainstem center for orientation. The superior colliculus also receives information from the frontal eye fields. The superior colliculus then signals the PPRF and/or the midbrain reticular formation. The PPRF controls voluntary horizontal saccades by activating the abducens nucleus, which then activates the oculomotor nucleus. The midbrain reticular formation controls vertical saccades by activating cranial nerves III and IV (Figure 16-13, *A*). Adjusting the relative levels of activity of the PPRF and the midbrain reticular formation controls diagonal saccades.

Saccades can be generated voluntarily (e.g., a person decides to look up) and can also be elicited by a variety of stimuli, including visual, tactile, auditory, or nociceptive. For example, a fast-moving object in the peripheral vision elicits reflexive movements of the eyes and head toward the stimulus. Control of reflexive saccades is less complex than control of voluntary saccades. Reflexive horizontal saccades are initiated

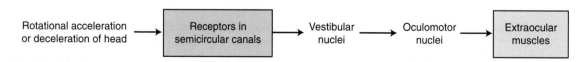

**Fig. 16-9 The generation of the vestibulo-ocular reflex.** Blue indicates sensory receptors and pink indicates movement.

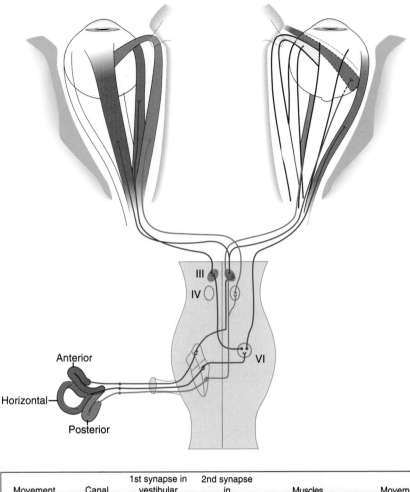

| Movement of face | Canal stimulated | 1st synapse in vestibular nucleus | 2nd synapse in nucleus of: | Muscles activated: | Movement of the eyes |
|---|---|---|---|---|---|
| Face tilts down | Anterior | Superior | CN III | Ipsilateral superior rectus<br>Contralateral inferior oblique | Up |
| Face turns right or left | Horizontal | Medial | CN III, VI | Ipsilateral medial rectus<br>Contralateral lateral rectus | Horizontal |
| Face tilts up | Posterior | Medial | CN III, IV | Ipsilateral superior oblique<br>Contralateral inferior rectus | Down |

**Fig. 16-10 The connections between receptors in the semicircular canals and the nuclei of the nerves to the extraocular muscles are shown.** For simplicity, only excitatory connections are shown. The inhibitory connections *(not shown)* adjust the activity of nerves to antagonistic extraocular muscles, so that their activity is inversely proportional to the activity of the agonist muscles.

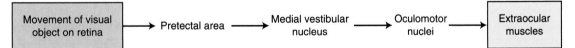

**Fig. 16-11 The generation of the optokinetic reflex.** Blue indicates sensory input and pink indicates motor output.

by the superior colliculus, then are directly signaled to the abducens nucleus, then, via the medial longitudinal fasciculus, to the oculomotor nucleus. Reflexive vertical saccades are signaled directly to the oculomotor and trochlear nuclei. The different actions of the visually guided system, the VOR, and the smooth pursuit system can be demonstrated by the following task. Reach forward and place your index finger about 1.5 feet in front of you. Compare the visual clarity when you move your finger from side to side rapidly versus when the finger is held steady and you move your head rapidly from side to side.

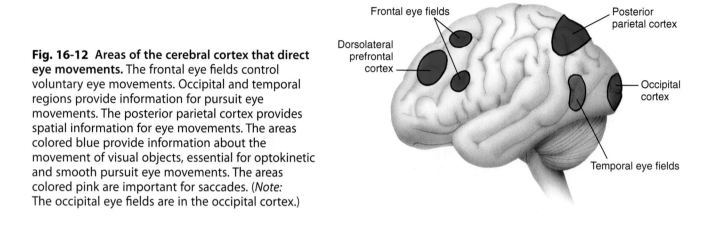

**Fig. 16-12 Areas of the cerebral cortex that direct eye movements.** The frontal eye fields control voluntary eye movements. Occipital and temporal regions provide information for pursuit eye movements. The posterior parietal cortex provides spatial information for eye movements. The areas colored blue provide information about the movement of visual objects, essential for optokinetic and smooth pursuit eye movements. The areas colored pink are important for saccades. (*Note:* The occipital eye fields are in the occipital cortex.)

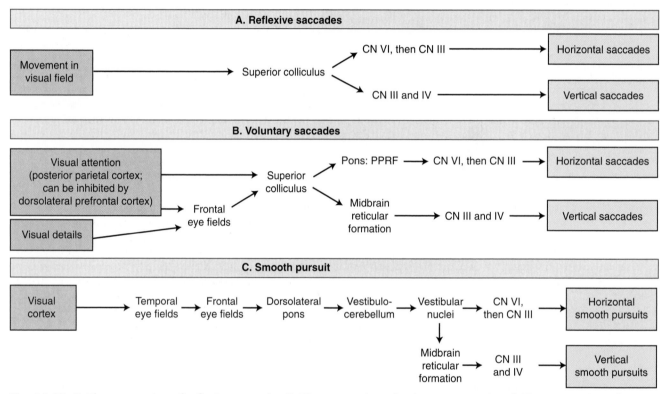

**Fig. 16-13 A,** The generation of reflexive saccades. **B,** The generation of voluntary saccades. **C,** The generation of smooth pursuit eye movements. *CN,* Cranial nerve; *PPRF,* paramedian pontine reticular formation. Blue indicates sensory/perceptual information; pink indicates movement.

Next, keep your head still while you move your finger from side to side slowly. Explain the difference in ability to see details.*

Smooth pursuit eye movements are used to follow a moving object. If you watch someone walk across the room, smooth pursuit movements maintain the direction of gaze so that the image is maintained on the fovea. Commands for smooth pursuit movement originate in the visual cortex. In sequence, signals are transmitted via the temporal eye fields, frontal eye fields, dorsolateral pons, vestibulocerebellum, and then vestibular nuclei to the nucleus of cranial nerve VI (abducens nerve) and/or to the midbrain reticular formation. The nucleus of cranial nerve VI connects with cranial nerve III via the medial longitudinal fasciculus. Activation of cranial nerve VI and part of cranial nerve III activates the appropriate rectus muscles to produce horizontal pursuit movements. The midbrain reticular formation activates ocular motor neurons to produce vertical pursuit movements (Figure 16-13, *B*). A moving visual

---

*The difference in clarity is due to the ability of the nervous system to adjust eye movements based on anticipated head location (when the head moves) versus the slower process of adjusting after visual information indicates loss of the target (when the finger moves rapidly). Thus the difference in the ability to see details results from rapid feedforward adjustments versus using the slow visual feedback process. Slow finger movements allow enough time to process and use visual feedback to control eye movements.

stimulus is essential for the production of smooth pursuit movements.

During reading, the pupils are directed toward the midline to allow the image to fall on corresponding areas of the retinas. This convergence is part of the accommodation discussed in Chapter 14. Control of eye movement is summarized in Table 16-2.

Involuntary back-and-forth movements of the eyes, including the involuntary eye movements that occur during or after rapid rotation of the head, are called *nystagmus*. The direction of nystagmus is named according to the direction of saccadic eye movements. Thus, if the fast movements are toward the right, the nystagmus is called *right-beating nystagmus. Physiologic nystagmus* is a normal response that can be elicited in an intact nervous system by rotational or temperature stimulation of the semicircular canals (see "Examining the Vestibular System" later in this chapter) or by moving the eyes to the extreme horizontal position. Pathologic nystagmus, a sign of nervous system abnormality, is discussed with disorders of the eye movement system.

> **◎ Clinical Pearl**
>
> Nystagmus (except nystagmus elicited by moving the eyes to the extreme horizontal position) indicates that the vestibular system senses head rotation and the eyes are moving to adjust for the rotation.

## PERCEPTION: INHIBITORY VISUAL-VESTIBULAR INTERACTION IN THE CEREBRAL CORTEX

During vection, activity in the vestibular cortex is inhibited. Similarly, activation of the vestibular cortex inhibits visual areas of the cortex.[2] Try turning your head and eyes slowly from one side of the room to the other side. Compare the visual detail with that observed when you make the same movement quickly. When vestibular activity increases, visual details are suppressed.

## DISORDERS OF THE VESTIBULAR AND VISUAL SYSTEMS

In either system, disorders may affect the receptors, the cranial nerves, brainstem nuclei, tracts within the central nervous system, or associated cortical areas. A complete lesion affecting receptors or the cranial nerve dedicated to that system produces total ipsilateral loss of sensory input for that system. Thus, in the vestibular system a complete peripheral lesion causes ipsilateral loss of vestibular information. In the visual system, a complete lesion in the retina or the optic nerve causes ipsilateral blindness. Lesions of these systems within the brain cause more variable outcomes, depending on the location and the extent of the lesion.

### Disorders of the Vestibular System

The most common symptom of vestibular system dysfunction is vertigo, an illusion of motion. People may falsely perceive movement of themselves or their surroundings. Vertigo occurs with both peripheral and central disorders and arises from disturbance of spatial orientation in the vestibular cortex. Vertigo is always caused by a sudden imbalance of vestibular signals, secondary to a lesion of the vestibular apparatus, vestibular nerve, vestibular nuclei, or vestibulocerebellum. Vestibular disorders may also cause pathologic nystagmus, which is typically more severe in peripheral than in central lesions. However, pathologic nystagmus is fatigable and habituates in most peripheral disorders but does not fatigue or habituate in central disorders. Pathologic nystagmus results from unbalanced inputs to the vestibulo-ocular reflex circuits. Another frequent symptom of vestibular disorders is disequilibrium, a perception of imbalance. Ataxia may occur with vestibular disorders. Vestibular ataxia must be differentiated from cerebellar and from sensory ataxia (see "Examining the Vestibular System" later in this chapter). In vestibular lesions, abnormal vestibulospinal, corticospinal, and reticulospinal tract activity causes the disequilibrium and ataxia. Nausea and vomiting may also occur, via connections that activate the reticular formation.

**TABLE 16-2**   CONTROL OF EYE MOVEMENT

| Neural Control System | Purpose | Type of Movement | Origin of Command |
|---|---|---|---|
| Vestibulo-ocular during rapid head movements | To keep the gaze fixed on a target | Reflex conjugate | Vestibular nuclei |
| Optokinetic | To keep the gaze fixed on a target during slow head movements | Reflex conjugate | Visual cortex |
| Smooth pursuit | To maintain the gaze on a moving target | Voluntary conjugate | Visual cortex |
| Saccadic | To rapidly move the eyes to a new target | Voluntary conjugate | Frontal eye fields |
| Vergence | To align the eyes on a near target | Voluntary disconjugate | Visual cortex |

When a person moves relative to the environment, or when objects in the environment move, a continuous stream of visual information flows across the retinas. Normally this information is suppressed, and there is no optokinetic effect on equilibrium. However, people with vestibular disorders may experience severe disequilibrium and disorientation in these situations. This is illustrated by the "grocery store effect," in which the intensity of optical flow provokes disequilibrium and disorientation. Walking in a busy mall or walking near traffic can elicit similar effects on equilibrium and orientation. To maintain orientation and control of posture, a person with a vestibular disorder may need to move slowly and devote conscious attention to staying upright.

## Peripheral Vestibular Disorders

Peripheral vestibular disorders typically cause recurring periods of vertigo, accompanied by moderate to severe nausea. Nystagmus almost always accompanies peripheral vertigo. Because the auditory and vestibular structures are in close proximity in the inner ear, diminished hearing and/or tinnitus are frequently present. No other neurologic findings are associated with peripheral vestibular disorders. Peripheral vestibular disorders include benign paroxysmal positional vertigo, vestibular neuritis, Ménière's disease (Table 16-3), traumatic injury, and perilymph fistula. Certain drugs may also cause peripheral vestibular damage.

### Benign Paroxysmal Positional Vertigo

Benign paroxysmal positional vertigo (BPPV) is an inner ear disorder that causes acute onset of vertigo and nystagmus. The term *benign* indicates not malignant, *paroxysmal* means a sudden onset of a symptom or a disease, and *positional* denotes head position as the provoking stimulus. In BPPV, a rapid change in head position results in vertigo and nystagmus that subside in less than 2 minutes, even if the provoking head position is sustained. Activities that frequently provoke BPPV include getting into or out of bed, bending over to look under a bed, reaching up to retrieve something from a high shelf ("top shelf vertigo"), and turning over in bed (Pathology 16-1).

The cause of BPPV is displacement of otoconia from the macula into a semicircular canal. In most cases, the posterior semicircular canal is affected. The otoconia may be displaced secondary to trauma or infection that affects the vestibular apparatus. However, BPPV appears to occur spontaneously in some elderly people. When the head is upright, the otoconia settle in a gravity-dependent position in the posterior semicircular canal. When the head is moved quickly into a provoking position, the otoconia fall to a new position within the canal. Their movement generates an abnormal flow of the endolymph, bending the cupula and initiating unilateral signals in the vestibular nerve. If the provoking head position is maintained, vertigo fades as the endolymph stops moving. Balance deficits may accompany the vertigo. Frequently the balance disorder outlasts the brief spell of vertigo. Signs and symptoms of BPPV can be provoked using the Hallpike maneuver (Figure 16-14). Treatment to restore the otoconia to their correct position, the particle repositioning maneuver, begins with the Hallpike maneuver. If the right ear is affected, the Hallpike ends with the head rotated toward the right side. When the vertigo and nystagmus stop, the patient's head is rotated to the left side and the patient turns fully prone. The patient remains in the prone position for 10 to 15 seconds. While maintaining the head turned toward the left shoulder, the patient is assisted into a sitting position. Prokopakis and associates (2005)[3] reported that in 84% of patients, particle repositioning immediately eliminated BPPV, and 92% of patients reported that they were free of vertigo during the follow-up period (average follow-up, 46 months).

### Vestibular Neuritis

Vestibular neuritis is inflammation of the vestibular nerve, usually caused by a virus. Disequilibrium, spontaneous nystagmus, nausea, and severe vertigo persist for up to 3 days, then gradually the symptoms subside over approximately two weeks. Hearing is unaffected. Caloric testing (see the section "Testing Vestibulo-ocular Reflexes" in this chapter) shows decreased or absent response on the involved side. During the acute phase,

| **TABLE 16-3** | COMPARISON OF PERIPHERAL VESTIBULAR DISORDERS | | |
|---|---|---|---|
| | **Benign Paroxysmal Positional Vertigo** | **Vestibular Neuritis** | **Ménière's Disease** |
| Etiology | Otoconia in semicircular canals | Infection | Unknown |
| Speed of onset | Acute | Acute | Chronic |
| Duration of typical incident | <2 minutes | Severe symptoms for 2–3 days, gradual improvement over 2 weeks | 0.5–24 hours |
| Prognosis | If untreated, improves in weeks or months; if treated with particle repositioning maneuver, often cured immediately | Improves after 3–4 days; usually resolves over 2 weeks as the viral infection is cleared | Some patients have only mild hearing loss and a few episodes of vertigo. Most have multiple episodes of vertigo and progressive loss of hearing. |
| Unique signs | Elicited by change of head position | None | Associated with hearing loss, tinnitus, and feeling of fullness in the ear |

| **PATHOLOGY 16-1** | BENIGN PAROXYSMAL POSITIONAL VERTIGO (BPPV) |
|---|---|
| Pathology | Otoconia freed from macula float into a semicircular canal, usually into the posterior semicircular canal; when a quick head movement causes the otoconia to fall to a new gravity-dependent position, movement of the otoconia produces abnormal fluid flow in the semicircular canal, stimulating hair cells in the cupula and creating abnormal signals in the vestibular nerve |
| Etiology | Often traumatic; may occur after a viral infection that affects the peripheral vestibular system or spontaneously |
| Speed of onset | Rapid |
| Signs and symptoms | Vertigo lasting less than 2 minutes provoked by moving the head into specific positions |
| Consciousness | Brief interference with orientation and concentration |
| Communication and memory | Normal |
| Sensory | Normal somatosensation; illusion of environment or self-moving |
| Autonomic | Nausea |
| Motor | Poor balance and trouble walking[4] |
| Region affected | Peripheral nervous system; inner ear |
| Demographics | Incidence = 0.6% per year[5]<br>Lifetime prevalence = 2.4%.[5] Incidence tends to increase with age. Oghalai and associates (2000)[6] reported that in a cross-sectional study, 9% of elderly people had unrecognized BPPV. |
| Prognosis | Physical repositioning maneuvers immediately effective in most people and are more effective than exercises[7] |

medication may be used to suppress the nausea, vertigo, and vomiting.

### Ménière's Disease

Ménière's disease causes a sensation of fullness in the ear, tinnitus, severe acute vertigo, nausea, vomiting, and hearing loss. Ménière's disease is associated with abnormal fluid pressure in the inner ear, causing expansion of the scala media (this expansion is called *endolymphatic hydrops*), but whether this is a cause or an effect of the disease is unknown. The incidence is 190 cases per 100,000 people, with a female-to-male ratio of 1.9 : 1.[8] Drugs that suppress vertigo are useful during acute attacks. In extreme cases, the vestibular nerve may be surgically severed to relieve symptoms. Destruction of the labyrinth by injection of drugs that damage the inner ear may also be used to control nausea and vomiting.

### Traumatic Injury

Traumatic injury to the head may cause concussion of the inner ear, fracture of the bone surrounding the vestibular apparatus and nerve, or pressure changes in the inner ear. Any of these injuries can compromise vestibular function.

### Perilymph Fistula

Perilymph is the fluid in the space between the bone and the membranous labyrinth in the inner ear. Perilymph fistula occurs when an opening is present between the middle and inner ear, allowing perilymph to leak from the inner ear into the middle ear. This leakage produces the abrupt onset of hearing loss, with tinnitus and vertigo. Most cases are secondary to trauma. Diagnosis requires an incision and endoscopic examination.

### Bilateral Lesions of the Vestibular Nerve

Bilateral lesions of the vestibular nerve interfere with reflexive eye movements in response to head movement. People with bilateral vestibular nerve lesions initially complain of oscillopsia. *Oscillopsia* is the illusion of visual objects bouncing when the head is moving. The world seems to bounce up and down as they walk because normal reflexive adjustments for head movement are decreased (decreased VOR). Over time, the nervous system adapts to the change, and people report less difficulty with disorienting movements of the visual field.

Certain antibiotics, specifically gentamicin and streptomycin, may damage both the cochlea and the vestibular apparatus in susceptible people. The effects are typically bilateral. Hearing loss, disequilibrium, and oscillopsia are common. Vertigo is infrequent because the vestibular apparatus damage is usually symmetric and thus the balance between the right and left vestibular signals is normal.

## Central Vestibular Disorders

Central vestibular disorders result from damage to the vestibular nuclei or their connections within the brain. Central disorders typically produce milder symptoms than peripheral disorders. Nystagmus may occur. Lesions that interfere with vestibular nuclei produce signs and symptoms similar to those of unilateral vestibular lesions: nystagmus, vertigo, and disequilibrium. However, because central lesions are rarely limited to only the vestibular nuclei, these lesions produce additional signs, depending on the involvement of other structures. Any brainstem signs, including sensory and/or motor loss, double vision, Horner's syndrome, clumsiness

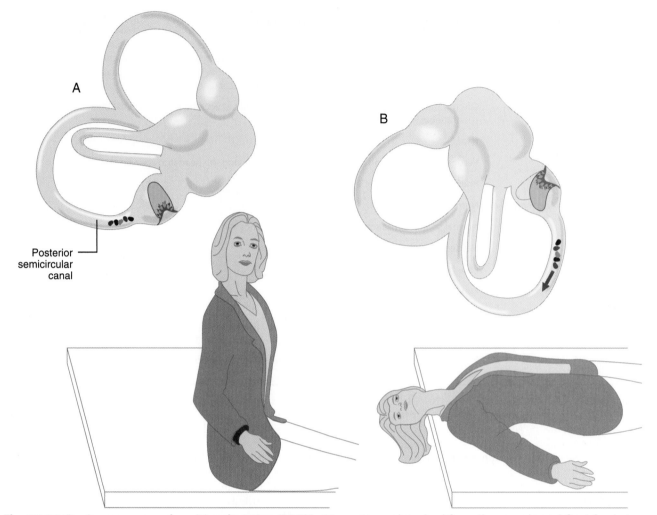

**Fig. 16-14 Benign paroxysmal positional vertigo (BPPV).** Otoconia are detached from the macula and float freely in a semicircular canal. Most commonly, the posterior semicircular canal is affected. **A,** Position of the semicircular canals when a person is sitting with the head turned 45 degrees to the right. Note the otoconia in the posterior canal. **B,** To determine whether otoconia are present in the posterior semicircular canal, the Hallpike maneuver is used. The Hallpike maneuver tests for BPPV by provoking maximal movement of the otoconia. The maneuver is performed by turning the person's head 45 degrees to the right (or left), then passively moving the person quickly from a sitting position to a supine position with the head turned and the neck extended 30 degrees. Free-floating otoconia in the posterior semicircular canal fall away from the cupula in response to gravity, creating movement of the endolymph that continues after the head is stationary. Continued movement of the endolymph bends the cupula, producing signals in the vestibular nerve that elicit vertigo and nystagmus. When the endolymph stops moving, the vertigo and nystagmus subside. Thus the Hallpike maneuver tests for BPPV by provoking maximal movement of otoconia.

when the trunk is supported (i.e., sitting or lying down), or dysarthria, are indications of a central lesion. Continuous (lasting all day) severe vertigo persisting longer than 3 days with mild nausea and vomiting usually indicates a central nervous system dysfunction. Pure vertical positional nystagmus and horizontal or vertical double vision also indicate a central lesion.[9]

Lesions in the vestibulothalamocortical pathway or the vestibular cortex create an abnormal perception of vertical without vertigo. No vertigo occurs because the signals in the vestibular nuclei are symmetric. The vestibular cortex is located in the parieto-insular cortex and receives input from both semicircular canals and otolithic organs.[10] People with lesions that affect the

vestibular system superior to the vestibular nuclei experience head tilt, misidentification of vertical, and lateropulsion. Lateropulsion is pushing toward one side of the body when sitting and/or standing. Lesions of the vestibular cortex may produce lateropulsion.[11] Lateropulsion also occurs in dorsolateral medullary syndrome (Wallenberg's syndrome[12]) via damage to the vestibular nuclei, inferior cerebellar peduncle, or spinocerebellar tracts.

Common causes of central vestibular disorders include ischemia or a tumor in the brainstem/cerebellar region, cerebellar degeneration, multiple sclerosis, or Arnold-Chiari malformation. Migraine may cause vestibular dysfunction. The diagnosis of migrainous vertigo (also known as *vestibular*

**TABLE 16-4** DIFFERENTIATING BETWEEN PERIPHERAL AND CENTRAL VESTIBULAR DISORDERS

| Symptom | Peripheral Nervous System | Central Nervous System |
|---|---|---|
| Nystagmus | Almost always present; typically unidirectional, not vertical | Frequently present; may be vertical, unidirectional, or multidirectional |
| Cochlear nerve symptoms | May have tinnitus, decreased hearing | Uncommon |
| Brainstem region signs | None | May have motor or sensory deficits, Babinski's sign, dysarthria, limb ataxia, or hyperreflexia |
| Nausea and/or vomiting | Moderate to severe | Mild |
| Oscillopsia | Mild unless the lesion is bilateral | Severe |

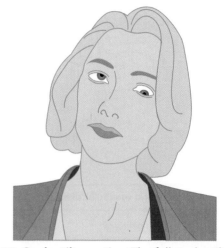

**Fig. 16-15 Ocular tilt reaction.** The full ocular tilt reaction consists of a triad of signs: lateral head tilt, skew deviation of the eyes, and ocular rotation. The drawing shows part of the ocular tilt reaction toward the left: left lateral head tilt, left eye looking downward, and right eye looking upward. The rotation of both eyes to the left is not visible in the illustration.

*migraine*) is based on vertigo symptoms that do not fit other syndromes, plus a history of migraine, a family history of migraine, and susceptibility to motion sickness.[13] Migrainous vertigo usually occurs as an isolated symptom, not coincident with headache, and a typical episode lasts for minutes or hours.[14] People with a migraine history have a 34% incidence of abnormal vestibular function during nonsymptomatic times.[13] Vestibular rehabilitation decreases imbalance and the severity of dizziness in people with migrainous vertigo.[15] Table 16-4 lists signs and symptoms that differentiate peripheral from central vestibular disorders.

### Unilateral Vestibular Loss

Unilateral vestibular loss causes problems with posture, eye movement control, and nausea, because signals from the damaged side are not correctly balanced with signals from the intact side. A peripheral lesion that interferes with otolithic function on one side causes an imbalance because information from the otoliths on the normal side is not balanced by information from the otoliths on the lesioned side. Acute imbalance in otolithic information affects the vestibulospinal system, producing a tendency to fall toward the side of the lesion. After compensation by the central vestibular system, the direction of falling is variable.

Unilateral semicircular canal lesions are associated with nystagmus and an asymmetric VOR. The nystagmus beats away from the impaired side and is never vertical. After a few days, central compensation may completely suppress the nystagmus during visual fixation. Unlike resolution of nystagmus, the VOR remains asymmetric as long as the semicircular canals are impaired.[9]

A central lesion that damages the vestibular nuclei on one side causes unbalanced signals because the vestibular nuclei are operating normally on one side and the signals are decreased or lost from the vestibular nuclei on the damaged side. Unilateral central lesions produce a tendency to fall toward the side of the lesion and nystagmus beating away from the side of the lesion.

A unilateral lesion affecting the otoliths or the vestibular nuclei may produce a complete or partial ocular tilt reaction.[16] The ocular tilt reaction (OTR; Figure 16-15) is a triad of signs consisting of:
- Head tilt
- Ocular torsion
- Skew deviation of the eyes

Head tilt is lateral flexion of the head caused by a misperception of vertical. Due to unbalanced vestibular information, the person perceives true vertical as being tilted. For example, if asked to identify when a lighted rod is upright in a dark room, the person will report that the rod is upright when it is actually tilted. Ocular torsion is the rotation of the eyes around the axis of the pupil. Both eyes rotate downward toward the downward side of the head. Skew deviation of the eyes is the upward direction of one eye combined with downward deviation of the other eye.

### Bilateral Vestibular Loss

Bilateral loss of otolith input eliminates a person's internal sense of gravity. Therefore the person must rely on visual and proprioceptive cues for spatial orientation. This creates difficulty walking in the dark and walking on uneven surfaces. Because no asymmetry of vestibular information occurs, no vertigo is present.[17]

Bilateral loss of semicircular canal input causes failure of the VOR. When the person walks, the world appears to bounce up and down. When the person turns the head, vision is blurry and unstable. This lack of visual stabilization due to lack of the afferent limb of the VOR is oscillopsia. People with chronic vestibular dysfunction often have stiffness of the neck and shoulders. This stiffness may result from attempts to stabilize the head, to lessen vertigo or oscillopsia. Figure 16-16 sum-

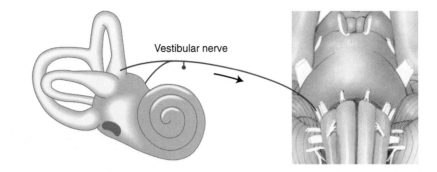

| Peripheral vestibular disorders | Central vestibular disorders (causes of central vertigo) |
|---|---|
| Acoustic neuroma | Arnold-Chiari malformation |
| Benign paroxysmal positional vertigo | Brainstem stroke or tumor affecting vestibular nuclei |
| Ototoxicity: usually bilateral, | Cerebellar tumor or stroke |
|     caused by certain antibiotics | Medication side effect |
| Perilymph fistula | Vestibular migraine |
| Ramsay-Hunt syndrome | Multiple sclerosis |
| Vertebrobasilar artery compression | Temporal lobe seizure |
| Vestibular neuritis | Transient ischemic attack |

**Fig. 16-16** Peripheral and central vestibular disorders.

marizes the more common causes of peripheral and central vestibular lesions.

## Disorders of the Visual System

Consequences of damage along the retinogeniculocortical pathway vary according to the location of the lesion (Figure 16-17). Clinically, visual losses are described by referring to the visual field deficit. Interruption of the optic nerve results in total loss of vision in the ipsilateral eye. *Bitemporal hemianopsia* is loss of information from both temporal visual fields, caused by damage to fibers in the center of the optic chiasm interrupting the axons from the nasal half of each retina. *Homonymous hemianopsia* is the loss of visual information from one hemifield. A complete lesion of the pathway anywhere posterior to the optic chiasm, in the optic tract, lateral geniculate, or optic radiations, results in loss of information from the contralateral visual field because all visual information posterior to the chiasm is from the contralateral visual field.

Following complete, bilateral loss of visual cortex function, some people retain the ability to orient their head position or point to objects, despite being cortically blind. *Cortically blind* means that the person has no awareness of any visual information. The ability of a cortically blind individual to orient or point to visual objects is called *blind sight*. Blind sight is possible because the ability to vaguely perceive light and dark is retained in the visual system. Blind sight is contingent on intact function of the retina and pathways from the retina to the superior colliculus.

## Disorders of the Eye Movement System

Abnormalities of eye movement occur with lesions involving:
• Cranial nerves that control extraocular muscles
• Strength of extraocular muscles

• Medial longitudinal fasciculus
• Vestibular system
• Cerebellum
• Eye fields in the cerebral cortex

Eye movement disorders that result from cranial nerve lesions were discussed in Chapter 14. In addition to the disorders listed in Chapter 14, problems with directing gaze may result from weakness of the extraocular muscles. For example, if the lateral rectus is weak, the position of the pupil in forward gaze will be directed medially. If the disorder is acute, double vision will occur because images of objects will not coincide on the retinas. If the disorder is chronic, the nervous system may suppress vision from the deviant eye, and double vision will be absent. However, with suppression of vision from one eye, the person will lose depth perception.

Difficulty aligning the eyes is called *tropia* or *phoria*. Tropia is a deviation of one eye from forward gaze when both eyes are open. Phoria is a deviation from forward gaze, apparent only when the person is looking forward with one eye (the other eye is covered). The person with a phoria is able to align both eyes accurately when binocular fusion is available. *Binocular fusion* is the blending of the image from each eye to become a single perception.

A variety of lesions cause abnormal eye movements. If the medial longitudinal fasciculus is affected, eye movements will not be coordinated with each other or with movements of the head. Damage to the vestibular system or to the cerebellum can cause pathologic nystagmus, abnormal oscillating eye movements that occur with or without external stimulation. Lesions of the vestibular system or cerebellum may also produce a deficient VOR, leading to inadequate gaze stabilization. Damage to a frontal eye field results in temporary ipsilateral gaze deviation, that is, the eyes look toward the damaged side. Recovery occurs because frontal eye field control of eye movement is controlled bilaterally. Damage to a parieto-occipital eye field

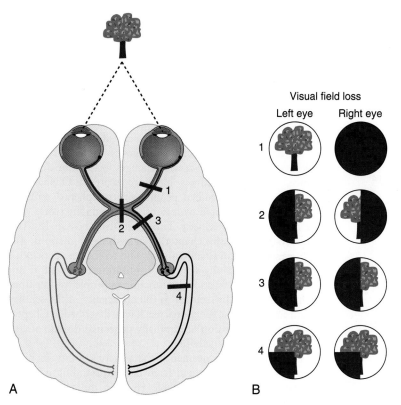

A

B

**Fig. 16-17 Results of lesions at various locations in the visual system. A,** Locations of the lesions. **B,** Visual field loss with each lesion. A lesion at location 1, the optic nerve, causes loss of vision from the right eye. A lesion at location 2, the middle of the optic chiasm, causes bitemporal hemianopsia, loss of the temporal visual field from both eyes. Any lesion that completely interrupts tracts posterior to the optic chiasm, including the lesion at location 3, the optic tract, causes loss of vision from the contralateral visual field of both eyes. An incomplete lesion of tracts posterior to the optic chiasm, as shown at location 4, causes partial loss of vision from the contralateral visual field.

Visual field loss

Left eye  Right eye

1

2

3

4

causes inadequate pursuit eye movements.[18] Although the lag of eye movements behind a moving target cannot be seen by an examiner, the disorder is visible because of the compensatory saccades that are required to catch up with a moving object.

## MOTION SICKNESS

Motion sickness—nausea, headache, anxiety, and vomiting sometimes experienced in moving vehicles—may be caused by a conflict between different types of sensory information[19] or by postural instability. For example, when one reads in a car moving at a constant speed, information in central vision and from the vestibular apparatus indicates that one is not moving, yet peripheral vision is reporting movement. Seasickness may be caused by a conflict between visual and vestibular information.[20] Optical simulation of normal body sway by vibration of ships, airplanes, or automobiles interacts with actual body sway in susceptible people to cause a perceptual mismatch between movement of the body and subconscious visual information from the vibration of moving vehicles.[21]

## EXAMINING THE VESTIBULAR SYSTEM

### Differentiation of Dizziness Complaints

Patients reporting dizziness are often describing quite different experiences. The clinician must distinguish among the following (Box 16-1):
- Vertigo (illusion of movement)
- Near syncope (feeling of impending faint)

**BOX 16-1  DIFFERENTIAL DIAGNOSIS OF DIZZINESS**

- Feeling faint for a few seconds usually indicates cardiopulmonary disorders.
- Feeling light-headed usually indicates psychological disorders but may be cardiovascular or hypoglycemic.
- Disequilibrium usually indicates neurologic disorders but may be a drug side effect.
- Vertigo typically indicates vestibular disorders.

- Disequilibrium (loss of balance)
- Light-headedness (inability to concentrate)

The differential diagnosis of these conditions is important because the cause and treatment of each are different. Vertigo indicates a vestibular origin, but the other symptoms typically do not indicate vestibular disorders. Near syncope is commonly caused by cardiovascular disorders. Disequilibrium results from somatosensory deficits, basal ganglia disorders, cerebellar dysfunction, drug use, complete loss of vestibular function, or tumor in the brainstem/cerebellar region. Light-headedness is associated with psychological disorders, including affective and anxiety disorders, but may be cardiovascular or hypoglycemic. Indications that the disorder is psychological include symptoms unaffected by head movements, lack of ataxia during a dizzy spell, and reproduction of symptoms with hyperventilation.

When taking a patient's history, often the most accurate information can be elicited by avoiding use of the terms *vertigo* and *dizziness*. Instead, encourage the patient to describe

**TABLE 16-5    FREQUENCY OF SPECIFIC CAUSES OF DIZZINESS**

| | Cause | Frequency, %* |
|---|---|---|
| Peripheral vestibular | Benign paroxysmal positional vertigo | 16 |
| | Inflammation of the inner ear (labyrinthitis) | 9 |
| | Ménière's disease | 5 |
| | Other (e.g., ototoxicity) | 14 |
| Central vestibular | Cerebrovascular | 6 |
| | Tumor | <1 |
| | Other (e.g., multiple sclerosis, migraine) | 3 |
| Psychological | Psychological disorder | 11 |
| | Hyperventilation | 5 |
| Nonvestibular, nonpsychological | Presyncope | 6 |
| | Disequilibrium | 5 |
| | Other (e.g., metabolic disorder, anemia) | 13 |
| Unknown | | 13 |

Data from Kroenke K, Hoffman RM, Einstadter D, et al: How common are various causes of dizziness? A critical review. *Southern Med J* 93:160–167, 2000; quiz 168.

*The percentages add up to more than 100% because dizziness was attributed to more than one cause in some patients.

precisely what he or she feels. If prompts are necessary, ask whether the patient feels faint, if the surroundings seem to be moving, if the patient feels unsteady, or if the patient is unable to concentrate. The frequencies of specific causes of dizziness are listed in Table 16-5.

If a patient has a vestibular disorder, the most important question to answer is whether the lesion is peripheral or central. Key questions that provide diagnostic information in vestibular disorders include inquiries regarding the provoking conditions and the frequency, duration, and severity of symptoms. Examination of the vestibular system includes self-reports in addition to tests:

- Postural control
- Transitional movements
- Gait
- Coordination
- Sensation (proprioception, vibration, hearing)
- Head position test for benign paroxysmal positional vertigo
- The vestibulo-ocular reflex

Self-report measures are intended to assess the impact of signs and symptoms on daily activities. A typical question is, "Do you feel confident walking in a busy store?"

### Testing Postural Control, Transitional Movements, and Gait

Postural tests can be used to assess vestibular system function (see "Postural Control" in Table 11-7). However, none of these tests can identify the cause of equilibrium problems. Postural tests may be static or dynamic. Static tests include Romberg's test and stationary posturography. These tests do not evaluate the ability of the subject to prepare for or adapt to challenges to equilibrium. Dynamic tests include tilt boards and dynamic posturography. As discussed in Chapter 11, these tests only assess reactions to externally imposed displacements. The clinical usefulness of stationary posturography (the sensory organization test, discussed in Chapter 11 and illustrated in Figure 11-23) is controversial, because changes on the sensory organization test do not correlate with changes in functional performance, nor with dizziness handicap scores.[22] O'Neill and colleagues (1998)[23] studied people with peripheral vestibular hypofunction and stable symptoms. Posturography scores were compared with gait velocity, Timed Get Up and Go Test (see Table 16-7 later in this chapter), gait with head rotations, gait with eyes closed, and tandem gait. The researchers concluded that the posturography sensory organization test alone is not useful for assessing balance and function in people with vestibular hypofunction. In contrast to the artificiality of the sensory organization test, the functional reach test (described in Chapter 11) assesses anticipation of internally generated displacements, as typically occur in daily life.

For transitional movements, the patient's ability to move from sitting to standing and from floor to standing is tested. For gait, tests are listed in Table 16-7. In the gait tests, the clinician assesses symptoms, loss of balance, and/or changes in gait.

### Lower Limb Coordination Tests and Ataxia

Tandem walking and the heel-to-shin test examine lower limb coordination. For the heel-to-shin test, the supine patient places the heel on the opposite knee, then slides the heel down to the ankle. To differentiate vestibular from cerebellar and from sensory ataxia, the following criteria are used:

- *Vestibular ataxia* is unique in being gravity dependent. Limb movements are normal when the person is lying down but are ataxic during walking. Stance is more stable with the eyes open than with the eyes closed. In supported sitting, rapid alternating movements (finger or toe tapping, pronation/supination) are normal. Vertigo and nystagmus are associated with vestibular ataxia.
- *Cerebellar ataxia* is evident regardless of whether the person is standing, sitting, or lying down. The ataxia may interfere with the ability to sit or stand without support. Typically, cerebellar ataxia produces inability to stand with feet together, regardless of whether the eyes are open or closed. Vertigo and nystagmus may be associated with cerebellar ataxia.
- *Sensory ataxia* is characterized by impaired vibratory and position sense, decreased or lost ankle reflexes, and lack of nystagmus and lack of vertigo.

### Sensation Testing

Sensation testing is used to localize a lesion. Hearing, proprioception, and vibration are tested. Tests for hearing were discussed in Chapter 14. Impaired hearing associated with vestibular signs and symptoms indicates that a lesion is likely to be located in the periphery. Because impaired proprioception can cause imbalance, proprioception and vibration tests (described in Chapter 7) are used to distinguish between lesions of the conscious proprioception pathways and vestibular lesions.

## Head Position Test for Benign Paroxysmal Positional Vertigo

The *Hallpike maneuver* is the most commonly used test for posterior and anterior canal BPPV. The maneuver rapidly inverts the posterior semicircular canal. In people with BPPV, this causes abnormal flow of the endolymph, provoking vertigo and nystagmus. The patient, with knees straight, is sitting on a plinth. The clinician places his or her hands on the sides of the patient's head, then asks the patient to keep looking at the clinician's nose the entire time. The clinician turns the patient's head 45 degrees from the sagittal plane. Then the patient is moved rapidly into a supine position with the head still turned 45 degrees from sagittal and the neck extended about 30 degrees (see Figure 16-14). Vertigo and nystagmus in response to the Hallpike maneuver indicate BPPV. According to El-Kashlan and Telian (2000),[24] the nystagmus evoked in BPPV is characterized by:

- Latency before onset; nystagmus begins several seconds after the movement is completed
- Intensifying, then fading
- Lasting 20 to 30 seconds, even if the patient remains in the provoking position
- Fatigability: with repetition of the provoking position, vertigo and nystagmus decrease and may disappear

To test for BPPV, the head must be held in the provoking position for at least 30 seconds. Because the posterior semicircular canal is in the most gravity-dependent position when a patient is upright or supine, BPPV most often affects the posterior canal. When the patient is placed in the provoking position, posterior canal BPPV will produce torsional nystagmus with a down-beating vertical component. If BPPV affects the left ear, the rotary nystagmus is clockwise; if the right ear is affected, the rotation is counterclockwise.

In less than 15% of BPPV cases, the anterior or horizontal semicircular canals are involved.[25] Anterior canal involvement produces a torsional nystagmus with an up-beating vertical component.[24] If the horizontal canal is involved, lateral head turn in the supine position produces a pure horizontal nystagmus.

## Testing Vestibulo-ocular Reflexes

The gain of the VOR depends on the frequency of the stimulus. Thus, testing with a frequency of 0.5 to 5.0 Hz is optimal, because the purpose of the VOR during natural situations is to stabilize gaze while a person is walking and turning the head. The VOR may be tested five ways: (1) by passive, rapid head thrusts, (2) by testing dynamic visual acuity, (3) by use of a rotating chair, (4) by caloric testing, and (5) by electronystagmography. The VOR can be tested by passively moving an individual's head and observing associated eye movements. The passive head turns should be rapid, unpredictable, and small amplitude (10 degrees to 20 degrees). A normal response is stable gaze. If the VOR is decreased or absent, a corrective saccade will be used after the head movement to compensate for loss of the visual target during the head movement. Passive head thrusts provide high-frequency and high-acceleration stimuli, similar to signals generated when a person is walking and turning the head.

Dynamic visual acuity tests the patient's ability to read an eye chart while the head is moving. The clinician passively rotates the patient's head at a frequency of 2 Hz, matching the cadence of a metronome to maintain accurate timing. Patients with an intact neural system will have less than one line loss of accuracy during head movements compared with their acuity when the head is stable. Patients with an abnormal VOR will have loss of acuity of two or more lines on the eye chart during head rotation.[26] The three other methods for testing the VOR are performed in vestibular specialty clinics. These tests include the rotating chair test, the caloric test, and electronystagmography.

The VOR can be tested with the individual seated in a rotating chair. With the head in neutral position, when the individual is rotated to the left, the eyes will move slowly to the right, as if to maintain fixation on an object in the visual field. When the eyes reach the extreme right, they shift quickly to the left, then resume moving to the right. When the head is rotated to the left, pursuit eye movements are toward the right, and saccades are toward the left.

If a person rotates quickly several revolutions to the left, then abruptly stops rotating, the direction of slow and fast eye movements reverses, that is, the eyes repeatedly move slowly to the left and then quickly to the right. This reversal of eye movement is due to the inertia of the fluid continuing to flow within the horizontal canals after the head stops moving. The fluid movement bends the cupulae in the opposite direction to their bend during acceleration, producing reversal of eye movements. Despite frequent use of the rotating chair test to evaluate the VOR, this test typically uses frequencies of movement that are too low and too predictable to accurately test the ability of the VOR to compensate for head turning while a person is walking.[27]

Another method of testing the VOR is the caloric test. Nontherapist specialists perform this test. A small amount of cold (30° C) or warm (44° C) water is instilled into the external ear canal. The temperature change induces a convective current in the endolymph of the adjacent horizontal semicircular canal. Nausea and vomiting may result from the vestibular action on autonomic function. In a conscious patient, the mnemonic COWS summarizes the saccadic (fast) movements of the eyes: cold opposite, warm same. This indicates that when cold water is instilled, the fast eye movements are toward the opposite side, and when warm water is used, the fast eye movements are toward the same side. Caloric stimulation is uniquely valuable in allowing unilateral assessment of the semicircular canal function (primarily the horizontal canal). However, caloric stimulation produces low frequency and low velocity signals in the vestibular nerve; thus the results of this test do not correlate well with VOR function during natural activities.[28]

Electronystagmography (ENG) is the recording of eye movements. Surface electrodes near the eyes detect changes in extraocular muscle electrical potentials during eye movements. ENG can be used to evaluate pursuit and saccadic eye movements and nystagmus elicited by changes in head position or by caloric tests. Figure 16-18 illustrates ENG, rotary chair with rotary drum, and caloric testing.

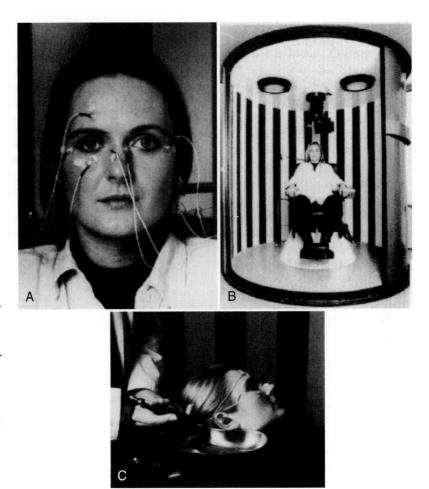

**Fig. 16-18** Electronystagmography (ENG), the recording of involuntary eye movements to evaluate patients with dizziness, vertigo, or balance problems. **A,** Placement of electrodes. **B,** Rotary chair with vertically striped rotary drum. Eye movements can be recorded while the chair is rotating or the surrounding drum is rotating, to distinguish between responses to head rotation or rotation of visual stimuli. **C,** Caloric irrigation with ENG. Cool or warm water is placed in the external auditory canal, inducing flow of fluid in the adjacent horizontal semicircular canal. This test isolates the function of one horizontal canal without stimulating the other horizontal canal. *(Used with permission from Brandt T, Strupp M: General vestibular testing.* Clin Neurophysiol *116:406–426, 2005.)*

## EXAMINING THE VISUAL AND EYE MOVEMENT SYSTEMS

Methods for testing the visual system and convergence were described in Table 14-7. The ability to direct gaze can be tested by three tests that involve observing eye movements when one eye is covered or uncovered: the cover test, the cover-uncover test, and the alternate cover test. The patient is seated and asked to look at a distant object in central vision. To test for tropia, the cover test is used. The clinician covers the patient's left eye. If the right eye remains directed at the target, the response is normal. If the right eye moves to look at the target, the right eye is tropic (Figure 16-19). To test for phoria, the cover-uncover test is used. The left eye is covered for approximately 10 seconds (to prevent fusion), and then uncovered. At the instant the left eye is uncovered, the left eye is observed for any movement. If the left eye does not move, the response is normal. If the left eye moves to look at the target, the left eye is phoric. Another test for phoria is the alternate cover test. In the alternate cover test, the cover is moved from one eye to the other several times. The cover remains over one eye for several seconds, then is quickly moved to cover the other eye. This technique prevents fusion. The eye that is uncovered is observed for

movement. If the uncovered eye remains steady, the response is normal. If the uncovered eye moves, the uncovered eye is phoric. The following tests examine eye movements.

Moving a vertically striped piece of cloth across the visual field tests the optokinetic reflex. This should produce pursuit eye movements in the direction of target movement, alternating with rapid eye movements to fixate the next target. The pursuit phase tests ipsilateral parieto-occipital pathways. Saccadic movements test the contralateral frontal lobe.

Asking the patient to move the eyes in response to verbal instructions from the examiner can test voluntary saccades. Damage to the frontal lobe interferes with this movement. To test pursuit eye movements, the patient is asked to keep the head still and follow the clinician's finger in the six directions shown in Figure 14-3, *C*. The eyes should move smoothly, and the movements should be well coordinated. Problems with pursuit movements indicate lesions in the parieto-occipital region. The effects of lesions on eye movements are summarized in Table 16-6. Tables 16-7 and 16-8 summarize tests used to examine the vestibular and visual systems. Tables 16-9 and 16-10 review how to distinguish among four categories of dizziness: feeling faint, feeling light-headed, disequilibrium, and vertigo, and the common causes of each of these symptoms.

Type of dizziness, timing of dizziness, and hearing status are critical factors in diagnosing dizziness.[29] Figures 16-20 through 16-23 provide flowcharts for differential diagnoses of dizziness complaints.

## REHABILITATION IN VESTIBULAR DISORDERS

Rehabilitation does not directly affect central dysfunctions of the vestibular system and is ineffective for active Ménière's disease. However, patients with certain central vestibular disorders may benefit from learning new ways of moving. Rehabilitation is effective for BPPV, unilateral vestibular loss or dysfunction and bilateral vestibular loss, and central vestibular disorders that benefit from movement retraining. Exercises are designed to promote movement retraining, habituation, or substitution to improve function. Movement retraining consists of practicing and modifying movements as appropriate. Habituation is exposure to positions or movements that produce symptoms, followed by relaxation until symptoms abate. Provocative stimuli are repeated frequently until the nervous system adapts to the stimuli. Habituation is effective for BPPV and unilateral vestibular loss. Substitution (also called *compensation*) consists of using alternative sensory inputs or motor responses or using predictive/anticipatory strategies. To compensate for bilateral vestibular loss, people learn to substitute visual and somatosensory cues and anticipation for absent or unreliable vestibular information. See Cohen (2006)[36] for a review of recent prospective studies of the effects of therapy on vertigo and balance disorders in patients with dizziness.

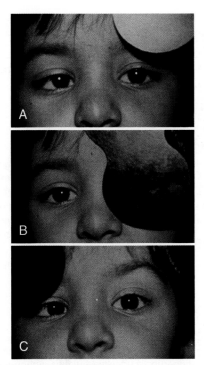

**Fig. 16-19  Cover testing.** With both eyes uncovered **(A)**, the left eye looks forward at the target and the right eye deviates toward the midline. For the cover test **(B)**, the examiner covers one eye and then the other eye. In this patient, the right tropia corrects temporarily when the left eye is covered. When the right eye is covered then uncovered, the tropia is present **(C)**. *(From Perkin GD: Mosby's color atlas and text of neurology, ed 2, London, 2002, Mosby.)*

**TABLE 16-6   EFFECTS OF LESIONS ON EYE MOVEMENTS**

| Location of Lesion | Effect on Resting Eye Position | Ability to Voluntarily Direct Eyes Past Midline | Double Vision |
|---|---|---|---|
| Vestibular nerve or vestibular nuclei | Contralateral nystagmus | Normal | No |
| Frontal eye fields | Both eyes deviated ipsilaterally | Unable to direct eyes past midline contralaterally | No |
| Pontine paramedian reticular formation | Both eyes deviated contralaterally | Unable to direct eyes past midline ipsilaterally | No |
| Abducens nucleus | Both eyes deviated contralaterally | Unable to direct eyes past midline ipsilaterally | No |
| Abducens nerve | Ipsilateral eye deviated medially | Normal | Yes |
| Medial longitudinal fasciculus | Ipsilateral eye deviated laterally | If the lesion is between the abducens and oculomotor nuclei, unable to adduct the ipsilateral eye past midline | Yes |

**TABLE 16-7　EXAMINATION OF THE BALANCE SYSTEM**

|  | Test | Procedure | Interpretation |
|---|---|---|---|
| Subjective reports | Rating scales | Patient rates vertigo, oscillopsia, and/or disequilibrium on a rating scale (0–10) or by marking a line (labeled "no vertigo" at left end and "most severe vertigo imaginable" at right end) to indicate severity of symptoms | Normal: rating of zero. Abnormal: ratings above zero |
|  | Dizziness Handicap Inventory[30] | 25-Item questionnaire; patient self-reports the impact of symptoms on everyday activities | Authors of the study report that a change of more than 17 points in the total score indicates a significant change in self-perceived disability. |
|  | Subjective visual vertical | In a completely dark room, patient moves a dimly illuminated bar to vertical | Normal: bar aligned within 2 degrees of true vertical. Aligning the bar more than 2 degrees from true vertical usually indicates a unilateral vestibular lesion.[31] |
|  | Activities–Specific Balance Confidence Scale[32] | 16 questions. Example: "How confident are you that you will not lose your balance or become unsteady when you walk in a crowded mall where people rapidly walk past you?" | Scored as a percentage, with 100% being completely confident |
| Past pointing test |  | Patient alternately touches the tip of the examiner's finger, then reaches overhead with extended arm. The examiner holds his or her finger directly in front of the patient at about arm's length. Patient makes four attempts with eyes open, then four attempts with eyes closed | Normal: patient is able to touch the examiner's fingertip accurately every time. Abnormal: when eyes are closed, patient's finger consistently drifts to one side of the examiner's finger. The side of drift is consistent with both hands. Indicates an acute unilateral vestibular lesion. If performance is equally inaccurate with both eyes open and eyes closed, indicates a cerebellar disorder. |
| Gait | Stops Walking When Talking Test[33] | Walk with the patient and ask a question | If the patient stops walking to answer the question, walking requires more conscious attention than normal, and the patient is at risk for falls. |
|  | Dynamic gait test[34] | 8 tasks. Tests gait at different speeds, with horizontal and vertical head turns, pivot turns, obstacles, and stairs | Test provides specific commands for the patient and scoring criteria. Four of the tasks are listed below. |
|  | With eyes open and eyes closed | Subject walks with eyes open or closed | Normal: little difference in gait whether eyes are open or closed. Abnormal: if gait is worse with eyes closed than with eyes open, this indicates that vision is substituting for impaired somatosensory information. If gait is ataxic, regardless of whether vision is available or not, a brainstem or cerebellar lesion is likely. |
|  | While turning the head right and left on command, or while moving the head up and down | Subject responds to commands while continuing to walk | Tests the ability of the vestibulomotor system to compensate for head movements (vestibulospinal tracts and vestibulo-ocular reflexes [VORs]). A person with a normal vestibular system can perform this task easily. A person with a vestibular lesion will tend to lose balance (due to abnormal input to vestibulospinal tracts) and have difficulty with visual orientation (inadequate VOR). |
|  | Stopping quickly on command, making a quick pivot turn on command, or navigating an obstacle course | Subject responds to commands or avoids obstacles while continuing to walk | Tests the ability to anticipate changes in postural control |
|  | While carrying an object | Subject walks while carrying books or a cup filled with water. | Tests the ability to make adjustments for changes in center of gravity and/or for increased cognitive demands |

**TABLE 16-7** EXAMINATION OF THE BALANCE SYSTEM—cont'd

| | Test | Procedure | Interpretation |
|---|---|---|---|
| Evaluation of balance system | Mini-Balance Evaluation Systems Test (Mini-BESTest[35]) | 14 test items; includes: sit-to-stand, rise to toes, stand on one leg, stepping forward and backward, lateral stepping, standing on firm surface, standing on foam with eyes closed, standing on incline with eyes closed, walking with changes in speed, head turns, pivot turns, and over obstacles | Test provides specific commands for the patient and scoring criteria. |
| Timed functional test | Get Up and Go Test | Quick screening of gait speed and control in turning; patient rises from a chair, walks 3 meters, turns around, walks back to the chair, and sits down. The timed Get Up and Go test includes timing the test. | Normal: requires less than 30 seconds. Abnormal: adults who require longer than 30 seconds to complete the test are likely to be dependent in mobility and in activities of daily living. |
| Positional testing | Hallpike maneuver | Patient long sitting (knees extended) on plinth. Examiner asks patient to keep looking at the examiner's nose. Examiner turns patient's head 45 degrees left or right, then quickly moves patient into a supine position with the head still turned 45 degrees and the neck extended 30 degrees. | Tests for benign paroxysmal positional vertigo (BPPV). Normal: no nystagmus or vertigo in the end position. BPPV: after a few seconds, nystagmus and vertigo begin and last 20–30 seconds. |

**TABLE 16-8** EXAMINATION OF THE EYE ALIGNMENT AND EYE MOVEMENT SYSTEM

| | | Procedure | Interpretation |
|---|---|---|---|
| Eye alignment | | Examiner observes the position of the patient's eyes while the patient looks straight ahead at a distant object. | Some eye misalignments are severe and can be observed simply by looking at the patient's eyes while the patient looks at a distant object. |
| | Cover test | To test eye alignment using the cover test, cover one of the patient's eyes and observe the other eye for movement. | Normal: eye that is not covered does not move. Abnormal: eye that is not covered moves. This indicates a tropia. Tropia may be congenital or acquired. Tropia results from paresis of one or more of the extraocular muscles of one eye or a lesion of cranial nerve III, IV, or VI. Acute tropia causes double vision. |
| | Cover-uncover test | Cover one of the patient's eyes for about 10 seconds. Watch the covered eye for movement as it is quickly uncovered. | Normal: no movement. Abnormal: eye that is covered then uncovered moves. This is a phoria. |
| | Alternate cover test | The cover is moved from one eye to the other several times. The cover remains over one eye for several seconds, then is quickly moved to cover the other eye. | Movement of an eye when it is uncovered indicates a phoria. |
| | Spontaneous nystagmus | Patient is looking at a distant object straight ahead. | Normal: no movement of the eyes. Abnormal: involuntary back-and-forth movements of the eyes; indicates a lesion of the vestibular, smooth pursuit, or optokinetic system, or the cerebellum |

*Continued*

**TABLE 16-8    EXAMINATION OF THE EYE ALIGNMENT AND EYE MOVEMENT SYSTEM—cont'd**

| | | | |
|---|---|---|---|
| Eye movement | | *Note:* test visual fields before testing eye movements (see Table 14-7). | |
| | Voluntary saccades | Ask the patient to look in the directions indicated in Figure 14-3, *C.* | Normal: smooth, conjugate, full-range movements. Assuming normal strength of extraocular muscles, abnormal responses include: 1. Both eyes deviated ipsilaterally; patient unable to direct eyes past midline contralaterally. Indicates acute or subacute lesion of the frontal eye field. Deficit is temporary because the contralateral frontal eye field can compensate. 2. Both eyes deviated contralaterally; patient unable to direct eyes past midline ipsilaterally. Lesion of the pontine paramedian reticular formation 3. One eye unable to adduct past midline; other eye moves normally. Indicates a lesion of the medial longitudinal fasciculus between abducens and oculomotor nucleus (internuclear ophthalmoplegia; see Chapter 14) |
| | Pursuits | Ask the patient to keep the head still and follow the movement of your finger. Move your finger slowly in the directions indicated in Figure 13-3, *C.* | Normal: smooth, conjugate eye movements. Abnormal: nystagmus and/or double vision. Assuming normal-strength extraocular muscles and intact oculomotor neurons, abnormal results indicate a lesion in the parieto-occipital cortex, cerebellum, or brainstem. |
| | Convergence | Convergence is adduction of the eyes. Ask the patient to look at the tip of a pen as it is slowly moved from about 2 feet away toward the patient's nose. | Normal: both eyes are directed toward the pen tip until the pen is within 10 cm (4 inches) of the nose. Abnormal: only one eye moves toward the midline. The other eye moves outward. Indicates defective perception or central nervous system control of visual fusion, or dysfunction of oculomotor neurons or ocular muscles |
| | Physiologic nystagmus | Patient looks at a striped moving target (optokinetic nystagmus), undergoes caloric testing, or moves the eyes to an extreme position. | Normal: Back-and-forth eye movements in response to any of these stimuli |
| | Pathologic nystagmus | Observe eyes when: 1. Patient is looking straight forward with eyes closed. Eyes are closed to eliminate visual fixation. 2. Patient looks in the directions indicated in Figure 13-3, *C.* | 1. Symmetric nystagmus usually is congenital. Jerk nystagmus—fast in one direction, slow in the opposite direction—usually indicates a unilateral vestibular lesion. 2. If nystagmus occurs only in a single direction, this indicates weakness of an extraocular muscle or a lesion affecting an oculomotor neuron. If nystagmus occurs in several directions, this usually indicates a drug effect, but it may indicate a cerebellar or central vestibular disorder. Central nystagmus does not suppress with fixation and may change direction with gaze. Peripheral vestibular nystagmus is inhibited by fixation and increases in amplitude when gaze is directed toward the direction of nystagmus. |
| | | 3. Test for position-evoked nystagmus by using the Hallpike maneuver (see Figure 16-14). | 3. Nystagmus and vertigo occur following a latency of a few seconds and last 20–30 seconds. |
| | Optokinetic eye movements | Ask the patient to look at a vertically striped cloth, then move the cloth horizontally | Normal: the eyes follow a stripe, then make a quick saccade to the next stripe. Abnormal: problems with slow phase indicate abnormal pursuit mechanisms; problems with fast phase indicate problems with generating saccades. |
| | Dynamic visual acuity | Patient reads Snellen chart while turning head left and right at a 2 Hz frequency | Normal: maximum of one line decrease in visual acuity. Bilateral vestibular deficit: decrease in visual acuity of two or more lines |
| | VOR to rapid head thrusts | Ask patient to look at examiner's nose. Examiner rotates patient's head passively, rapidly, about 10 degrees to the left and to the right | Normal: eyes remain fixed on examiner's nose. Abnormal: eyes move away from examiner's nose, and a corrective saccade must be used to regain the target. Abnormal response to rapid head thrusts indicates a vestibular disorder. |

*VOR,* Vestibulo-ocular reflex.

**TABLE 16-9** TESTS FOR DIFFERENTIAL DIAGNOSIS OF DIZZINESS COMPLAINTS

| | Tests | Interpretation |
|---|---|---|
| Screening | Hearing test | If hearing is impaired on same side as a vestibular lesion, usually indicates that vestibular lesion is peripheral |
| | Cranial nerves V and VII | Checks for involvement of brainstem or area adjacent to junction of cerebellum and pons |
| | Hyperventilation | If symptoms are reproduced, indicates a psychological component to dizziness |
| | Compare blood pressure supine vs. blood pressure after supine to stand | Orthostatic hypotension is a drop in blood pressure >20/10 mm Hg for 3 minutes following move from supine to standing. |
| | Check for carotid, subclavian bruits | Presence of bruits indicates arterial disease. |
| | Proprioception and vibration sense | Impairment of these senses can produce ataxia and disequilibrium. |
| Laboratory (see text for descriptions of laboratory tests) | Caloric irrigation<br>Rotary chair<br>Electronystagmography (ENG)<br>Dynamic posturography—sensory organization test | Tests function of a single horizontal semicircular canal<br>Quantifies eye movements in response to rotation; abnormal responses indicate vestibular, brainstem, or cerebellar lesions<br>Quantifies nystagmus, pursuits, saccades, optokinetic nystagmus<br>Tests ability to maintain balance when visual and somatosensory information is altered; provides no information about site of lesion; clinical usefulness is controversial (see text) |

**TABLE 16-10** DIZZINESS EVALUATION

| Patient's Report | Specific Sign(s) | Likely Diagnosis |
|---|---|---|
| Feeling faint for a few seconds | Blurred vision or loss of consciousness when moving from supine to standing | Postural hypotension |
| | Dizziness, blurred vision, slurred speech, nystagmus, or loss of consciousness during vertebral artery test (patient supine; examiner slowly extends, rotates, and laterally flexes the patient's cervical spine to each side) | Vertebral artery compression |
| Feeling light-headed | Lasts longer than a few minutes | Low blood sugar |
| | Lasts only a few minutes and is associated with perioral and distal extremity tingling, tunnel vision, chest pain/tightness, and/or anxiety | Psychological, or medication side effect |
| | Provoked by anxiety, affective disorders, or pain | Vasovagal syncope or presyncope |
| | Provoked ONLY by coming to sitting or standing | Postural hypotension |
| | Associated with irregular heart rate, paresis, blurred vision, and/or confusion | Cardiopulmonary disease |
| Disequilibrium (perception of losing balance without vertigo or feeling faint) | Impaired somatosensation; patient feels more unsteady in the dark than when adequate lighting is available | Peripheral neuropathy, vitamin B deficiency, or multiple sclerosis |
| | Ataxia | Vascular disorder, tumor, alcohol abuse, or anticonvulsant drugs |
| | Impaired vestibulo-ocular reflexes (VORs) and oscillopsia. Cannot drive, cannot read signs when walking | Vestibular neuritis or damaged labyrinths; aminoglycosides (streptomycin, gentamicin, etc.) can damage vestibular receptors |
| | Positive VOR to rapid head thrusts (corrective saccade occurs) | Peripheral vestibular loss |
| | Negative VOR to rapid head thrusts, perceptual tilt, skew deviation, lateral head/body tilt | If signs are severe, central vestibular loss; if signs are mild, acute vestibular loss |
| | Abnormal cranial nerve tests, especially II–VIII | Brainstem vascular disorder or tumor or basilar migraine |
| | Musculoskeletal impairment | Deconditioning, poor postural alignment, multiple sclerosis |
| | Provoked by transportation | Motion sensitivity |

*Continued*

**TABLE 16-10**    DIZZINESS EVALUATION—cont'd

| Patient's Report | Specific Sign(s) | Likely Diagnosis |
| --- | --- | --- |
| Vertigo (false perception of movement; often associated with pallor, sweating, nausea, vomiting) | Episode lasts less than 1 minute; positive vertebral compression test in sitting | Arterial compression or cervical facet pathology |
| | Lasts less than 1 minute; nystagmus with head positional tests | Benign paroxysmal positional vertigo (BPPV) or central vestibular disorder |
| | Episode lasts longer than 1 minute; continuous symptoms, including persistent disequilibrium, during an episode; symptoms are worst during first 1–2 hours of an episode | Ménière's or migraine |
| | Longer than 12 hours of intermittent episodes provoked by head movement | Unilateral vestibular loss (e.g., neuronitis) |
| | Continuous vertigo with nystagmus, decreased hearing, and tinnitus | Acoustic neuroma |
| | Continuous vertigo without nystagmus | Systemic disease or drug effect |
| | Provoked by transportation | Motion sensitivity |

Developed from Sloane PD, Coeytaux RR, Beck RS, Dallara J: Dizziness: state of the science. *Ann Intern Med* 134:823–832, 2001; Hanley K, O'Dowd T: Symptoms of vertigo in general practice: a prospective study of diagnosis. *Br J Gen Pract* 52:809–812, 2002; and Chawla N, Olshaker JS: Diagnosis and management of dizziness and vertigo. *Med Clin North Am* 90:291–304, 2006.

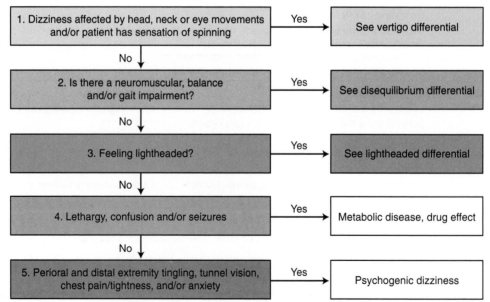

**Fig. 16-20 Dizziness.** The differential begins at top left. The first item to assess is whether symptoms are affected by head, neck, or eye movements, or whether the patient has a sensation of spinning. A "yes" response, to the right in the flowchart, directs the examiner to the vertigo differential. If the response to the first item is "no," proceed down to the second item. For each item, a "yes" response leads to the right, and a "no" response directs the examiner down the chart to the next item. Colored shapes indicate questions or tests; white rectangles indicate diagnoses.

**Vertigo differential**

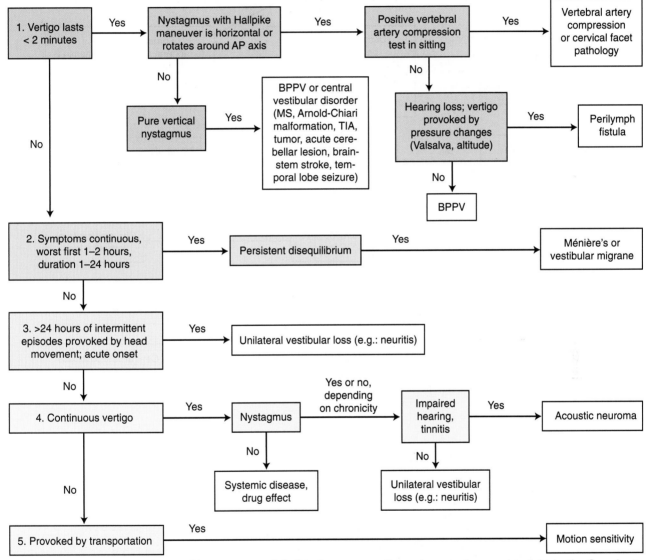

**Fig. 16-21 Vertigo.** The differential begins at top left. "Yes" responses direct the examiner to the right in the flowchart; "no" responses direct the examiner down to the next item. Colored rectangles indicate questions or tests; white rectangles indicate diagnoses.

**Disequilibrium differential**

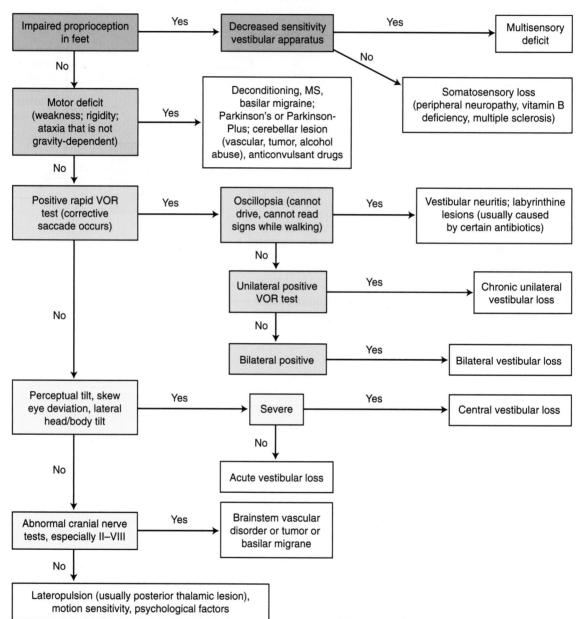

**Fig. 16-22  Disequilibrium.** The differential begins at top left. "Yes" responses direct the examiner to the right in the flowchart; "no" responses direct the examiner down to the next item. Colored rectangles indicate questions or tests; white rectangles indicate diagnoses.

**Feeling lightheaded differential**

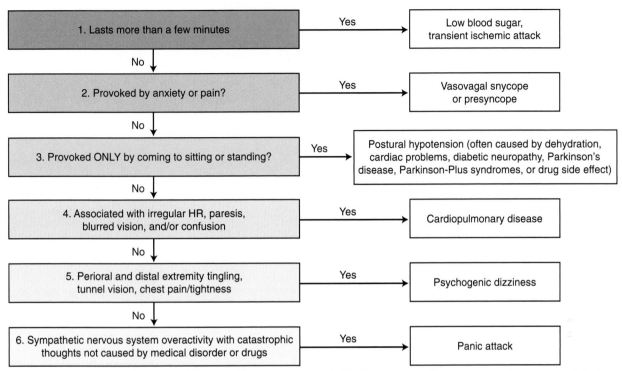

Fig. 16-23 **Light-headedness.** The differential begins at top left. "Yes" responses direct the examiner to the right in the flowchart; "no" responses direct the examiner down to the next item. Colored rectangles indicate questions or tests; white rectangles indicate diagnoses.

## SUMMARY

The vestibular labyrinth in the inner ear is the peripheral receptor for the vestibular system. Vestibular signals are essential for postural control and for coordination of movements, including eye movements. Vestibular signals contribute to awareness of head orientation and to actively orienting the head and body relative to gravity and to movement.

Visual information from a visual hemifield is processed in the contralateral visual cortex. From the primary visual cortex, information flows dorsally in the action stream and ventrally in the perception stream. Gaze stabilization is achieved by the vestibulo-ocular and optokinetic reflexes. Direction of gaze is accomplished by saccades, smooth pursuits, and vergence eye movements.

For appropriate diagnosis and intervention, clinicians must distinguish between peripheral and central vestibular disorders, and must recognize a variety of disorders affecting the visual system and the eye movement system.

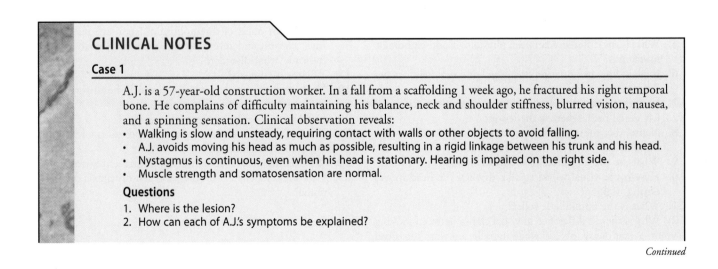

## CLINICAL NOTES

### Case 1

A.J. is a 57-year-old construction worker. In a fall from a scaffolding 1 week ago, he fractured his right temporal bone. He complains of difficulty maintaining his balance, neck and shoulder stiffness, blurred vision, nausea, and a spinning sensation. Clinical observation reveals:
- Walking is slow and unsteady, requiring contact with walls or other objects to avoid falling.
- A.J. avoids moving his head as much as possible, resulting in a rigid linkage between his trunk and his head.
- Nystagmus is continuous, even when his head is stationary. Hearing is impaired on the right side.
- Muscle strength and somatosensation are normal.

### Questions
1. Where is the lesion?
2. How can each of A.J.'s symptoms be explained?

*Continued*

## CLINICAL NOTES—cont'd

### Case 2

B.F., a 37-year-old woman, presents with the following signs and symptoms on the right:
- Loss of sensation from the face
- Loss of voluntary movement of the face
- Ataxia of the limbs
- Inability to move the right eye toward the right
- Deafness

In addition, pain and temperature sensations are impaired from the left side of the body, and she has vertigo, nystagmus, and vomiting. The onset of symptoms has been gradual over the last 6 months, but unremitting.

#### Questions

1. Where is the lesion?
2. What is the most likely etiology?

### Case 3

K.W. is a 27-year-old man who abruptly sustained the following losses 2 days ago:
- The ability to localize pain, temperature, touch, and proprioceptive information from the right side of his body
- Voluntary motor control of the right side of his body
- The ability to see objects in his right visual field

#### Questions

1. What are possible locations of lesions that would explain the visual loss?
2. Given the combination of visual, motor, and somatosensory loss, where is the most likely location of the lesion?

## REVIEW QUESTIONS

1. Describe how rotational acceleration of the head stimulates the endings of the vestibular nerve. Describe the mechanism for converting head position relative to gravity into neural signals.
2. What does "each pair of semicircular canals produces reciprocal signals" mean?
3. Name the tracts that use information from the vestibular nuclei to control posture.
4. What tract conveys signals that coordinate eye and head movements?
5. What is the difference between physiologic and pathologic nystagmus?
6. Explain how information from the left visual field reaches the right visual cortex.
7. If a person can see but cannot recognize an object in the left visual field, where is the lesion?
8. Name the sources of information used to direct eye movements.
9. What are the objectives of eye movements?
10. How is the visual world stabilized when the head moves during walking?
11. What is the optokinetic reflex?
12. Why is there a difference in visual clarity between looking at a stationary object while rapidly moving the head and looking at a rapidly moving object with the head stationary?
13. Normally, what happens to the perception of visual details when the head is quickly turned?
14. What symptom is most common in peripheral vestibular disorders?
15. If a person has hearing loss, tinnitus, vertigo, and nystagmus, where is the lesion?
16. What is BPPV?
17. The abrupt onset of disequilibrium, spontaneous nystagmus, nausea, and severe vertigo, persisting up to 3 days, indicates what disorder?
18. What is oscillopsia?
19. How can peripheral vestibular disorders be distinguished from central vestibular disorders?
20. Describe the ocular tilt reaction.
21. What is the location of a lesion that produces a left homonymous hemianopsia?
22. What is the difference between a phoria and a tropia?
23. How are cerebellar, vestibular, and sensory ataxia differentiated?

# References

1. Della Santina CC, Carey JP: Principles of applied vestibular physiology. In Paul W, Flint PW, Haughey BH, et al, editors: *Cummings otolaryngology: head & neck surgery*, ed 5, St Louis, 2010, Mosby.

2. Bense S, Stephan T, Bartenstein P, et al: Fixation suppression of optokinetic nystagmus modulates cortical visual-vestibular interaction. *Neuroreport* 16:887–890, 2005.

3. Prokopakis EP, Chimona T, Tsagournisakis M, et al: Benign paroxysmal positional vertigo: 10-year experience in treating 592 patients with canalith repositioning procedure. *Laryngoscope* 115:1667–1671, 2005.

4. Roberts JC, Cohen HS, Sangi-Haghpeykar H: Vestibular disorders and dual task performance: impairment when walking a straight path. *J Vestib Res* 21:167–174, 2011.

5. Lee SH, Kim JS: Benign paroxysmal positional vertigo. *J Clin Neurol* 6:51–63, 2010.

6. Oghalai JS, Manolidis S, Barth JL, et al: Unrecognized benign paroxysmal positional vertigo in elderly patients. *Otolaryngol Head Neck Surg* 122:630–634, 2000.

7. Hillier SL, McDonnell M: Vestibular rehabilitation for unilateral peripheral vestibular dysfunction. *Cochrane Database Syst Rev* (2):CD005397, 2011.

8. Alexander TH, Harris JP: Current epidemiology of Ménière's syndrome. *Otolaryngol Clin North Am* 43:965–970, 2010.

9. Magaziner JL, Walker MF: Dizziness, vertigo, motion sickness, syncope and near syncope, and disequilibrium. In Fiebach NH, Kern DE, Thomas PA, et al, editors: *Principles of ambulatory medicine*, ed 7, Philadelphia, 2007, Lippincott Williams & Wilkins.

10. Nieuwenhuys R, Voogd J, van Huijzen C: *The vestibular system. In The human central nervous system*, ed 4, Berlin, 2008, Springer, p 729.

11. Pérennou DA, Mazibrada G, Chauvineau V, et al: Lateropulsion, pushing and verticality perception in hemisphere stroke: a causal relationship? *Brain* 131:2401–2413, 2008.

12. Cnyrim CD, Rettinger N, Mansmann U, et al: Central compensation of deviated subjective visual vertical in Wallenberg's syndrome. *J Neurol Neurosurg Psychiatry* 78:527–528, 2007.

13. Casani AP, Sellari-Franceschini S, Napolitano A, et al: Otoneurologic dysfunctions in migraine patients with or without vertigo. *Otol Neurotol* 30:961–967, 2009.

14. Karatas M: Vascular vertigo: epidemiology and clinical syndromes. *Neurologist* 17:1–10, 2011.

15. Cha YH: Migraine-associated vertigo: diagnosis and treatment. *Semin Neurol* 30:167–174, 2010.

16. Leigh RJ, Rucker JC: Eye movements. In Tasman W, Jaeger EA, editors: *Duane's ophthalmology*, Philadelphia, 2011, Lippincott Williams & Wilkins.

17. Shepard NT, Solomon D: Functional operation of the balance system in daily activities. *Otolaryngol Clin North Am* 33:455–469, 2000.

18. Wong AMF: Ocular motor disorders caused by lesions in the cerebrum. In *Eye movement disorders*, New York, 2007, Oxford University Press, p 190.

19. Bonato F, Bubka A, Ishak S, et al: The sickening rug: a repeating static pattern that leads to motion-sickness-like symptoms. *Perception* 40:493–496, 2011.

20. Bos JE, MacKinnon SN, Patterson A: Motion sickness symptoms in a ship motion simulator: effects of inside, outside, and no view. *Aviat Space Environ Med* 76:1111–1118, 2005.

21. Dong X, Yoshida K, Stoffregen TA: Control of a virtual vehicle influences postural activity and motion sickness. *J Exp Psychol Appl* 17:128–138, 2011.

22. Badke MB, Miedaner JA, Shea TA, et al: Effects of vestibular and balance rehabilitation on sensory organization and dizziness handicap. *Ann Otol Rhinol Laryngol* 114:48–54, 2005.

23. O'Neill DE, Gill-Body KM, Krebs DE: Posturography changes do not predict functional performance changes. *Am J Otol* 19:797–803, 1998.

24. El-Kashlan HK, Telian SA: Diagnosis and initiating treatment for peripheral system disorders: imbalance and dizziness with normal hearing. *Otolaryngol Clin North Am* 33:563–578, 2000.

25. Cakir BO, Ercan I, Cakir ZA, et al: What is the true incidence of horizontal semicircular canal benign paroxysmal positional vertigo? *Otolaryngol Head Neck Surg* 134:451–454, 2006.

26. Walker MF, Zee DS: Bedside vestibular examination. *Otolaryngol Clin North Am* 33:495–506, 2000.

27. Chiu CM, Huang SF, Tsai PY, et al: Computer-aided vestibular autorotational testing of the vestibulo-ocular reflex in senile vestibular dysfunction. *Comput Methods Programs Biomed* 97:92–98, 2010.

28. Park HJ, Shin JE, Lim YC, et al: Clinical significance of vibration-induced nystagmus. *Audiol Neurootol* 13:182–186, 2008.

29. Kentala E, Rauch SD: A practical assessment algorithm for diagnosis of dizziness. *Otolaryngol Head Neck Surg* 128:54–59, 2003.

30. Jacobson GP, Newman CW: The development of the Dizziness Handicap Inventory. *Arch Otolaryngol Head Neck Surg* 116:424–427, 1994.

31. Tusa RJ: The dizzy patient: disturbances of the vestibular system. In Tasman W, Jaeger EA, editors: *Duane's ophthalmology*, Philadelphia, 2011, Lippincott Williams & Wilkins.

32. Powell LE, Meyers AM: The Activities-Specific Balance Confidence (ABC) scale. *J Gerontol A Biol Sci Med Sci* 50A:M28-34, 1995.

33. Andersson AG, Kamwendo K, Seiger A, Appelros P: How to identify potential fallers in a stroke unit: validity indexes of 4 test methods. *J Rehabil Med* 38:186–191, 2006.

34. Shumway-Cook A, Baldwin M, Polissar NL, Gruber W: Predicting the probability for falls in community-dwelling older adults. *Phys Ther* 77:812–819, 1997.

35. Franchignoni F, Horak F, Godi M, et al: Using psychometric techniques to improve the Balance Evaluation Systems Test: the mini-BESTest. *J Rehabil Med* 42:323–331, 2010.

36. Cohen HS: Disability and rehabilitation in the dizzy patient. *Curr Opin Neurol* 19:49–54, 2006.

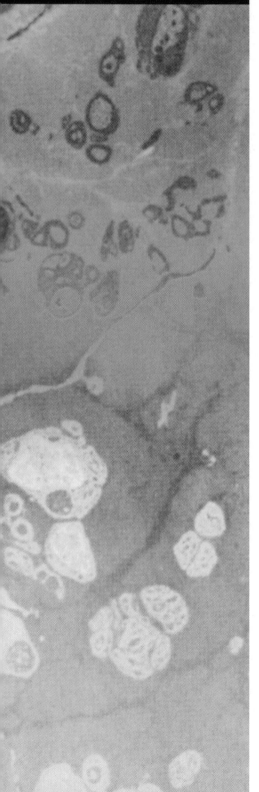

# 17

# Cerebrum

Laurie Lundy-Ekman, PhD, PT

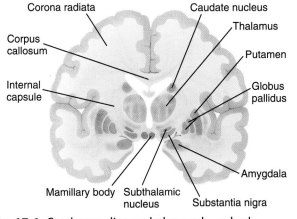

**Fig. 17-1** Cerebrum: diencephalon and cerebral hemispheres. Coronal section.

Labels in figure: Corona radiata, Corpus callosum, Internal capsule, Mamillary body, Subthalamic nucleus, Caudate nucleus, Thalamus, Putamen, Globus pallidus, Amygdala, Substantia nigra

Perception, moving voluntarily, using language and nonverbal communication, understanding spatial relationships, using visual information, making decisions, consciousness, emotions, mind-body interactions, and remembering all rely on systems in the cerebrum. These complex activities require extensive networks of neural connections, some involving brainstem circuits.

The cerebrum consists of the diencephalon and the cerebral hemispheres. The diencephalon is in the center of the cerebrum, superior to the brainstem, and is almost entirely enveloped by the cerebral hemispheres (Figure 17-1). In the intact adult brain, only a small part of the diencephalon is visible: the region between the optic chiasm and the cerebral peduncles, marked by the mammillary bodies. The cerebral hemispheres include both subcortical structures and the cerebral cortex. The subcortical structures include subcortical white matter, basal ganglia, and amygdala. The cerebral cortex is the gray matter on the external surface of the hemispheres. The collection of diencephalic, subcortical, and cortical structures involved with emotional and some memory functions is the limbic system.

## DIENCEPHALON

The diencephalon includes all structures with the term *thalamus* in their names. The thalamus proper, the largest subdivision of the diencephalon, receives information from the basal ganglia, the cerebellum, and all sensory systems except olfactory. The thalamus processes the information and then relays the information to specific areas of the cerebral cortex. Other areas in the diencephalon are named for their locations relative to the thalamus, not for similarities of function. Thus the hypothalamus is inferior and anterior to the thalamus, the epithalamus is superior and posterior to the thalamus, and the subthalamus is directly inferior to the thalamus.

### Thalamus

The thalamus is a large, egg-shaped collection of nuclei located bilaterally above the brainstem. A Y-shaped sheet of white matter (intramedullary lamina) divides the nuclei of each thalamus into three groups: anterior, medial, and lateral. The lateral group is further subdivided into dorsal and ventral tiers. All nuclei in these groups are named for their location. For example, the ventral anterior nucleus is the most anterior nucleus of the ventral tier.

Additional thalamic nuclei—intralaminar, reticular, and midline—are not included in the three major groups. Intralaminar nuclei are found within the white matter of the thalamus. The reticular and midline nuclei form thin layers of cells on the lateral and medial surfaces of the thalamus (Figure 17-2).

The thalamus acts as a selective filter for the cerebral cortex, directing attention to important information by regulating the flow of information to the cortex. Thus, overall, the thalamus regulates the activity level of cortical neurons. Individual thalamic nuclei can be classified into three main functional groups:
- Relay nuclei convey information from the sensory systems (except olfactory), the basal ganglia, or the cerebellum to the cerebral cortex.
- Association nuclei process emotional and some memory information or integrate different types of sensations.
- Nonspecific nuclei regulate consciousness, arousal, and attention.

Relay nuclei receive specific information and serve as relay stations by sending the information directly to localized areas of the cerebral cortex. For example, the ventral posteromedial nucleus receives somatosensory information from the face and relays the information to the somatosensory cortex. All relay nuclei are found in the ventral tier of the lateral nuclear group.

Association nuclei connect reciprocally to large areas of the cortex, that is, axons from association nuclei project to the cerebral cortex, and axons from the same cerebral cortical regions project to the association nuclei. Examples include the anterior nucleus, with reciprocal connections to areas of the cortex involved in emotions, and the pulvinar nucleus, reciprocally connected with parietal, temporal, and occipital cortices. Association nuclei are found in the anterior thalamus, medial thalamus, and dorsal tier of the lateral thalamus.

Nonspecific nuclei receive multiple types of inputs and project to widespread areas of the cortex. This functional group includes the reticular, midline, and intralaminar nuclei, important in consciousness and arousal. Table 17-1 lists the functions and connections of the thalamic nuclei.

### Hypothalamus

The hypothalamus is essential for individual and species survival because the hypothalamus integrates behaviors with visceral functions. For example, small areas in the hypothalamus coordinate eating behavior with digestive activity. Electrical stimulation of these hypothalamic areas causes an animal to search for and ingest food as long as the stimulation is applied. At the same time, peristalsis and blood flow increase throughout the intestine. Bilateral destruction of the areas associated with eating behaviors results in refusal of food, causing starvation even when food is readily available. The following functions are orchestrated by the hypothalamus:
- Maintaining homeostasis: adjustment of body temperature, metabolic rate, blood pressure, water intake and excretion, and digestion
- Eating, reproductive, and defensive behaviors
- Emotional expression of pleasure, rage, fear, and aversion

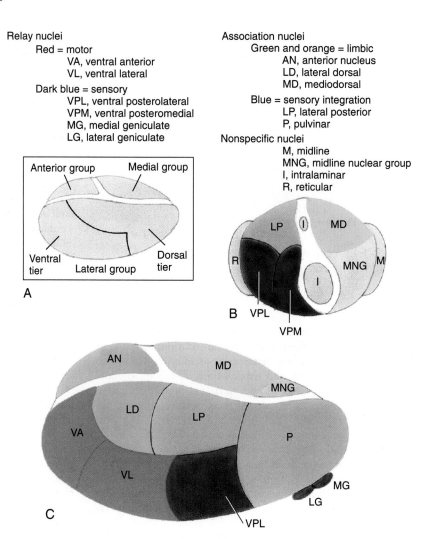

**Fig. 17-2 Thalamus. A,** Three major groups of nuclei. **B,** Coronal section through the thalamus. **C,** Nuclei of the thalamus.

| TABLE 17-1 | THALAMIC NUCLEI | | | | |
|---|---|---|---|---|---|
| **Functional Classification** | **Nuclei** | **Function** | **Afferents** | | **Efferents** |
| Relay nuclei | Ventral anterior | Motor | Globus pallidus | | Motor planning areas |
| | Ventral lateral | Motor | Dentate | | Motor cortex, motor planning areas |
| | Ventral posterolateral | Somatic sensation from body | Spinothalamic and medial lemniscus paths | | Somatosensory cortex |
| | Ventral posteromedial | Somatic sensation from face | Sensory nucleus trigeminal nerve | | Somatosensory cortex |
| | Medial geniculate | Hearing | Inferior colliculus | | Auditory cortex |
| | Lateral geniculate | Vision | Optic tract | | Visual cortex |
| Association nuclei | Anterior | Limbic | Reciprocal with limbic cortex | | |
| | Mediodorsal | Limbic | Reciprocal with limbic cortex | | |
| | Lateral dorsal | Limbic | Reciprocal with limbic cortex | | |
| | Lateral posterior | Sensory integration | Reciprocal with parietal cortex | | |
| | Pulvinar | Sensory integration | Reciprocal with parietal, occipital, and temporal cortices | | |
| Nonspecific nuclei | Midline | Limbic | Viscera | | Hypothalamus, amygdala, cerebral cortex |
| | Intralaminar | Limbic, arousal | Ascending reticular system | | Widespread areas of cortex |
| | Reticular | Adjusts thalamic activity | Interconnections with other thalamic nuclei | | |

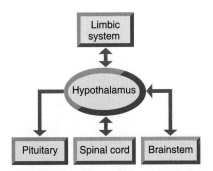

**Fig. 17-3** Interactions of the hypothalamus.

- Regulation of circadian (daily) rhythms, including sleep-wake cycles, in concert with other brain regions
- Endocrine regulation of growth, metabolism, and reproductive organs

These functions are carried out by hypothalamic regulation of pituitary gland secretions (hormones) and by efferent neural connections with the cortex (via the thalamus), limbic system, brainstem, and spinal cord (Figure 17-3).

## Epithalamus

The major structure of the epithalamus is the pineal gland, an endocrine gland innervated by sympathetic fibers. The pineal gland helps regulate circadian rhythms and influence the secretions of the pituitary gland, adrenals, parathyroids, and islets of Langerhans.

## Subthalamus

The subthalamus is located superior to the substantia nigra of the midbrain. Functionally, the subthalamus is part of the basal ganglia circuit, involved in regulating movement. The subthalamus facilitates basal ganglia output nuclei.

## SUBCORTICAL STRUCTURES

### Subcortical White Matter

All white matter, whether located in the spinal cord or the brain, consists of myelinated axons. In the cerebrum, the white matter is deep to the cortex and thus is called *subcortical*. Subcortical white matter fibers are classified into three categories, depending on their connections (Figure 17-4):
- Projection
- Commissural
- Association

### Projection Fibers

Projection fibers extend from subcortical structures to the cerebral cortex and from the cerebral cortex to the spinal cord, brainstem, basal ganglia, and thalamus. Almost all projection fibers travel through the internal capsule, a section of white matter bordered by the thalamus posteromedially, the caudate anteromedially, and the lentiform nucleus laterally

(Figure 17-5). Similar to the stems of a bouquet of flowers, the axons of projection neurons are gathered into a small bundle, the internal capsule. Above the internal capsule, the axons spread apart to form the corona radiata, connecting with all areas of the cerebral cortex.

Regions of the internal capsule are the anterior limb, genu (from the Latin for "knee," indicating a bend), and posterior limb. The anterior limb, lateral to the head of the caudate, contains corticopontine fibers and fibers interconnecting thalamic and cortical limbic areas. The most medial part of the internal capsule, the genu, contains cortical fibers that project to cranial nerve motor nuclei and to the reticular formation. The posterior limb is located between the thalamus and the lenticular nucleus, with additional fibers traveling posterior and inferior to the lenticular nucleus (retrolenticular and sublenticular fibers). The posterior limb consists of corticospinal and thalamocortical projections (Figure 17-4, *C*). The thalamocortical projections relay somatosensory, visual, auditory, and motor information to the cerebral cortex. Because axons from so many areas are together in the internal capsule, small lesions in the internal capsule have consequences disproportionate to their size.

### Commissural Fibers

Unlike projection fibers connecting cortical and subcortical structures, commissural fibers connect homologous areas of the cerebral hemispheres. The largest group of commissural fibers is the corpus callosum (see Figure 17-4, *A,B*), which links many areas of the right and left hemispheres. Fibers of the other two commissures, anterior and posterior, link the right and left temporal lobes.

### Association Fibers

Association fibers connect cortical regions within one hemisphere (see Figure 17-4, *A,D,E*). The short association fibers connect adjacent gyri, and the long association fibers connect lobes within a single hemisphere. For example, the cingulum connects frontal, parietal, and temporal lobe cortices. Additional long association fiber bundles are listed in Table 17-2.

### Basal Ganglia

- As noted in Chapter 11, the basal ganglia are vital for normal motor function. The basal ganglia sequence movements, regulate muscle tone and muscle force, and select and inhibit specific motor synergies. In addition to their motor functions, the basal ganglia are involved in cognitive functions,[1] participating in the following:
- Executive function (goal-directed behavior)
- Sustained attention
- Ability to change behavior as task requirements change (behavioral flexibility and control loop)
- Motivation

Motivation is centered in the ventral striatum. The ventral striatum is the inferior part of the junction between the caudate and the putamen (see Figure 11-1). The ventral striatum serves to link motivation and behavior. Specifically, ventral striatum activity is essential for the generation of locomotion, and for increasing the frequency of rewarded behaviors.[2]

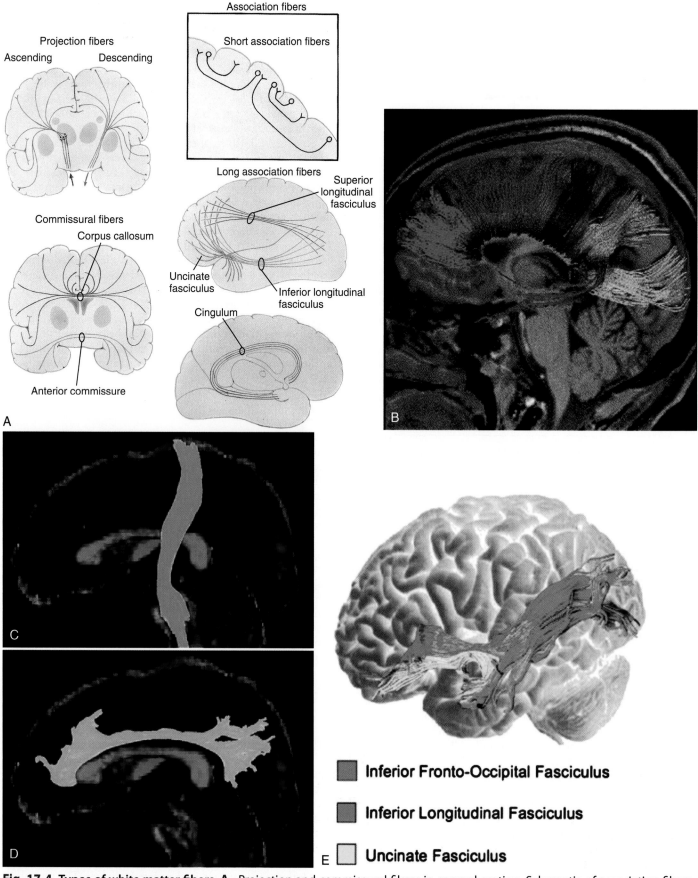

**Fig. 17-4 Types of white matter fibers. A,** Projection and commissural fibers in coronal section. Schematic of association fibers. **B,** Diffusion tensor image (DTI) of corpus callosum. The colors indicate connectivity of the callosal neurons. *Blue,* Primary motor cortex; *yellow,* occipital lobe; *green,* prefrontal cortex; *black,* premotor cortex and supplementary motor area; *orange,* posterior parietal cortex; *red,* primary somatosensory cortex; *purple,* temporal lobe. *(With permission from Hofer S, Frahm J: Topography of the human corpus callosum revisited—comprehensive fiber tractography using diffusion tensor magnetic resonance imaging. Neuroimage 32:989–994, 2006.)* **C,** Projection fibers: corticospinal tract. **D,** Dorsal cingulate bundle. *(C and D with permission from Wahl M, Yi-Ou L, Ng J, et al: Microstructural correlations of white matter tracts in the human brain. Neuroimage 51:531–541, 2010.)* **E,** Long association fibers. *(From Catani M, Mesulam M: The arcuate fasciculus and the disconnection theme in language and aphasia: history and current state. Cortex 44:953–961, 2008.)*

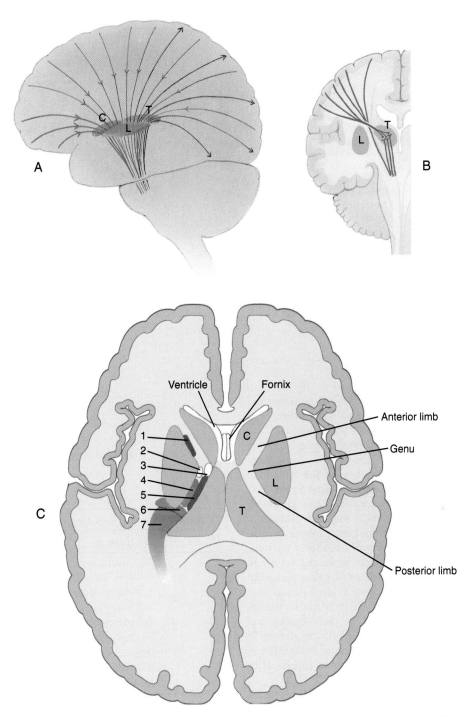

**Fig. 17-5  Internal capsule.** Only the fibers projecting beyond the cerebrum are illustrated. Green, frontopontine fibers; red, motor fibers; blue, sensory fibers. **A,** Schematic view of the left internal capsule. The superior parts of the caudate (C) and lenticular (L) nuclei and the thalamus (T) have been removed. **B,** Coronal section showing internal capsule. **C,** Horizontal section through the internal capsule. The limbs of the capsule are indicated on the right; the fiber tracts passing through are indicated on the left. The white areas of the internal capsule on the left contain thalamocortical fibers. Fiber tracts: (1) frontopontine, (2) corticoreticular, (3) corticobrainstem, (4) ascending sensory, (5) corticospinal, (6) auditory radiation, and (7) optic radiation.

**TABLE 17-2**    SUBCORTICAL WHITE MATTER

| Type of Fibers | Examples |
| --- | --- |
| Projection | Thalamocortical<br>Corticospinal<br>Corticobrainstem |
| Commissural | Corpus callosum<br>Anterior commissure<br>Posterior commissure |
| Association | Short association fibers (connect adjacent gyri)<br>Cingulum (connects frontal, parietal, and temporal lobe cortices)<br>Uncinate fasciculus (connects frontal and temporal lobe cortices)<br>Superior longitudinal fasciculus (connects cortices of all lobes)<br>Inferior longitudinal fasciculus (connects temporal and occipital lobes) |

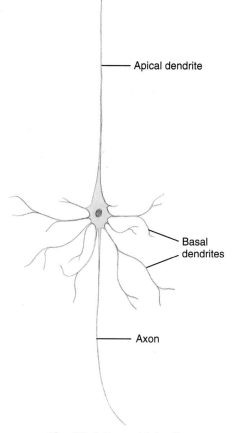

**Fig. 17-6** Pyramidal cell.

## CEREBRAL CORTEX

The cerebral cortex is a vast collection of cell bodies, axons, and dendrites covering the surface of the cerebral hemispheres. The most common types of cortical neurons are pyramidal, fusiform, and stellate cells. Pyramidal cells have an apical dendrite that extends toward the surface of the cortex, several basal dendrites extending laterally from the base of the soma, and one axon (Figure 17-6). Although some pyramidal cells have short axons that synapse without leaving the cortex, almost all pyramidal cell axons travel through white matter as projection, commissural, or association fibers. Thus most pyramidal cells are output cells for the cerebral cortex. Fusiform cells are spindle-shaped and are also output cells, projecting mainly to the thalamus. Stellate (granule) cells are smaller than pyramidal cells, remain within the cortex, and serve as interneurons.

The cerebral cortex contains layers, differentiated by the size and connectivity of constituent cells. In the olfactory and medial temporal cortex, only three layers of cells are present. In the remainder of the cerebral cortex, six layers of cells are found (Figure 17-7). These six layers, numbered from superficial to deep, are listed in Table 17-3.

This list of cortical layers is a generalization; different areas of the cerebral cortex have distinctive arrangements of cells. For example, although layers II through V can be distinguished in the visual cortex, stellate cells predominate in these four layers. In 1909, Brodmann[3] published a map of the cortex that distinguished 52 histologic areas (Figure 17-8). Brodmann's areas are commonly used to designate cortical locations.

### Mapping of the Cerebral Cortex

People undergoing brain surgery have allowed neurosurgeons to stimulate and record from various areas of the cerebral cortex. During these surgeries, patients were fully conscious. Some experiments consist of placing recording electrodes on the surface of the brain and then stimulating various parts of the

**TABLE 17-3**    LAYERS OF THE CEREBRAL CORTEX

| Name | Description |
| --- | --- |
| I | Molecular layer; mainly axons and dendrites; contains few cells |
| II | External granular layer; many small pyramidal and stellate cells |
| III | External pyramidal layer; pyramidal cells |
| IV | Internal granular layer; mainly stellate cells |
| V | Internal pyramidal layer; predominantly pyramidal cells, with stellate and other interneurons |
| VI | Multiform layer; primarily fusiform cells |

body to determine whether the cortical area being recorded responds to the stimulus. For example, when the surgeon touches the patient's fingertip, only a small, specific area of the cortex, located in a consistent position of the cortex among various people, responds.

Other experiments involve mild electrical stimulation of the cortex. In these experiments, stimulation may elicit movements of a part of the body or may cause the patient to recall a particular situation.

Imaging techniques can be used to investigate brain function without invasive procedures. For example, brain activity

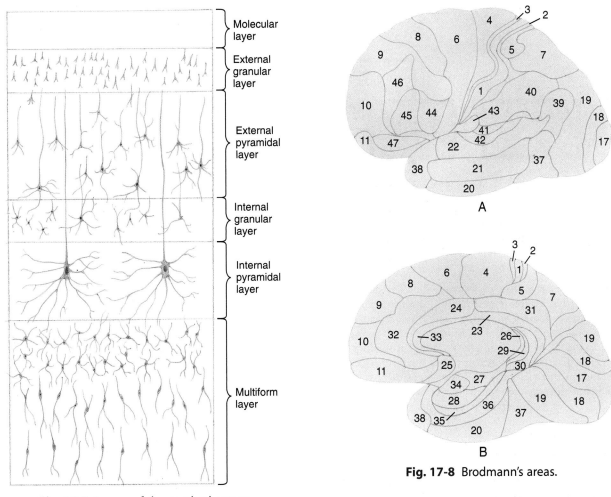

**Fig. 17-7** Layers of the cerebral cortex.

Molecular layer

External granular layer

External pyramidal layer

Internal granular layer

Internal pyramidal layer

Multiform layer

**Fig. 17-8** Brodmann's areas.

can be recorded and analyzed while a person is having a conversation.

## Localized Functions of the Cerebral Cortex*

Different areas of the cerebral cortex are specialized to perform a variety of functions. Based on their functions, five categories of cortex have been identified:

- The primary sensory cortex discriminates among different intensities and qualities of sensory information.
- The secondary sensory cortex performs more complex analysis of sensation.
- The motor planning areas organize movements.
- The primary motor cortex provides descending control of motor output.
- The association cortex controls behavior, interprets sensation, and processes emotions and memories.

Each type of cortex may play a role in response to a stimulus. For example, when one sees a bell, the primary visual cortex

discriminates its shape and its brightness from the background. The secondary visual cortex analyzes the color of the bell. The association cortex may recall the name of the object, what sound the bell makes, and specific memories associated with bells. The association cortex also participates in the decision of what to do with the bell. If the decision is to lift the bell, premotor areas plan the movement, then the primary motor cortex sends commands to neurons in the spinal cord. The flow of cortical activity from the primary sensory cortex to cortical motor output is illustrated in Figure 17-9. This figure provides a simplified schematic that applies only to movement generated in response to an external stimulus. An equally plausible alternative would begin with a decision in the association cortex leading to movement.

## PRIMARY SENSORY AREAS OF THE CEREBRAL CORTEX

Primary sensory areas receive sensory information directly from the ventral tier of thalamic nuclei. Each primary sensory area discriminates among different intensities and qualities of one type of input. Thus there are separate primary sensory areas for somatosensory, auditory, visual, and vestibular information.

---

*In neuroscience, the term *localization of function* is used to connote that an area contributes to the performance of a specific neural activity. Neural functions are achieved by networks of neurons, not by isolated centers.

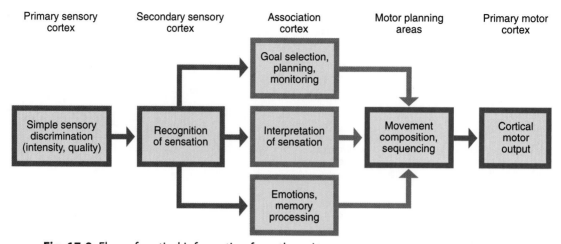

**Fig. 17-9** Flow of cortical information from the primary sensory cortex to motor output.

Most primary sensory areas are located within and adjacent to landmark cortical fissures (Figure 17-10). The primary somatosensory cortex is located within the central sulcus and on the adjacent postcentral gyrus. The primary auditory cortex is located in the lateral fissure and on the adjacent superior temporal gyrus. The primary visual cortex is within the calcarine sulcus and on the adjacent gyri. Only the primary vestibular cortex is not close to a landmark fissure; instead, the primary vestibular cortex is posterior to the primary somatosensory cortex.

### Primary Somatosensory Cortex

The primary somatosensory cortex receives information from tactile and proprioceptive receptors via a three-neuron pathway: peripheral afferent/dorsal column neuron, medial lemniscus neuron, and thalamocortical neuron. Although crude awareness of somatosensation occurs in the ventral posterolateral and ventral posteromedial nuclei of the thalamus, neurons in the primary somatosensory cortex identify the location of stimuli and discriminate among various shapes, sizes, and textures of objects. The cortical termination of nociceptive and temperature pathways is more widespread than the discriminative tactile and proprioceptive information and thus is not limited to the primary somatosensory cortex.

### Primary Auditory and Primary Vestibular Cortices

The primary auditory cortex receives information from the cochlea of both ears via a pathway that synapses in the inferior colliculus and medial geniculate body before reaching the cortex (see Chapter 14). The primary auditory cortex provides conscious awareness of the intensity of sounds. The primary vestibular cortex receives information regarding head movement and head position relative to gravity by a vestibulothalamocortical pathway (see Chapter 16).

### Primary Visual Cortex

Visual information travels to the cortex via a pathway from the retina to the lateral geniculate body of the thalamus, then to the primary visual cortex. Individual neurons in the primary visual cortex are specialized to distinguish between light and dark, various shapes, locations of objects, and movements of objects.

## SECONDARY SENSORY AREAS

Secondary sensory areas analyze sensory input from both the thalamus and the primary sensory cortex. Secondary sensory areas contribute to the analysis of one type of sensory information. For example, if one picks up a pen, the primary somatosensory cortex registers that the object is small, smooth, and cylindrical. The secondary somatosensory area recognizes the object as a pen, although a different area of the cortex is required to name the object. Secondary somatosensory areas integrate tactile and proprioceptive information obtained from manipulating an object. Neurons in the secondary somatosensory area provide stereognosis by comparing somatosensation from the current object with memories of other objects.

The secondary visual cortex analyzes colors and motion, and its output to the tectum directs visual fixation, the maintenance of an object in central vision. The secondary auditory cortex compares sounds with memories of other sounds and then categorizes the sounds as language, music, or noise. Secondary sensory areas are illustrated in Figure 17-11.

## PRIMARY MOTOR CORTEX AND MOTOR PLANNING AREAS OF THE CEREBRAL CORTEX

The primary motor cortex is located in the precentral gyrus, anterior to the central sulcus. The primary motor cortex is the source of most neurons in the corticospinal tract and controls contralateral voluntary movements, particularly the fine movements of the hand and face. Because the primary motor cortex is unique in providing precise control of hand and lower face movements, a much greater proportion of the total area of the primary motor cortex is devoted to neurons that control these parts of the body than is devoted to the trunk and proximal limbs, where more gross motor activity is required. The hand, foot, and lower face representations in the motor cortex are entirely contralateral. In contrast, many muscles that tend to

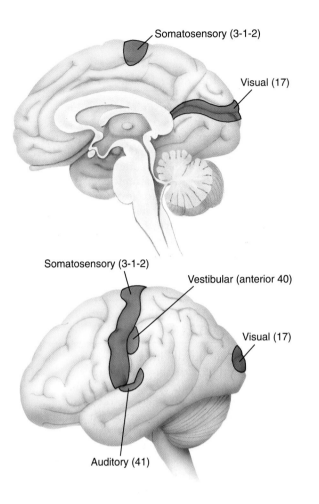

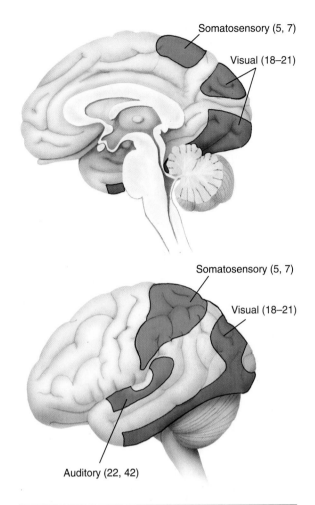

| Cortical Area | Function |
|---|---|
| Primary somatosensory | Discriminates shape, texture, or size of objects |
| Primary auditory | Conscious discrimination of loudness and pitch of sounds |
| Primary visual | Distinguishes intensity of light, shape, size, and location of objects |
| Primary vestibular | Discriminates among head positions and head movements |

**Fig. 17-10 Primary sensory areas of the cerebral cortex.** Corresponding Brodmann's areas are indicated in parentheses.

| Cortical Area | Function |
|---|---|
| Secondary somatosensory | Stereognosis and memory of the tactile and spatial environment |
| Secondary visual | Analysis of motion, color; control of visual fixation |
| Secondary auditory | Classification of sounds |

**Fig. 17-11 Secondary sensory areas of the cerebral cortex.** Corresponding Brodmann's areas are indicated in parentheses.

be active bilaterally simultaneously—muscles of the back, for example—are controlled by the primary motor cortex on both sides.

The cortical motor planning areas (Figure 17-12) include:
- Supplementary motor area
- Premotor area
- Broca's area
- Area corresponding to Broca's area in the opposite hemisphere

## Motor Planning Areas

The cortex anterior to the primary motor cortex consists of three areas: supplementary motor area, premotor area, and Broca's area (or, on the contralateral side, the area corresponding to Broca's area). The supplementary motor cortex, located anterior to the lower body region of the primary motor cortex, is important for initiation of movement, orientation of the eyes and head, and planning bimanual and sequential movements. The premotor area, located anterior to the upper body region of the primary motor cortex, controls trunk and girdle muscles via medial upper motor neurons. Thus the premotor area stabilizes the shoulders during upper limb tasks and the hips during walking.

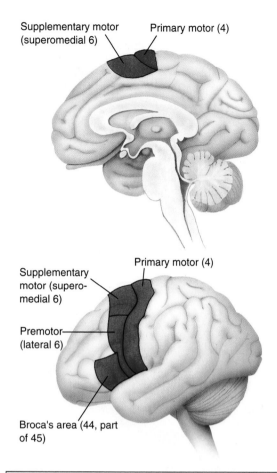

**Fig. 17-12 Motor areas of the cerebral cortex.** Corresponding Brodmann's areas are indicated in parentheses.

| Motor Areas | Function |
|---|---|
| Primary motor cortex | Voluntarily controlled movements |
| Premotor area | Control of trunk and girdle muscles, anticipatory postural adjustments |
| Supplementary motor area | Initiation of movement, orientation planning, bimanual and sequential movements |
| Broca's area | Motor programming of speech (usually in the left hemisphere only) |
| Area analogous to Broca's in opposite hemisphere | Planning nonverbal communication (emotional gestures, tone of voice; usually in the right hemisphere) |

Broca's area, anteroinferior to the premotor area and anterior to the face and throat region of the primary motor cortex, is usually in the left hemisphere. Broca's area is responsible for planning movements of the mouth during speech and the grammatical aspects of language. An area analogous to Broca's area, in the opposite hemisphere, plans nonverbal communication, including emotional gestures and adjusting the tone of

voice. These areas will be considered further in a later section on communication.

## Connections of the Motor Areas

Premotor and supplementary motor areas and Broca's area receive information from secondary sensory areas. Both the primary motor cortex and motor planning areas receive information from the basal ganglia and cerebellum, relayed by the thalamus. The primary motor cortex receives somatosensory information relayed by the thalamus and from the primary somatosensory cortex and motor instructions from the motor planning areas. Cortical motor output, including corticospinal tracts, corticobrainstem tracts, corticoreticular tracts, corticopontine tracts, and cortical projections to the putamen, originates in the primary motor and primary somatosensory cortex and motor planning areas.

## ASSOCIATION AREAS OF THE CEREBRAL CORTEX

Areas of cortex not directly involved with sensation or movement are called the *association cortex*. Three areas of cortex are designated as association cortex (Figure 17-13):
- Dorsolateral prefrontal association cortex
- Parietotemporal association cortex, at the junction of the parietal, occipital, and temporal lobes
- Ventral and medial dorsal prefrontal association cortex
Enormously complex abilities are localized in the association areas: personality, integration and interpretation of sensations, processing of memory, and generation of emotions. Damage to these areas causes specific deficits. For example, damage to the ventral prefrontal cortex can alter personality characteristics, while, damage to other cortical areas has little effect on personality. Thus, although the neurophysiology of personality is not understood, personality is localized to the ventral prefrontal cortex. Similarly, cognitive intelligence, as measured by intelligence tests, and integration and interpretation of sensations are localized in the parietotemporal association areas. Conscious emotions are localized in the limbic association areas.

The prefrontal cortex is divided into five areas named for their anatomic location: dorsolateral, medial dorsal, and ventral prefrontal cortex and anterior dorsal and rostral anterior cingulate cortex.

## Dorsolateral Prefrontal Cortex

Dorsolateral prefrontal cortex functions include self-awareness and executive functions (also called *goal-oriented behavior*). Executive functions include the following:
- Deciding on a goal
- Planning how to accomplish the goal
- Executing a plan
- Monitoring execution of the plan
Executive function includes the processes of working memory, judgment, planning, abstract reasoning, dividing attention, and sequencing activity. Decisions ranging from the trivial to the momentous are made in the dorsolateral prefrontal area; what to wear, whether to buy a new house, and whether to have children are decided in and carried out by instructions

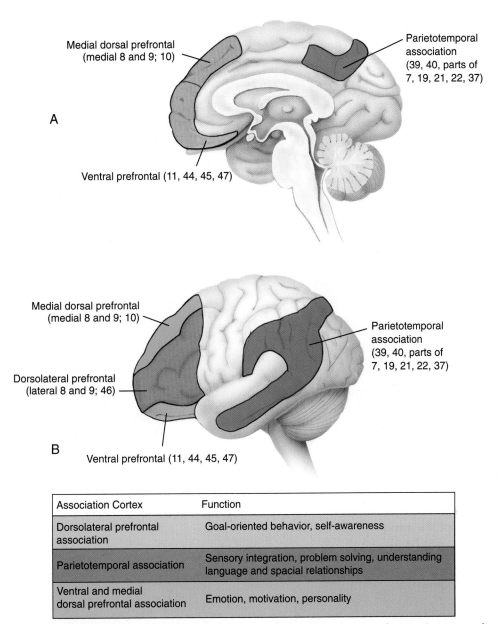

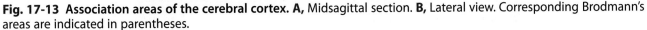

| Association Cortex | Function |
|---|---|
| Dorsolateral prefrontal association | Goal-oriented behavior, self-awareness |
| Parietotemporal association | Sensory integration, problem solving, understanding language and spacial relationships |
| Ventral and medial dorsal prefrontal association | Emotion, motivation, personality |

**Fig. 17-13** **Association areas of the cerebral cortex. A,** Midsagittal section. **B,** Lateral view. Corresponding Brodmann's areas are indicated in parentheses.

from the dorsolateral prefrontal cortex. The dorsolateral prefrontal cortex is also part of the system that decides what behaviors to avoid, inhibiting socially inappropriate behaviors. The dorsolateral prefrontal cortex is part of the executive loop (see Figure 11-5), connects extensively with secondary sensory areas in the parietal, occipital, and temporal lobes and with limbic areas.

## Parietotemporal Association Cortex

Cognitive intelligence is primarily a function of the parietotemporal association areas, in the posterior parietal and temporal cortices. Here, problem solving and comprehension of communication and of spatial relationships occur. The spatial coordinate system of this area is essential for constructing an image of one's own body and for planning movements.

## Ventral and Medial Dorsal Prefrontal Association Cortex

The third, and final, cortical association area is the ventral and medial dorsal prefrontal cortex. This cortex is involved in impulse control, personality, and reactions to surroundings. The ventral prefrontal association area connects with areas regulating mood (subjective feelings) and affect (observable demeanor). The ventral prefrontal cortex includes the orbital cortex (located superior to the eyes) and the ventromedial prefrontal cortex. The medial dorsal prefrontal cortex perceives others' emotions and makes assumptions about what other people believe and their intentions.[4]

## EMOTIONS AND BEHAVIOR

An emotion is a short-term subjective experience. A mood is a sustained, subjective, ongoing emotional experience. Emotions color our perceptions and influence our actions. For example, a person vexed by a difficult problem may misinterpret a question about progress in solving the problem as a threat and may become angry. The person's facial expressions and abrupt, choppy movements indicating anger are easy to recognize.

Immediate responses to a threat include somatic, autonomic, and hormonal changes, including increased muscle tension and heart rate, dilation of the pupils, and cessation of digestion. However, emotions also shape our lives in more subtle ways because emotions signal the nonconscious evaluation of a situation.

Five structures recognize emotional stimuli and generate and perceive emotions. These structures are the amygdala, area 25, the mediodorsal nucleus of the thalamus, the ventral striatum, and the anterior insula (Figure 17-14).

The amygdala generates feelings of fear and disgust and interprets facial expressions, body language, and social signals. Thus the amygdala is essential for social behavior[5] and is important for emotional learning.[6] All sensory systems provide

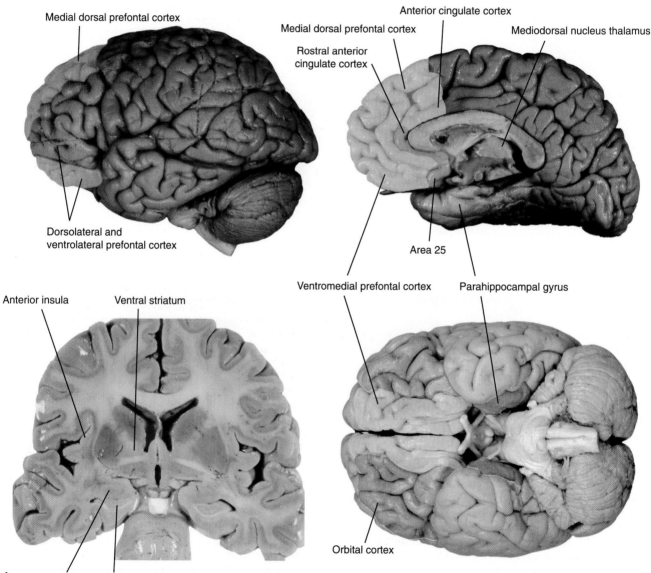

**Fig. 17-14 Areas of the brain involved in emotions.** Orange indicates structures that recognize emotional stimuli, generate and perceive emotions, and regulate autonomic aspects of emotions. Light green structures automatically regulate emotions. Yellow structures are involved in both automatic and voluntary regulation of emotions, and dark green structures voluntarily regulate emotions. *(Image top right modified from Nolte J. The Human Brain: An Introduction to its Functional Anatomy, ed 6. St. Louis, 2009, Mosby. All other images modified from copyright 1994, University of Washington. From Digital Anatomist Interactive Brain Atlas and the Structural Informatics Group.)*

| Function | Structure | Specific function |
|---|---|---|
| Indentify emotional significance of stimuli, generate and perceive emotions, regulate autonomic aspects of emotions | Amygdala | Detects emotional and social cues, generates feelings of fear and disgust |
| | Area 25 and Mediodorsal nucleus thalamus | Generate sad mood and depression |
| | Ventral striatum | Reward oriented behavior and responses to conditioned stimuli |
| | Anterior insula | Awareness of emotions and of stimuli inside the body |
| Automatic emotional regulation (cortical regions are part of the behavioral flexibility and control basal ganglia loop) | Rostral anterior cingulate cortex | Direct attention away from emotion; motivated behavior |
| | Orbital cortex | Use of rewards to guide behavior; inhibits undesirable behavior |
| | Hippocampus | Resolve goal conflicts |
| | Parahippocampal gyrus | Detect novel stimuli |
| Automatic and voluntary emotional regulation (part of the limbic basal ganglia loop, connects with the ventral striatum and pallidum) | Medial dorsal prefrontal cortex | Perception of other's emotions and infer other's beliefs and intentions |
| | Ventromedial prefrontal cortex | Sad mood, value assessment of objects, reward associations, elicits visceral responses |
| | Ventrolateral prefrontal cortex | Guilt, recall of personal memories |
| | Dorsal anterior cingulate cortex | Goal-directed behavior, expressing emotions, error monitoring |
| Voluntary emotional regulation (part of the executive basal ganglia loop) | Dorsolateral prefrontal cortex | Executive (goal-directed) function; self-awareness |

B

**Fig. 17-14, cont'd**

information to the amygdala. The amygdala is an almond-shaped collection of nuclei deep in the anterior temporal lobe.

Area 25 and the mediodorsal thalamus generate sad mood and depression.[7] Area 25 is the cingulate cortex inferior to the genu of the corpus callosum.

The ventral striatum determines reward-oriented behavior and responses to conditioned stimuli.[8] The ventral striatum is the region where the caudate and the putamen blend. The anterior insula provides awareness of emotions and of stimuli inside the body.[9] Structures that recognize, generate, and perceive emotions are all deep within the cerebrum, except area 25, which is medially located.

In addition to the brain areas directly involved in emotions, multiple areas attempt to control which emotions are experienced, and how emotions are experienced and expressed. This emotional regulation increases or decreases the duration and intensity of emotions. Often this regulation is automatic (i.e., implicit, not conscious). Examples include ignoring, leaving, or denying an emotional situation, sustaining particular beliefs about a situation, and controlling behavior after an emotion has been generated.[10] The dissociation of automatic and voluntary regulation is obvious in people with orbital cortex lesions, who are able to identify undesirable behaviors (e.g., sharing personal information with strangers) but in real situations engage in undesirable behaviors (actually share personal information with strangers).[11]

Automatic regulation of emotions uses a ventromedial system comprising four cortical areas plus the hippocampus.[12] The rostral cingulate cortex directs attention away from emotional stimuli. The ventromedial prefrontal cortex is involved in sad mood, determining the value of objects, and linking rewards with specific stimuli, and it elicits autonomic nervous system activity.[13] The ventromedial prefrontal cortex is active in determining the value of donations to charity.[14] The orbital cortex uses rewards to guide behavior and inhibits undesirable behaviors.[11] If I say something inappropriate, the orbital cortex recognizes the social error, generates feeling embarrassed, and makes it less likely that I will repeat the behavior in the future. The parahippocampal cortex detects novel stimuli, including unrecognized faces.[12] The hippocampus evaluates and resolves goal conflicts.[12] For example, the hippocampus is involved in deciding whether to eat ice cream or keep a resolution to lose weight.

Voluntary regulation of emotions occurs when a person consciously decides to control his or her emotions, for example, by choosing not to express anger toward the boss when being unfairly blamed for a coworker's failure. The dorsolateral prefrontal cortex partially provides voluntary regulation of emotions. Several additional dorsolateral cortical areas provide both automatic and voluntary emotional regulation: the medial dorsal and ventrolateral prefrontal cortex and the dorsal anterior cingulate cortex.[12] Emotion is intimately tied to decision making.[15]

## DECISION MAKING

Part of our decision-making process involves imagining consequences and then attending to resultant emotional signals from the visceral, muscular, and hormonal systems and from neurotransmitters.[15] These emotional signals are based on prior experience and provide "gut feelings" about the actions being contemplated. When I was an undergraduate, my roommate was dating a man, Ted Bundy, who made me feel frightened. I quickly learned to avoid him. Several years later, he was identified as a serial killer. Despite not knowing why I felt frightened, I made the decision to avoid him on the basis of visceral sensations. The theory that emotions are crucial for sound judgment is called the *somatic marker hypothesis*.[15] Emotional signals, elicited by activity in the ventromedial prefrontal cortex, do not make decisions but are considered in the decision process. Emotional and social intelligence, the ability to manage personal and social life, requires the ventromedial prefrontal cortex, the amygdala, and the anterior insula.[16]

Making decisions depends on a stimulus coding system, an action selection system, and an expected reward system.[17] The stimulus coding system is located in the ventral prefrontal cortex, which determines the value of a stimulus. The action selection system includes the anterior cingulate, lateral prefrontal, and parietal cortices. These areas determine what to do next: pack for the trip, call the airline, or go for a run. The expected reward system involves the ventral striatum, the amygdala, and the insula.[17]

The limbic loop (discussed in Chapter 11) is active when making a decision with an uncertain outcome.[18] For example, the outcome of investing in the stock market is uncertain. The limbic loop is concerned with seeking pleasure.[8,19,20] Thus this loop often sabotages diet resolutions and is the key player in addictive behavior (discussed further in Chapter 18).

When making social decisions, the behavioral flexibility and control loop is active (Figure 17-15). This loop recognizes social disapproval, self-regulates behavior, selects relevant information from irrelevant,[21] maintains attention, and is important to stimulus-response learning.[22-27] During a somber occasion, the behavioral flexibility and control loop keeps a person's behavior subdued and restrained. During a festive occasion, the behavioral flexibility and control loop allows the same person to be much louder and more expressive. Figure 17-16 illustrates the decision-making limbic and behavioral flexibility and control loops.

## PSYCHOLOGICAL AND SOMATIC INTERACTIONS

Thoughts and emotions influence the functions of all organs. Neurotransmitters and hormones regulated by the brain modulate immune system cells, and cytokines (chemicals secreted by white blood cells, including tumor necrosis factor and interleukins) regulate the neuroendocrine system (Figure 17-17). An individual's reaction to experiences can disrupt homeostasis; this is called a *stress response*. When an individual feels threatened, the stress response increases strength and energy to deal with the situation. Three systems create the stress response:

- Somatic nervous system: motor neuron activity increases muscle tension
- Autonomic nervous system: sympathetic activity increases blood flow to muscles and decreases blood flow to the skin, kidneys, and digestive tract
- Neuroendocrine system: sympathetic nerve stimulation of the adrenal medulla causes the release of epinephrine into the bloodstream. Epinephrine increases the cardiac rate and the strength of cardiac contraction, relaxes intestinal smooth muscle, and increases the metabolic rate.

About 5 minutes after the initial response to stress, the hypothalamus stimulates the pituitary to secrete adrenocorticotropic hormone, causing the release of cortisol from adrenal glands. Cortisol mobilizes energy (glucose), suppresses immune responses, and serves as an anti-inflammatory agent. As the stress response ends, homeostasis gradually returns. Unfortunately, often the stress response does not terminate because stress is maintained by circumstances or by the individual's thinking patterns. For example, a social slight that would go unnoticed by one person may cause another person to extensively contemplate why he was snubbed and how he should respond.

Excessive amounts of cortisol are associated with stress-related diseases, including colitis, cardiovascular disorders, and adult-onset diabetes. Excessive cortisol also causes emotional instability and cognitive deficits.[28]

In healthy married couples, hostile behaviors provoke more severe adverse immunologic changes and slow the rate of healing compared with supportive behaviors. Hostile couples used contempt, criticism, and other negative behaviors during a discussion of conflict-producing marital issues. The healing rate of hostile couples was only 60% of that of couples who were mutually supportive during discussion of marital

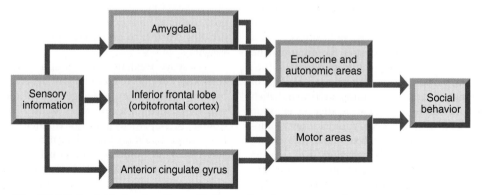

**Fig. 17-15** Social behavior: flow of information from sensory input to motor output.

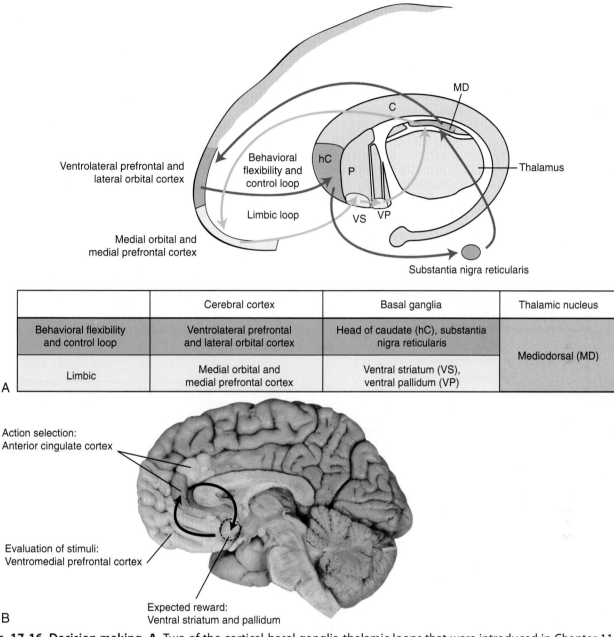

**Fig. 17-16 Decision making. A,** Two of the cortical-basal ganglia-thalamic loops that were introduced in Chapter 11. The posterior two thirds of the lenticular nucleus have been removed so that the entire thalamus is visible. This figure is a copy of part of Figure 11-5. C, Caudate; P, putamen. **B,** Some of the decision-making areas on a midsagittal section. The dotted line around the ventral striatum and pallidum indicates that these structures are deep inside. *(Modified from copyright 1994, University of Washington. From Digital Anatomist Interactive Brain Atlas and the Structural Informatics Group.)*

conflicts.[29] Mutually supportive partners used more humor, self-disclosure, and relationship-enhancing statements.[30]

When the stress response is prolonged, persistently high levels of cortisol continue to suppress immune function. Immune suppression is advantageous for decreasing inflammation and regulating allergic reactions and autoimmune responses. However, chronic stress–induced immune suppression reduces skin resistance to viruses, bacteria, and fungi.[31] Thus, the effects of the stress response can be beneficial or damaging, depending on the situation and whether the response is prolonged. Figure 17-18 illustrates the consequences

of prolonged psychological stress. As noted in the figure, immune cells respond to neurotransmitters, neurohormones, and neuropeptides.

Researchers are beginning to analyze ways that immune function can be improved. Short-term benefits of hypnotic relaxation have been demonstrated in medical and dental students 3 days before an examination. Students who practiced relaxation more frequently were more protected from the immune decrement that often accompanies acute stress.[32] Thus, cognition, emotions, and immune activity are intertwined. Another component in this complex is how records of new experiences are formed and used to guide subsequent activities. Memory functions involve many areas of the brain, as the following section illustrates.

## MEMORY

At least three different types of memory have been identified (Table 17-4):
- Working
- Declarative
- Procedural

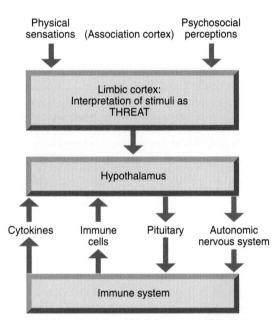

Fig. 17-17 **Chemical signaling between the nervous system and the immune system in response to stress.** Cytokines are nonantibody proteins that participate in the immune response (e.g., interferons, interleukins).

Working memory is temporary storage and manipulation of information. Declarative memory is easily declared: facts, events, concepts, and locations. Procedural memory involves knowing the procedures, that is, knowledge of how to perform actions and skills.

### Working Memory

Working memory maintains goal-relevant information for a short time. Working memory is essential for language, problem solving, mental navigation, and reasoning. During a conversation, you listen to the person speaking, are aware of emotional and social cues, and simultaneously plan what you want to say and what you want to do next. Extricate yourself from the conversation? Invite the person to dinner? Plan your route to the gym? When you are driving, you are able to plan and rapidly update your route when a street or bridge is closed and simultaneously converse with people in the car and with people on the speaker phone. This complex mental multitasking requires working memory and is central to cognition. The prefrontal cortex and the parietotemporal association cortex maintain, manipulate, and update information in working memory. Longer storage of language-based memory information requires declarative memory.

| TABLE 17-4 | THREE TYPES OF MEMORY | | |
|---|---|---|---|
| | **Working Memory** | **Declarative** | **Procedural** |
| Information | Goal-relevant information for a short time | Facts, events, concepts, and locations | Skilled movements and habits |
| Location | Prefrontal and parietotemporal association cortex | Dorsolateral prefrontal cortex and medial temporal lobe | Frontal cortex, thalamus, and basal ganglia |

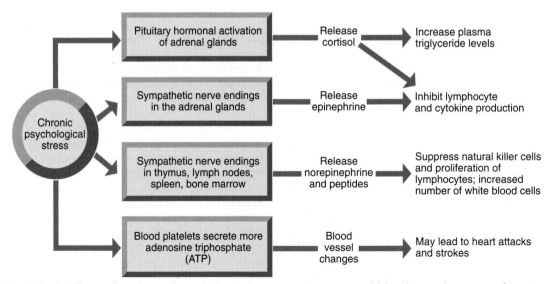

Fig. 17-18 Effects of prolonged psychological stress on immune and blood-vascular system function.

## Declarative Memory

Declarative memory refers to recollections that can be easily verbalized. Declarative memory is also called conscious or explicit memory.

A famous case of unintended consequences of a surgery to relieve severe epilepsy contributed significantly to our understanding of memory. The patient, H.M., suffered severe, frequent seizures. Because his seizures originated in the medial temporal lobes, this area of his brain was removed bilaterally when he was 27 years old. The epilepsy improved, but his memory was permanently damaged. Over the 55 years he lived subsequent to the surgery, H.M. was unable to remember any new people, facts, or events from 1 year before the surgery through the end of his life. He could not recall text he read minutes ago, nor could he remember people he had met repeatedly subsequent to the operation. Earlier memories were intact, and he was able to learn new skills.[33] His perception, personality, and cognitive skills other than declarative memory were unaffected. These outcomes indicate that the medial temporal lobe reorganizes memory for storage but that declarative memories are not stored in the medial temporal lobe.

Declarative memory requires attention during recall. Declarative memory has three stages:
- Encoding
- Consolidation
- Retrieval

Encoding processes information into a memory representation. Encoding is enhanced by paying attention, emotional arousal, linking new information to other information, and reviewing. Being distracted or uninterested interferes with encoding.

Consolidation stabilizes memories. This stabilization has two forms: synaptic and systems. Synaptic consolidation involves long-term potentiation (discussed in Chapter 4) and requires a few hours. Systems consolidation is medial temporal lobe processing that reorganizes memory information across large neuronal networks.[34]

A probable circuit of neural activity leading to the development of declarative memory is shown in Figure 17-19. Declarative memory begins with perceptual information in the parietotemporal association area that is encoded in the medial temporal lobe. The medial temporal lobe includes the hippocampus, fornix, amygdala, and surrounding cerebral cortex. The hippocampus is named for its fancied resemblance, in coronal section, to the shape of a seahorse. The hippocampus is formed by the gray and white matter of two gyri rolled together in the medial temporal lobe. The fornix is an arch-shaped fiber bundle connecting the hippocampus with the mammillary body and the anterior nucleus of the thalamus. Electrical stimulation of the medial temporal lobe cortex causes people to report that it seems as if a past event or experience was occurring during the stimulation, despite their awareness of actually being in surgery.[35]

The dorsolateral prefrontal cortex exerts voluntary control over the medial temporal lobe, processing, selecting, and organizing information for storage; accessing stored information[36]; and analyzing language content. To retrieve a memory, the dorsolateral prefrontal cortex generates cues that are used to search memories encoded in the medial temporal lobe.[37] Once the memory is retrieved, the dorsolateral prefrontal cortex maintains and verifies the memory.

As memories age, activation of brain areas during recall changes. Smith and Squire (2009)[20] confirmed that in neurologically intact people, recalling newer memories (in this study, 1 to 12 years ago) depends more upon activity in the medial temporal lobe; recall of older memories (in this study, 13 to 30 years ago) requires more activity in the prefrontal, parietal, and lateral temporal cortices.

## Procedural Memory

Procedural memory refers to recall of skills and habits. This type of memory is also called skill, habit, nonconscious memory, or implicit memory. Implicit memory produces changes in performance without conscious awareness. The distinction between declarative memories and procedural memories can be clarified by recalling memories of riding a bicycle. Declarative memories describe the location, terrain, companions on the ride, the weather, and other features of the ride. Procedural memories are not conscious. Thus if you ask bicycle riders how they restore the bicycle to upright when the bicycle begins to fall to the left, most will say by leaning right. However, this would make the bicycle tilt farther to the left. What the rider actually does is turn the handlebars to the left, restoring the center of gravity between the two wheels. Thus the typical rider accurately performs the effective movement to prevent falling without being conscious of how the fall is prevented.

Procedural memory also includes perceptual and cognitive skill learning. Perceptual skills include object, pattern, and face recognition. Cognitive skills include reasoning and logic.

Practice is required to store procedural memories. Once the skill or habit is learned, less attention is required while performing the task. For example, the initially difficult skill of driving a car in traffic becomes automatic with practice.

For learning motor skills, three learning stages have been identified:
- Cognitive
- Associative
- Automatic

During the cognitive stage, the beginner is trying to understand the task and to find out what works. Often beginners verbally guide their own movements. For example, people learning to use crutches often talk their way through descending stairs: "First the crutches, then the cast, then the right leg …" During the associative stage, the person refines the movements selected as most effective. Movements are less variable and less dependent on cognition. During the automatic stage, the movement or perception requires less attention. When movements are automatic, attention can be devoted to having a conversation or to other activities while the movements are being executed.

Learning a motor sequence involves the motor and parietal cortex and the striatum.[38] The representation of the learned movement sequences appears to be located in the supplementary motor area and the putamen/globus pallidus.[39] Motor adaptation, the ability to adjust movements to environmental changes, involves the cerebellum and the parietal and motor cortices.[38]

| Function | Structure |
|---|---|
| Declarative memory processing | Medial temporal lobe:<br>Medial temporal cortex<br>Hippocampus |
| Declarative memory processing | Amygdala |
| Perceptual integration | Parietotemporal association cortex |
| Organization and categorization of information | Dorsolateral prefrontal cortex |

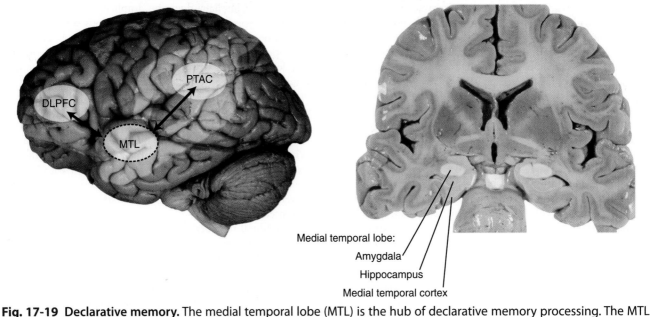

Medial temporal lobe:
Amygdala
Hippocampus
Medial temporal cortex

**Fig. 17-19 Declarative memory.** The medial temporal lobe (MTL) is the hub of declarative memory processing. The MTL processes integrated perceptual information from the parietotemporal association cortex (PTAC). The dorsolateral prefrontal cortex organizes and categorizes information for the MTL. The MTL includes the amygdala, the hippocampus, and the surrounding medial temporal cortex. The amygdala is yellow to correspond to the amygdala in Figure 17-14. The MTL has a dotted outline because the amygdala, the hippocampus, and the fornix are deep in the temporal lobe, and the medial temporal cortex is medial to the view. *(Modified from copyright 1994, University of Washington. From Digital Anatomist Interactive Brain Atlas and the Structural Informatics Group.)*

The abilities of H.M., the man with both medial temporal lobes removed, illustrate the dissociation of declarative and procedural memories. He was able to learn new motor skills but could not consciously remember that he had learned them. Thus his procedural memory was intact, despite his total loss of ability to consciously recall having practiced a task. H.M.'s communication abilities were intact because different brain areas are responsible for communication than for procedural memories.

## COMMUNICATION

People use both language and nonverbal methods to communicate. In approximately 95% of adults, the cortical areas responsible for understanding language and producing speech are found in the left hemisphere[40,41] (Figure 17-20). The distinction between language, a communication system based on symbols, and speech, the verbal output, is clinically important because different regions of the brain are responsible for each function.

Comprehension of spoken language occurs in Wernicke's area, a subregion of the left parietotemporal cortex. Broca's area, in the left frontal lobe, provides instructions for language output. These instructions consist of planning the movements to produce speech and providing grammatical function words, such as the articles *a, an,* and *the.* The contributions of the cortical and subcortical areas involved in normal conversation are shown in Figure 17-21.

In contrast to the auditory neural networks used during conversation, reading requires intact vision, secondary visual areas for visual recognition of written symbols, and connections

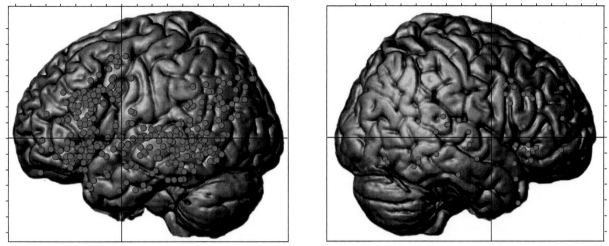

**Left hemisphere**                    **Right hemisphere**

**Fig. 17-20** **Peaks of activation in the left and right hemispheres during vocabulary and meaning of language tasks.** Data are summarized from 128 neuroimaging studies. The left hemisphere is significantly more active than the right for language tasks, and the right hemisphere primarily provides attention and working memory processing of verbal information. *(With permission from Vigneau M, Beaucousin V, Hervé PY, et al: What is right-hemisphere contribution to phonological, lexico-semantic, and sentence processing? Insights from a meta-analysis.* Neuroimage *54:577–593, 2011.)*

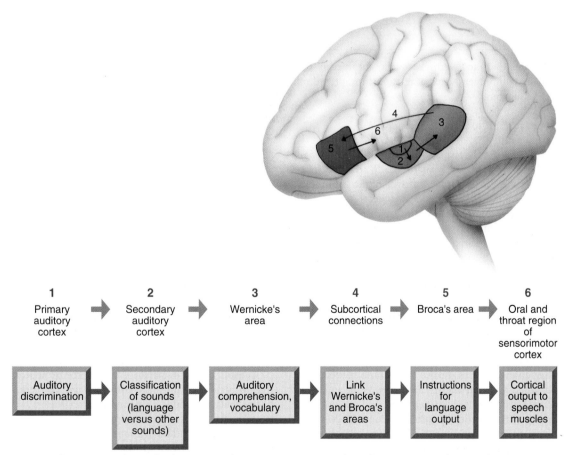

| 1 | 2 | 3 | 4 | 5 | 6 |
|---|---|---|---|---|---|
| Primary auditory cortex | Secondary auditory cortex | Wernicke's area | Subcortical connections | Broca's area | Oral and throat region of sensorimotor cortex |
| Auditory discrimination | Classification of sounds (language versus other sounds) | Auditory comprehension, vocabulary | Link Wernicke's and Broca's areas | Instructions for language output | Cortical output to speech muscles |

**Fig. 17-21** Flow of information during conversation, from hearing speech to replying.

with an intact Wernicke's area for interpreting the symbols. Writing requires motor control of the hand in addition to connections with Wernicke's and Broca's areas. Broca's area provides the grammatical relationship between words when writing, and Wernicke's area provides formulation of language.

Given that the right hemisphere typically does not process language, what do the contralateral areas corresponding to Wernicke's and Broca's areas contribute? In most people, activity in these areas of the right hemisphere is associated with nonverbal communication. Gestures, facial expressions, tone of voice, and posture convey meanings in addition to a verbal message. In the right hemisphere, the area corresponding to Wernicke's area is vital for interpreting nonverbal signals from other people. The right hemisphere area corresponding to Broca's area provides instructions for producing nonverbal communication, including emotional gestures and intonation of speech.

## PERCEPTION

Perception is the interpretation of sensation into meaningful forms. Perception is an active process, requiring interaction among the brain, the body, and the environment. For example, eye movements are essential for visual perception, and manipulating objects improves the ability to recognize objects via tactile input. Perception involves memory of past experiences, motivation, expectations, selection of sensory information, and active search for pertinent sensory information. The thalamus and many additional areas of the cerebrum are involved in perception.

### Spatial Perception

The area corresponding to Wernicke's area, located in the right hemisphere, comprehends spatial relationships, providing schemas of the following:
- The body
- The body in relation to its surroundings
- The external world

The body schema, also known as the body image, is a mental representation of how the body is anatomically arranged (e.g., with the hand distal to the forearm). Schemas of the self in relation to the surroundings enable us to locate objects in space and to navigate accurately, finding our way within rooms and hallways and outside. Schemas of the external world provide the information necessary to plan a route from one site to another.

## USE OF VISUAL INFORMATION

Visual information processed by the secondary visual cortex flows in two directions: dorsally, in an action stream to the frontal lobe via the posterior parietal cortex, and ventrally, in a perceptual stream to the temporal lobe (Figure 17-22). Information in the action stream is used to adjust limb movements. For example, when a person reaches for a cup, visual information in the dorsal stream is used to orient the hand and position the fingers appropriately during the reach. In contrast, information in the perceptual stream is used to identify objects, as in recognizing the cup. The two streams operate independently. People with damage in the dorsal stream have problems with

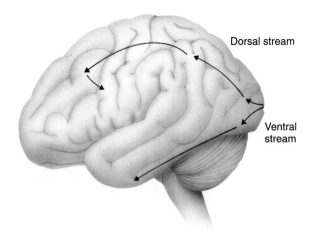

**Fig. 17-22** Use of visual information by the cerebral cortex: the action stream (dorsal) and the perceptual stream (ventral).

visually guided movements but no difficulty identifying objects, and those with damage in the ventral stream cannot identify objects by sight but are able to use visual information to adjust their movements.

## CONSCIOUSNESS

Waking and sleeping, paying attention, and initiating action are the province of the consciousness system. Various aspects of consciousness require different subsystems. Aspects of consciousness include the following:
- General level of arousal
- Attention
- Selection of object of attention, based on goals
- Motivation and initiation for motor activity and cognition

Each of these aspects of consciousness is associated with activity of specific neurotransmitters produced by brainstem neurons[42] and delivered to the cerebrum by the reticular activating system (see Chapter 15). The neurotransmitters are serotonin, norepinephrine, acetylcholine, and dopamine. Serotonin is widely distributed throughout the cerebrum and modulates the general level of arousal. Norepinephrine contributes to attention and vigilance via locus coeruleus projections primarily to sensory areas. Acetylcholine activation of the anterior cingulate cortex[42] contributes to voluntary direction of attention toward an object. Finally, dopamine contributes to the initiation of motor or cognitive actions, based on cognitive activity. Figure 17-23 summarizes the function and distribution of each brainstem neurotransmitter involved in consciousness.

Although the brainstem is the source of neurotransmitters that regulate consciousness, consciousness also requires activity of the thalamus and the cerebral cortex. The intralaminar thalamic nuclei are essential for arousal, awareness, thinking, and motor behavior.[43] Thus, lesions of the brainstem, thalamus, and/or cerebral cortex may result in the alterations of consciousness listed in Chapter 15.

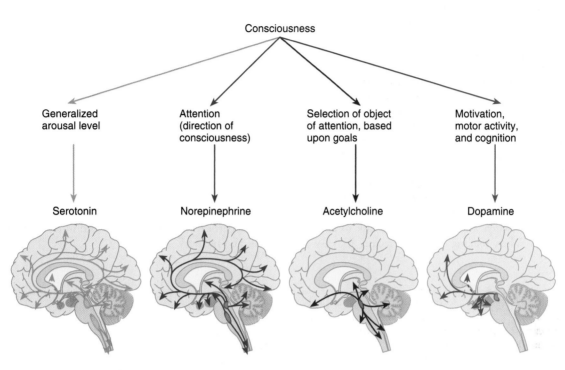

CONSCIOUSNESS SYSTEMS

DISTRIBUTION OF NEUROTRANSMITTER

| Transmitter | | Serotonin | Norepinephrine | Acetylcholine | Dopamine |
|---|---|---|---|---|---|
| Origin | | Raphe nuclei | Locus coeruleus and medial reticular zone | Pedunculopontine nucleus | Substantia nigra and ventral tegmental area |
| Limbic | Amygdala | | | | |
| | ventral striatum septal area | | | | |
| Basal forebrain | | | | | |
| Neocortex | | | | | |
| | | | | | Frontal only |
| Thalamus | | | | | |
| Striatum | | | | | |
| Cerebellar cortex | | | | | |

**Fig. 17-23 Function and distribution of neurotransmitters involved in consciousness.** Neurotransmitters are produced in the brainstem and are delivered to the cerebrum by the reticular activating system. Colored boxes below each neurotransmitter indicate that the neurotransmitter is distributed to the indicated brain area.

## Limits of Attention

The amount of attention is limited. Information that is not attended is not processed, so if you're driving and talking on the phone but not looking for pedestrians while turning, tragedy can result. As tasks become more automatic, less attention is required. When first learning to drive, the number and

coordination of tasks seem overwhelming. After much practice, the coordination becomes nearly automatic, and the driver can be aware of traffic, pedestrians, bicyclists, road repair crews, rerouting, and plans for the destination.

Sometimes attention must be divided among tasks that can be performed simultaneously, as when adjusting the car's speed according to the anticipated trajectory of other vehicles while talking with a passenger. In the clinic, dual tasks are used to assess the ability to divide attention. An example is the Stops Walking When Talking test.[44] To pass this test, the person is able to walk and talk simultaneously; inability to continue walking while talking indicates fall risk.[44] Sometimes attention is selective, requiring effort to inhibit competing information. An example is listening only to the person you're conversing with in a café with numerous other conversations proceeding at the same time.

Attention is also limited by the amount of effort available. If someone is talking softly and monotonously for an hour, the ability to maintain attention is challenged. If the listener is extremely interested in the topic and the speaker is an expert on the topic, attention may be maintained. However, if the listener is fatigued or disinterested, distractions will be readily attended to and the speaker forgotten.

The ability to switch attention from one task to another is also limited. When making half of a recipe, it's easy to make a mistake in the conversion while attending to the processes of measuring and mixing, and thus end up with the amount of salt required for a full recipe rather than half of the recipe. One also has to remember what steps have been performed and what steps remain: Was the baking powder already added?

## SUMMARY

Subcortical structures are involved in the nonconscious regulation of sensory, autonomic, and motor functions. Distinct areas of the cerebral cortex are devoted to analyzing sensation, planning and controlling movements, communicating, controlling behavior, and performing intellectual activities. Both cortical and subcortical structures are involved in consciousness, emotions, and memory.

## REVIEW QUESTIONS

1. What neural connections would be lost with lesions of each of the thalamic relay nuclei?
2. Why is compression of or damage to the hypothalamus potentially life threatening?
3. What signs would follow destruction of the genu region of the internal capsule?
4. What are the five functional categories of the cerebral cortex?
5. Draw a flowchart of the cortical areas activated to comply with the request, "Please pass the salt."
6. What is *executive function,* and where is executive function located in the brain?
7. What does the parietotemporal association cortex do?
8. Where are impulse control, personality, and reactions to surroundings represented in the brain?
9. Explain the somatic marker hypothesis.
10. What is the behavioral flexibility and control loop?
11. What are the effects of excessive, prolonged stress?
12. What is the role of the medial temporal lobe in memory?
13. Which structures are important for learning and storing procedural memories?
14. Bob is reading intently when he hears someone call his name. He looks up and begins a conversation with a friend. What brain areas contribute to Bob's ability to maintain his attention while reading, then disengage from reading and shift his attention to his friend?
15. When you are finding your way to a new restaurant, what part of your cortex is essential?
16. How do we use visual information in the ventral stream?
17. What are the factors that limit attention?

## References

1. Cropley VL, Fujita M, Innis RB, et al: Molecular imaging of the dopaminergic system and its association with human cognitive function. *Biol Psychiatry* 59:898–907, 2006.
2. Meredith GE, Baldo BA, Andrzejewski ME, et al: The structural basis for mapping behavior onto the ventral striatum and its subdivisions. *Brain Struct Funct* 213:17–27, 2008.
3. Brodmann K: *Vergleichende lokalisationslehre der grosshirnrinde in ihren prinzipien dargestellt auf grud des zellenbaues,* Leipzig, 1909, Barth.
4. Peelen MV, Atkinson AP, Vuilleumier P: Supramodal representations of perceived emotions in the human brain. *J Neurosci* 30: 10127–10134, 2010.
5. de Gelder B: Towards the neurobiology of emotional body language. *Nat Rev Neurosci* 7:242–249, 2006.
6. LaBar KS, Cabeza R: Cognitive neuroscience of emotional memory. *Nat Rev Neurosci* 7:54–64, 2006.
7. Anand A, Lia Y, Wang Y, et al: Resting state corticolimbic connectivity abnormalities in unmedicated bipolar disorder and unipolar depression. *Psychiatry Res* 171:189–198, 2009.
8. Sesack SR, Grace AA: Cortico-basal ganglia reward network: microcircuitry. *Neuropsychopharmacology* 35:27–47, 2010.
9. Giuliani NR, Drabant EM, Bhatnagar R, et al: Emotion regulation and brain plasticity: expressive suppression use predicts anterior insula volume. *Neuroimage* 58:10–15, 2011.
10. Mauss IB, Bunge SA, Gross JJ: Automatic emotion regulation. *Social and Personality Psychology Compass* 1:146–167, 2007.
11. Beer JS, John OP, Scabini D, et al: Orbitofrontal cortex and social behavior: integrating self-monitoring and emotion-cognition interactions. *J Cogn Neurosci* 18:871–879, 2006.
12. Phillips ML, Ladouceur CD, Drevets WC: A neural model of voluntary and automatic emotion regulation: implications for understanding the pathophysiology and neurodevelopment of bipolar disorder. *Mol Psychiatry* 13:829–857, 2007.
13. Price JL, Drevets WC: Neurocircuitry of mood disorders. *Neuropsychopharmacology* 35:192–216, 2010.
14. Hare TA, Camerer CF, Knoepfle DT, et al: Value computations in ventral medial prefrontal cortex during charitable decision making incorporate input from regions involved in social cognition. *J Neurosci* 30:583–590, 2010.
15. Bechara A, Damasio AR: The somatic marker hypothesis: a neural theory of economic decision. *Games Econ Behav* 52:336–372, 2005.

16. Bar-On R, Tranel D, Denburg N, et al: Exploring the neurological substrate of emotional and social intelligence. *Brain* 126:1790–1800, 2003.

17. Gleichgerrcht E, Ibáñez A, Roca M, et al: Decision-making cognition in neurodegenerative diseases. *Nat Rev Neurol* 6:611–623, 2010.

18. Hsu M, Bhatt M, Adolphs R, et al: Neural systems responding to degrees of uncertainty in human decision-making. *Science* 310:1680–1683, 2005.

19. Kringelbach ML: The human orbitofrontal cortex: linking reward to hedonic experience. *Nat Rev Neurosci* 6:691–702, 2005.

20. Smith CN, Squire LR: Medial temporal lobe activity during retrieval of semantic memory is related to the age of the memory. *J Neurosci* 29:930–938, 2009.

21. Badre D, Poldrack RA, Paré-Blagoev EJ, et al: Dissociable controlled retrieval and generalized selection mechanisms in ventrolateral prefrontal cortex. *Neuron* 47:907–918, 2005.

22. Benoit M, Robert PH: Neural basis of behavior. In Whitaker HA, editor: *Concise encyclopedia of brain and language*, Amsterdam, 2010, Elsevier, pp 79–84.

23. Bonelli RM, Cummings JL: Frontal-subcortical circuitry and behavior. *Dialogues Clin Neurosci* 9:141–151, 2007.

24. Heatherton TF: Neuroscience of self and self-regulation. *Annu Rev Psychol* 62:363–390, 2011.

25. Piech RM, Lewis J, Parkinson CH, et al: Neural correlates of affective influence on choice. *Brain Cogn* 72:282–282, 2010.

26. Dove A, Manly T, Epstein R, et al: The engagement of mid-ventrolateral prefrontal cortex and posterior brain regions in intentional cognitive activity. *Hum Brain Mapp* 29:107–119, 2008.

27. Guyer AE, Lau JY, McClure-Tone EB, et al: Amygdala and ventrolateral prefrontal cortex function during anticipated peer evaluation in pediatric social anxiety. *Arch Gen Psychiatry* 65:1303–1312, 2008.

28. Young AH: Cortisol in mood disorders. *Stress* 7:205–208, 2004.

29. Kiecolt-Glaser JK, Loving TJ, Stowell JR, et al: Hostile marital interactions, proinflammatory cytokine production, and wound healing. *Arch Gen Psychiatry* 62:1377–1384, 2005.

30. Gouin JP, Kiecolt-Glaser JK: The impact of psychological stress on wound healing: methods and mechanisms. *Immunol Allergy Clin North Am* 31:81–93, 2011.

31. Dhabhar FS: A hassle a day may keep the pathogens away: the fight-or-flight stress response and the augmentation of immune function. *Integr Comp Biol* 49:215–236, 2009.

32. Kiecolt-Glaser JK, Marucha PT, Atkinson C, et al: Hypnosis as a modulator of cellular immune dysregulation during acute stress. *J Consult Clin Psychol* 69:674–682, 2001.

33. Vakalopoulos C: Neuropharmacology of cognition and memory: a unifying theory of neuromodulator imbalance in psychiatry and amnesia. *Med Hypotheses* 66:394–431, 2006.

34. Winocur G, Moscovitch M: Memory transformation and systems consolidation. *J Int Neuropsychol Soc* 17:766–780, 2011.

35. Penfield W: Functional localization in temporal and deep sylvian areas. *Res Publ Assoc Res Nerv Ment Dis* 36:210–226, 1958.

36. Blum S, Hebert AE, Dash PK: A role for the prefrontal cortex in recall of recent and remote memories. *Neuroreport* 17:341–344, 2006.

37. Rutishauser U, Schuman EM, Mamelak AN: Activity of human hippocampal and amygdala neurons during retrieval of declarative memories. *Proc Natl Acad Sci U S A* 105:329–334, 2008.

38. Orban P, Peigneux P, Lungu O, et al: Functional neuroanatomy associated with the expression of distinct movement kinematics in motor sequence learning. *Neuroscience* 179:94–103, 2011.

39. Poldrack RA, Sabb FW, Foerde K, et al: The neural correlates of motor skill automaticity. *J Neurosci* 25:5356–5364, 2005.

40. Selnes O, Whitaker HA: Anatomical asymmetries versus variability of language areas of the brain. In Whitaker HA, editor: *Concise encyclopedia of brain and language*, Amsterdam, 2010, Elsevier, pp 37–40.

41. Vigneau M, Beaucousin V, Hervé P-Y, et al: What is right-hemisphere contribution to phonological, lexico-semantic, and sentence processing? Insights from a meta-analysis. *Neuroimage* 54:577–593, 2011.

42. Zeman A: Consciousness: concepts, neurobiology, terminology of impairments, theoretical models and philosophical background. In Young GB, Wijdicks EFM, editors: *Handbook of clinical neurology*, vol 90, 3rd series, Disorders of consciousness, Amsterdam, 2008, Elsevier, pp 3–31.

43. Benarroch EE: The midline and intralaminar thalamic nuclei: anatomic and functional specificity and implications in neurologic disease. *Neurology* 71:944–949, 2008.

44. Lundin-Olsson L, Nyberg L, Gustafson Y: "Stops walking when talking" as a predictor of falls in elderly people. *Lancet* 349:617, 1997.

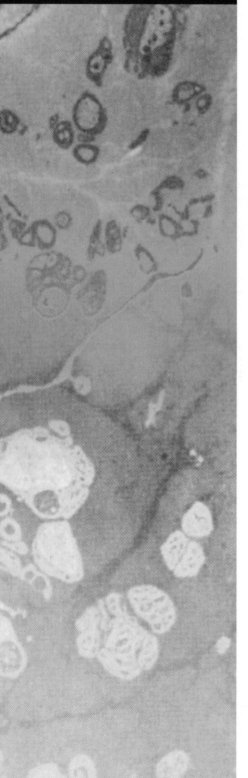

# 18 Cerebrum: Clinical Applications

Laurie Lundy-Ekman, PhD, PT

I am a 39-year-old woman. Before my stroke, I was very athletic. I ran every day. Two years ago, I was at work, filling orders at a shoe warehouse, when I developed an excruciating headache. Before this, I never had headaches. My sister, who worked with me, asked if I needed an ambulance. I didn't think I needed an ambulance for a headache, so she drove me to a local emergency medical clinic. In the car on the way to the clinic, I had seizures. An aneurysm (a dilation of part of a wall of an artery, where the arterial wall is abnormally thin) had burst in my brain, causing bleeding into my brain. I underwent surgery to repair the damaged artery. People told me the doctor was amazed that I survived, and he repaired a second aneurysm during the surgery, so that it would not rupture later. I had another surgery to insert a shunt about 2 weeks later because fluids were not draining normally from my brain.

I don't remember anything about the 2 months following the surgery. The stroke never affected my sensation or language abilities. The first thing I remember is that I couldn't recall how to chew or swallow. I couldn't plan the movements. I had to slowly figure out by trial and error how to eat by myself. Now I can do many things independently, except transfers and walking. Keeping my balance is difficult and fatiguing. When I am sitting, I use my arms for balance. My legs are very weak; I can move them a little when I'm lying down, but I cannot move them when I'm standing. I have had physical therapy since my hospitalization, focusing on balance, transfers, standing, and assisted walking. I take Dilantin to prevent seizures. I also take the antidepressants amitriptyline hydrochloride and nortriptyline hydrochloride.

Amitriptyline hydrochloride also acts as an aid for sleeping, which I need because I am not active enough to get tired.

The stroke has profoundly altered my life. Before the stroke, I was vigorous, healthy, and independent. Now I live in a convalescent home, I use a wheelchair, and I need help to get into and out of the wheelchair. I think about when I could walk before the stroke, and I am planning on walking again.

*—Janet Abernathy*

**Janet's hemorrhage affected the anterior communicating artery, depriving both anterior cerebral arteries of blood flow. In similar cases, the following occurs: Because the anterior caudate and the ventromedial part of the frontal lobes are damaged bilaterally, motivation and emotional expression are severely impaired. People become inactive and apathetic owing to the brain injury; they do not independently initiate any self-care or other activities. Emotional expression is absent in their speech and behavior. The initial difficulty with chewing and swallowing can be caused by damage to medial frontal cortical areas involved in planning movements and by edema interfering with signals in the internal capsule genu (see Figure 17-4). The edema subsequently resolves, allowing cortical signals to reach cranial nerve nuclei in the brainstem, but partially overcoming the difficulties with motor planning requires substitution from other brain areas. The medial frontal lobe lesion interrupts upper motor neurons (UMNs) to the lower limbs, causing both lower limbs to be paretic. Because the lateral cerebrum is not affected (middle cerebral artery is intact), upper limb and trunk function and language and communication are normal.**

This chapter begins with disorders of the deep cerebral structures: thalamus, subcortical white matter, and basal ganglia, and then covers dysfunctions of specific areas of the cerebral cortex. The second part considers cerebral functions that involve several areas of cerebral cortex and specific deep cerebral structures. These functions include control of emotional behavior, memory, communication, spatial understanding, use of visual information, and ability to maintain upright posture. The third part covers diseases and disorders affecting cerebral function. Psychological signs, symptoms, and disorders are discussed in the fourth section. The final section comprises information on testing of cerebral function.

## SITES OF DAMAGE TO CEREBRAL SYSTEMS

### Thalamic Injury

Thalamic lesions involving the relay nuclei interrupt ascending pathways, severely compromising or eliminating contralateral sensation. Usually proprioception is most affected. Rarely, a thalamic pain syndrome ensues after damage to the thalamus, producing severe contralateral pain that may occur with or without provoking external stimuli. Neuronal loss in the intra-laminar nuclei produces moderate to severe disability or a veg-etative state.[1] Intralaminar nuclei are most frequently damaged by Parkinson's disease, thalamic stroke, or traumatic brain injury.[1]

### Subcortical White Matter Lesions

Occlusion or hemorrhage of arteries supplying the *internal capsule* is common. Because the internal capsule is composed of many projection axons, even a small lesion may have severe consequences. For example, a lesion the size of a nickel could interrupt the posterior limb and adjacent gray matter. This would prevent messages in corticospinal and thalamocortical fibers from reaching their destinations, resulting in the following:
• Contralateral decrease in voluntary movement
• Contralateral loss of conscious somatosensation
If the lesion extended more posteriorly, into the retrolen-ticular and sublenticular parts of the capsule, conscious vision from the contralateral visual field would be lost because optic radiation fibers would be interrupted.

### Callosotomy

Remarkable outcomes occur when the huge fiber bundle con-necting the hemispheres, the *corpus callosum,* is surgically severed. Surgery (callosotomy) is performed in cases of intrac-table epilepsy when the excessive neuronal activity that charac-terizes epilepsy cannot be controlled by medication or surgical damage of a single cortical site. Callosotomy is usually success-ful in preventing excessive firing from spreading from one hemisphere to the other, thus limiting the seizure to one hemi-sphere. Although people with callosotomies are rarely seen for rehabilitation, because callosotomies are performed infrequently and because recovery is usually spontaneous, results of callo-sotomies illustrate differences in function between cerebral hemispheres.

Initially, after recovery from surgery, many people with cal-losotomies report conflicts between their hands: the left hand will begin a task, and the right hand will interfere with the left hand's activity. A physical therapist working with a person post callosotomy reported to the doctor, "You should have seen Rocky yesterday—one hand was buttoning up his shirt, and the other hand was coming along right behind it undoing the buttons!"[2] Typically, these competitive hand movements resolve with time. Following recovery, compensation occurs, allowing the person with a "split brain" to interact normally in social situations and to perform normally on most traditional neuro-logic examinations. Specialized tests designed to assess the per-formance of a single hemisphere are required to demonstrate abnormalities.

The most commonly used specialized tests involve assess-ment of vision and stereognosis. Results from right-handed people with callosotomies are summarized here. When words are presented briefly to the right visual field, people are able to read the words. However, when words are flashed in the left visual field, people are unable to read them and often report seeing nothing.

For somatosensory tests, people handle objects that are out of sight. For example, when handling a comb in the right hand, a person with a callosotomy is able to name and verbally describe the comb, yet is unable to demonstrate using the comb. If the comb is handled by the left hand, the same person is able to demonstrate its use but is unable to name it.

Why the great disparity in the abilities of the separated hemispheres? Information presented to the right visual field or the right hand projects to the language-dominant left hemi-sphere, so the person is able to name and describe the word or object. Information from the left visual field or the left hand is processed in the right cerebral hemisphere, which excels at comprehending space, manipulating objects, and perceiving shapes. Thus the person is able to manipulate the object appro-priately but cannot name or verbally describe the object because, in most people, the right hemisphere does not process language.

### Caudate/Ventral Striatum Disorders

In contrast to the movement disorders associated with lenticular dysfunction (see Chapter 11), lesions or dysfunctions of the caudate/ventral striatum rarely cause motor disorders but instead cause behavioral disturbances. The most common behavioral abnormality secondary to caudate/ventral striatum damage is apathy, with loss of initiative, spontaneous thought, and emotional responses.[3] Conversely, excessive activity of the circuit connecting the caudate, anterior cingulate cortex, and ventral prefrontal cortex is correlated with obsessive-compulsive disorders,[4] discussed in the psychological disorders section.

## DISORDERS OF SPECIFIC AREAS OF THE CEREBRAL CORTEX

### Primary Sensory Areas: Loss of Discriminative Sensory Information

Lesions of the primary sensory areas impair the ability to dis-criminate intensity and quality of stimuli, severely interfering with the capacity to use the sensations. Lesions of the primary somatosensory cortex interfere most with the localization of tactile stimuli and with proprioception. Crude awareness of touch and thermal stimuli is not affected in lesions of the primary somatosensory cortex, because crude awareness occurs in the thalamus. Also, lesions confined to the primary somato-sensory cortex do not compromise localization of pain. Pain information is processed in the secondary somatosensory cortex, the insula, and the anterior cingulate cortex rather than in the primary somatosensory cortex.[5]

Because auditory information has extensive bilateral projec-tions to the cortex, a lesion in the primary auditory cortex only interferes with the ability to localize sounds (see Chapter 14).

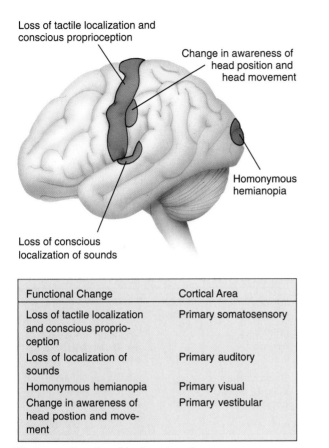

**Fig. 18-1** Results of lesions in primary sensory areas.

| Functional Change | Cortical Area |
| --- | --- |
| Loss of tactile localization and conscious proprio-ception | Primary somatosensory |
| Loss of localization of sounds | Primary auditory |
| Homonymous hemianopia | Primary visual |
| Change in awareness of head postion and move-ment | Primary vestibular |

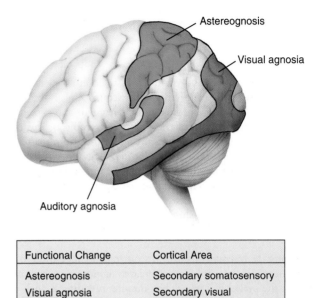

| Functional Change | Cortical Area |
| --- | --- |
| Astereognosis | Secondary somatosensory |
| Visual agnosia | Secondary visual |
| Auditory agnosia | Secondary auditory |

**Fig. 18-2** Results of lesions in secondary sensory areas.

Lesions in the primary vestibular cortex interfere with conscious awareness of head position and movement. Primary visual cortex lesions cause contralateral homonymous hemianopia (see Chapter 16). The consequences of lesions in primary sensory areas are illustrated in Figure 18-1.

## Secondary Sensory Areas: Agnosia

*Agnosia* is the general term for the inability to recognize objects when using a specific sense, even though discriminative ability with that sense is intact. Agnosia subtypes include:
• Astereognosis
• Visual agnosia
• Auditory agnosia

## Astereognosis

*Astereognosis* is the inability to identify objects by touch and manipulation despite intact discriminative somatosensation. A person with astereognosis would be able to describe an object being palpated but would not recognize the object by touching and manipulating it. Astereognosis results from lesions in the secondary somatosensory area. A person with astereognosis affecting the information from one hand may avoid using that hand as a result of perceptual changes if information from the other hand is processed normally.

## Visual Agnosia

Similarly, lesions in the secondary visual area interfere with the ability to recognize objects in the contralateral visual field, although the capacity for visual discrimination remains intact. *Visual agnosia* is the inability to visually recognize objects despite having intact vision. A person with visual agnosia can describe the shape and size of objects using vision but cannot identify the objects visually.

A highly specific type of visual agnosia is *prosopagnosia*. People with this rare condition are unable to visually identify people's faces, despite being able to correctly interpret emotional facial expressions and being able to visually recognize other items in the environment. Only visual recognition is defective; people can be identified by their voices or by mannerisms. Prosopagnosia is usually associated with bilateral damage to the inferior secondary visual areas (part of the ventral stream).

## Auditory Agnosia

Destruction of the secondary auditory cortex spares the ability to perceive sound but deprives the person of recognition of sounds. If the lesion destroys the left secondary auditory cortex, the person is unable to understand speech (see later section). Destruction of the right auditory cortex interferes with interpretation of environmental sounds.[6] For example, a person cannot distinguish between the sound of a doorbell and the sound of footsteps. The areas of cortex involved in agnosias are illustrated in Figure 18-2.

**◎ Clinical Pearl**

Agnosia results from damage to secondary sensory areas.

## Motor Planning Areas: Apraxia, Motor Perseveration, and Broca's Aphasia

*Apraxia* can be considered motor agnosia; the knowledge of how to perform skilled movement is lost.[7] In apraxia, a person is unable to perform a movement or a sequence of movements despite intact sensation, normal muscle strength and coordination, and understanding of the task. An example is brushing one's teeth with a dry toothbrush, then putting toothpaste on the brush. Another example is putting socks on over shoes. Apraxia occurs as a result of damage to the premotor or supplementary motor areas or the inferior parietal lobe.[7] A subtype of apraxia, *constructional apraxia,* interferes with the ability to comprehend the relationship of parts to the whole. This deficit impairs the ability to draw and to arrange objects correctly in space.

*Motor perseveration* is the uncontrollable repetition of a movement. For example, a person may continue to lock and unlock the brakes of a wheelchair despite intending to lock the brakes. Motor perseveration is more associated with the amount of neural damage than with damage to a specific site.[8]

*Broca's aphasia* is difficulty expressing oneself using language or symbols. A person with Broca's aphasia is impaired in both speaking and writing. Broca's aphasia occurs with damage to Broca's area and will be discussed further in a later section.

## Primary Motor Cortex: Loss of Movement Fractionation and Dysarthria

Damage to the primary motor cortex is characterized by contralateral paresis and loss of fractionation of movement. The worst effects are distal: people with complete destruction of the primary motor cortex cannot voluntarily move their contralateral hand, lower face, and/or foot because movements of these parts of the body are controlled exclusively by the contralateral primary motor cortex.

*Dysarthria* is a speech disorder resulting from spasticity or paresis of the muscles used for speaking. Two types of dysarthria can be distinguished: spastic and flaccid. Damage to upper motor neurons causes *spastic dysarthria,* which is characterized by harsh, awkward speech. In contrast, damage to lower motor neurons (cranial nerves IX, X, and/or XII) causes paresis of speech muscles, producing *flaccid dysarthria.* Flaccid dysarthria is breathy, soft, and imprecise speech. In pure dysarthria, only the production of speech is impaired; language generation and comprehension are unaffected. The difficulty involves the mechanics of producing sounds accurately, not finding words or grammar. Lesions in areas of cortex that produce motor disorders are illustrated in Figure 18-3.

### ◎ *Clinical Pearl*

The four A's for remembering cerebral cortex disorders are aphasia, apraxia, agnosia, and astereognosis. These disorders indicate damage to specific areas of the cerebral cortex.

## Dorsolateral Prefrontal Association Cortex: Loss of Executive Functions and Divergent Thinking

Although physical therapy and occupational therapy do not focus on remediation of association cortex deficits, these deficits

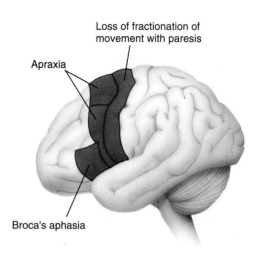

| Functional Change | Motor Areas |
|---|---|
| Paresis, loss of fine motor control, spastic dysarthria | Primary motor cortex |
| Apraxia | Premotor area |
| Apraxia | Supplementary motor area |
| Broca's aphasia or difficulty producing nonverbal communication | Broca's area (usually in left hemisphere) or analogous area in opposite hemisphere |

**Fig. 18-3** Results of lesions in motor areas of the cerebral cortex.

may have a profound influence on compliance and outcomes. Apathy and lack of goal-directed behavior are typical of people with lesions in the dorsolateral prefrontal area. People with damage to this region have difficulty with executive functions: choosing goals, planning, executing plans, and monitoring the execution of a plan. Lack of initiative may interfere with the ability to live independently and to be employed. In extreme cases, the person may not attend to basic needs, including eating and drinking. The behavior of people with dorsolateral prefrontal damage may be misinterpreted as uncooperative, when actually they have lost the neural capacity to initiate goal-directed action.

Lesions in the dorsolateral prefrontal cortex have little effect on intelligence as measured by conventional intelligence tests. People with prefrontal damage are able to perform paper-and-pencil problem-solving tasks nearly as well as they were able to before the damage occurred. This may be because conventional intelligence tests assess convergent thinking, or the ability to choose one correct response from a list of choices. In people with prefrontal lesions, divergent thinking, the ability to conceive of a variety of possibilities, is impaired.[9] For example, if asked to list possible uses of a stick, they perform much worse than people without brain damage. Despite the ability to perform normally on conventional intelligence tests, people with prefrontal lesions function poorly in daily life because they lack goal orientation and behavioral flexibility because of loss of executive functions and limited divergent thinking.

Dorsolateral prefrontal syndrome consists of inability to initiate behavior, apathy, flat affect, perseveration, and lack of cognitive flexibility.

## Parietotemporal Association Areas: Problems With Communication, Understanding Space, and Directing Attention

Parietotemporal association areas are specialized for communication and for comprehending space. Damage to this area in the left hemisphere causes Wernicke's aphasia, a language disturbance. Damage to the same area in the right hemisphere causes deficits in directing attention, comprehending space, and understanding nonverbal communication. Detailed discussion of these areas and disorders is deferred to a later section. Results of lesions in the association cortex are illustrated in Figure 18-4.

## Ventral and Medial Dorsal Prefrontal Association Cortex: Personality and Emotional Changes

The ventral prefrontal association cortex (VPAC) includes the ventrolateral prefrontal, orbital, and ventromedial prefrontal cortex. Damage to these areas interferes with the emotional response to inferred emotional events, that is, people with VPAC are impaired in feeling empathy, embarrassment, guilt, and regret.[10] Damage to the VPAC leads to inappropriate and risky behavior.[11] People with these lesions have intact intellectual abilities but use poor judgment, are impulsive, and have difficulty conforming to social conventions.

Bechara and associates (2002)[12] reported that people with damage to the ventral prefrontal association cortex are unable to make sound decisions in an experimental card game. Unlike people with intact nervous systems or those with brain damage to other areas, people with lesions in the ventral prefrontal association cortex showed no elevation of galvanic skin response before picking a card from a high-risk deck. People with intact VPAC had an elevated galvanic skin response before selecting cards from a high-risk deck, and based on somatic marker

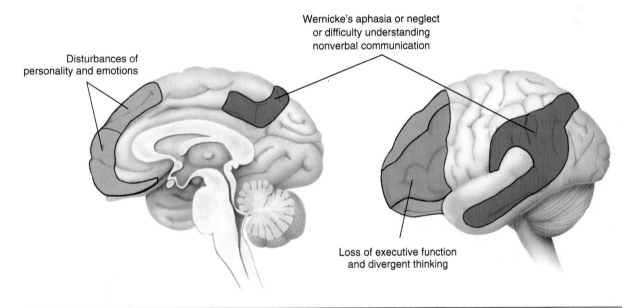

| Functional change | Association cortex |
|---|---|
| Loss of executive function and divergent thinking | Dorsolateral prefrontal association |
| Inability to handle new information effectively; concrete thinking, inability to distinguish relevant from irrelevant information, difficulty generalizing information, become upset with even minor changes in routine | Parietotemporal association |
| Wenicke's aphasia | Parietotemporal association usually in left hemisphere |
| Neglect and/or difficulty understanding nonverbal communication | Parietotemporal association usually in right hemisphere |
| Disturbances of personality and emotions | Ventral and medial dorsal prefrontal association |

**Fig. 18-4** Results of lesions in the association cortex.

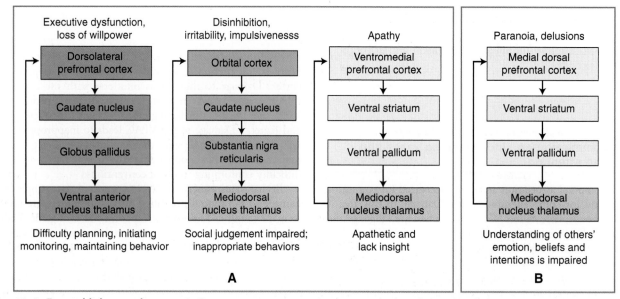

**Fig. 18-5 Frontal lobe syndromes. A,** Damage to structures in the cortico-basal ganglia-thalamic circuit causes the dysfunctions cited above the circuit, and more information about the syndrome is listed below the circuit. **B,** Abnormal processing in the circuit causes the dysfunctions and signs and symptoms listed.

signals from sympathetic nervous system activation (sweaty palms, nervous stomach, neck muscle tension), they quickly gravitated toward selecting from the low-risk deck to minimize their losses. People with VPAC lesions, absent somatic marker signals of risk, increasingly preferred to select from the high-risk deck, quickly losing all the play money. Thus a possible explanation of the inappropriate behavior is lack of a sense of risk, that is, no emotional concern about outcomes.

Medial dorsal prefrontal cortex is involved in self-control[13] and in perceiving others' emotions and inferring others' beliefs and intentions.[14] In people with schizophrenia who wrongly ascribe emotions, intentions, and beliefs to other people, the medial dorsal prefrontal cortex is less active than normal.[15] Figure 18-5 summarizes the prefrontal syndromes.

> ### ◉ Clinical Pearl
>
> Ventral prefrontal syndrome (also known as *orbital syndrome*) consists of disinhibition, lack of concern about consequences, impulsiveness, and inappropriate behaviors. The medial dorsal prefrontal cortex makes inferences about what other people are feeling, thinking, and intending to do, and contributes to self-control.

## DECISION MAKING AND SOMATIC MARKER DYSFUNCTION

Making good decisions depends on a balance between an emotional, impulsive, immediate system centered in the amygdala and a dorsolateral prefrontal rational cortex.[16] The somatic marker circuitry in the ventromedial and orbital prefrontal cortex integrates emotional and rational information to guide behavior.[17]

The role of the amygdalae in decision making is illustrated by a woman with damage to both amygdalae.[18] She never feels afraid, even when threatened with a knife or a gun. Police reports support her recall of crime experiences. The researchers note that she fails to detect threats and to learn to avoid dangerous situations. During a trip to a pet store with the researchers, she repeatedly asked to touch venomous snakes.[18] She has difficulty recognizing the fear conveyed by people's facial expressions, and she makes poor social and personal decisions. Despite these deficits, her memory for facts and events and her ability to feel other emotions are completely intact. Phelps (2006)[19] concludes that the amygdala has a role in social learning and in behavior associated with personal interactions.

In lesions that affect the somatic marker circuitry, poor judgment and defective social intelligence cause severe problems in social function, employment, interpersonal relationships, and social status. Although executive functions and cognitive intelligence are intact, people with lesions in the somatic marker circuitry fail to learn from their mistakes.[20] This occurs because brain areas that make decisions about behavior are separate from the areas that make decisions about goals and from areas essential for cognitive intelligence. Social intelligence depends on integration of information from structures that process emotions with analytic information, whereas executive functions require the dorsolateral prefrontal cortex and the parietal cortex.[21,22]

Damasio (1994)[23] reported that a man with damage to the ventral prefrontal cortex was unable to choose between two dates for a return appointment. For nearly a half hour, the man considered the pros and cons of the dates without approaching a conclusion. When told to come on the second date, he quickly accepted the suggestion. According to Damasio, in the absence of emotional cues that some considerations were more important than others, and without the sense that the decision was trivial, the man with ventral prefrontal damage was unable to make decisions. In other circumstances, that is, driving on icy roads, the same man performed well because he remained calm even when witnessing accidents. The ventral prefrontal syndrome consists of disinhibition, impulsivity, and emotional lability.[24]

## EMOTIONAL LABILITY

Changes in the expression of emotion may occur following brain lesions. Emotional lability (also called *labile affect*) is abnormal, uncontrolled expression of emotions.

Emotional lability has three aspects:

1. Abrupt mood shifts, usually to anger, depression, or anxiety
2. Involuntary, inappropriate emotional expression in the absence of subjective emotion (pathologic laughter or crying)
3. Emotion is triggered by nonspecific stimuli unrelated to the emotional expression

The emotional expression may or may not be congruent with the person's mood. For example, the person may laugh uncontrollably while he or she is feeling sad, or may cry excessively when feeling only slightly sad. The prevalence of emotional lability in a variety of neurologic conditions is listed in Table 18-1.

**TABLE 18-1   PREVALENCE OF EMOTIONAL LABILITY IN NEUROLOGIC CONDITIONS**

| Neurologic Condition | Percent With Emotional Lability |
|---|---|
| Amyotrophic lateral sclerosis | 50% |
| Alzheimer's disease | 39% |
| Multiple sclerosis | 46% |
| Parkinson's disease | 24% |
| Stroke | 28% |
| Traumatic brain injury | 48% |

Data from Work SS, Colamonico JA, Bradley WG, et al: Pseudobulbar affect: an under-recognized and under-treated neurological disorder. *Adv Ther* 28:586–601, 2011.

## THE REWARD PATHWAY AND MOTIVATIONAL DISORDERS

The reward pathway comprises dopamine neurons from the ventral tegmental area in the midbrain to the ventral striatum.[25,26] All natural stimuli that reinforce behavior and all drugs of abuse increase dopamine in the ventral striatum.[27] Thus dopamine is the motivation neurotransmitter.[28]

The ability of a drug to increase dopamine in the ventral striatum predicts whether the drug is addictive in a specific person. *Addiction* is loss of behavioral control in response to a stimulus combined with continued use of a substance regardless of negative consequences. People who are addicted to alcohol, cocaine, methamphetamine, heroin, or nicotine have lower levels of certain dopamine receptor types than people without drug addictions; whether this is a cause or an effect of drug abuse is unknown. In the reward pathway, amphetamines promote the release of dopamine and norepinephrine; cocaine blocks the reuptake of dopamine; heroin and morphine block the release of inhibitory transmitters; and nicotine activates acetylcholine receptors that depolarize ventral tegmental area dopamine neurons.[29] The action of alcohol is more complex: alcohol initially causes release of dopamine, opioid peptides, and gamma-aminobutyric acid (GABA).[30] Dopamine and opioid peptides elicit feelings of pleasure. GABA reduces social inhibition and motor control. Large quantities of alcohol decrease the release of those transmitters and increase the release of corticotropin-releasing factor (CRF). CRF activates the amygdala, causing anxiety, and anxiety is involved in the decision to drink again.[31] In addition to the reward pathway pathology in addiction, prefrontal cortex executive function is diminished and orbital cortex activity is enhanced, causing impaired decision making with more impulsive behavior and less concern for long-term consequences.[32] The reward pathway and the projections of the ventral striatum are illustrated in Figure 18-6. The risk for drug addiction depends on the interplay of genetics, mental disorders, developmental stage of the person, social environment, and how the drug is taken.

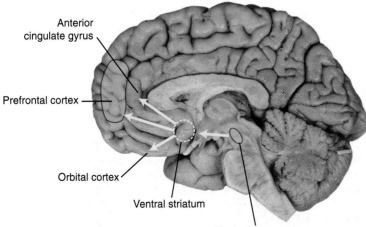

**Fig. 18-6 The reward pathway from the ventral tegmental area to the ventral striatum.** The ventral striatum projects to the orbital cortex, anterior cingulate cortex, and prefrontal cortex. Photograph courtesy of John W. Sundsten, Department of Biological Structures, University of Washington. *(Modified from copyright 1994, University of Washington. From Digital Anatomist Interactive Brain Atlas and the Structural Informatics Group.)*

## DECLARATIVE MEMORY FAILURE: AMNESIA

*Amnesia* is the loss of declarative memory. Retrograde amnesia involves loss of memories for events that occurred before the trauma or disease that caused the condition. In H.M. (see Chapter 17), after removal of both hippocampi, his past memories were intact, but he could not remember events that occurred after the surgery. This loss of memory for events following the event that caused the amnesia is called *anterograde amnesia.*

People with amnesia retain the ability to form new preferences, despite lacking cognitive awareness of the preferences. A patient with postencephalitic amnesia was studied to determine whether he would learn to distinguish among different response patterns of staff members. Three staff members consistently provided different responses to his request for special foods: positive, negative, and neutral. When asked whom he would ask for special foods, he indicated the staff member who responded positively to his requests, although he was totally unable to show familiarity with any of the staff members.[33] The patient's behavior demonstrated his ability to unconsciously recall the staff member who would provide him with special foods.

The dissociation of declarative and procedural memory is important clinically. People with severe declarative memory deficits following head trauma learn new motor skills at the same rate as people without declarative memory deficits, despite their inability to consciously recall having practiced the tasks.[34] Motor, perceptual, and cognitive skills and habits can be learned even when declarative memory fails.[34]

## LANGUAGE DISORDERS

Disorders of language can affect spoken language (*aphasia*), comprehension of written language (*alexia*), and/or the ability to write (*agraphia*). Because aphasia has the most severe impact on communication during treatment, the following discussion focuses on aphasia. Common types of aphasia are Broca's, Wernicke's, conduction, and global.

*Broca's aphasia* is defined as difficulty expressing oneself using language. The ability to understand language except grammatical function words (prepositions, pronouns, conjunctions) and an ability to control the muscles used in speech for other purposes (swallowing, chewing) are not affected. People with Broca's aphasia may not produce any language output, or they may be able to generate habitual phrases, such as "Hello. How are you?" or make brief meaningful statements, and may be able to produce emotional speech (obscenities, curses) when upset. People with Broca's aphasia usually are aware of their language difficulties and are frustrated by their inability to produce normal language. Usually writing is as impaired as speaking. The ability to understand spoken language except grammatical function words and to read is spared. Motor, expressive, and nonfluent types of aphasia are synonymous with Broca's aphasia.

In *Wernicke's aphasia,* language comprehension is impaired. People with Wernicke's aphasia easily produce spoken sounds, but the output is meaningless. An example of a meaningless phrase repeated by one of my patients is "Wishrab lamislar blagg." For a person with Wernicke's aphasia, listening to other people speak is equally meaningless, despite the ability to hear

normally. The inability to produce and understand language may be analogous to when a person with an intact native language encounters an unknown foreign language. Wernicke's aphasia also interferes with the ability to comprehend and produce symbolic movements, as in sign language.[35] Because the ability to comprehend language is impaired, people with Wernicke's aphasia have alexia (inability to read), inability to write meaningful words, and paraphasia. *Paraphasia* is the use of unintended words or phrases. Paraphasia ranges from word substitution to the use of nonsensical, unrecognizable words. An example of word substitution is saying or writing "captain of the school" instead of "principal." Unlike people with Broca's aphasia, people with Wernicke's aphasia often appear to be unaware of the disorder. Synonyms for Wernicke's aphasia include receptive, sensory, and fluent aphasia, although language output is also abnormal.

*Conduction aphasia* results from damage to the neurons that connect Wernicke's and Broca's areas. In the most severe form, the speech and writing of people with conduction aphasia are meaningless. However, their ability to understand written and spoken language is normal. In mild cases, only substitution paraphasia occur.

The most severe form of aphasia is *global aphasia,* an inability to use language in any form. People with global aphasia cannot produce understandable speech, comprehend spoken language, speak fluently, read, or write. Global aphasia is usually secondary to a large lesion damaging much of the lateral left cerebrum: Broca's area, Wernicke's area, intervening cortex, adjacent white matter, caudate, and anterior thalamus. Common types of aphasia are summarized in Table 18-2.

## DISORDERS OF NONVERBAL COMMUNICATION

Damage to the right cortex in the area corresponding to Broca's area may cause the person to speak in a monotone, to be unable to effectively communicate nonverbally, and to lack emotional facial expressions and gestures. These consequences are sometimes referred to as *flat affect.* If the area corresponding to Wernicke's is damaged on the right side, the person has difficulty understanding nonverbal communication. Thus the person may be unable to distinguish between hearing "Get out of here" spoken jokingly and "GET OUT OF HERE!" spoken in anger. As noted earlier, the area corresponding to Wernicke's area is also important for body image and for understanding the relationship between self and the environment. Damage to the area corresponding to Wernicke's area may cause neglect.

## NEGLECT

The tendency to behave as if one side of the body and/or one side of space does not exist is called *neglect.* People with neglect fail to report or respond to stimuli present on the contralesional side. Neglect usually affects the left side of the body because the right parietal area is necessary for directing attention, and the area analogous to Wernicke's in the right hemisphere comprehends spatial relationships.[36] In people with left neglect, underactivity of damaged right brain attention areas is associated with hyperactivity in the left brain attention system.[37] Neglect may be misinterpreted by others as confusion or lack

**TABLE 18-2    COMMUNICATION DISORDERS**

| Name | Synonyms | Characteristics | Comprehend Spoken Speech | Speak Fluently | Produce Meaningful Language | Normal Use of Grammatical Words | Read | Write | Structures Involved |
|---|---|---|---|---|---|---|---|---|---|
| Dysarthria | None | Lacks motor control of speech muscles | Yes | No | Yes, although difficult to understand | Yes | Yes | Yes | Lower motor neurons or corticobrainstem neurons |
| Broca's aphasia | Motor, expressive, or nonfluent aphasia | Grammatical omissions and errors, short phrases, effortful speech | Yes, except grammatical function words | No | Yes, although grammatical words missing | No | Yes | No | Broca's area, usually in left hemisphere |
| Wernicke's aphasia | Sensory, receptive, or fluent aphasia | Cannot comprehend language; speaks fluently but unintelligibly | No | Yes | No | No | No | No | Wernicke's area, usually in left hemisphere |
| Conduction aphasia | Disconnection aphasia | Understands language; language output unintelligible | Yes | Yes | No | No | Yes | No | Neurons connecting Wernicke's area with Broca's area |
| Global aphasia | Total aphasia | Cannot speak fluently; cannot communicate verbally; cannot understand language | No | No | No | No | No | No | Wernicke's area, Broca's area, and the intervening cortical and subcortical areas |

of cooperation. Neglect can be personal or spatial. Aspects of personal neglect include the following:

- Unilateral lack of awareness of sensory stimuli
- Unilateral lack of personal hygiene and grooming
- Unilateral lack of movement of the limbs

Personal neglect results from failure to direct attention, affecting awareness of one's own body parts. Therefore personal neglect is also called *hemi-inattention.* Some people with personal neglect are able to localize light touch and to distinguish between sharp and dull if a stimulus is presented unilaterally, but fail to respond to stimulation on one side when both sides of the body are stimulated concurrently. This phenomenon is called *bilateral simultaneous extinction* (see Chapter 7).

A form of denial, *anosognosia,* occurs in some people with severe hemiparesis and personal neglect. People with anosognosia deny their inability to use the paretic limbs, claiming they could clap their hands or climb a ladder. However, when asked what the experimenter would be able to do if he had exactly the same impairments as theirs, people with anosognosia who claimed they could perform the tasks reported that the experimenter would be impaired or unable to do the same task.[38] Some people with anosognosia believe the impaired limb belongs to someone else.[39] In anosognosia, the lesion is often in the right anterior insula, an area devoted to representation of self and distinguishing between self and others.[39]

Spatial neglect is characterized by a unilateral lack of understanding of spatial relationships, resulting in a deranged internal representation of space. In an intriguing investigation of spatial neglect, Bisiach and Luzzatti (1978)[40] asked two people with neglect to describe from memory what they would see when looking at the main square in Milan from the steps of the cathedral, and then to describe the same scene looking across the square at the cathedral. When describing the view from the steps of the cathedral, both people consistently mentioned buildings on the right side of the visualized scene. When asked to mentally change their perspective, imagining looking at the cathedral, both described buildings on the right side and omitted buildings they had described moments earlier. Similarly, one of my patients, who had been a successful artist, painted the right half of a scene, leaving the left half of the canvas blank. She claimed the painting was finished and appeared perplexed when questioned about the missing parts of the boy in the painting. When I inverted the canvas to show her that the painting was incomplete, she began a new, different painting on the fresh canvas, oblivious to the image on the left side. Figure 18-7 illustrates aspects of spatial neglect.

Some aspects of neglect are currently unexplained. Bisiach and Berti (1989)[41] have shown that when a person with spatial neglect was asked to copy three figures, he completed both the right and left figures but drew only half of the central figure. Attentional theories of neglect would predict that the person would omit the left figure, not part of the central figure.

Manifestations of spatial neglect include problems with:

- Navigation
- Construction
- Dressing

One aspect of a deficit in understanding spatial relationships is difficulty with finding the correct route to a location. People with spatial neglect may have difficulty finding their way even within a single room. People with spatial neglect may catch part of a wheelchair on an object and continue to try to move forward, unaware of the object interfering with the intended movement. An inpatient with severe neglect at the hospital I worked at tried to drive himself home. Fortunately, he didn't make it to the street, although he did total three cars on his left side in the parking lot. When security personnel reached him, he was still flooring the accelerator despite his car's inability to move the wrecked mass of the other three cars, and he was unaware of any problem.

Decreased comprehension of spatial relationships also causes construction apraxia and difficulty with drawing and assembling. *Dressing apraxia* is difficulty with dressing due to an inability to correctly orient clothing to the body.

People with neglect may have only one sign (e.g., lack of awareness of people or objects on their left) or any combination of signs. In most cases, neglect follows damage to the right cortex in the parietal lobe, the superior temporal lobe, or the area corresponding to Wernicke's area.[42] Thus neglect is a complex phenomenon, with different presentations and diverse causes.

## INABILITY TO USE VISUAL INFORMATION

Visual information is used independently in the ventral and dorsal visual streams.[43] The ventral stream is involved with perception and identification of visual objects, and the dorsal stream contributes to actions based on visual input. For example, a woman with damage to the ventral stream was profoundly unable to consciously recognize the shape, orientation, or size of objects, yet she was able to pick up the unrecognized objects using a normal approach and anticipatory positioning of her hand and fingers. If she saw a glass of water, she could not identify it using vision. But if she reached for the glass, her hand was oriented correctly, and the space between the thumb and fingers was appropriate to grasp the glass. Thus despite visual agnosia, use of visual information for controlling movement was normal. The opposite impairment was noted in another woman with damage in the parietal lobe: she was unable to adjust her reach and hand orientation appropriately to the size and shape of objects, yet she was able to describe and visually identify the objects. Thus, optic ataxia does not affect the ability to consciously perceive visual information.

## LATEROPULSION

Approximately 10% of people post stroke exhibit the unusual behavior of lateropulsion. *Lateropulsion* is a powerful pushing away from the less paretic side in sitting, during transfers, during standing, and during walking. The patient extends the nonparetic arm and leg and pushes, creating a high risk for falls. People who present with this behavior are extremely resistant to attempts to passively adjust their posture to a symmetric position. This problem is sometimes called *pusher syndrome* or *contratraversive pushing.* Lateropulsion appears to be a response to a specific deficit in sensing postural alignment relative to gravity due to a lesion of the posterior thalamus[44] causing spatial inattention[45] or a medullary lesion affecting the vestibular nuclei. At 1 week post stroke, 63% of people demonstrated lateropulsion; however, only 21% of those persisted in pushing

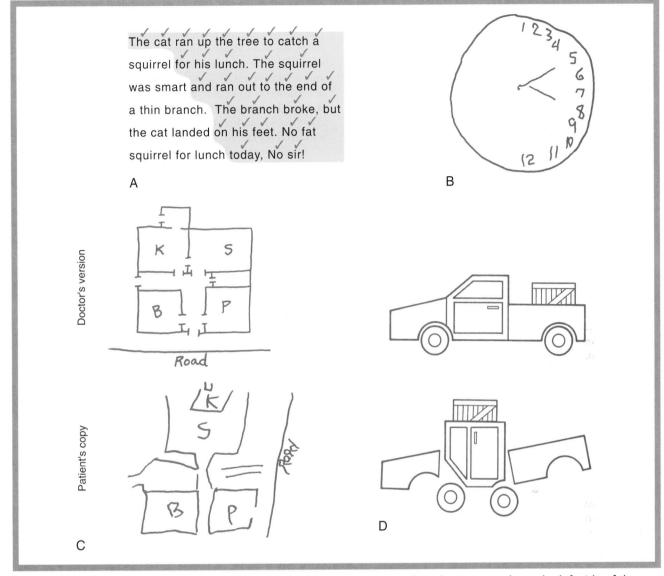

**Fig. 18-7 Signs indicating neglect. A,** Patient is asked to read a paragraph and misses words on the left side of the text. **B,** When asked to draw a clock, the patient draws a circle yet places all or most of the numbers on the right side for the clock face. **C,** Compare the doctor's version of a house floor plan with the patient's version. **D,** Patient is unable to duplicate a block construction while looking at a model. *(From Haines DE: Fundamental neuroscience for basic and clinical applications, ed 3, Philadelphia, 2006, Churchill Livingstone.)*

at 3 months. Motor recovery requires more time in people with lateropulsion, but they do attain significant motor and functional recovery.[46] Karnath and colleagues (2002)[47] report that lateropulsion has a good prognosis: 6 months after stroke, the pathologic pushing is usually resolved.

## DISEASES AND DISORDERS AFFECTING CEREBRAL FUNCTION

### Loss of Consciousness

At any age, a blow to the head may cause temporary loss of consciousness. Loss of consciousness results from movement of the cerebral hemispheres relative to the brainstem, causing torque of the brainstem, and from an abrupt increase in intracranial pressure. Consciousness may also be impaired by large, space-occupying lesions of the cerebrum, located in the diencephalon or exerting pressure on the brainstem.

### Impaired Attention

The ability to pay attention is limited by the total amount of attention available and by abilities to orient, divide, select, sustain, and switch attention. *Orienting* is the ability to locate specific sensory information from among many stimuli.[48] Most people orient to another person's eyes when conversing. Children with autism fail to orient to others' eyes.[49] *Divided attention* is the ability to attend to two or more things simultaneously. The ability to divide attention is assessed with dual tasks. *Dual tasks* are frequently used during therapy, both to assess the ability to perform tasks simultaneously and as a treatment technique. An example is asking a person to respond to questions while he or she continues walking. People post stroke, with traumatic head injury, with Parkinson's disease, or with Alzheimer's benefit from walking training combined with cognitive tasks to improve divided attention.[50-52] Walking requires attention even in healthy young adults.[53]

*Selective attention* is the ability to attend to important information and ignore distractions. Deficits in selective attention make it difficult to concentrate on a specific task. People with severe traumatic brain injury have deficits in selective, total, sustained, and switching attention.[54] An example of impaired selective attention is being unable to focus on a conversation when other conversations are occurring nearby. *Sustained attention* is the ability to continue an activity over time. Many tasks, including reading a book, driving a car, having a conversation, and building furniture, require persistent attentiveness. *Switching attention* is the ability to change from one task to another. If you are intently thinking about an urgent problem and receive a phone call, it can be difficult to pay attention to the person calling. Another example is transferring information from a piece of paper to a computer spreadsheet. People with an attention switching deficit have difficulty transferring attention from one task to a different task, and thus make many errors on the second task, or they become so frustrated that they can't continue with the second task. Figure 18-8 illustrates cortical areas associated with various aspects of attention.

## Attention Deficit Hyperactivity Disorder

Difficulty sustaining attention with onset during childhood is called *attention deficit hyperactivity disorder (ADHD)*. People with ADHD display developmentally inappropriate inattention and impulsiveness. Their attention deficit affects every aspect of attention.[55] Deficits in executive function, working memory, and the dopamine reward pathway cause difficulty maintaining attention when they are uninterested in a task. However, people with ADHD can concentrate on tasks that interest them.

Specific cerebral structures and the reward pathway show abnormalities in ADHD. In unmedicated children with ADHD, circuits that link the prefrontal cortex to the striatum, parietal cortex, and cerebellum, and the parietal cortex to the temporal cortex, are abnormal.[56] Also in unmedicated children with ADHD, the volume of gray matter is reduced in the orbital cortex, the caudate nucleus, the ventral striatum, and the cerebellum.[57] Adults with ADHD show an inability to attend to boring or uninteresting tasks, an inability to delay gratification, and a preference for small immediate rewards over larger delayed rewards—signs of difficulties with the reward and motivation system.[58] In unmedicated adults with ADHD without a history of recreational drug use, dopamine deficits in the reward pathway (ventral tegmental area to ventral striatum) are associated with impaired attention.[58]

ADHD affects 2% to 6% of children and 2% to 4% of adults.[59,60] Girls with ADHD are more likely to be inattentive than boys.[61] Boys with ADHD tend to be hyperactive or impulsive. The disorder usually persists into adulthood, impairing social, academic, and work capabilities.[60] Heritability is estimated to be greater than 75%.[59] Stimulant medication improves all aspects of attention, although selective, divided, orienting,

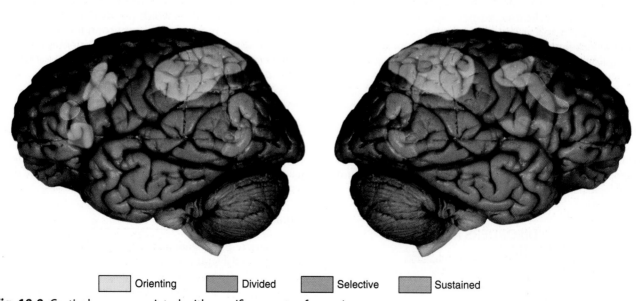

☐ Orienting    ■ Divided    ■ Selective    ☐ Sustained

**Fig. 18-8** Cortical areas associated with specific aspects of consciousness. *(Modified from copyright 1994, University of Washington. From Digital Anatomist Interactive Brain Atlas and the Structural Informatics Group.)*

and switching remain impaired relative to age- and gender-matched controls.[55] Stimulant medication improves social behavior, academic performance, and cognition in both children and adults.[55,62]

## Autism Spectrum Disorders

Characteristics of autism, Asperger's syndrome, and pervasive developmental disorder include a range of impaired social skills, restricted interests, and repetitive behaviors, as described in Chapter 5. Abnormal anatomy and connectivity of the limbic and striatal social brain systems are found in children and adults with autism spectrum disorders.[63] In people who develop autism, the brain grows abnormally rapidly for the first few years, beginning soon after birth; then the rate of brain development slows. The pattern as well as the pace of brain development is abnormal. An immune attack on brain proteins, in addition to genetic factors, may cause autism spectrum disorders.[64,65]

## Epilepsy

Epilepsy is characterized by sudden attacks of excessive cortical neuronal discharge interfering with brain function. Involuntary movements, disruption of autonomic regulation, illusions, and hallucinations may occur. Partial seizures affect only a restricted area of the cortex. Generalized seizures affect the entire cortex. The two main types of generalized seizures are absence seizures, identified by brief loss of consciousness without motor manifestations, and tonic-clonic seizures, which begin with tonic contraction of the skeletal muscles followed by alternating contraction and relaxation of muscles. Typically the tonic and clonic phases last about 1 minute each. After the seizure, the person is confused for several minutes and has no memory of the seizure. Causes of epilepsy range from genetic channelopathies to brain changes secondary to tumor, infection, stroke, traumatic brain injury, neurodegenerative disease, and febrile seizures.[66,67] The prevalence of epilepsy is 7 to 10 per 1000 people.[68] Epileptic seizures are not always medical emergencies (Box 18-1).

Treatments for epilepsy include drug therapy, brain surgery to remove the neurons most prone to excessive discharge or to interrupt connections between neurons, behavioral adjustments (regular sleep and stress coping strategies), and vagus nerve stimulation. Vagus nerve stimulation consists of attaching a pacemaker to the vagus nerve to deliver electrical pulses. The rationale is that vagal visceral afferents project diffusely in the central nervous system, and activation of these pathways has widespread beneficial effects on neuronal excitability.[69]

## Disorders of Intellect

Cognitive disability, dementia, and dyslexia all reduce the capability for understanding and reasoning. Common causes of cognitive disability are trisomy 21 and untreated phenylketonuria.

### Trisomy 21

*Trisomy 21,* also known as *Down syndrome,* is a genetic disorder caused by an extra copy of chromosome 21. People with trisomy 21 have round heads, slanted eyes, a fold of skin extending from the nose to the medial end of the eyebrow, and simian creases on the palms of their hands. The weight of the brain and the relative size of the frontal lobes are both reduced compared with normal brains. Prevalence has been reported as 12 cases per 10,000 live births.[70]

### Phenylketonuria

*Phenylketonuria* is an autosomal recessive defect in metabolism resulting in retention of a common amino acid, phenylalanine. The accumulation of phenylalanine results in demyelination and, later, neuronal loss. If the condition is diagnosed in infancy (by blood and urine tests), nervous system damage may be prevented by a diet low in phenylalanine.

### Dementia

In contrast to cognitive disability, dementia usually occurs late in life. *Dementia* is generalized mental deterioration, characterized by disorientation and impaired memory, judgment, and intellect. Many different causes may lead to dementia. Among the most common causes of dementia are multiple infarcts, Alzheimer's disease, diffuse Lewy body disease, Parkinson's dementia, and chronic traumatic encephalopathy. Multiple infarcts in the cerebral hemispheres result in focal neurologic signs, in addition to deterioration in intellectual function.

*Alzheimer's disease* causes progressive mental deterioration consisting of memory loss, confusion, and disorientation. Typically, symptoms become apparent after age 60, and death follows in 5 to 10 years. Initially the disease presents with signs of forgetfulness, progressing to an inability to recall words, and finally to failure to produce and comprehend language. People with Alzheimer's disease become lost easily due to motion blindness.[71] Motion blindness is an inability to interpret the flow of visual information. For example, when a person walks forward, objects in the visual field flow past the person in a radial pattern. People with Alzheimer's disease are unable to interpret the direction of motion of objects in their visual field. They cannot tell whether objects are moving toward or away from them, or whether they are moving relative to objects. This inability interferes with using visual information to guide self-movement and may explain the tendency to wander and to become lost. Another difficulty experienced by almost 40% of people with Alzheimer's disease is uncontrollable emotional outbursts that are unrelated to their true emotional state

---

**BOX 18-1   SEIZURES AS MEDICAL EMERGENCIES**

A seizure is a medical emergency if:
- The cause of the seizure is unknown, that is, the person has not been identified as having epilepsy or another seizure disorder
- The person is diabetic, injured, or pregnant
- The seizure lasts longer than 5 minutes, or a second seizure begins after the first
- Consciousness does not return
- The seizure occurred in water

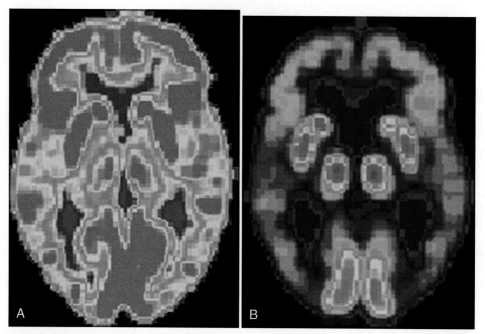

**Fig. 18-9  Positron emission tomography (PET) scans of a normal brain and an Alzheimer's brain.** Red and yellow indicate areas of high neural activity; blue and purple represent low neural activity. *(Courtesy Alzheimer's Disease Education and Referral Center, a service of the National Institute on Aging.)*

(emotional lability).[72] In late-stage Alzheimer's disease, people fail to dress, groom, or feed themselves.

The cause of cognitive loss in Alzheimer's disease is dysfunction affecting brain endothelial cells (cells that line the interior of blood vessels). Altered vascular endothelial cells cause blood-brain barrier malfunction and release factors that are injurious or toxic to neurons, creating chronic inflammation that results in Alzheimer's.[73,74] Later in the disease process, extracellular soluble amyloid-beta assembly and an abnormal form of tau protein within neurons accumulate. Late signs of Alzheimer's disease include severe atrophy of the cerebral cortex, amygdala, and hippocampus. Figure 18-9 compares the neural activity of a normal brain versus a brain with Alzheimer's disease.

The prevalence of Alzheimer's in people aged 70 years or older is 8.7%.[75] The incidence increases with increasing age, reaching 41% in people aged 100 years or older.[76] Virtually all people with trisomy 21 develop cellular-level changes similar to those in Alzheimer's disease by age 40, although in most cases behavioral changes are not obvious because the previous level of cognitive function was low. People with trisomy 21 have the trisomy of chromosome 21 in all cells. In contrast, people with Alzheimer's disease have some genetically normal cells and other cells with trisomy 21.[77] Skin biopsy for an enzyme involved in Alzheimer's disease shows promise as a diagnostic method.[78]

The three remaining types of dementia were introduced in Chapter 11 and are briefly reviewed here. *Diffuse Lewy body disease* is characterized by progressive cognitive decline, memory impairments, and deficits in attention, executive function, and visuospatial ability. Fluctuating alertness and cognition, visual hallucinations, and parkinsonism may also occur.[79] Parkinson's dementia primarily affects planning, goal orientation, and decision making.[80] Chronic traumatic encephalopathy (CTE) occurs following repeated head trauma. CTE causes behavioral

and personality changes, memory impairment, parkinsonism, and speech and gait abnormalities.[81]

## Learning Disabilities

In contrast to the generalized intellectual deficits of cognitive disability and dementia, learning disabilities arise from failure to develop specific types of intelligence. The most common learning disability is dyslexia, a condition of inability to read at a level commensurate with the person's overall intelligence. People with dyslexia have difficulty reading, writing, and spelling words, yet their conversational and visual abilities are normal. They can interpret visual objects and illustrations without difficulty. Some cases of dyslexia have been traced to abnormalities of a gene on chromosome 6.

## Traumatic Brain Injury

Traumatic brain injury is mild in about 80% of cases.[82] A single mild traumatic brain injury (concussion) usually causes no long-term cognitive abnormalities[83] (Pathology 18-1). Mild traumatic brain injury, often called a *concussion,* is distinguished by a brief loss of consciousness, a transitory post-traumatic amnesia, or a brief period of confusion following head trauma. Following concussion, a minority of people (about 15%) develop postconcussion syndrome, a lingering set of disorders that at 1 year post most frequently includes poor cognitive function, difficulty with concentration, and irritability. Postconcussion syndrome is associated with psychological and litigation factors, not with neurologic factors.[82,83]

Most moderate to severe traumatic brain injuries occur in motor vehicle accidents. The impact tends to damage the orbital, anterior, and inferior temporal regions and to cause

| PATHOLOGY 18-1 | TRAUMATIC BRAIN INJURY DUE TO BLUNT TRAUMA WITHOUT FRACTURE |
|---|---|
| Pathology | Diffuse axonal injury; contusion, hemorrhage, swelling, and/or laceration |
| Etiology | Trauma |
| Speed of onset | Acute |
| Signs and symptoms | |
|    Personality | Decreased goal-directed behavior (executive functions) if dorsolateral prefrontal cortex involved; impulsiveness and other inappropriate behaviors if ventral prefrontal cortex damaged; low tolerance for frustration; emotional lability and delusions (caused by temporal lesions that interrupt limbic connections with sensory inputs) |
|    Cognitive | Slow mental processing; decreased cognitive flexibility |
|    Consciousness | May be impaired temporarily or for a prolonged period; often have difficulty directing attention (distractibility) and attending to several things simultaneously |
|    Communication and memory | Communication usually normal; declarative memory impairments may be temporary or prolonged |
|    Sensory | May be impaired |
|    Autonomic | May have problems with autonomic regulation secondary to damage to or compression of the brainstem and/or hypothalamus |
|    Motor | Perseveration of movements; degree of motor impairment depends on severity of injury; paresis/paralysis; spasticity; contracture; balance, posture, gait, speech, swallowing, eye movement disorders |
| Region affected | Most frequently affects the anterior frontal, ventral frontal, and temporal lobes |
| Demographics | For traumatic brain injury (including open head injury and closed injuries with and without fractures), the incidence is 215 per 100,000 persons[82]; males are 1.4 times as likely as females to suffer traumatic brain injury; the highest overall incidence of traumatic brain injury occurs in the <4 year age group (1256 per 100,000); however, highest rates of hospitalization and death occur in the >85 year age group (339 per 100,000 and 57 per 100,000, respectively).[86] Prevalence of disability caused by traumatic brain injury is 20 per 1000 people.[87] |
| Prognosis | Mortality rate before and during hospitalization is 23 per 100,000 population per year[88]; severity of injury and age at time of injury determine outcome. Five to seven years after head injury, 24% had died; of the survivors, 19% were severely disabled, 33% were moderately disabled, and 47% had a good recovery.[89] Ratings of disability and recovery were based on the Glasgow Coma Scale–Extended. In addition to duration of amnesia, items include eye opening, verbal responses, and motor responses, with scores ranging from spontaneous to no response. For example, on the eye opening item, the person might open his or her eyes spontaneously, or might not open the eyes in response to a loud voice or a painful stimulus. |

diffuse axonal injury. Diffuse axonal injury results from stretch injury to the membrane of an axon. This injury allows excessive calcium influx, producing cytoskeletal collapse that disrupts anterograde axonal transport. Organelles collect at the damaged site, the axon swells at the site of injury, and the axon eventually breaks.[84] The distal axon degenerates. Axonal injury primarily affects the basal ganglia, superior cerebellar peduncle, corpus callosum, and midbrain.

Because frontal, temporal, and limbic areas are typically damaged, people show poor judgment, decreased executive functions (planning, initiating, monitoring behavior), memory deficits, slow information processing, attentional disorders, and poor divergent thinking. Inability to effectively use new information results in concrete thinking, an inability to appropriately apply rules, and trouble distinguishing relevant from irrelevant information. Because judgment is impaired, people with traumatic brain injury are at significant risk for problems with substance abuse, aggression, and inappropriate sexual behaviors. Other problematic behaviors secondary to traumatic brain injury may include agitation, emotional lability, lack of self-awareness, lack of empathy, lack of motivation, and inflexibility. Imbalance may also be a persistent problem: physically well-recovered men with traumatic brain injury have impaired balance, agility, and coordination.[85]

Traumatic brain damage in infants is most frequently attributable to accidental falls, but brain damage consequent to most falls is relatively minor. More severe brain injury usually requires greater force than a typical fall—forces that sometimes are generated when an infant is violently shaken. Trauma from shaking is due to the impact of the brain's striking the skull repeatedly. Soon after the incident, cerebral edema may increase the infant's head circumference and cause bulging of the anterior fontanelle. Brain scans show hemorrhage and edema. The outcomes of shaken baby syndrome are: 17.7% die, 22% have severe disability, 31% have moderate disability, and 29% have good recovery.[90] The incidence of shaken baby syndrome is 14

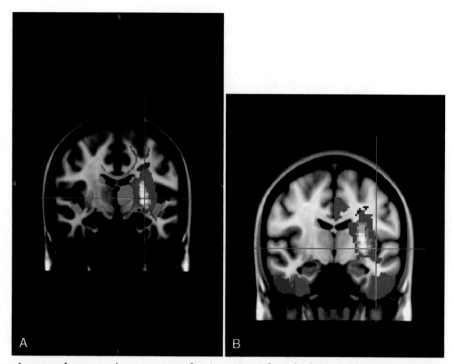

**Fig. 18-10 Changes in neural connections post stroke.** Location of stroke lesions shown in red to white. Lesions are in the area of the internal capsule/basal ganglia. **A,** Gray matter regions with reduced connections in patients relative to controls *(light blue significant differences, dark blue area shows trends).* Pink indicates white matter areas with reduced connection. **B,** Green indicates gray matter areas with increased connection relative to controls. *(Both images are from Crofts JJ, Higham DJ, Bosnell R: Network analysis detects changes in the contralesional hemisphere following stroke.* Neuroimage *54:167, 2011.)*

per 100,000 live births.[90] Survivors may exhibit motor signs similar to those of developmental delay or cerebral palsy and have a pattern of cognitive deficits similar to that seen in adults with traumatic brain injury.[91]

## Alien Hand Syndrome

Alien hand syndrome is involuntary, uncontrollable movement of the upper limb. The limb may elevate when the person is walking, may unintentionally grasp objects, and may interfere with movements of the unaffected hand. In the earlier section on callosotomy, a case was cited of an alien hand that undid buttons that were buttoned by the unaffected hand. Although callosotomy may cause alien hand syndrome, the syndrome also occurs with damage to a variety of cortical and subcortical structures.[92] The most common psychological responses to alien hand syndrome are frustration, perplexity, annoyance, and anger.[93] Kikkert and coauthors (2006)[93] recommend visual feedback and sensory stimulation for alien hand associated with right hemisphere damage, and cognitive therapy to treat the anxiety and anger associated with left hemisphere alien hand.

## Stroke

The neurologic outcome of interruption of blood flow to the cerebrum depends on the etiology, location, and size of the infarct or hemorrhage. Infarcts occur when an embolus or thrombus lodges in a vessel, obstructing blood flow. Figure 18-10 illustrates the changes in neural connections post stroke.

## Signs and Symptoms of Stroke

Signs and symptoms of stroke depend on the location and size of the lesion; a small insult to the cortex may produce no symptoms, and the same size or a smaller lesion in the brainstem could cause death. Large hemorrhages or edema secondary to large infarcts can cause death regardless of location by compressing vital structures. Each of the following acute neurologic deficits has been reported to affect more than 25% of people surviving brain infarctions: hemiparesis, ataxia, hemianopia, visual-perceptual deficits, aphasia, dysarthria, sensory deficits, memory deficits, and problems with bladder control. Chapter 19 presents localization of deficits in the context of the vascular supply.

Although hemiplegia and hemisensory deficits resulting from stroke often appear to be unilateral, "uninvolved side" is usually a misnomer. Pai and associates (1994)[94] report that people with right hemiparesis who were able to walk independently (some with assistive devices) were able to successfully transfer and maintain their weight to the nonparetic side in only 48% of trials and to the paretic side in only 20% of trials. Ipsilateral hand function is also affected: compared with control subjects, people with hemiplegia have significantly impaired dexterity ipsilateral to the lesion.[95] See Chapter 10 for mechanisms of ipsilateral involvement in cerebral stroke.

**TABLE 18-3** EFFECTS OF MIDDLE CEREBRAL ARTERY STROKE

| Affected Brain Area | Signs and Symptoms |
| --- | --- |
| Left hemisphere stroke | Hemiparesis or hemiplegia and hemisensory loss affecting right side of body and face<br>Language and/or speech disorders<br>Difficulty understanding and producing language<br>Dysarthria<br>Cautious behavior, hesitant to try new tasks |
| Right hemisphere stroke | Hemiparesis or hemiplegia and hemisensory loss affecting left side of body and face<br>Left neglect<br>Impulsive behavior, unaware of deficits<br>May drive with devastating results<br>May walk without necessary cane or brace<br>Unintentional fabrication of information caused by deficits in recognizing errors and memory and by disinhibition<br>Because language is intact, other people may think the person is much more capable than he/she is<br>Unable to comprehend and produce emotional content of speech |

Effects of middle cerebral artery stroke affecting the right versus the left hemisphere are summarized in Table 18-3.

## Recovery From Stroke

In physical and occupational therapy, an ongoing controversy is the long-term effectiveness of compensation, remediation, and motor control approaches to stroke rehabilitation. Compensation approaches emphasize performing tasks using the paretic limb with an adapted approach or using the nonparetic limb to perform the task. Compensation approaches assume that damaged neural mechanisms cannot be restored, so external aids or environmental supports are used to assist patients in daily activities. For example, the ankle on the paretic side might be braced to allow early ambulation.

Remediation approaches attempt to decrease the severity of the neurologic deficits. Here the assumption is that activation or stimulation of damaged processes will result in change at both behavioral and neural levels. Using the remediation approach, the therapist might use hands-on techniques to inhibit muscle tone and work on a sequence of activities from supine to upright before gait training. During gait training, the therapist might move the client's hips.

Motor control approaches emphasize task specificity, that is, practicing the desired task in a specific context. If the goal is independent walking, walking is practiced, rather than preparatory activities like standing balance or lateral weight transfers in standing. Using the motor control approach, the client might walk an obstacle course with the therapist guarding for loss of balance.

Current research indicates that intensive, task-specific therapy produces significantly better motor function compared with the remediation approach.[96-98] Chan and colleagues (2006)[99] reported that a task-specific program combined with patient self-identification of their own problems in performance produced significantly improved balance, self-care, ability to perform instrumental activities of daily living (laundry, taking public transportation, and cleaning a floor), and integration into the community than a conventional, remediation approach in people an average of 3 to 4 months post stroke.

---

**BOX 18-2    TYPES OF BRAIN TUMORS**

**Malignant**
Astrocytoma (from astrocytes; some are benign)
Glioblastoma multiforme (from glial cells)
Oligodendroglioma (from oligodendrocytes)
Ependymoma (from ependymal cells)
Medulloblastoma (from neuroectodermal cells)
Lymphoma (from lymphatic tissue)
Metastatic (commonly arise from lung, skin, kidney, colon, or breast)

**Benign**
Meningioma (from arachnoid)
Adenoma (from epithelial tissue)
Acoustic neuroma (from Schwann cells)

---

## Tumors

A *tumor* is a spontaneous abnormal growth of tissue that forms a mass. Signs and symptoms produced by brain tumors are usually due to compression and thus are determined by the location and size of the tumor. Brain tumors frequently cause mild to moderate intermittent headaches. The headaches are aggravated by changes in position or by abrupt increases in intracranial pressure (coughing, sneezing, or straining to empty bowels increases intrathoracic pressure, followed by an increase in aortic pressure that subsequently raises intracranial pressure) and are accompanied by nausea and vomiting.

Tumors that arise in the brain are named for the type of cell involved (Box 18-2). Most primary central nervous system tumors are derived from glia and therefore are called *gliomas*.

The incidence of central nervous system (CNS) tumors (both malignant and benign) is 25 per 100,000 adults per year,

**TABLE 18-4    PSYCHOLOGICAL DISORDERS**

| Disorder | Hyperactive Regions | Hypoactive Regions |
|---|---|---|
| Bipolar disorder | Amygdala, ventral striatum, hippocampus | Orbital and dorsomedial prefrontal cortex |
| Depression | Area 25 | |
| Obsessive-compulsive disorder (OCD) | Orbital and anterior cingulate cortex, and ventral striatum | Dorsolateral prefrontal cortex |
| Schizophrenia | Amygdala and hippocampus/parahippocampal region (delusions and hallucinations) | Dorsolateral prefrontal cortex (cognitive disorders). Ventrolateral prefrontal cortex and ventral striatum (lack of pleasure, flat affect, lack of speech); dorsomedial prefrontal cortex (delusions and hallucinations) |
| Anxiety disorders including post-traumatic stress disorder | Amygdala, medial prefrontal cortex, hippocampus, and insular cortex | Ventromedial prefrontal and rostral anterior cingulate cortex |

and 4.8 per 100,000 children per year.[100] In adults, nonmalignant tumors are twice as common as malignant tumors; in children, 65% of CNS tumors are malignant.[100] Prognosis depends on the histology, size, and location of the tumor, the age of the patient, and the effectiveness of surgical, chemical, and radiation therapy.

## Psychological Disorders and Psychiatric Signs/Symptoms in Neurologic Disorders

In this section, two psychological disorders that may impact therapy—somatoform and personality disorders—are discussed first. Then, psychiatric signs and symptoms that occur in both primary psychological disorders and in neurologic disorders are considered. Schizophrenia is the final topic.

### Somatoform and Personality Disorders

In *somatoform disorders,* emotional distress is subconsciously converted into physical symptoms. People with somatoform disorders use their symptoms to avoid emotional conflicts or to manipulate other people. Common symptoms of somatoform disorders include back pain, joint pain, aching of the extremities, trouble walking, muscle weakness, gastrointestinal problems, nonexertional shortness of breath, problems with swallowing, double vision, and blurred vision. Somatoform disorders are distinct from malingering because no external gain can be identified. In malingering, the person intentionally exaggerates or feigns symptoms for external gain. For example, receiving time off from work, access to drugs, and/or financial incentives may motivate a person who is malingering.

*Personality disorders* have more pervasive effects on the individual than somatoform disorders. People with personality disorders have inflexible, maladaptive patterns of inner experience and behavior. The three general types are eccentric, acting out, and fearful. People with personality disorders may be prone to rapid mood swings, excessive sensitivity to the judgment of other people, passive resistance to instructions (e.g., "losing" a home exercise program, talking excessively to avoid practicing tasks during therapy), and/or ambiguous complaints.

Treatment provided by occupational and physical therapists for people with these disorders should focus on improving activities of daily living, work, leisure activities, and physical function. Psychological counseling is outside the scope of occupational and physical therapy practice. Referral of the patient to a mental health professional may be beneficial.

### Psychiatric Signs, Symptoms, and Disorders

Psychiatric signs and symptoms include delusions, hallucinations, mania, depression, anxiety, and obsessive-compulsive thoughts and behaviors. These symptoms occur in psychiatric disorders (Table 18-4) and in neurologic conditions.

*Delusions* are false beliefs despite evidence to the contrary. Delusions range from thinking someone is stealing money, to believing that the television is specifically talking to them, to believing that some people have taken the physical appearance of others. The first type of simple delusion is common in delirium, Alzheimer's disease, and vascular dementia. The more complicated delusions occur in schizophrenia and may be induced by medication in Parkinson's disease.

*Hallucinations* are sensory perceptions experienced without corresponding sensory stimuli. Visual hallucinations occur with ocular/optic nerve abnormalities, migraine, delirium, schizophrenia, mania, depression, and temporal lobe seizures.[101] Auditory hallucinations are more common in primary psychological disease but can occur in neurologic disorders.[102]

*Mania* is excessive excitement, euphoria, delusions, and overactivity. Racing thoughts, disregard for consequences, and energetic behaviors typify mania. Drugs, including steroids, stimulants, and antidepressants, can induce mania. Mania also occurs in *bipolar disorder,* a disease characterized by elevated or irritable mood alternating with depression. People with bipolar disorder have greater amygdala, ventral striatum, and hippocampus response to emotional stimuli than do healthy individuals, regardless of whether their mood is manic, depressed, or normal.[103] The orbital and dorsomedial prefrontal cortices are hypoactive compared with normal.[103] Bipolar disorder has a lifetime prevalence of approximately 2.0% in the general population.[104]

Rarely, mania can be caused by brain lesions on the right side that affect structures in the behavioral flexibility and control loop (see Figure 17-16), including ventrolateral prefrontal and lateral orbital cortices, the caudate head, or the mediodorsal thalamic nucleus.[105] People with right temporal lobectomies report increased happiness.[106]

*Depression,* a syndrome of hopelessness and a sense of worthlessness, with aberrant thoughts and behavior, has been linked to neurotransmitter and neural activity abnormalities rather than to structural abnormalities. People with depression have reduced levels of serotonin metabolites in their cerebrospinal fluid. Drugs that effectively treat depression enhance the effectiveness of serotonin transmission. Drugs for depression include monoamine oxidase (MAO) inhibitors, tricyclic antidepressants, and selective serotonin reuptake inhibitors (SSRIs). MAO degrades catecholamines, so inhibiting MAO raises levels of norepinephrine, serotonin, and epinephrine. The main effect of tricyclic antidepressants is increased activity of serotonin and $\alpha$1-(norepinephrine) receptors, and decreased activity of central beta receptors (norepinephrine). SSRIs, including Prozac (fluoxetine), which selectively inhibits serotonin uptake, prolong the availability of serotonin in synapses.

Area 25, in the anterior cingulate cortex, increases activity with sad mood.[107] Area 25 neurons project to the dorsal raphe nuclei in the brainstem, influencing mood by adjusting serotonin neurotransmitter levels throughout the brain.[108] Area 25 has extensive connections throughout the anterior brain. When area 25 is overactive, signals to the prefrontal cortex interfere with thinking and executive functions. Signals to the ventral striatum interfere with reward pathways and contribute to lack of pleasure. Signals to the brainstem and the hypothalamus cause difficulty with motivational, nutritional, metabolic, and endocrine function. Signals to the medial temporal lobe hinder memory processing.[107] Area 25 also reciprocally connects with the amygdala, which registers fear and negative emotions.[109] Effective treatment of depression reduces activity in area 25.[103]

Changes in emotions and moods may occur with damage to the prefrontal cortex and/or to the temporal lobe. Left prefrontal cortex damage tends to produce unusually severe depression.[106] Similarly, people with left temporal lobectomies report increased depression.[106] Depression frequently occurs in dementia, Parkinson's disease, multiple sclerosis, and epilepsy. The lifetime prevalence of major depressive disorder is 23%.[110]

*Anxiety* is a feeling of tension or uneasiness that accompanies anticipating danger. The autonomic system is overactive, skeletal muscles are tense, and the person is excessively alert. The five anxiety disorders are: *generalized anxiety disorder* (excessive worry over daily events), *social anxiety disorder* (excessive self-consciousness and worry in social settings), panic disorder, obsessive-compulsive disorder (OCD), and post-traumatic stress disorder (PTSD). The lifetime prevalence of any anxiety disorder is 28.8%.[110]

*Panic disorder* is an episode of intense fear that begins abruptly and lasts 10 to 15 minutes. Symptoms include pounding heart, rapid heart rate, sweating, feeling of choking, difficulty breathing, nausea, feeling faint or light-headed, and fear of fainting, going crazy, or dying. In addition to psychological disorders, panic attacks can be caused by seizure activity, vestibular disorders, cardiac disorders, or drugs.[111-113]

*Obsessive-compulsive disorder* is characterized by persistent upsetting thoughts and the use of compulsive behavior in response to the obsessive thoughts. Common examples include fear of germs and repeated excessive hand washing. In comparison with controls, people with OCD have decreased activity in dorsal, cognitive prefrontal areas combined with increased activity in ventral, emotion-related prefrontal-striate circuits, and increased amygdala activity.[114] Orbital cortex and striatal lesions, Parkinson's disease, Parkinson-Plus syndromes, and Tourette's disorder are also associated with OCD. *Tourette's disorder* comprises motor and vocal tics, the involuntary production of movements and sounds. The tics are usually preceded by a strong urge, and typically can be suppressed temporarily. Caudate nucleus volumes are smaller in people with Tourette's than in control subjects.[115] The prevalence is 1% of the population, and most cases are mild.[115]

*Post-traumatic stress disorder* is an anxiety disorder that can develop in survivors of war, physical and sexual assault, abuse, accidents, disasters, and other serious trauma. People with PTSD re-experience the original event in flashbacks or nightmares, avoid stimuli linked to the trauma, and are hyperaroused. Hyperarousal interferes with sleeping and concentrating and is associated with angry outbursts. The amygdala (fear perception), the insula (perceives internal body conditions), and the medial prefrontal cortex (perception of others' beliefs and intentions) are overactive in people with PTSD compared with controls.[116,117] In PTSD, the ventromedial prefrontal and rostral anterior cortices are underactive and fail to adequately inhibit emotional regions.[116] The estimated prevalence of PTSD is 8% in the adult population.[118]

## Schizophrenia

Schizophrenia is a group of disorders consisting of disordered thinking, delusions, hallucinations, lack of motivation, apathy, and social withdrawal. Executive function, including planning, goal orientation, and behavioral inhibition, is impaired. Poor working memory interferes with considering possible alternatives, leading to externally driven behavior.[119]

The syndrome involves both anatomic and neurotransmitter abnormalities. The frontal and temporal lobes and the amygdala and hippocampus are smaller in people with schizophrenia than in normal people. Functional connection abnormalities between the dorsolateral prefrontal cortex and the inferior temporal cortex and visual areas, and between the inferior frontal cortex and the posterior parietal cortex may explain the delusions and disorganization symptoms.[120,121] Drugs that block the reuptake of serotonin or that block dopamine receptors reduce symptoms in many people with schizophrenia. Thus abnormality of neurotransmitter regulation may contribute to the symptoms of schizophrenia. Aerobic exercise training improves memory function and hippocampal volume in people with schizophrenia.[122] The incidence of schizophrenia is approximately 1% of the population.[123]

## NEURAL PROSTHESES

Neural prostheses are devices that substitute for diseased or injured parts of the nervous system to enhance function. Neural prostheses include deep brain stimulation and brain-computer interfaces.

## Deep Brain Stimulation

Deep brain stimulation (DBS) is most frequently used in Parkinson's disease, and that use was discussed in Chapter 11. Dystonia responds well to DBS.[124] DBS to the ventral striatum or area 25 is frequently effective for treatment-resistant depression.[125,126] Treatment-resistant obsessive-compulsive disorder also responds to DBS.[127] DBS is considered an experimental treatment for adults with severe treatment-resistant Tourette's syndrome.[128] Most frequent DBS adverse events involve bleeding, infection, mental status decline, gait and other motor problems, seizure, speech and language disorders, and mania.[129] However, quality of life is the same in people who experience DBS adverse events as in those who do not have adverse events.[129]

## Brain-Computer Interfaces

Brain-computer interface (BCI) technology analyzes signals from the brain to determine the person's intended action, then generates commands to move a computer cursor or a mechanical limb. In people with quadriplegia, recordings from a microarray of electrodes implanted into the motor cortex can be used to point and click a computer cursor.[130] Electroencephalographic (EEG) signals from electrodes over the scalp can reliably acquire signals during motor imagery in elderly subjects with normal neuromuscular systems.[131] The intent is to use this technology with people post stroke, to give feedback about cortical activation during motor imagery, and to improve rehabilitation outcome.[131] EEG signals also accurately infer lower limb joint angle kinematics and trajectories during normal walking,[132] indicating possible future brain-computer interface use in gait rehabilitation.

# TESTING CEREBRAL FUNCTION

Therapists often briefly assess cerebral function. Part of this assessment may include evaluating the level of consciousness. Normal consciousness requires intact function of the ascending reticular activating system, thalamus, and thalamic projections to the cerebral cortex, in addition to the cerebral cortex. Functions that are localized in the cerebral cortex include language, orientation, declarative memory, abstract thought, identification of objects, motor planning, and comprehension of spatial relationships (Table 18-5). Consciousness and language are

---

**TABLE 18-5    EVALUATION OF MENTAL FUNCTION**

| Function | Test | Interpretation |
| --- | --- | --- |
| Consciousness level | Observe the person's interaction with the environment. Levels of consciousness are classified as follows:<br>Alert: attends to ordinary stimuli<br>Lethargic: tends to lose track of conversations and tasks; falls asleep if little stimulation is provided<br>Obtunded: becomes alert briefly in response to strong stimuli; cannot answer questions meaningfully<br>Stupor: alert only during vigorous stimulation<br>Coma: little or no response to stimulation | Levels of consciousness depend on neural activity in the ascending reticular activating system, thalamus, thalamic projections to the cerebral cortex, and cerebral cortex |
| Language and speech | Evaluate the spontaneous use of words, grammar, and fluency of speech | Disorders may be caused by any form of aphasia, or by dysarthria. Brain areas involved may be Broca's area, Wernicke's area, connections between Broca's and Wernicke's areas, premotor and/or motor cortex, corticobrainstem fibers, or motor cranial nerves |
|  | Comprehension: ask the person to answer a question similar to the following: "Is my brother's sister a man or a woman?" | Difficulty may be due to receptive aphasia or a hearing disorder. Brain areas involved may include Wernicke's area or peripheral or central auditory structures |
|  | Naming: ask the person to identify objects (pencil, watch, paper clip) and body parts (nose, knee, eye) | If the person can produce automatic social speech (e.g., "Hello, how are you?") but cannot name objects, the difficulty may be due to dysfunction of Wernicke's area (Wernicke's aphasia) |
|  | Reading: ask the person to read a simple paragraph aloud. Then ask questions about the paragraph | Assuming that the person has intact speech, difficulty may be due to alexia, dyslexia, short-term memory deficit, visual deficit, or illiteracy. Wernicke's area is the site of dysfunction in alexia |
|  | Writing: ask the person to write answers to simple questions | Difficulty may be due to agraphia, visual deficit, impaired motor control of the upper limb, or illiteracy. Wernicke's area is the site of dysfunction in agraphia |

**TABLE 18-5**   EVALUATION OF MENTAL FUNCTION—cont'd

| Function | Test | Interpretation |
|---|---|---|
| *All of the following tests require language abilities. Some, as noted, also require intact speech.* | | |
| Orientation | Assess the person's orientation to person, place, and time. Questions similar to the following may be used:<br>*Person*<br>What is your name?<br>Where were you born?<br>Are you married?<br>*Place*<br>Where are we now?<br>What city and state are we in?<br>*Time*<br>What time is it?<br>What day of the week is this?<br>What year is this? | Test assumes intact speech abilities. These questions assess declarative memory. Questions about the person assess long-term memory, and questions about time and place assess short-term memory. Difficulty with these questions may indicate dysfunction of the hippocampus; a language or speech disorder; or a generalized cortical processing disorder, due to drug toxicity, psychosis, or extreme anxiety |
| Declarative memory | Short-term memory: tell the person that you are going to check his or her memory by asking him or her to remember three words for a few minutes. Give the person three unrelated words, and have him or her repeat the words. Then converse about other topics, and after 3 minutes, ask what the three words were. People with intact short-term memory can recall all three words. Examples of words used include *clock, telephone, shoe*<br>Recent memory: ask the person about activities in the past several days. Examples include: What did you have for breakfast? Who visited you yesterday?<br>Long-term memory: ask the person to name U.S. presidents, about historical events, or about his or her school and work experience | Test requires speech abilities. Declarative memory problems occur with damage to the hippocampus or with temporary disruptions of cerebral function, as may occur during psychosis, with extreme anxiety, or following acute head trauma |
| Interpretation of proverbs | Ask the person to explain what a proverb means. For example, "What does 'A rolling stone gathers no moss' mean?" | Test requires speech abilities. A concrete answer, for example, "It means that a rock that keeps moving does not grow moss," indicates difficulty with abstract thinking |
| Calculation | Serial 7's: Ask the person to subtract 7 from 100 and to keep subtracting 7 from each result. Ask the person simple addition, subtraction, multiplication, or division problems. For example, "What is $6 \times 30$?" | Test requires speech abilities. Difficulty may indicate problems with maintaining attention, or a problem with abstract thinking |
| Stereognosis | Ask the person to close his or her eyes, then place a small object in the person's hand and ask him or her to identify it. Objects may include a paper clip, a key, or a coin | Test requires speech abilities. Astereognosis indicates damage to the secondary somatosensory area of the cerebral cortex |
| Visual identification | Show the person an object and ask him or her to identify it | Test requires speech abilities. If the person cannot identify the object visually but can identify the object by touch or another sense, the disorder is visual agnosia. Visual agnosia is caused by damage to secondary visual areas in the cerebral cortex of the occipital lobe |
| Motor planning | Ask the person to demonstrate hair brushing, using a screwdriver, or buttoning a shirt | Assuming intact sensation, understanding of the task, and motor control, inability to produce specific movements indicates apraxia. Apraxia usually occurs as a result of damage to the premotor or supplementary motor areas |

*Continued*

**TABLE 18-5** EVALUATION OF MENTAL FUNCTION—cont'd

| Function | Test | Interpretation |
|---|---|---|
| Comprehension of spatial relationships | Activities of daily living: observe the person eating a meal; ask him or her to put on an article of clothing; or ask him or her to perform a grooming task or to get into and out of a bed or a chair | Difficulty may indicate motor impairment, neglect, or a generalized decline in cerebral function. Asymmetry of performance usually indicates neglect. Neglect occurs with damage to the area that corresponds to Wernicke's area |
| | Ask the person to copy a simple drawing, or to draw a person, a clock, a house, or a flower from memory | Difficulty may indicate motor impairment, neglect, constructional apraxia, or a generalized decline in cerebral function. Asymmetry of performance usually indicates neglect. Neglect occurs with damage to the area that corresponds to Wernicke's area. If most parts of the drawing are present but are not in correct spatial relationship to each other, and if the drawing improves when the subject is copying a model, the deficit is constructional apraxia. In constructional apraxia, the lesion is typically in the parietal or frontal lobe of the language-dominant hemisphere |
| | Visual scanning: ask the person to read a paragraph aloud, or to cross out specific characters in a printed array (e.g., cross out all of the small stars in an array of large and small stars) | Assuming that visual acuity and visual fields are adequate, omission of words or parts of words located on the left side of the paragraph or failing to cross out all of the specified characters on the left side of a visual array indicates visual neglect |
| | Body scheme drawing: give the person a blank piece of paper and ask him or her to draw a person | Asymmetry in the drawing of a person (for example, omitting part of the left side of the body or providing less detail on the left side of the body) indicates neglect associated with damage to the right parietal lobe |
| Concept of relationship of body parts | Ask the person to point to a body part on command, or to imitate the examiner in pointing to parts of his or her own body | Bilateral inaccuracy or failure to point to body parts indicates a specific deficit in conception of the relationship of body parts to the whole body. The lesion is usually in the parietal or the posterior temporal lobe of the left hemisphere |
| Orientation to vertical position | Hold a cane vertically, and then move it to a horizontal position. Give the cane to the person and ask him or her to return it to the original position | If the cane is not vertical, orientation to vertical position is impaired. The lesion may be in the right parietal lobe, in the posterior thalamus, or in the vestibular system |
| Ability to attend to bilaterally simultaneous stimulation | Touch: ask the person to say "yes" if he or she feels a touch. Lightly touch both sides of the body simultaneously. If the person says "yes," ask where the touch was felt | If the person is able to correctly report touch or visual objects presented to the left of his or her midline, but is unaware of these stimuli when the stimuli are presented bilaterally, the person has sensory extinction, a form of unilateral neglect |
| | Vision: show the person two objects, one in the right visual field and one in the left visual field. Ask the person to name the objects | |

assessed first because the other tests, except for comprehension of spatial relationships, require that the person be alert and able to understand language. The message that the therapist wants the person to copy a drawing to assess comprehension of spatial relationships may be conveyed by gestural cues.

Difficulties with certain tests of mental function indicate lesions in specific parts of the cerebral cortex. For example, Broca's aphasia indicates damage to Broca's area. Difficulty with other tests does not implicate any specific part of the cerebral cortex, but instead indicates more generalized dysfunction. The significance of difficulty with each test is listed in Table 18-5, in the "Interpretation" column. For patients with moderate to severe speech and/or language difficulties, consultation with a speech/language pathologist is recommended.

## SUMMARY

Functions and lesions of the four lobes of the cerebrum are considered first, followed by a discussion of the parietotemporal cortex and cerebral lesions.

Frontal lobes control motor function, initiation of activity, planning of nonverbal communication, goal-oriented behavior, judgment, interpretation of emotion, attention, flexibility in problem solving, social behavior, and motivation. Lesions cause Broca's aphasia (damage in language-dominant hemiphere), impaired production of nonverbal communication (area analogous to Broca's area), and hemiplegia. Dorsolateral prefrontal association cortex lesions interfere with initiation and monitoring of goal-oriented behavior and divergent thinking. Ventral prefrontal lesions produce disinhibited behavior, poor judgment, and disturbances of personality and emotions.

Parietal lobes process sensation and provide perception related to body schema. Parietal lobe lesions may cause contralateral somatosensory loss, hemiplegia, homonymous hemianopia, agnosia, astereognosis, and apraxia.

Occipital lobes process vision, including spatial relationships of visual objects and analysis of motion and color, and control visual fixation. Lesions in the primary visual cortex produce homonymous hemianopia. Lesions in the secondary visual cortex cause visual agnosia. Disorders of the occipital lobe can also cause visual hallucinations or loss of visual fixation.

Temporal lobes process auditory information, classify sounds, and process emotion and memory. Lesions cause loss of localization of sounds, auditory agnosia, impaired long-term memory, and disturbances of personality and emotions.

The parietotemporal association cortex is involved in sensory integration, communication, understanding of spatial relationships, and convergent problem solving. Lesions in the left parietotemporal association cortex can produce disorders of language (Wernicke's aphasia). Lesions in the right parietotemporal cortex may cause contralateral neglect, difficulty understanding nonverbal communication, and anosognosia (denial of deficits).

Consciousness, attention, control of movements, motivation, memory, intellect, sensation, perception, communication, all forms of behavior, personality, and emotions all rely on the cerebrum. Cerebral function is diverse and adaptable. Cerebral dysfunction can be devastating, as in severe brain injury or schizophrenia. Cerebral compensation for injury can also be remarkable, because people recover from cerebral injuries and disorders.

## CLINICAL NOTES

### Case 1

A famous case in the right-to-die debate involved Karen Quinlan. After ingesting a tranquilizer, an analgesic, and alcohol, she suffered cardiopulmonary arrest that permanently damaged her brain. She became the focus of a conflict between doctors intent on keeping her alive and her parents, who requested that she be allowed to die because no hope for recovery existed. A court ordered the doctors to remove her ventilator. However, she continued to breathe without the ventilator and survived in a vegetative state for 9 more years. She never regained consciousness. Although her brain damage was assumed to be in the cerebral cortex, subsequent analysis of her brain showed that the cortex was relatively intact, and that the region with severe damage was the thalamus.[133]

#### Questions

1. Why does thalamic damage interfere with consciousness?
2. What other structures are required for consciousness?

### Case 2

H.A. is a 47-year-old woman who is recovering from surgery to remove a benign tumor in the optic chiasm region. One day post surgery, the therapist arrives to assess the patient. The therapist notes that the patient is unconscious and has no bedcovers, the air conditioning is on full, and fans are placed to blow across the patient's body, yet the temperature of the patient's skin is unusually warm. When the therapist arrives the next day, the patient is warmly covered, the heater is on, and the room temperature is near 90° F, yet the patient's skin temperature is cool.

#### Questions

1. What is the hospital staff trying to do by manipulating the room temperature?
2. What part of H.A.'s brain is not functioning optimally?

### Case 3

K.L. is a 72-year-old man who has been transferred to rehabilitation 2 weeks after sustaining a cerebrovascular accident on the left side. He complains of weakness of his right limbs and of being unable to button his clothing or tie his shoes. Right hand movements are clumsy. On the right side of his body, K.L. is unable to localize tactile stimuli or to distinguish between passive flexion and extension of his joints. He is able to correctly report whether he was touched or not, and whether a stimulus is sharp or dull.

#### Question

Where is the lesion?

*Continued*

## CLINICAL NOTES—cont'd

### Case 4

R.B. is a 19-year-old boy who was rescued, unconscious, after falling from a 40 foot cliff. One day later, he regained consciousness. Strength, position sense, touch localization, and two-point discrimination were normal on both sides. R.B. was easily able to identify unseen objects in his left hand but was totally unable to recognize the same objects using his right hand. Although he was right-handed before the accident, after the accident he used his left hand whenever possible.

#### Questions

1. Name the deficit in ability to recognize an object by palpation.
2. Why does R.B. avoid using his right hand?

### Case 5

F.S., a 26-year-old schoolteacher, sustained head trauma and multiple femoral fractures in a traffic accident. She was comatose for 3 days. On regaining consciousness, sensation, movement, and her ability to communicate were intact. However, she seemed listless and did not initiate conversations or activities. F.S. was unable to learn a partial weight-bearing gait, flailing the crutches rather than bearing weight on them. She appeared totally apathetic, even about her situation and her family.

#### Question

Where is the lesion?

### Case 6

B.G., a 34-year-old stockbroker, suffered multiple fractures of the frontal skull in a motorcycle accident. After recovery from surgical repair, he was hemiparetic on the right side. Muscle strength on the right expressed as a percentage of strength on the left was as follows: girdle muscles, 80%; elbow/knee, 50%; and distal muscles, 0%. With an ankle-foot orthosis and a cane, he was able to walk with minimal assistance. However, he frequently attempted to walk independently without the cane or orthosis, and he fell each time. He began to make tactless comments and became impulsive, frequently grabbing or pushing people and objects. After 3 days in rehabilitation, he left the hospital against medical advice. A friend drove him to work. Within an hour he was fired because of his behavior toward coworkers and was readmitted to the hospital.

#### Question

Where is the lesion?

### Case 7

Critchley (1953)[134] reported a patient who seemed normal but put a tea bag in the teapot, set the pot on the stove, and poured cold water into a cup. She lit a match, put the match to the gas burner, blew out the match, and turned on the gas.

#### Question

Name the disorder.

### Case 8

H.M., a 66-year-old man, is 5 days post stroke. He is able to walk using a step-to gait, with minimal assist for balance. He is unable to voluntarily move his right arm. The right arm is adducted at the shoulder, and the elbow, wrist, and fingers are flexed. His speech is strained, harsh, and slow, and some sounds are produced incorrectly, as in "Ow are oo? I am fime." His ability to produce and understand language and his writing are entirely normal.

#### Questions

1. Name the communication disorder.
2. Where is the lesion?

### Case 9

V.M., a 72-year-old woman, was admitted to the hospital with right hemisensory loss, hemiplegia, and communication problems. She greeted visitors with a halting, effortful, and garbled "Hello, how you?" Language output was marred by poor articulation and omission of grammatical function words. She appeared extremely

## CLINICAL NOTES—cont'd

frustrated by her inability to express herself. Her attempts at writing left-handed also showed omission of grammatical function words. She was able to easily follow simple verbal or written commands, indicating intact ability to comprehend language.

### Questions
1. Where is the lesion?
2. Name the communication disorder.

### Case 10

P.D., an 86-year-old man, was referred to physical therapy following a total hip replacement 1 week ago. Two days ago, while his wife was visiting him in the hospital, he abruptly began to speak nonsense in a conversational tone as if he were speaking normally. His speech was a mixture of jargon and English. For example, he insisted, "I get creekons, tallings, and you must uffners." He became agitated when his wife didn't understand him, and he was unable to understand her questions. With hospital staff, he continued to speak freely in his mixture of jargon and English. He showed no indication of comprehending spoken or written language, nor any awareness that his language output was defective. Communication was strictly limited to gestures. No other signs or symptoms are evident. In therapy today, he was cooperative if the therapist pantomimed the desired movements. If the therapist tried to instruct him verbally, he became withdrawn and uncooperative.

### Questions
1. Name the communication disorder.
2. Where is the lesion?

### Case 11

A.G., a 68-year-old man, is 2 weeks post right cerebrovascular accident. In all situations, he ignores the left side of his body and objects and people on his left. He never looks toward the left, does not respond to touch or pinprick on his left side, does not eat food from the left side of a plate, does not move his left limbs, does not shave the left side of his face, nor dress his left side. Last week, two fingers on his left hand were lacerated while caught in his wheelchair spokes. Although the entrapped fingers prevented the wheelchair from moving, A.G. continued to try to move forward until stopped by the therapist. Gait requires maximal assistance because he does not bear full weight on the left leg and attempts to take steps using only the right leg, dragging the left leg behind. He becomes lost easily, and his attempts to copy drawings are distorted because he omits features that should be included on the left side of the drawing.

### Questions
1. Name the disorder.
2. What specific subtypes of the disorder does AG have?

### Case 12

A 32-year-old man was hit on the side of the head by a baseball 1 week ago. He complains of clumsiness in picking up objects, although he has no difficulty visually identifying objects. When he reaches for objects, he does not orient the position of his hand to the object; for example, when reaching for a pen held by the examiner, he uses a forearm pronated approach, regardless of whether the pen is vertical or horizontal. In reaching for a cup, he does not adjust the opening between fingers and thumb to the size of the cup.

### Questions
1. What is this condition called?
2. What area(s) of the brain is (are) damaged?

### Case 13

H.L. is a 17-year-old boy who sustained a closed head injury in an auto accident 1 month ago. H.L. was comatose for 2 weeks. During week 3, he became responsive to simple commands but was mute. Now H.L. talks, he believes he is at home, and he cannot report the correct year or month despite daily reminders of time and place. He does not initiate any activities unless prompted. H.L. is frequently verbally and physically aggressive. All limb movements are ataxic and dysmetric. Coming from sit to stand and gait require moderate assistance due to balance impairments, bilateral weakness, and poor coordination.

### Question
What areas of the brain are impaired?

## REVIEW QUESTIONS

1. What is the most likely location of a lesion in a person with loss of conscious somatosensation and voluntary movement on the left side of the body and face and loss of conscious vision from the left visual field?
2. Define each of the following terms and identify the area of the cortex most commonly damaged with each sign: astereognosis, visual agnosia, apraxia, and spastic dysarthria.
3. A person unable to understand nonverbal communication and exhibiting signs of left neglect probably has a lesion where?
4. Is Broca's aphasia an upper motor neuron disorder?
5. Describe the reward pathway. What happens when the reward pathway is activated?
6. What is emotional lability?
7. A person with severe traumatic brain injury is likely to have problems with what aspects of attention?
8. What is the difference between dysarthria and aphasia?
9. A 64-year-old woman has right hemiparesis, hemisensory loss, Broca's aphasia, and intact vision. Where is the most likely site for the lesion?
10. When working with a person who has global aphasia, what type of communication is most effective?
11. J.H. is 2 weeks post stroke. Although she has been in the same hospital room for 10 days, she cannot find the bathroom or the hallway. What is the name for this problem?
12. Define depression.
13. What is the pathology in post-traumatic stress disorder?

## References

1. Benarroch EE: The midline and intralaminar thalamic nuclei: anatomic and functional specificity and implications in neurologic disease. *Neurology* 71:944–949, 2008.
2. Bogen JE: The callosal syndromes. In Heilman KM, Valenstein E, editors: *Clinical neuropsychology*, New York, 1993, Oxford University Press, pp 337–407.
3. Herrero MT, Barcia C, Navarro JM: Functional anatomy of thalamus and basal ganglia. *Childs Nerv Syst* 18:386–404, 2002.
4. Saxena S, O'Neill J, Rauch SL: The role of cingulate cortex dysfunction in obsessive-compulsive disorder. In Vogt BA, editor: *Cingulate neurobiology and disease*, Oxford, UK, 2009, Oxford University Press, pp 587–617.
5. Peyron R, Laurent B, García-Larrea L: Functional imaging of brain responses to pain: a review and meta-analysis. *Neurophysiol Clin* 30:263–288, 2000.
6. Kaga K, Kaga M, Tamai F, Shindo M: Auditory agnosia in children after herpes encephalitis. *Acta Otolaryngol* 123:232–235, 2003.
7. Chawla J, Jacobs DH: Apraxia and related syndromes, 2009. Available at: http://emedicine.medscape.com/article/1136037. Accessed Dec. 20, 2011.
8. Ruchinskas RA, Giuliano AJ: Motor perseveration in geriatric medical patients. *Arch Clin Neuropsychol* 18:455–461, 2003.
9. Goel V, Vartanian O: Dissociating the roles of right ventral lateral and dorsal lateral prefrontal cortex in generation and maintenance of hypotheses in set-shift problems. *Cereb Cortex* 15:1170–1177, 2005.
10. Young L, Bechara A, Tranel D, et al: Damage to ventromedial prefrontal cortex impairs judgment of harmful intent. *Neuron* 65:845–851, 2010.
11. Bechara A: Risky business: emotion, decision-making, and addiction. *J Gambl Stud* 19:23–51, 2003.
12. Bechara A, Tranel D, Damasio H, et al: The somatic marker hypothesis and decision-making. In Boller F, Grafman J, editors: *Handbook of neuropsychology: frontal lobes*, ed 2, Amsterdam, 2002, Elsevier, pp 117–143.
13. Kühn S, Gallinat J, Brass M: "Keep calm and carry on": structural correlates of expressive suppression of emotions. *PLoS One* 6:e165–e169, 2011.
14. Peelen MV, Atkinson AP, Vuilleiumier P: Supramodal representations of perceived emotions in the human brain. *J Neurosci* 30:10127–10134, 2010.
15. Park IH, Ku J, Lee H, et al: Disrupted theory of mind network processing in response to idea of reference evocation in schizophrenia. *Acta Psychiatr Scand* 123:43–54, 2011.
16. Noël X, Bechara A, Brevers D, et al: Alcoholism and the loss of willpower: a neurocognitive perspective. *J Psychophysiol* 24:240–248, 2010.
17. Roiser JP, de Martino B, Tan GC, et al: A genetically mediated bias in decision making driven by failure of amygdala control. *J Neurosci* 29:5985–5991, 2009.
18. Feinstein JS, Adolphs R, Damasio A, et al: The human amygdala and the induction and experience of fear. *Curr Biol* 21:34–38, 2011.
19. Phelps EA: Emotion and cognition: insights from studies of the human amygdala. *Annu Rev Psychol* 24:27–53, 2006.
20. Bar-On R, Tranel D, Denburg NL, Bechara A: Exploring the neurological substrate of emotional and social intelligence. *Brain* 126:1790–1800, 2003.
21. Collette F, Hogge M, Salmon E, Van der Linden M: Exploration of the neural substrates of executive functioning by functional neuroimaging. *Neuroscience* 139:209–221, 2006.
22. Coricelli G, Dolan RJ, Sirigu A: Brain, emotion and decision making: the paradigmatic example of regret. *Trends Cogn Sci* 11:258–265, 2007.
23. Damasio AR: *In Descartes' error: emotion, reason, and the human brain*, New York, 1994, G. P. Putnam's Sons.
24. Chow TW: Personality in frontal lobe disorders. *Curr Psychiatry Rep* 2:446–451, 2000.
25. Arias-Carrión O, Stamelou M, Murillo-Rodríguez E, et al: Dopaminergic reward system: a short integrative review. *Int Arch Med* 3:24, 2010.
26. Sesack SR, Grace AA: Cortico-basal ganglia reward network: microcircuitry. *Neuropsychopharmacology* 35:27–47, 2010.
27. Beaulieu JM, Gainetdinov RR: The physiology, signaling, and pharmacology of dopamine receptors. *Pharmacol Rev* 63:182–217, 2011.
28. Haber SN, Knutson B: The reward circuit: linking primate anatomy and human imaging. *Neuropsychopharmacology* 35:4–26, 2010.
29. Maldonado JR: An approach to the patient with substance use and abuse. *Med Clin North Am* 94:1169–1205, 2010.
30. Crabbe JC, Harris RA, Koob GF: Preclinical studies of alcohol binge drinking. *Ann N Y Acad Sci* 1216:24–40, 2011.
31. Lowery EG, Thiele TE: Pre-clinical evidence that corticotropin-releasing factor (CRF) receptor antagonists are promising targets for pharmacological treatment of alcoholism. *CNS Neurol Disord Drug Targets* 9:77–86, 2010.
32. Ross S, Peselow E: Pharmacotherapy of addictive disorders. *Clin Neuropharmacol* 32:277–289, 2009.

33. Damasio AR, Tranel D, Damasio HD, et al: Amnesia caused by herpes simplex encephalitis, infarctions in basal forebrain, Alzheimer's disease, and anoxia/ischemia. In Boller F, Grafman J, editors: *Handbook of neuropsychology*, vol 3, Amsterdam, 1989, Elsevier, pp 149–166.

34. Squire LR, Bayley PJ, Smith CN: Amnesia, declarative and non-declarative memory. In Whitaker HB, editor: *Concise encyclopedia of brain and language*, Amsterdam, 2010, Elsevier, pp 30–35.

35. Gordon N: The neurology of sign language. *Brain Dev* 26:146–150, 2004.

36. Hillis AE: Neurobiology of unilateral spatial neglect. *Neuroscientist* 12:153–163, 2006.

37. Corbetta M, Kincade MJ, Lewis C, et al: Neural basis and recovery of spatial attention deficits in spatial neglect. *Nat Neurosci* 8:1603–1610, 2005.

38. Marcel AJ, Tegnér R, Nimmo-Smith I: Anosognosia for plegia: specificity, extension, partiality and disunity of bodily unawareness. *Cortex* 40:19–40, 2004.

39. Fotopoulou A, Pernigo S, Maeda R, et al: Implicit awareness in anosognosia for hemiplegia: unconscious interference without conscious re-representation. *Brain* 133:3564–3577, 2010.

40. Bisiach E, Luzzatti C: Unilateral neglect of representational space. *Cortex* 14:129–133, 1978.

41. Bisiach E, Berti A: Unilateral misrepresentation of distributed information: paradoxes and puzzles. In Brown WJ, editor: *Neuropsychology of visual perception*, Hillsdale, NJ, 1989, Erlbaum.

42. Medina J, Kannan V, Pawlak MA, et al: Neural substrates of visuospatial processing in distinct reference frames: evidence from unilateral spatial neglect. *J Cogn Neurosci* 21:2073–2084, 2009.

43. Goodale MA, Króliczak G, Westwood DA: Dual routes to action: contributions of the dorsal and ventral streams to adaptive behavior. *Prog Brain Res* 149:269–283, 2005.

44. Ticini LF, Klose U, Nägele T, et al: Perfusion imaging in Pusher syndrome to investigate the neural substrates involved in controlling upright body position. *PLoS One* 4:e573–e577, 2009.

45. Barra J, Marquer A, Joassin R, et al: Humans use internal models to construct and update a sense of verticality. *Brain* 133:3552–3563, 2010.

46. Danells CJ, Black SE, Gladstone DJ, McIlroy WE: Poststroke pushing: natural history and relationship to motor and functional recovery. *Stroke* 35:2873–2878, 2004.

47. Karnath HO, Johannsen L, Broetz D, et al: Prognosis of contraversive pushing. *J Neurol* 249:1250–1253, 2002.

48. Fan J, Gu X, Guise KG, et al: Testing the behavioral interaction and integration of attentional networks. *Brain Cogn* 70:209–220, 2009.

49. Dawson G, Webb SJ, McPartland J: Understanding the nature of face processing impairment in autism: insights from behavioral and electrophysiological studies. *Dev Neuropsychol* 27:403–424, 2005.

50. Brauer SG, Morris ME: Can people with Parkinson's disease improve dual tasking when walking? *Gait Posture* 31:229–233, 2010.

51. Pichierri G, Wolf P, Murer K, et al: Cognitive and cognitive-motor interventions affecting motor functioning of older adults: a systematic review. *BMC Geriatr* 11:29, 2011.

52. Rand D, Eng JJ, Liu-Ambrose T, et al: Feasibility of a 6-month exercise and recreation program to improve executive functioning and memory in individuals with chronic stroke. *Neurorehabil Neural Repair* 24:722–729, 2010.

53. Yogev-Seligmann G, Hausdorff JM, Giladi N: The role of executive function and attention in gait. *Mov Disord* 23:329–342, 2008; quiz 472.

54. Mathias JL, Wheaton P: Changes in attention and information-processing speed following severe traumatic brain injury: a meta-analytic review. *Neuropsychology* 21:212–223, 2007.

55. Tucha O, Tucha L, Kaumann G, et al: Training of attention functions in children with attention deficit hyperactivity disorder. *Atten Defic Hyperact Disord* 3:271–283, 2011.

56. Nagel BJ, Bathula D, Herting M, et al: Altered white matter microstructure in children with attention-deficit/hyperactivity disorder. *J Am Acad Child Adolesc Psychiatry* 50:283–292, 2011.

57. Soliva JC, Carmona S, Fauquet J, et al: Neurobiological substrates of social cognition impairment in attention-deficit hyperactivity disorder: gathering insights from seven structural and functional magnetic resonance imaging studies. *Ann N Y Acad Sci* 1167:212–220, 2009.

58. Volkow ND, Wang GJ, Kollins SH, et al: Evaluating dopamine reward pathway in ADHD: clinical implications. *JAMA* 302:1084–1091, 2009.

59. Wang KS, Liu X, Zhang Q, et al: Parent-of-origin effects of FAS and PDLIM1 in attention-deficit/hyperactivity disorder. *J Psychiatry Neurosci* 36:1001–1073, 2011.

60. Ginsberg Y, Hirvikoski T, Lindefors N: Attention deficit hyperactivity disorder (ADHD) among longer-term prison inmates is a prevalent, persistent and disabling disorder. *BMC Psychiatry* 10:112, 2010.

61. Staller J, Faraone SV: Attention-deficit hyperactivity disorder in girls: epidemiology and management. *CNS Drugs* 20:107–123, 2006.

62. Buitelaar JK, Casas M, Philipsen A, et al: Functional improvement and correlations with symptomatic improvement in adults with attention deficit hyperactivity disorder receiving long-acting methylphenidate. *Psychol Med June* 1:1–10, 2011. [Epub ahead of print]

63. McAlonan GM, Cheung V, Cheung C, et al: Mapping the brain in autism: a voxel-based MRI study of volumetric differences and intercorrelations in autism. *Brain* 128:268–276, 2005.

64. Goines P, Van de Water J: The immune system's role in the biology of autism. *Curr Opin Neurol* 23:111–117, 2010.

65. Hallmayer J, Cleveland S, Torres A, et al: Genetic heritability and shared environmental factors among twin pairs with autism. *Arch Gen Psychiatry* 2011 Jul 4. [Epub ahead of print]

66. Löscher W, Brandt C: Prevention or modification of epileptogenesis after brain insults: experimental approaches and translational research. *Pharmacol Rev* 62:668–700, 2010.

67. Mantegazza M, Rusconi R, Scalmani P, et al: Epileptogenic ion channel mutations: from bedside to bench and, hopefully, back again. *Epilepsy Res* 92:1–29, 2010.

68. Linehan C, Kerr MP, Walsh PN, et al: Examining the prevalence of epilepsy and delivery of epilepsy care in Ireland. *Epilepsia* 51:845–852, 2010.

69. Rosenfeld WE, Roberts DW: Tonic and atonic seizures: what's next—VNS or callosotomy? *Epilepsia* 50(Suppl 8):25–30, 2009.

70. Shin M, Besser LM, Kucik JE, et al: Prevalence of Down syndrome among children and adolescents in 10 regions of the United States. *Pediatrics* 124:1565–1571, 2009.

71. Tsai PH, Mendez M: Akinetopsia in the posterior cortical variant of Alzheimer disease. *Neurology* 73:731–732, 2009.

72. Work SS, Colamonico JA, Bradley WG, et al: Pseudobulbar affect: an under-recognized and under-treated neurological disorder. *Adv Ther* 28:586–601, 2011.

73. Altman R, Rutledge J: The vascular contribution to Alzheimer's disease. *Clin Sci (Lond)* 119:407–421, 2010.

74. Grammas P: Neurovascular dysfunction, inflammation and endothelial activation: implications for the pathogenesis of Alzheimer's disease. *J Neuroinflamm* 8:26, 2011.

75. Rocca WA, Petersen RC, Knopman DS, et al: Trends in the incidence and prevalence of Alzheimer's disease, dementia, and cognitive impairment in the United States. *Alzheimers Dement* 7:80–93, 2011.

76. James BD, Schneider JA: Increasing incidence of dementia in the oldest old: evidence and implications. *Alzheimers Res Ther* 2:9, 2010.

77. Granic A, Padmanabhan J, Norden M, et al: Alzheimer Abeta peptide induces chromosome mis-segregation and aneuploidy, including trisomy 21: requirement for tau and APP. *Mol Biol Cell* 21:511–520, 2010.

78. Khan TK, Alkon DL: Early diagnostic accuracy and pathophysiologic relevance of an autopsy-confirmed Alzheimer's disease peripheral biomarker. *Neurobiol Aging* 31:889–900, 2010.

79. Gaig C, Valldeoriola F, Gelpi E, et al: Rapidly progressive diffuse Lewy body disease. *Mov Disord* 26:1316–1323, 2011.

80. Ceravolo R, Rossi C, Kiferle K, et al: Nonmotor symptoms in Parkinson's disease: the dark side of the moon. *Future Neurol* 5:851–871, 2010.

81. McKee AC, Cantu RC, Nowinski CJ, et al: Chronic traumatic encephalopathy in athletes: progressive tauopathy after repetitive head injury. *J Neuropathol Exp Neurol* 68:709–735, 2009.

82. Williams WH, Potter S, Ryland H: Mild traumatic brain injury and postconcussion syndrome: a neuropsychological perspective. *J Neurol Neurosurg Psychiatry* 81:1116–1122, 2010.

83. Greiffenstein MF: Clinical myths of forensic neuropsychology. *Clin Neuropsychol* 23:286–296, 2009.

84. Henderson FC, Geddes JF, Vaccaro AR, et al: Stretch-associated injury in cervical spondylotic myelopathy: new concept and review. *Neurosurgery* 56:1101–1113, 2005; discussion 1101–13.

85. Rinne MB, Pasanen ME, Vartiainen MV, et al: Motor performance in physically well-recovered men with traumatic brain injury. *J Rehabil Med* 38:224–229, 2006.

86. Faul M, Xu L, Wald MM, Coronado VG: *Traumatic brain injury in the United States: emergency department visits, hospitalizations and deaths 2002–2006*, Atlanta, Ga, 2010, Centers for Disease Control and Prevention, National Center for Injury Prevention and Control.

87. Hirtz D, Thurman DJ, Gwinn-Hardy K, et al: How common are the "common" neurologic disorders? *Neurology* 68:326–337, 2007.

88. Dawodu ST: Traumatic brain injury (TBI): definition, epidemiology, pathophysiology. Available at: emedicine.medscape.com/article/326510-overview. Accessed June 13, 2011.

89. Whitnall L, McMillan TM, Murray GD, Teasdale GM: Disability in young people and adults after head injury: 5–7-year follow up of a prospective cohort study. *J Neurol Neurosurg Psychiatry* 77:640–645, 2006.

90. Fanconi M, Lips U: Shaken baby syndrome in Switzerland: results of a prospective follow-up study, 2002–2007. *Eur J Pediatr* 169:1023–1028, 2010.

91. Barlow KM, Thomson E, Johnson D, Minns RA: Late neurologic and cognitive sequelae of inflicted traumatic brain injury in infancy. *Pediatrics* 116:e174–e185, 2005.

92. Bartolo M, Zucchella C, Pichiecchio A, et al: Alien hand syndrome in left posterior stroke. *Neurol Sci* 32:483–486, 2011.

93. Kikkert MA, Ribbers GM, Koudstaal PJ: Alien hand syndrome in stroke: a report of 2 cases and review of the literature. *Arch Phys Med Rehabil* 87:728–732, 2006.

94. Pai Y-C, Rogers M, Hedman LD, Hanke TA: Alterations in weight-transfer capabilities in adults with hemiparesis. *Phys Ther* 74:647–659, 1994.

95. Noskin O, Krakauer JW, Lazar RM, et al: Ipsilateral motor dysfunction from unilateral stroke: implications for the functional neuroanatomy of hemiparesis. *J Neurol Neurosurg Psychiatry* 79:401–406, 2008.

96. Langhammer B, Stanghelle JK: Can physiotherapy after stroke based on the Bobath concept result in improved quality of movement compared to the motor relearning programme? *Physiother Res Int* 16:69–80, 2011.

97. Masiero S, Armani M, Rosati G: Upper-limb robot-assisted therapy in rehabilitation of acute stroke patients: focused review and results of new randomized controlled trial. *J Rehabil Res Dev* 48:355–366, 2011.

98. Rose D, Paris T, Crews E, et al: Feasibility and effectiveness of circuit training in acute stroke rehabilitation. *Neurorehabil Neural Repair* 25:140–148, 2011.

99. Chan DY, Chan CC, Au DK: Motor relearning programme for stroke patients: a randomized controlled trial. *Clin Rehabil* 20:191–200, 2006.

100. Kohler BA, Ward E, McCarthy BJ, et al: Annual report to the nation on the status of cancer, 1975–2007, featuring tumors of the brain and other nervous system. *J Natl Cancer Inst* 103:714–736, 2011.

101. Ffytche DH: Visual hallucinatory syndromes: past, present, and future. *Dialogues Clin Neurosci* 9:173–189, 2007.

102. Nicolson SE, Mayberg HS, Pennell PB, et al: Persistent auditory hallucinations that are unresponsive to antipsychotic drugs. *Am J Psychiatry* 163:1153–1159, 2006.

103. Phillips ML, Ladouceur CD, Drevets WC: A neural model of voluntary and automatic emotion regulation: implications for understanding the pathophysiology and neurodevelopment of bipolar disorder. *Mol Psychiatry* 13:829–857, 2003.

104. Dell'Osso B, Buoli M, Riundi R, et al: Clinical characteristics and long-term response to mood stabilizers in patients with bipolar disorder and different age at onset. *Neuropsychiatr Dis Treat* 5:399–404, 2009.

105. Santos CO, Caeiro L, Ferro JM, et al: Mania and stroke: a systematic review. *Cerebrovasc Dis* 32:11–21, 2011.

106. Demaree HA, Everhart DE, Youngstrom EA, Harrison DW: Brain lateralization of emotional processing: historical roots and a future incorporating emotional dominance. *Behav Cogn Neurosci Rev* 4:3–20, 2005.

107. Hamani C, Mayberg H, Stone S, et al: The subcallosal cingulate gyrus in the context of major depression. *Biol Psychiatry* 69:301–308, 2011.

108. Mauss IB, Bunge SA, Gross JJ: Automatic emotion regulation. *Social and Personality Psychology Compass* 1:146–167, 2007.

109. Bellani M, Baiano M, Brambilla P: Brain anatomy of major depression II: focus on amygdala. *Epidemiol Psychiatr Sci* 20:33–36, 2011.

110. Kessler RC, Berglund P, Demler O, et al: Lifetime prevalence and age-of-onset distributions of DSM-IV disorders in the National Comorbidity Survey Replication. *Arch Gen Psychiatry* 62:593–602, 2005.

111. Colucci RA, Silver MJ, Shubrook J: Common types of supraventricular tachycardia: diagnosis and management. *Am Fam Physician* 82:942–952, 2010.

112. Evcimen H, Kushon D, Jensen S: Nonepileptic hallucinations in use of levetiracetam. *Psychosomatics* 48:548–549, 2007.

113. Mirsattari SM, Gofton TE, Chong DJ: Misdiagnosis of epileptic seizures as manifestations of psychiatric illnesses. *Can J Neurol Sci* 38:487–493, 2011.

114. van den Heuvel OA, Mataix-Cols D, Zwitser G, et al: Common limbic and frontal-striatal disturbances in patients with obsessive compulsive disorder, panic disorder and hypochondriasis. *Psychol Med* 41:2399–2410, 2011.

115. Jimenez-Shahed J: Tourette syndrome. *Neurol Clin* 27:737–755, 2009.

116. Lanius RA, Vermetten E, Loewenstein RJ, et al: Emotion modulation in PTSD: clinical and neurobiological evidence for a dissociative subtype. *Am J Psychiatry* 167:640–647, 2010.

117. Shin LM, Liberzon I: The neurocircuitry of fear, stress, and anxiety disorders. *Neuropsychopharmacology* 35:169–191, 2010.

118. Kaloupek DG, Chard KM, Freed MC, et al: Common data elements for posttraumatic stress disorder research. *Arch Phys Med Rehabil* 91:1684–1691, 2010.

119. Manoach DS: Cognitive deficits in schizophrenia. In Whitaker HB, editor: *Concise encyclopedia of brain and language,* Amsterdam, 2010, Elsevier, pp 132–140.

120. Henseler I, Falkai P, Gruber O: Disturbed functional connectivity within brain networks subserving domain-specific subcomponents of working memory in schizophrenia: relation to performance and clinical symptoms. *J Psychiatr Res* 44:364–372, 2010.

121. Kang SS, Sponheim SR, Chafee MV, et al: Disrupted functional connectivity for controlled visual processing as a basis for impaired spatial working memory in schizophrenia. *Neuropsychologia* 2011 Jun 16. [Epub ahead of print]

122. Pajonk FG, Wobrock T, Gruber O, et al: Hippocampal plasticity in response to exercise in schizophrenia. *Arch Gen Psychiatry* 67:133–143, 2010.

123. McGrath JJ, Susser ES: New directions in the epidemiology of schizophrenia. *Med J Aust* 190(4 Suppl):S7–S9, 2009.

124. Tagliati M, Krack P, Volkmann J, et al: Long-term management of DBS in dystonia: response to stimulation, adverse events, battery changes, and special considerations. *Mov Disord* 26(Suppl 1):S54–S62, 2011.

125. Bewernick BH, Hurlemann R, Matusch A, et al: Nucleus accumbens deep brain stimulation decreases ratings of depression and anxiety in treatment-resistant depression. *Biol Psychiatry* 67:110–116, 2010.

126. Mohr P, Rodriguez M, Slavíčková A, et al: The application of vagus nerve stimulation and deep brain stimulation in depression. *Neuropsychobiology* 64:170–181, 2011.

127. Howland RH, Shutt LS, Berman SR, et al: The emerging use of technology for the treatment of depression and other neuropsychiatric disorders. *Ann Clin Psychiatry* 23:48–62, 2011.

128. Müller-Vahl KR, Cath DC, Cavanna AE, et al: European clinical guidelines for Tourette syndrome and other tic disorders. Part IV. Deep brain stimulation. *Eur Child Adolesc Psychiatry* 20:209–217, 2011.

129. Burdick AP, Fernandez HH, Okun MS, et al: Relationship between higher rates of adverse events in deep brain stimulation using standardized prospective recording and patient outcomes. *Neurosurg Focus* 29:E4, 2010.

130. Kim SP, Simeral JD, Hochberg LR, et al: Point-and-click cursor control with an intracortical neural interface system by humans with tetraplegia. *IEEE Trans Neural Syst Rehabil Eng* 19:193–203, 2011.

131. Kaiser V, Kreilinger A, Müller-Putz GR, et al: First steps toward a motor imagery based stroke BCI: new strategy to set up a classifier. *Front Neurosci* 5:86, 2011.

132. Presacco A, Goodman R, Forrester LW, et al: Neural decoding of treadmill walking from non-invasive, electroencephalographic (EEG) signals. *J Neurophysiol* 2011 Jul 13. [Epub ahead of print]

133. Kinney HC, Korein J, Panigrahy A, et al: Neuropathological findings in the brain of Karen Ann Quinlan: the role of the thalamus in the persistent vegetative state [see comments]. *N Engl J Med* 330:1469–1475, 1994.

134. Critchley M: The parietal lobes, London, UK, 1953, E. Arnold.

# 19   Support Systems: Blood Supply and Cerebrospinal Fluid System

Laurie Lundy-Ekman, PhD, PT

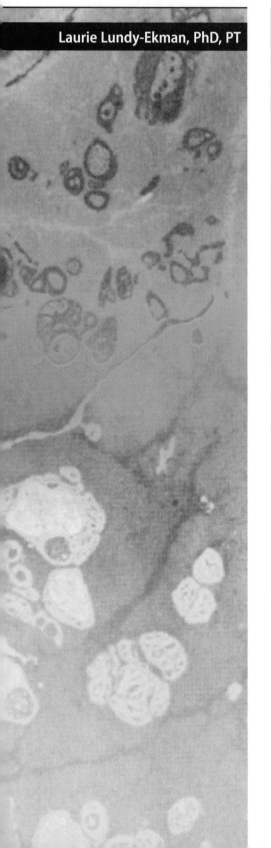

## Chapter Outline

I am a 51-year-old professor of neuroanatomy. I teach physical and occupational therapy students, medical students, dental students, and undergraduates. My particular interest, in both teaching and research, is recovery of function. For 10 years or so, I was doing research on recovery from spinal cord injury using rats, but the money dried up, and I haven't done research in several years.

I have had two strokes. The first stroke was when I was 3 years old. But it was misdiagnosed at the time (they thought I had polio), and I didn't know until my twenties that I had had a stroke. People certainly recover a lot better when they are young. The second stroke occurred when I was 41.

The first signs of this stroke were a very severe headache and (so I am told, since my memory of this time was wiped out) a collapse on my left side due to left hemiparesis. My wife asked me to move my left arm. I said, "My left arm is gone. All I've got is a big hole there." This was the first sign of left side neglect. I had no transient ischemic attacks or other warning signs of impending stroke.

When I was taken into a nearby emergency room, they immediately did a CAT scan, which showed a serious right hemisphere hemorrhage. I think I was also given a lumbar puncture and an angiogram. The physician threw up his hands at the results of the scans and placed me under a no-code order that night.

I had four major effects of the stroke. One, I had loss of proprioception, which was particularly noticeable. I could never tell where my left arm was without looking. I also had a patchy loss of touch and pain sensation (when starting dialysis, I would feel one needle going in but not the other), but I never got it mapped out. Two, I have left-side hemiparesis. I walk with a quad cane, and my left fingers are tonically flexed so that my left arm is not usable. Three, left-side neglect. At first I would bump into drinking fountains that I just didn't see. This was worst immediately after the stroke, when I missed the first word of every line I read. The neglect has gotten much better over time and is no longer a real problem. Four, I have short-term memory loss. For some reason, the short-term memory loss is worst with food. I can't remember what I eat each day, but otherwise the memory loss doesn't cause me much of a problem.

All of these problems have improved over time, so that they are no longer the problems they were. This is probably partly because I have learned how to get around them.

I received lots of physical therapy, including intensive PT during recovery right after the stroke (9 weeks inpatient, several months outpatient). Learning how to stand and transfer, as well as how to walk, was the most important. I have also received PT

after two fractures—one of the pelvis, and one of the hip. The therapy helped me get going again.

All of the physical therapy was very effective; I couldn't function without it! Working on my own, the best exercise I get is walking as much as possible. I do some other exercises, but not too often.

I take phenobarbital, 400 mL/day, to prevent seizures, but occasionally they happen and I have to increase the dosage. I had one grand mal (generalized tonic-clonic) seizure about 2 years after the stroke, but no subsequent grand mal seizures after being on this medication. I have had a number of minor atonic seizures, most of which caused no problems. My atonic seizures ("drop attacks") hit without any warning—I go along, minding my business, and suddenly find myself on the ground. I am never aware of falling, and I don't know whether I lose consciousness, but probably very briefly if so. Most of the time I fall like a rag doll (no muscle tone) and don't hurt myself. As soon as I am aware of being down, I have to figure out how to get up again, which I can't do myself. Fortunately, someone has always been around to help me up. Only twice have I had serious problems. Once, it hit me as I was getting in the shower, and I fell into the shower door, discovering on the way down that it was not shatterproof glass. I came to, lying in a sea of shards and bleeding profusely. I was lucky my wife was home, or I may not have made it. The other time was last February, when I collapsed while walking home from the bus stop one night and fractured my hip. That was nasty, requiring 4 months of hospitalization.

The biggest change due to the stroke was not a physical one but a mental one. I felt very positive, despite the stroke, and felt that life was really good! In addition I discovered new social skills that I never had before and had wonderfully creative thoughts drop in on me. These changes are described in my book *Life at a Snail's Pace*, published in 1995 by Peanut Butter Publishing in Seattle, Washington.

*—Dr. Roger Harris*

Four of the changes reported by Dr. Harris are common after a right hemisphere stroke affecting the middle cerebral artery. Loss of proprioception in the left upper limb follows loss of neurons in the upper limb area of the right somatosensory cortex. Damage to the primary motor cortex causes contralateral hemiparesis. Damage to the right parietotemporal cortex causes left neglect. Damage to the dorsolateral prefrontal interferes with working memory.[1] However, mood and sociability changes occur less frequently. Right hemisphere lesions sometimes also cause elevated mood, increased talkativeness, flight of ideas, and social disinhibition, particularly in males.[2]

Two fluid systems support the neurons and glial cells of the nervous system: the cerebrospinal fluid (CSF) system and the vascular system. The CSF system includes the ventricles, the meninges, and the CSF. The vascular system includes the arterial supply, veins and venous sinuses, and mechanisms to regulate blood flow.

## CEREBROSPINAL FLUID SYSTEM

The CSF system regulates the extracellular milieu and protects the central nervous system. CSF is formed primarily in the ventricles and then circulates through the ventricles and into the subarachnoid space (between the arachnoid and the pia

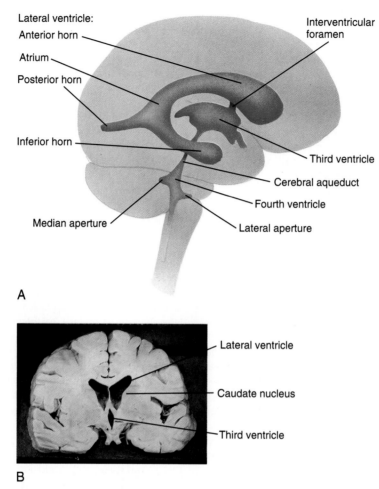

**Fig. 19-1  Ventricles. A,** Lateral view of the ventricles. **B,** Coronal section of the brain showing the lateral and third ventricles.

mater) before it is absorbed into the venous circulation. CSF supplies water, certain amino acids, and specific ions to the extracellular fluid and probably removes metabolites from the brain. CSF and extracellular fluid freely communicate in the brain. The meninges and the buoyancy of the fluid provide protection to the brain by absorbing some of the impact when the head is struck.

## Ventricles

CSF-filled spaces inside the brain form a system of four ventricles (Figure 19-1). The lateral ventricles are paired, one in each cerebral hemisphere. The C-shaped lateral ventricles consist of a body; an atrium; and anterior, posterior, and inferior horns. The spaces extend into each lobe of the hemispheres. Much of the outside wall of the lateral ventricle is formed by the caudate nucleus, and the tail of the caudate is above the inferior horn. Below the body of the lateral ventricle is the thalamus; above is the corpus callosum. The lateral ventricles connect to each other and to the third ventricle by the interventricular foramina (foramina of Monro).

The third ventricle is a narrow slit in the midline of the diencephalon; thus its walls are the thalamus and the hypothalamus. An interthalamic adhesion often crosses the center of the

third ventricle. A canal through the midbrain, the cerebral aqueduct (aqueduct of Sylvius), connects the third and fourth ventricles.

The fourth ventricle is a space posterior to the pons and medulla and anterior to the cerebellum. Inferiorly the fourth ventricle is continuous with the central canal of the spinal cord. The fourth ventricle drains into the subarachnoid space via three small openings: the two lateral foramina (foramina of Luschka) and a midline opening (foramen of Magendie).

## Meninges

Three layers of meninges cover the brain and spinal cord. From external to internal, these layers are the dura mater, the arachnoid, and the pia mater. The dura mater surrounds the brain and consists of an outer layer firmly bound to the inside of the skull and an inner layer. The inner layer attaches to the arachnoid. The two layers are fused except at the dural sinuses, which are spaces for the collection of venous blood and CSF. The inner layer of dura has two projections: the falx cerebri, separating the cerebral hemispheres, and the tentorium cerebelli, separating the cerebellum from the cerebral hemispheres. Spinal dura is continuous with the inner layer of brain dura.

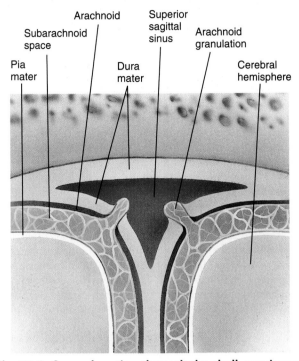

Pia mater · Subarachnoid space · Arachnoid · Dura mater · Superior sagittal sinus · Arachnoid granulation · Cerebral hemisphere

**Fig. 19-2 Coronal section through the skull, meninges, and cerebral hemispheres.** The section shows midline structures near the top of the skull. The three layers of meninges, the superior sagittal sinus, and arachnoid granulations are indicated.

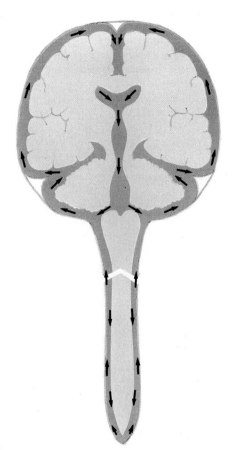

**Fig. 19-3** The flow of cerebrospinal fluid from the lateral ventricles, third ventricle, and fourth ventricle into the subarachnoid space surrounding the brain and spinal cord. Cerebrospinal fluid is reabsorbed into the venous sinuses.

The arachnoid is a delicate membrane loosely attached to the dura. Projections of arachnoid form arachnoid villi, which pierce the dura and protrude into the venous sinuses. The arachnoid villi allow CSF to flow into the sinuses. Clusters of arachnoid villi form arachnoid granulations (Figure 19-2).

Pia mater, the innermost layer, is tightly apposed to the surfaces of the brain and spinal cord. Arachnoid trabeculae (collagen fibers) connect the arachnoid and the pia mater, serving to suspend the brain in the meninges. The subarachnoid space, between the pia and the arachnoid, is filled with CSF. Extensions of the pia, the denticulate ligaments, anchor the spinal cord to the dura mater.

## Formation and Circulation of Cerebrospinal Fluid

Although some CSF is formed by extracellular fluid leaking into the ventricles, choroid plexuses in the ventricles secrete most of the CSF. A choroid plexus is a network of capillaries embedded in connective tissue and epithelial cells. Through three layers of cells (capillary wall, connective tissue, and epithelium), CSF is formed from blood by filtration, active transport, and facilitated transport of certain substances. These processes result in the formation of a fluid similar to plasma.

CSF flows from the lateral ventricles into the third ventricle via the interventricular foramina and from the third ventricle into the fourth via the cerebral aqueduct (Figure 19-3). CSF exits the fourth ventricle through the lateral and medial foramina, entering the subarachnoid space. Within the subarachnoid space, CSF flows around the spinal cord and brain. Finally, the CSF is absorbed through the arachnoid villi, which

project through the dura and into the venous sinuses. In the unidirectional flow of CSF into venous blood, all contents of the CSF (proteins, microorganisms) are included.

## Clinical Disorders of the Cerebrospinal Fluid System

Common disorders of the CSF system include epidural and subdural hematomas, hydrocephalus, and meningitis. Hematomas are usually a consequence of trauma. Normally only potential spaces exist between the dura and the skull, and between the dura and the arachnoid. Bleeding into either of these potential spaces can cause separation of the layers, resulting in an epidural or subdural hematoma. Epidural hematoma results from arterial bleeding between the skull and the dura mater. Most often an epidural hematoma occurs when the middle meningeal artery is torn by a fracture of the temporal or parietal bone. Because arteries bleed rapidly, signs and symptoms develop swiftly. After a blow to the head, the person may have a few hours of normal function and then may develop a worsening headache, vomiting, decreasing consciousness, hemiparesis, and Babinski's sign. In contrast, signs and symptoms of subdural hematoma gradually worsen over a prolonged period (days to months). Bleeding is slow in subdural hematoma because the hematoma is produced by venous bleeding, where the blood pressure is less than in arteries. Signs and symptoms are similar to those of epidural hematoma, with confusion being more prominent. Both types of hematoma are potentially life threatening because neural tissue is compressed and displaced.

If CSF circulation is blocked, pressure builds in the ventricles, causing hydrocephalus (Figure 19-4, *A*). Hydrocephalus

is an enlargement of the ventricles. In infants, the cranial bones have not yet fused, so the pressure causes the ventricles, hemispheres, and cranium to expand. Signs of hydrocephalus include a disproportionately large head size for age, a large anterior fontanel, poor feeding, inactivity, and downward gaze of the eyes (from compression of the oculomotor nerve center; Figure 19-4, *B*). Common causes of congenital hydrocephalus include failure of the fourth ventricle foramina to open, blockage of the cerebral aqueduct, cysts in the fourth ventricle (Dandy-Walker cysts), and the Arnold-Chiari malformation (see Chapter 5). Rarely, hydrocephalus may result from excessive production or inadequate reabsorption of CSF. In older children or adults, because the cranium cannot expand, excessive pressure in the ventricles compresses the nervous tissue, particularly the white matter. This commonly results in gait and balance impairments, incontinence, and headache. Frequently, frontal lobe functions are also involved (i.e., some features of emotions, planning, memory, and intellect). Language, spatial awareness, and declarative memory are spared. In progressive hydrocephalus, a shunt is implanted, usually draining a ventricle into the peritoneum (Figure 19-5). In most cases, the shunts remain in place permanently.

A technique alleged to evaluate and treat the CSF system is craniosacral therapy. Advocates of this therapy claim that CSF production is periodic, with each period of secretion followed by a period during which no CSF is produced. Fluid pressure changes purportedly produce a rhythmic movement of the dura that can be palpated.[3] Currently no evidence exists for the existence of craniosacral rhythm (pulse-like movement of CSF

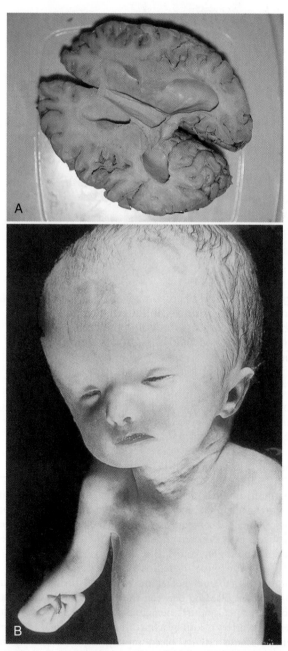

**Fig. 19-4  A,** Horizontal section showing enlarged ventricles characteristic of hydrocephalus. Note the displacement of white matter by excessive cerebrospinal fluid pressure. **B,** A child with hydrocephalus. The skull is enlarged. The fontanelle is depressed owing to excessive draining of CSF by a shunt (see Figure 19-5). *(B courtesy Children's Hospital Medical Center, Cincinnati, Ohio.)*

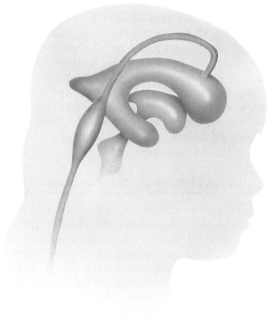

**Fig. 19-5  Placement of a shunt into the lateral ventricle to drain excessive cerebrospinal fluid.** The swelling in the shunt shows the location of a valve that prevents reverse flow of fluid in the shunt.

transmitted to the dura mater and to the body fascia),[4] and attempts to assess the rhythm have been demonstrated to be unreliable.[5-7]

The membranes of the cerebrospinal system may be affected by disease. Meningitis is inflammation of the membranes that surround the brain and/or spinal cord. Signs and symptoms include headache, fever, confusion, vomiting, and neck stiffness. Pain intensifies in the upright position, with head movement, and with sneezing or coughing. Photophobia may accompany meningitis. Bacterial or viral infection can cause meningitis.

## DISORDERS OF VASCULAR SUPPLY

Please review the vascular supply to the nervous system, covered in Chapter 1.

The functional areas of the cerebral cortex are shown with the cerebral arteries in Figure 19-6. Loss of blood supply in a specific area correlates with a specific loss of function. For example, loss of blood supply to Broca's area interferes with expressive speech.

Interrupting the blood flow to a part of the brain usually produces a focal loss of function, except in cases of subarachnoid hemorrhage. The effects of blood flow interruption range from a brief loss of function followed by complete recovery to permanent life-altering impairments and activity limitations to death. Episodes of focal functional loss following vascular incidents are classified according to both the pattern of progression and etiology. The patterns of progression from the time of onset include the following:

- Transient ischemic attack: a brief, focal loss of brain function, with full recovery from neurologic deficits within 24 hours. Transient ischemic attacks (TIAs) are believed to be due to ischemia. TIA is a medical emergency despite full recovery because 10% to 30% of people who have a TIA have a stroke within 3 months.[8]
- Completed stroke: neurologic deficits from vascular disorders that persist for longer than 1 day and are stable (not progressing or improving)

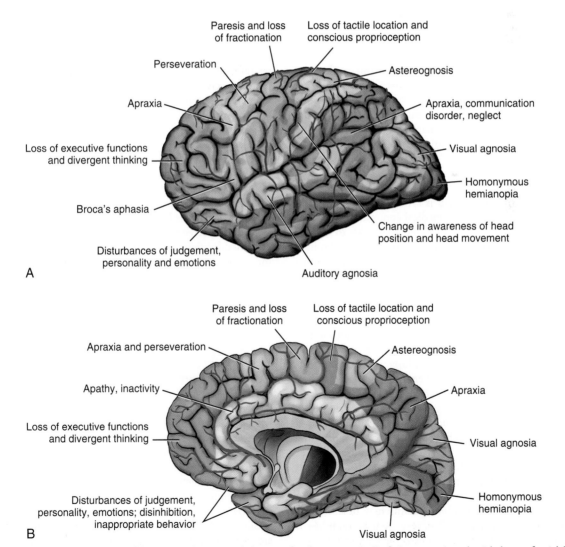

**Fig. 19-6  The arterial supply of functional areas of the cerebral cortex. A,** Deficits associated with loss of middle cerebral artery circulation. **B,** Deficits associated with loss of anterior and posterior cerebral artery circulation.

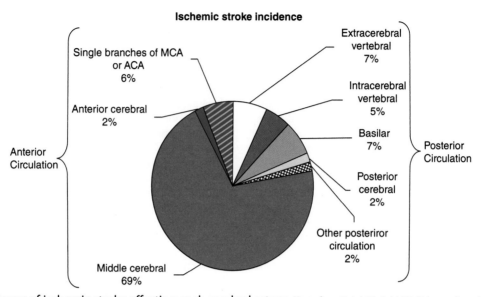

**Fig. 19-7** Incidence of ischemic stroke affecting each cerebral artery. *(Data from Baird AE, Jichici D, Talavera F, et al: Anterior circulation stroke, 2011. Available at: http://emedicine.medscape.com/article/1159900. Accessed Dec. 15, 2011; Caplan L, Wityk R, Pazdera L, et al: New England Medical Center Posterior Circulation Stroke Registry II: vascular lesions. Clin Neurol 1:31–49, 2005; Ng YS, Stein J, Ning M, et al: Comparison of clinical characteristics and functional outcomes of ischemic stroke in different vascular territories. Stroke 38:2309–2314, 2007.)*

- Progressive stroke: some people with ischemic stroke have deficits that increase intermittently over time. These are believed to be due to repeated emboli (blood clots that formed elsewhere and were transmitted by the blood to a new location) or continued formation of a thrombus (blood clot that stays where it formed).

## Types of Stroke

The term *cerebrovascular accident* is synonymous with stroke. Currently some members of the medical community are advocating "brain attack" as a lay term to replace stroke, to emphasize that prompt treatment may benefit some people who have strokes, just as prompt treatment is effective for some heart attacks. The two types of stroke are infarction and hemorrhagic.

### Brain Infarction

Brain infarction occurs when an embolus or thrombus lodges in a vessel, obstructing blood flow. Typically, an embolus abruptly deprives an area of blood, resulting in almost immediate onset of deficits. Sometimes the embolus breaks into fragments and is dislodged, resulting in quick resolution of deficits. More often, residual brain damage is permanent, resulting in prolonged and incomplete functional recovery. The most rapid spontaneous recovery from ischemic stroke occurs during the first and second weeks post stroke. Infarcts cause 80% of strokes. More than 90% of anterior circulation ischemic strokes affect the middle cerebral artery.[9] The incidence of ischemic stroke affecting each artery is shown in Figure 19-7.

Onset of signs from thrombic ischemia may be abrupt or may worsen over several days. Recovery from a thrombus is usually slow, and significant residual disability is common.

Obstructions of blood flow in small, deep arteries result in *lacunar infarcts*. Lacunae are small cavities that remain after the

necrotic tissue has been cleared away (Figure 19-8). Lacunar infarcts occur most often in the basal ganglia, internal capsule, thalamus, and brainstem. Signs of lacunar infarcts develop slowly and are often purely motor or purely sensory; good recovery is the norm.

Slow occlusion of an artery has a very different outcome from an abrupt occlusion. For example, if one internal carotid artery is slowly occluded, anastomotic connections and collateral circulation among the unaffected arteries may be adequate to maintain brain function. Less frequently, an abrupt internal carotid occlusion is fatal due to infarction of the anterior two-thirds of the cerebral hemisphere. The difference in outcome is explained by the time course of the occlusion, the location of the occlusion, blood pressure at the time of the occlusion, and individual variation in collateral connections. Gradual occlusion may allow the development of increased collateral circulation. Low blood pressure during the occlusion makes adequate perfusion of the brain less likely.

### Hemorrhage

Hemorrhage deprives the downstream vessels of blood, and the extravascular blood exerts pressure on the surrounding brain. Generally, hemorrhagic strokes present with the worst deficits within hours of onset; then improvement occurs as edema decreases and extravascular blood is removed. Figure 19-9 shows severe hemorrhage within the brain.

#### Subarachnoid Hemorrhage

Bleeding into the subarachnoid space usually causes sudden, excruciating headache with a brief (a few minutes) loss of consciousness. Unlike other hemorrhages, the initial findings often are not focal. Deficits from subarachnoid hemorrhage are progressive because of continued bleeding or secondary hydrocephalus. Vasospasm and infarction are common sequelae of

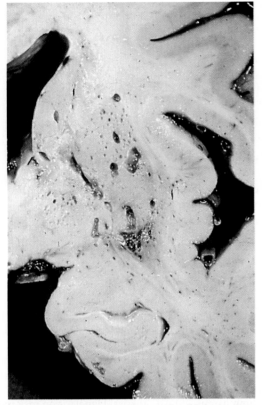

**Fig. 19-8 Coronal section of a cerebral hemisphere, with a lateral ventricle appearing near the top left corner.** The small cavities in the basal ganglia are lacunar infarcts, produced by occlusions of small, deep arteries. *(Courtesy Dr. Melvin J. Ball.)*

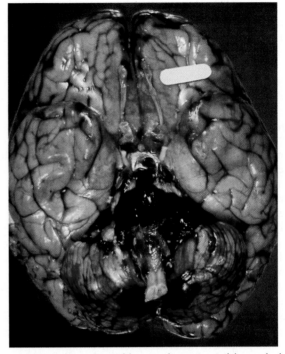

**Fig. 19-10** Subarachnoid hemorrhage is visible as dark areas, most prominent in the brainstem region. *(Courtesy Dr. Melvin J. Ball.)*

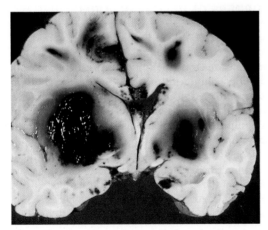

**Fig. 19-9 Multiple hemorrhages within the brain secondary to head trauma.** *(Courtesy Dr. Melvin J. Ball.)*

subarachnoid hemorrhage. Figure 19-10 shows a subarachnoid hemorrhage.

## Stroke Signs and Symptoms by Arterial Location

Pathology may involve the main arteries, smaller branches, the capillary network, or arteriovenous formations.

### Vertebral and Basilar Arteries

Twenty percent of ischemic strokes affect the brainstem/cerebellar region.[10] Because the vertebral arteries are subject to shear forces at the atlantoaxial joint, abrupt neck rotation or hyperextension can cause brainstem ischemia. Gouveia and associates (2009)[11] published a review of cases of strokes attributable to chiropractic manipulation and reported a maximum incidence of 5 strokes per 100,000 manipulations. The mechanism was vertebral artery dissection, a separation of the wall of the artery that allows bleeding into the wall of the artery. The chief symptom of vertebral artery dissection is pain, usually in the posterior neck or occiput and spreading to the shoulders.[12]

In vertebrobasilar artery ischemia, the most common signs are gait and limb ataxia, limb weakness, oculomotor palsies, and oropharyngeal dysfunction.[12] Other signs and symptoms that frequently occur are loss of vision, double vision, numbness, dizziness, vertigo, headache, and vomiting. Less than 1% of patients with vertebrobasilar ischemia have only a single presenting sign or symptom; thus isolated dizziness or brief loss of consciousness is unlikely to be caused by vertebrobasilar ischemia.[12]

Emboli in the intracranial vertebral arteries usually cause cerebellar infarction. The most common symptoms in acute cerebellar infarction are dizziness and/or vertigo, inability to sit upright without support, difficulty walking, nausea and vomiting, dysarthria, and headache.[13]

Complete occlusion of the basilar artery causes death due to ischemia of brainstem nuclei and tracts that control vital functions. Partial occlusions of the basilar artery can cause tetraplegia (descending motor tracts), loss of sensation (ascending sensory tracts), coma (reticular activating system), and cranial nerve signs. Severe partial occlusion of the basilar artery causes locked-in syndrome,[12] preserving consciousness but preventing voluntary movement below the neck and preventing speech.[14] Occlusion of a cerebellar artery causes ataxia.

## Cerebral Arteries

Occlusion of the cortical branches of the **anterior cerebral artery** results in personality changes (frontal lobe) with contralateral hemiplegia and hemisensory loss. The hemiplegia and hemisensory loss are more severe in the lower limb than in the face and upper limb because the medial sensorimotor cortex and adjacent white matter are affected. Lack of blood supply to the deep branches of the anterior cerebral artery results in motor dysfunction caused by damage of the anterior putamen and of frontopontine axons in the internal capsule.[15]

Occlusion of the cortical branches of the middle cerebral artery deprives the optic radiation and the lateral parts of the sensorimotor cortex and adjacent white matter of blood. This produces homonymous hemianopia combined with contralateral hemiplegia and hemisensory loss involving the upper limb and face more than the lower limb, because the neurons regulating movement and processing conscious sensation of the upper body are located in the lateral cerebral cortex. Language impairment is common if the lesion is in the language-dominant hemisphere (usually the left hemisphere). Difficulty understanding spatial relationships, neglect, and impairment of nonverbal communication often occur with lesions in the hemisphere that is nondominant for language (usually the right hemisphere).[15]

Deep branches of the **middle cerebral artery** (striate arteries) supply the striatum and the genu and limbs of the internal capsule. Loss of blood supply to the deep branches deprives axons passing through the internal capsule, producing contralateral hemiplegia that affects the upper and lower extremities and the face equally. Most ischemic strokes occlude the middle cerebral artery, often producing a stereotypic standing posture on the hemiparetic side: characteristic adduction at the shoulder, flexion at the elbow, and extension throughout the lower limb. Occlusion of the anterior choroidal artery, a branch off the internal carotid, produces contralateral hemiplegia and hemisensory loss with homonymous hemianopia by depriving axons in the posterior internal capsule of blood.[9]

Occlusion of the midbrain branches of the **posterior cerebral artery**[10] can result in contralateral hemiparesis (cerebral peduncle) and eye movement paresis or paralysis affecting the muscles innervated by the oculomotor nerve (oculomotor nerve and its controlling nuclei or descending neurons). Occlusion of the branches to the calcarine cortex results in cortical blindness affecting information from the contralateral visual field (see Chapter 16). Deep branches of the posterior cerebral artery supply much of the diencephalon and hippocampus. Lack of blood flow to the thalamus can cause thalamic syndrome, characterized by severe pain, contralateral hemisensory loss, and flaccid hemiparesis. Vascular compromise of the hippocampus interferes with declarative memory (see Chapter 17). Occlusion of the posterior choroidal branch prevents blood from reaching

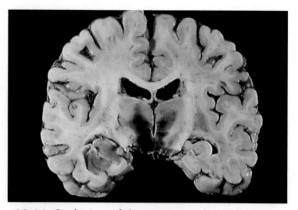

**Fig. 19-11** Occlusion of the posterior choroidal artery, producing necrosis in part of the thalamus. *(Courtesy Dr. Melvin J. Ball.)*

parts of the thalamus and hippocampus (Figure 19-11). Figure 19-12 summarizes the deficits that commonly occur following strokes in specific arteries.

The **watershed area** (Figure 19-13), the site of anastomoses among the distal branches of cerebral arteries, is vulnerable to ischemia. Lack of blood to the watershed region often causes upper limb paresis and paresthesias. Hypotension may result in decreased blood flow in the watershed area, thereby decreasing the effectiveness of the anastomoses.[10]

The effects of a stroke depend on the etiology, severity, and location.

## DISORDERS OF VASCULAR FORMATION

### Arteriovenous Malformations

Arteriovenous malformations are developmental abnormalities with arteries connected to veins by abnormal, thin-walled vessels larger than capillaries. The malformations usually do not cause signs or symptoms until they rupture; then the bleeding causes dysfunction due to lack of blood to the area the arteries normally supply and due to pressure exerted by the extravascular blood. Rupture of an arteriovenous malformation can cause subdural hematoma, intracerebral hemorrhage, or both, depending on the location of the malformation.

### Aneurysm

An aneurysm is a dilation of the wall of an artery or vein. These swellings have thin walls that are prone to rupture. Saccular aneurysms are most common, affecting only one side of the vessel wall. A berry aneurysm, a type of saccular aneurysm, is a small sac that protrudes from a cerebral artery and has a thin connection with the artery (Figure 19-14). Hemorrhage resulting from aneurysm rupture may be massive, causing sudden death, or causing a wide variety of signs and symptoms depending on the location and extent of the bleeding. The bleeding occurs into the subarachnoid space, producing subdural hematoma.

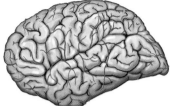
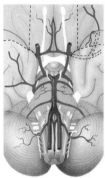

| Artery affected: | Somatosensory | Motor | Special senses and autonomic function | Emotions and behavior | Cognition, language, memory | Other |
|---|---|---|---|---|---|---|
| **Anterior cerebral artery** | Loss of sensation in lower limb | Apraxia; hemiplegia (lower limb more affected than upper limb and face); impaired gait | No changes | Flat affect; impulsiveness; perseveration; confusion; motor inactivity | Difficulty with divergent thinking | Urinary incontinence |
| **Middle cerebral artery** | Hemianesthesia affecting face and upper limb more than lower limb | Face and upper limb more impaired than lower limb; if striate arteries involved, lower limb paresis or paralysis in addition to face and upper limb impairment | Homonymous hemianopia | If right hemisphere (left hemiplegia): easily distracted, poor judgment, impulsiveness; if left hemisphere (right hemiplegia): apraxia, compulsiveness, overly cautious | Left MCA: Aphasia Right MCA: difficulty understanding spatial relationships, neglect, impairment of nonverbal communication, dressing apraxia, constructional apraxia | None |
| **Posterior cerebral artery** | Hemianesthesia; slow pain is preserved | Hemiparesis; if lesion near origin of artery; vertical gaze palsy, oculomotor nerve palsy, loss of medial deviation of the eyes with preserved convergence, vertical skew deviation of the eyes | Homonymous hemianopia; cortical blindness; hallucinations; lack of depth perception; impaired eye movements, except lateral and infero-medial eye movements; visual agnosia; limbs may show vasomotor and/or trophic abnormalities | Memory loss | Difficulty reading | None |
| **Basilar artery** | Bilateral sensory loss | Tetraplegia; abducens nerve palsy (palsy of lateral gaze); locked-in syndrome; oculomotor nerve palsy; decorticate or decerebrate rigidity; paresis or paralysis of muscles of the tongue, lips, palate, pharynx, and larynx | Vertigo, diplopia, vomiting, nausea, nystagmus, hearing loss, pupil constriction (involvement of descending sympathetic fibers in the pons; however, pupils may be reactive to light) | None | Reduced consciousness | Coma |

**Fig. 19-12** Depending on the distribution and severity of the occlusion or hemorrhage, various subsets of the signs listed would occur.

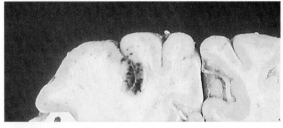

**Fig. 19-13** Coronal section near the top of the skull, showing an infarction in the watershed area. *(Courtesy Dr. Melvin J. Ball.)*

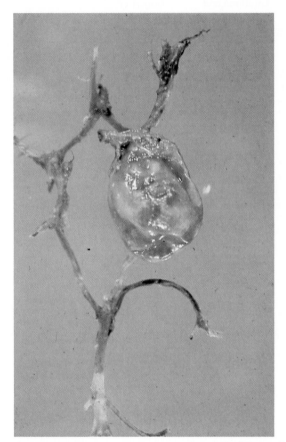

**Fig. 19-14** Large berry aneurysm at the end of the right internal carotid artery. *(Courtesy Dr. Melvin J. Ball.)*

## FLUID DYNAMICS

### Blood-Brain Barrier

The blood-brain barrier is a specialized permeability barrier between the capillary endothelium of the central nervous system and the extracellular space. The barrier is formed by tight junctions between the capillary endothelial cells that exclude large molecules (free fatty acids, proteins, specific amino acids). This exclusion is useful for preventing many pathogens from entering the central nervous system; however, the barrier also prevents certain drugs and protein antibodies from accessing the brain. For example, in the early stages of Parkinson's disease, dopamine delivered to the brain can ameliorate the signs and symptoms. However, dopamine cannot cross the blood-brain barrier. Therefore a metabolic precursor of dopamine, called L-dopa, is given to people with Parkinson's disease; L-dopa can cross the blood-brain barrier. Once L-dopa is in the brain, it is converted into dopamine. Currently, intentional disruption of the blood-brain barrier is an experimental method of delivering some medications to the central nervous system.

The blood-brain barrier is absent in areas of the brain that directly sample the contents of the blood or secrete into the bloodstream. These regions include parts of the hypothalamus and other specialized areas around the third and fourth ventricles. Specialized ependymal cells (tanycytes) separate leaky regions from the rest of the brain; these special cells may prevent proteins, viruses, and some drugs from entering the brain via leaky regions.

### Cerebral Blood Flow

Because the brain cannot store glucose or oxygen effectively, a consistent blood supply is essential. Oxygen consumption increases from brainstem to cerebral cortex, leaving the cerebral cortex more vulnerable to hypoxia than vital centers in the lower brainstem.[16,17] This differential oxygen requirement explains some incidents of persistent vegetative state. In some cases of persistent vegetative state, severe head trauma or anoxia destroys the cerebral and cerebellar cortices, yet the person survives because brainstem and spinal cord functions continue.[18]

Cerebral arteries autoregulate local blood flow, depending primarily on two factors: blood pressure and metabolites. The arteries dilate if blood pressure, oxygen, or pH levels are inadequate, or if carbon dioxide or lactic acid is excessive. Conversely, when blood pressure, oxygen, or pH levels are excessive, or carbon dioxide or lactic acid levels are below functional levels, the arteries constrict. A minor role in regulating arterial diameter is played by autonomic and other neuron systems within the brain; these mechanisms currently are not well understood. Autoregulation is vitally important to ensure adequate blood flow and to prevent brain edema.

### Cerebral Edema

Cerebral edema is the accumulation of excess tissue fluid in the brain. Concussion frequently causes cerebral edema because trauma allows fluid to leak from the damaged capillaries. Cardiac arrest and high altitude may also cause cerebral edema. High-altitude cerebral edema (HACE) is a frequently fatal form of altitude sickness. Signs and symptoms include headache, weakness, disorientation, memory loss, hallucinations, psychotic behavior, coma, and, less frequently, ataxia.[19] Edema is often progressive because the fluid pressure results in ischemia, causing arterioles to dilate, increasing capillary pressure, and producing more edema. Also, lack of oxygen to a region of the brain makes the capillaries more permeable; thus more fluid escapes into the extracellular compartment.[19] Edema can be alleviated by shunts or medications or, in the case of HACE, by moving to a lower altitude.

## INCREASES IN INTRACRANIAL PRESSURE

Cerebral edema, hydrocephalus, tumors, and other lesions that occupy space in the brain can cause an increase in intracranial pressure. Symptoms include vomiting and nausea (pressure on vagus nerve), headache (increased capillary pressure), drowsiness, frontal lobe gait ataxia, and visual and eye movement problems (pressure on optic and oculomotor nerves).

Space-occupying lesions may produce herniation (protrusion) of part of the brain. Pressure from hemorrhage, edema, or a tumor can cause displacement of brain structures with grave consequences.

### Uncal Herniation

Uncal herniation occurs when a space-occupying lesion in the temporal lobe displaces the uncus medially, forcing the uncus into the opening of the tentorium cerebelli. In turn, this compresses the midbrain, interfering with the function of the oculomotor nerve and consciousness (effect on ascending reticular activating system). Figure 19-15 shows an infarct secondary to uncal herniation.

### Central Herniation

Central herniation occurs when a space-occupying lesion in the cerebrum exerts pressure on the diencephalon, moving the diencephalon, midbrain, and pons inferiorly. This movement stretches the branches of the basilar artery, causing brainstem ischemia and edema. Bilateral paralysis ensues (as the result of damage to upper motor neurons), and consciousness and oculomotor control are impaired.

### Tonsillar Herniation

Pressure from an uncal herniation, a tumor in the brainstem/cerebellar region, hemorrhage, or edema may force the cerebellar tonsils (small lobes forming part of the inferior surface of the cerebellum) through the foramen magnum. Tonsillar herniation compresses the brainstem, interfering with vital signs, consciousness, and flow of CSF.

## LABORATORY EVALUATION OF CEREBRAL BLOOD FLOW

Blood flow to the brain can be evaluated by positron emission tomography (PET) scan or by angiography. A PET scan is a computer-generated image based on the metabolism of injected radioactively labeled substances (Figure 19-16). A PET scan records local variations in blood flow, reflecting neural activity. Angiography consists of injection of a radiopaque dye into a carotid or vertebral artery, followed by a sequence of x-rays (Figure 19-17). Typically the end of a plastic catheter inserted into the femoral artery is moved to the origin of the vessel to be visualized, and then the dye is injected. In the first series of x-rays, the arteries are visible; later, as the dye circulates, the veins are seen. Angiography is particularly useful for visualizing aneurysms, occlusions, and malformations of the arteriovenous system; however, thrombosis and embolization are risks with this invasive procedure.

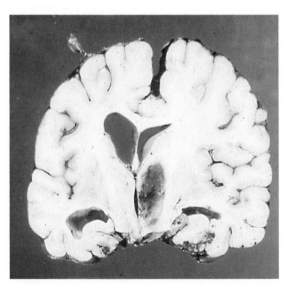

**Fig. 19-15  A large subdural hematoma displaced the right cerebral hemisphere, causing uncal herniation.** Note the distortion of the shape of the lateral ventricles, and that both lateral ventricles and the third ventricle are to the left of the midline. An infarct of the posterior cerebral artery occurred secondary to uncal herniation. *(Courtesy Dr. Melvin J. Ball.)*

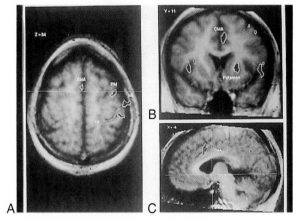

**Fig. 19-16  Positron emission tomography scan.** These scans show cortical areas that have significantly more regional blood flow during self-paced finger flexions than during visually triggered finger flexions or during rest. The colors indicate the level of metabolic activity: red is highest, orange is high, yellow is moderate, green is low, and blue is lowest. *CMA,* Cingulate motor cortex; *M1,* primary motor cortex; *PM,* premotor area; and *SMA,* supplemental motor area. The CMA is a region that has not been studied extensively. **A,** Horizontal section. Posterior to the central sulcus (CS), increased activation of the primary somatosensory cortex is visible. **B,** Coronal section. **C,** Midsagittal section. *(From Larsson J, Bulyas B, Roland PE: Cortical representation of self-paced finger movement. Neuroreport 7:466, 1996.)*

## VENOUS SYSTEM

The spinal cord and the lower medulla drain into small veins that run longitudinally. These veins drain into radicular veins, which then empty into the epidural venous plexus.

The major venous system of the brain consists of cerebral veins. These veins drain into dural sinuses (Figure 19-18) and eventually into the internal jugular vein (Figure 19-19). Cerebral veins interconnect extensively. Two sets of veins drain the cerebrum: superficial and deep. Superficial veins drain the cortex and adjacent white matter, then empty into the superior sagittal sinus or one of the sinuses around the inferior cerebrum. Deep cerebral veins drain the basal ganglia, diencephalon, and nearby white matter, then empty into the straight sinus. The superior sagittal and straight sinuses join at the confluence of the sinuses. The transverse sinuses arise from the confluence and connect with the internal jugular veins.

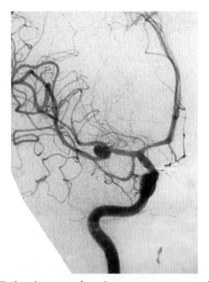

**Fig. 19-17** Angiogram showing an aneurysm arising from the middle cerebral artery.

## SUMMARY

CSF is produced in the ventricles as a filtrate of blood. CSF cushions the brain and spinal cord, provides nutrients and ionic balance in the CNS, and removes waste. CSF flows from the lateral ventricles to the third ventricle via the interventricular

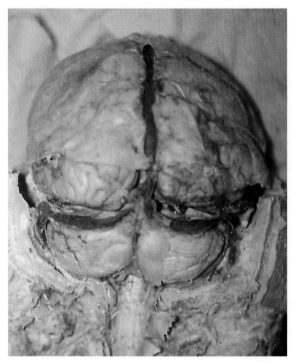

**Fig. 19-18 Posterior view of the dura mater covering the brain, with the dural (venous) sinuses exposed.** The superior sagittal sinus, between the superior parts of the cerebral hemispheres, and the transverse sinuses, between the cerebral and cerebellar hemispheres, are visible.

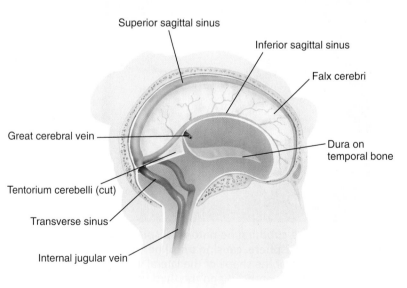

**Fig. 19-19 The venous system of the brain.** The venous sinuses eventually drain into the internal jugular vein.

foramina, then via the cerebral aqueduct into the fourth ventricle. The fourth ventricle has small openings that allow the flow of CSF into the subarachnoid space. CSF returns to the blood in the dural sinuses. The meninges protect the brain and confine the CSF. Disorders of the CSF system include epidural and subdural hematoma and hydrocephalus.

Blood is supplied to the brain via the vertebral and internal carotid arteries. The two vertebral arteries join to form the basilar artery, and the basilar artery divides to become the posterior cerebral arteries. The internal carotid has two large branches: the anterior and middle cerebral arteries. Strokes are classified according to the pattern of progression (transient ischemic attack, completed stroke, or progressive stroke), the cause (infarction, hemorrhage, subarachnoid hemorrhage), and the arterial location. Developmental disorders of vascular formation include arteriovenous malformations and aneurysms. The blood-brain barrier protects the brain from toxins, pathogens, and specific drugs. Blood flow in local areas is autoregulated by cerebral arteries. Cerebral edema and excessive intracranial pressure interfere with brain function and may be fatal.

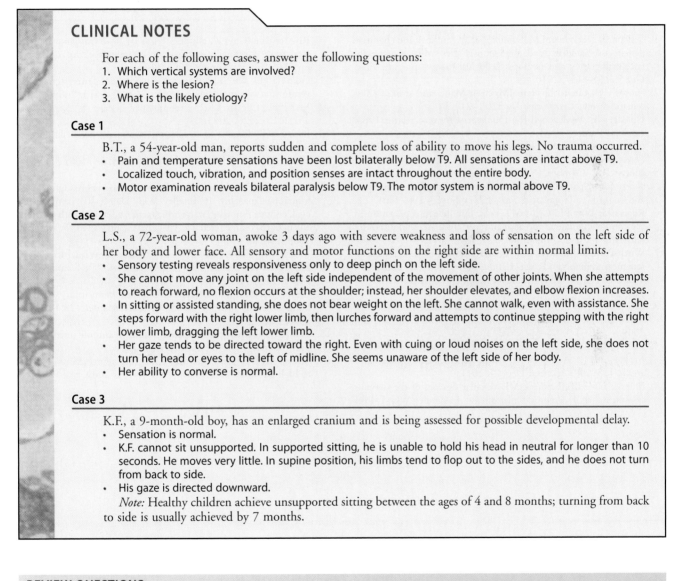

## CLINICAL NOTES

For each of the following cases, answer the following questions:
1. Which vertical systems are involved?
2. Where is the lesion?
3. What is the likely etiology?

### Case 1

B.T., a 54-year-old man, reports sudden and complete loss of ability to move his legs. No trauma occurred.
- Pain and temperature sensations have been lost bilaterally below T9. All sensations are intact above T9.
- Localized touch, vibration, and position senses are intact throughout the entire body.
- Motor examination reveals bilateral paralysis below T9. The motor system is normal above T9.

### Case 2

L.S., a 72-year-old woman, awoke 3 days ago with severe weakness and loss of sensation on the left side of her body and lower face. All sensory and motor functions on the right side are within normal limits.
- Sensory testing reveals responsiveness only to deep pinch on the left side.
- She cannot move any joint on the left side independent of the movement of other joints. When she attempts to reach forward, no flexion occurs at the shoulder; instead, her shoulder elevates, and elbow flexion increases.
- In sitting or assisted standing, she does not bear weight on the left. She cannot walk, even with assistance. She steps forward with the right lower limb, then lurches forward and attempts to continue stepping with the right lower limb, dragging the left lower limb.
- Her gaze tends to be directed toward the right. Even with cuing or loud noises on the left side, she does not turn her head or eyes to the left of midline. She seems unaware of the left side of her body.
- Her ability to converse is normal.

### Case 3

K.F., a 9-month-old boy, has an enlarged cranium and is being assessed for possible developmental delay.
- Sensation is normal.
- K.F. cannot sit unsupported. In supported sitting, he is unable to hold his head in neutral for longer than 10 seconds. He moves very little. In supine position, his limbs tend to flop out to the sides, and he does not turn from back to side.
- His gaze is directed downward.
  *Note:* Healthy children achieve unsupported sitting between the ages of 4 and 8 months; turning from back to side is usually achieved by 7 months.

## REVIEW QUESTIONS

1. What are the functions of the CSF?
2. Where is CSF located?
3. Why is a difference in the pattern of progression evident between an epidural hematoma and a subdural hematoma?
4. In an infant, an abnormally large head, inactivity, insufficient feeding, and downward gaze of both eyes may indicate what disorder?
5. Can hydrocephalus occur in adults?
6. What is the watershed area?
7. What is a transient ischemic attack?
8. What is a lacuna?
9. Partial occlusion of which artery can result in tetraplegia, loss of sensation, coma, and cranial nerve signs?
10. Hemiplegia and hemisensory loss more severe in the lower limb than in the upper limb and face indicate that what part of the brain is affected? What artery supplies this region?

11. Neglect, poor understanding of spatial relationships, and impairment of nonverbal communication are signs of damage to what part of the brain? Which artery supplies this region?
12. If hemiplegia and hemisensory loss affect the upper and lower limbs and the face equally, where is the lesion? Branches of what major artery supply this region?
13. Eye movement paresis with sparing of lateral and inferomedial eye movements combined with contralateral hemiplegia indicates a lesion located where? Which artery supplies this region?
14. What arteries supply the watershed area?
15. What is an arteriovenous malformation?
16. What is an aneurysm?
17. What is an uncal herniation?
18. What is a PET scan?

## References

1. Särkämö T, Tervaniemi M, Soinila S, et al: Auditory and cognitive deficits associated with acquired amusia after stroke: a magnetoencephalography and neuropsychological follow-up study. *PLoS One* 5:e151–e157, 2010.
2. Santos CO, Caeiro L, Ferro JM, et al: Mania and stroke: a systematic review. *Cerebrovasc Dis* 32:11–21, 2011.
3. Upledger JE, Vredevoogd JD: *Craniosacral therapy*, Seattle, 1983, Eastland Press.
4. Hartman SE: Cranial osteopathy: its fate seems clear. *Chiropr Osteopat* 14:10, 2006.
5. Moran RW, Gibbons P: Intraexaminer and interexaminer reliability for palpation of the cranial rhythmic impulse at the head and sacrum. *J Manipulative Physiol Ther* 24:183–190, 2001.
6. Rogers JS, Witt PL, Gross MT, et al: Simultaneous palpation of the craniosacral rate at the head and feet: intrarater and interrater reliability and rate comparisons. *Phys Ther* 78:1175–1185, 1998.
7. Wirth-Pattullo V, Hayes KW: Interrater reliability of craniosacral rate measurements and their relationship with subjects' and examiners' heart and respiratory rate measurements. *Phys Ther* 74:908–920, 1994.
8. Ross M, Nahab F: Management of transient ischemia attacks in the twenty-first century. *Emerg Med Clin North Am* 27:51–69, viii, 2009.
9. Baird AE, Jichici D, Talavera F, et al: Anterior circulation stroke, 2011. Available at: http://emedicine.medscape.com/article/1159900. Accessed Dec. 15, 2011.
10. Biller J, Love BB, Schneck MJ: Vascular diseases of the nervous system: ischemic cerebrovascular disease. In Bradley WG, Daroff RB, Fenichel G, et al, editors: *Neurology in clinical practice*, ed 5 (text with continually updated online reference, vol 2, part 3, pp 1165–1223), Munich, 2008, Elsevier.
11. Gouveia LO, Castanho P, Ferreira JJ: Safety of chiropractic interventions: a systematic review. *Spine* 34:e405–e413, 2009.
12. Savitz SI, Caplan LR: Vertebrobasilar disease. *N Engl J Med* 352:2618–2626, 2005.
13. Jensen MB, Louis EK: Management of acute cerebellar stroke. *Arch Neurol* 62:537–544, 2005.
14. Smith E, Delargy M: Locked-in syndrome. *Br Med J* 330:406–409, 2005.
15. Sandhu JS, Wakhloo AK: Neuroimaging: neuroangiographic functional anatomy. In Bradley WG, Daroff RB, Fenichel G, et al, editors: *Neurology in clinical practice*, ed 5 (text with continually updated online reference, vol 1, part 2, pp 639–657), Munich, 2008, Elsevier.
16. Bruno MA, Vanhaudenhuyse A, Schnakers C: Visual fixation in the vegetative state: an observational case series PET study. *BMC Neurol* 10:35–41, 2010.
17. Huang BY, Castillo M: Hypoxic-ischemic brain injury: imaging findings from birth to adulthood. *Radiographics* 28:417–439, 2008; quiz 617.
18. Bernat JL: Current controversies in states of chronic unconsciousness. *Neurology* 75(18 Suppl 1):S33–S38, 2010.
19. Wilson MH, Newman S, Imray CH: The cerebral effects of ascent to high altitudes. *Lancet Neurol* 8:175–191, 2009.

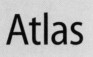

# Atlas

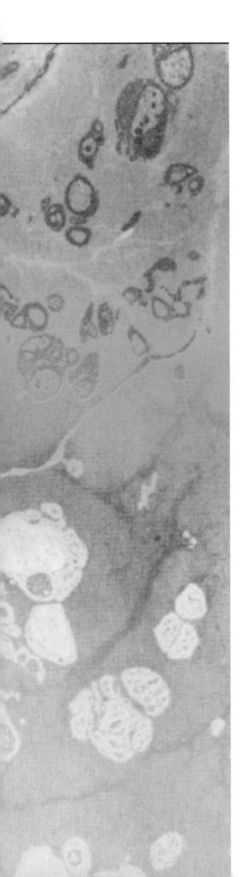

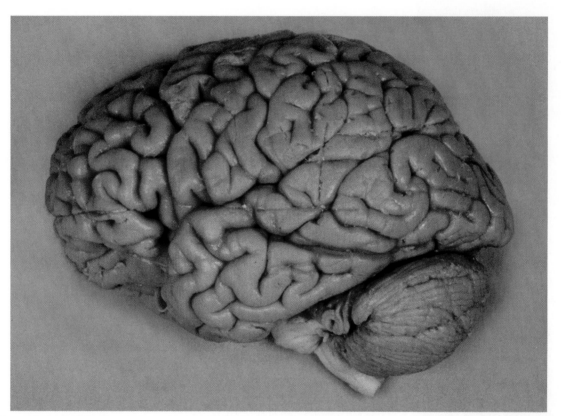

**Fig. A1** Lateral view of the brain. Anterior is to the left. Dotted lines indicate boundaries between areas that are not separated by the sulci. The orbital gyri are part of the frontal lobe. *(Copyright 1994, University of Washington. From Digital Anatomist Interactive Brain Atlas and the Structural Informatics Group.)*

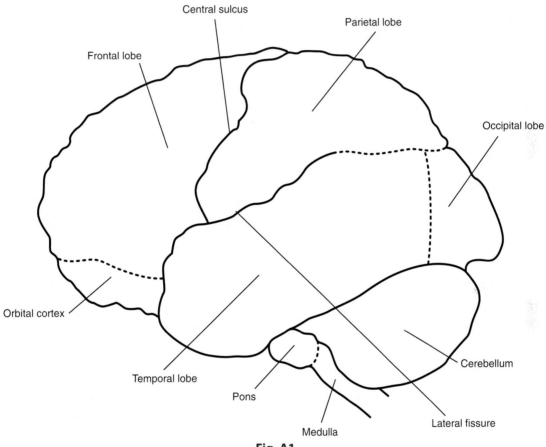

**Fig. A1**

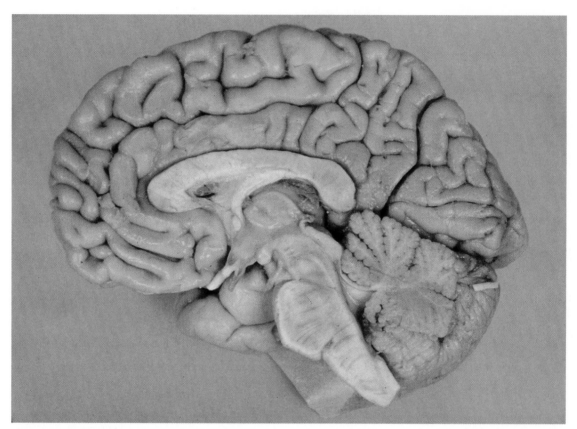

**Fig. A2** Midsaggital view of the brain. Anterior is to the left. *(Copyright 1994, University of Washington. From Digital Anatomist Interactive Brain Atlas and the Structural Informatics Group.)*

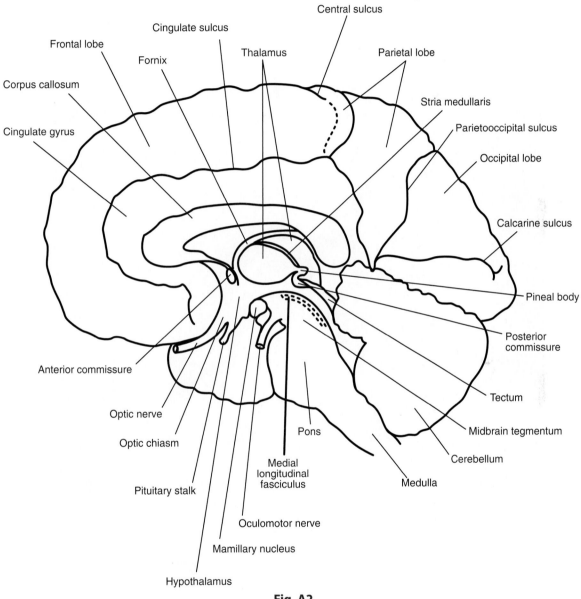

Central sulcus

Cingulate sulcus

Frontal lobe

Thalamus

Parietal lobe

Fornix

Corpus callosum

Stria medullaris

Cingulate gyrus

Parietooccipital sulcus

Occipital lobe

Calcarine sulcus

Pineal body

Posterior commissure

Anterior commissure

Tectum

Optic nerve

Midbrain tegmentum

Optic chiasm

Pons

Cerebellum

Pituitary stalk

Medial longitudinal fasciculus

Medulla

Oculomotor nerve

Mamillary nucleus

Hypothalamus

**Fig. A2**

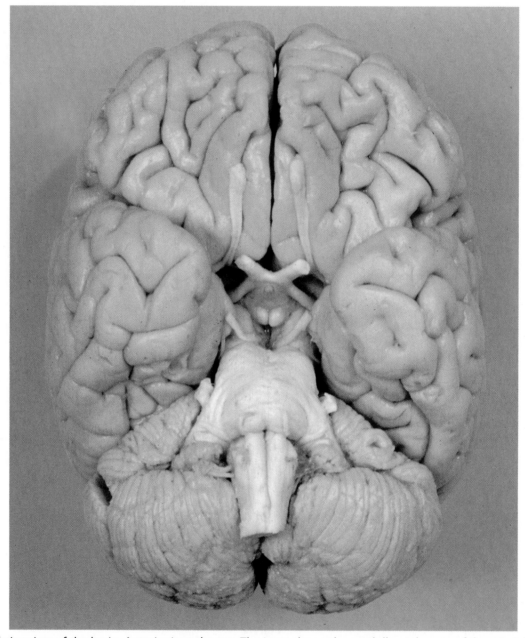

**Fig. A3** Inferior view of the brain. Anterior is at the top. The inset shows the medulla and some of the cranial nerves associated with the medulla. *(Copyright 1994, University of Washington. From Digital Anatomist Interactive Brain Atlas and the Structural Informatics Group.)*

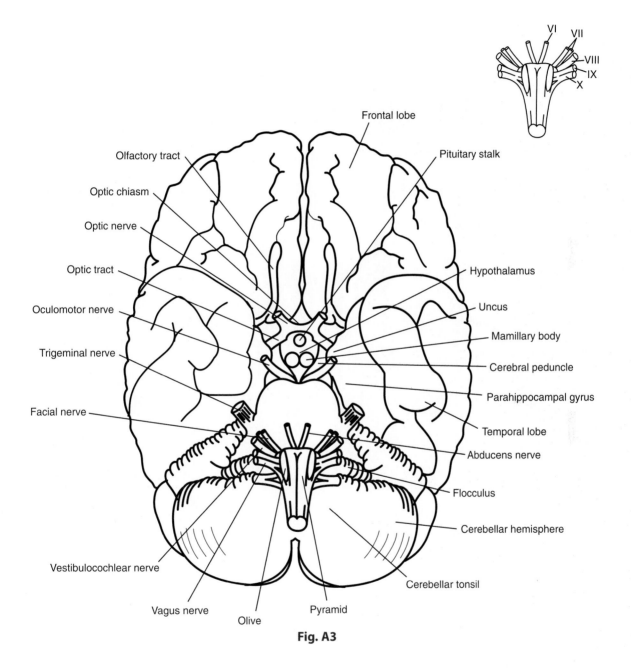

VI VII VIII IX X

Frontal lobe

Olfactory tract

Optic chiasm

Optic nerve

Optic tract

Oculomotor nerve

Trigeminal nerve

Facial nerve

Vestibulocochlear nerve

Vagus nerve

Olive

Pyramid

Pituitary stalk

Hypothalamus

Uncus

Mamillary body

Cerebral peduncle

Parahippocampal gyrus

Temporal lobe

Abducens nerve

Flocculus

Cerebellar hemisphere

Cerebellar tonsil

**Fig. A3**

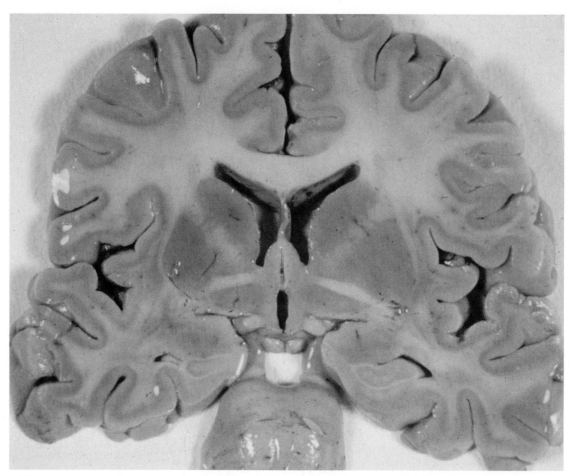

**Fig. A4** Oblique coronal section. See inset of a midsagittal section for the angle of the section. *(Copyright 1994, University of Washington. From Digital Anatomist Interactive Brain Atlas and the Structural Informatics Group.)*

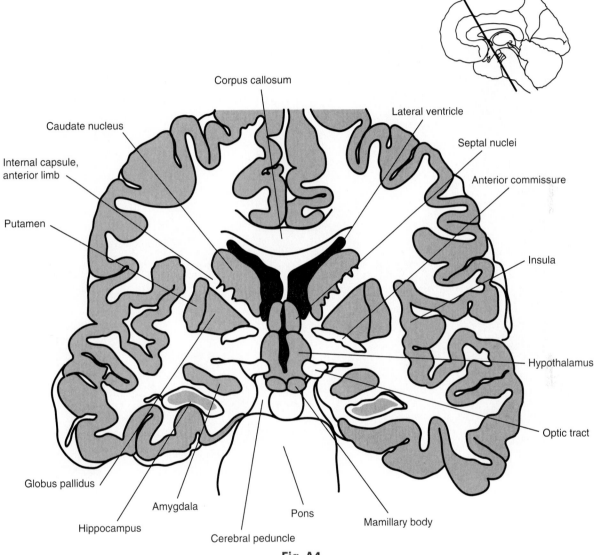

Corpus callosum

Lateral ventricle

Caudate nucleus

Septal nuclei

Internal capsule,
anterior limb

Anterior commissure

Putamen

Insula

Hypothalamus

Optic tract

Globus pallidus

Amygdala

Pons

Mamillary body

Hippocampus

Cerebral peduncle

**Fig. A4**

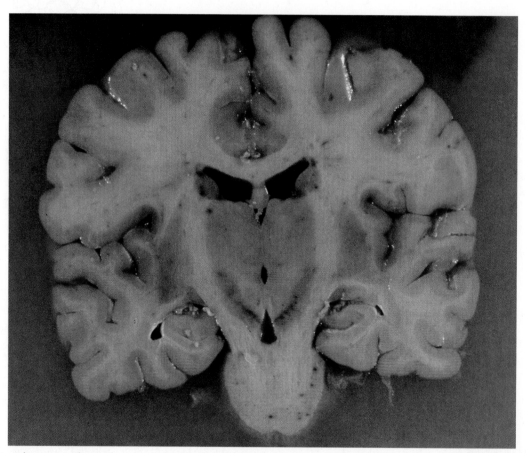

**Fig. A5** Coronal section, through putamen and globus pallidus. Note the direct continuation of the internal capsule into the cerebral penduncle. *(Copyright 1994, University of Washington. From Digital Anatomist Interactive Brain Atlas and the Structural Informatics Group.)*

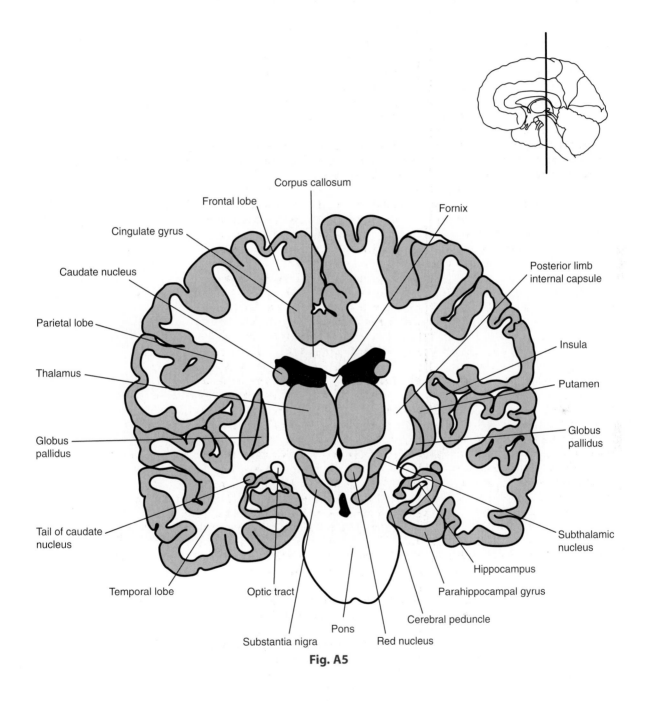

**Fig. A5**

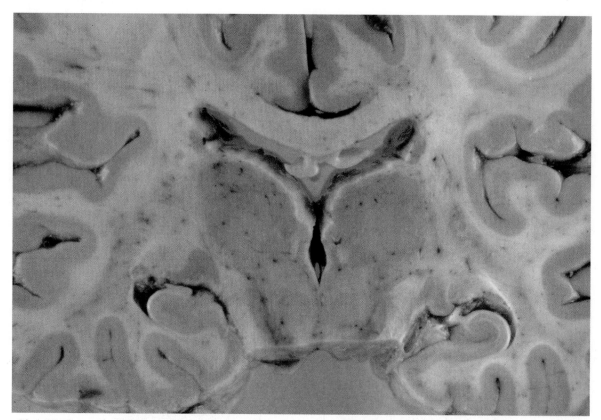

**Fig. A6** Coronal section, through posterior thalamus. *(Photograph courtesy Dr. Jeannette Townsend, University of Utah.)*

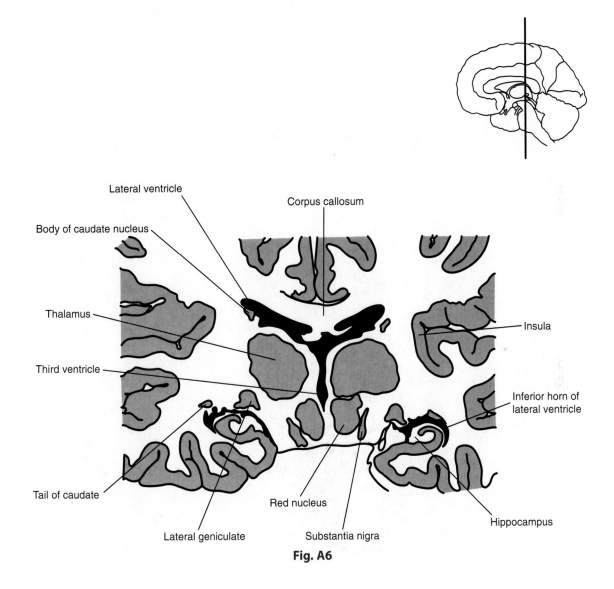

Lateral ventricle

Corpus callosum

Body of caudate nucleus

Thalamus

Insula

Third ventricle

Inferior horn of lateral ventricle

Tail of caudate

Red nucleus

Hippocampus

Lateral geniculate

Substantia nigra

**Fig. A6**

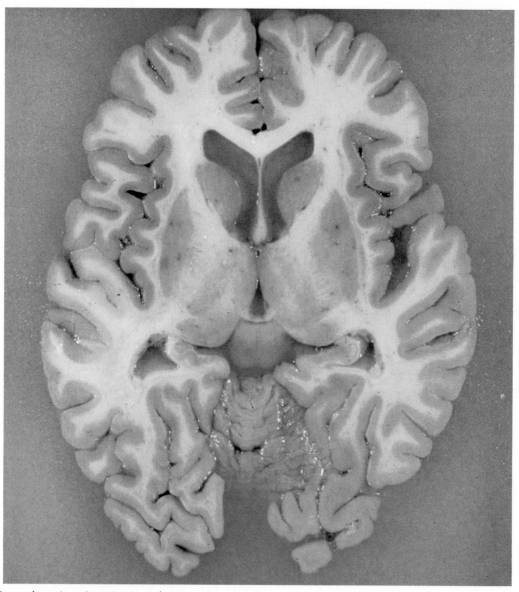

**Fig. A7** Horizontal section. Anterior is at the top. *(Copyright 1994, University of Washington. From Digital Anatomist Interactive Brain Atlas and the Structural Informatics Group.)*

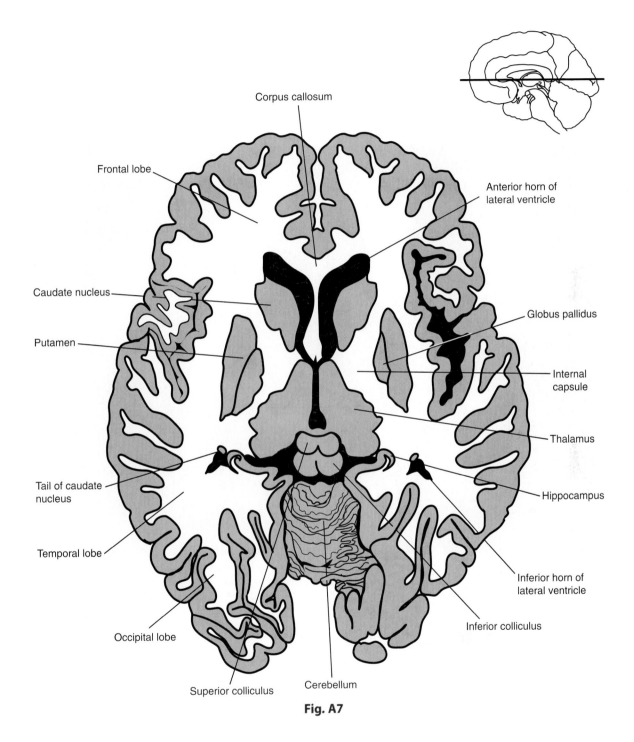

Corpus callosum

Frontal lobe

Anterior horn of
lateral ventricle

Caudate nucleus

Globus pallidus

Putamen

Internal
capsule

Thalamus

Tail of caudate
nucleus

Hippocampus

Temporal lobe

Inferior horn of
lateral ventricle

Occipital lobe

Inferior colliculus

Superior colliculus

Cerebellum

**Fig. A7**

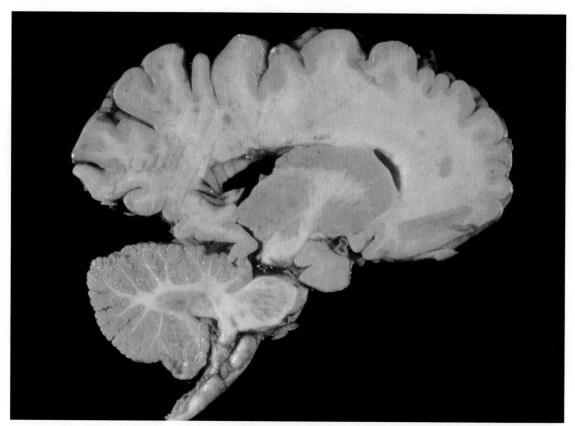

**Fig. A8** Sagittal section, lateral to the midline. Anterior is to the right. In the inset, the cerebellum has been removed to clearly show the location of the section. The section includes the cerebellum. *(Photograph courtesy Dr. Jeannette Townsend, University of Utah.)*

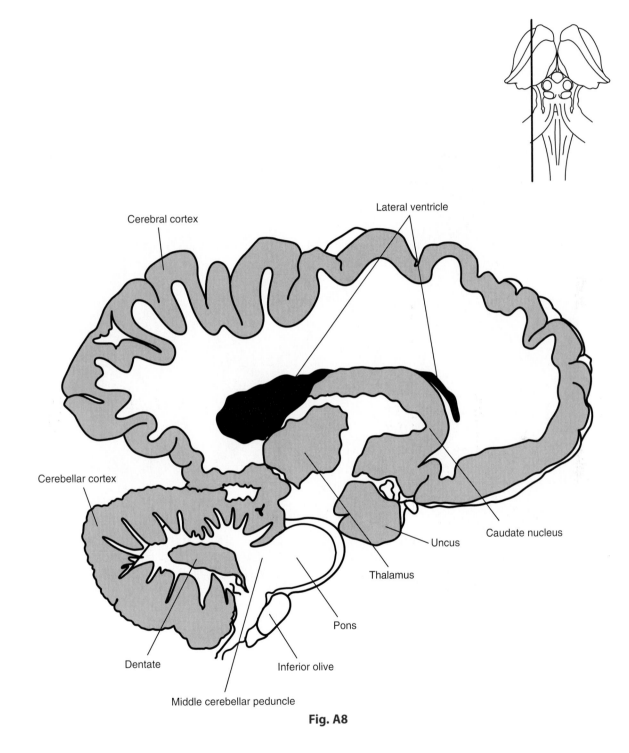

**Fig. A8**

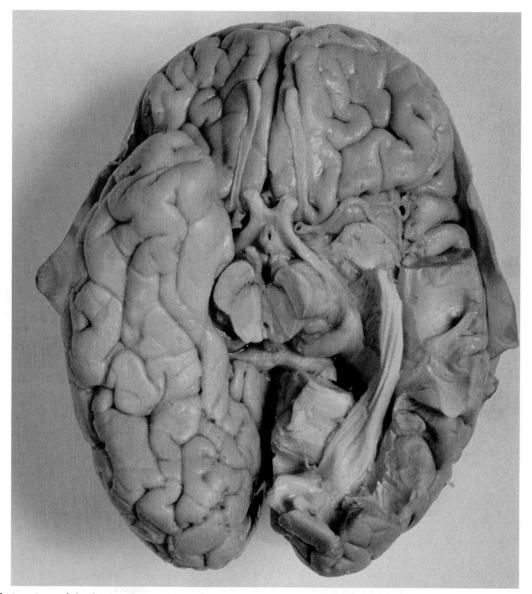

**Fig. A9** Inferior view of the brain. Anterior is at the top. The pons, medulla, and cerebellum have been removed. The temporal and occipital lobes have been partially removed to reveal the visual radiation. *(Copyright 1994, University of Washington. From Digital Anatomist Interactive Brain Atlas and the Structural Informatics Group.)*

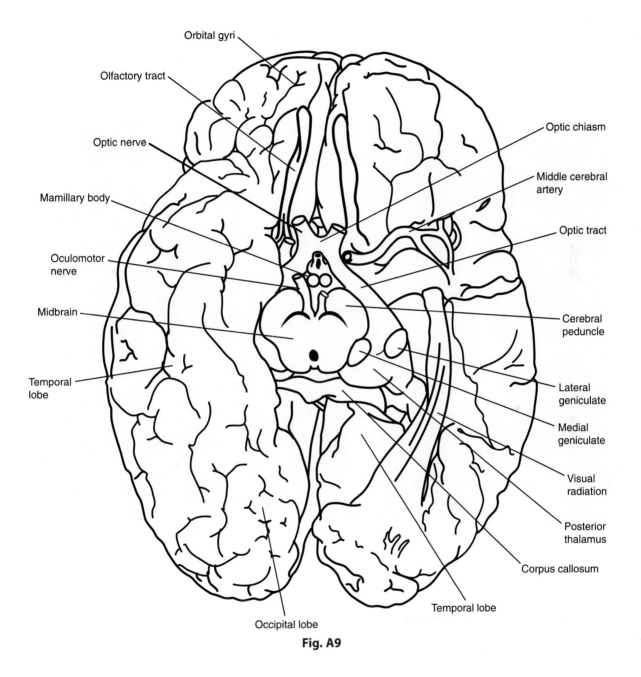

Orbital gyri

Olfactory tract

Optic nerve

Mamillary body

Oculomotor nerve

Midbrain

Temporal lobe

Optic chiasm

Middle cerebral artery

Optic tract

Cerebral peduncle

Lateral geniculate

Medial geniculate

Visual radiation

Posterior thalamus

Corpus callosum

Temporal lobe

Occipital lobe

**Fig. A9**

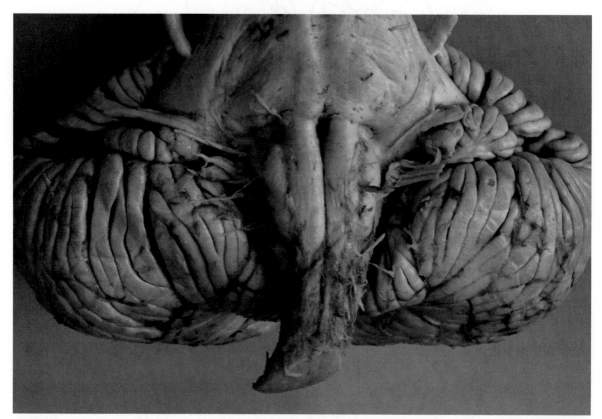

**Fig. A10** Anterior view of the pons, medulla, and cerebellum. On the specimen, only a fragment of the hypoglossal nerve is intact. In the illustration, the initial section of the hypoglossal nerve has been added on the right.

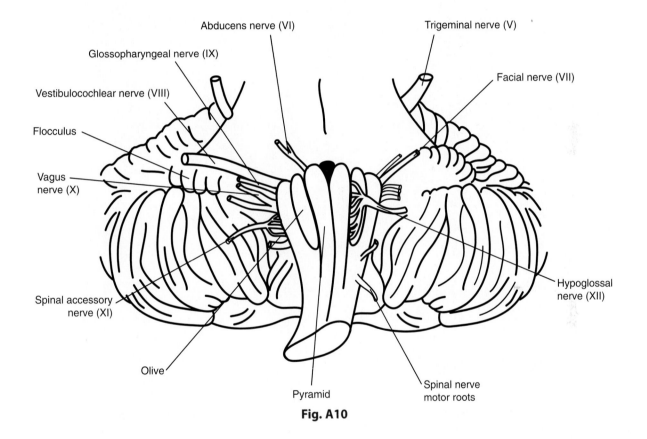

**Fig. A10**

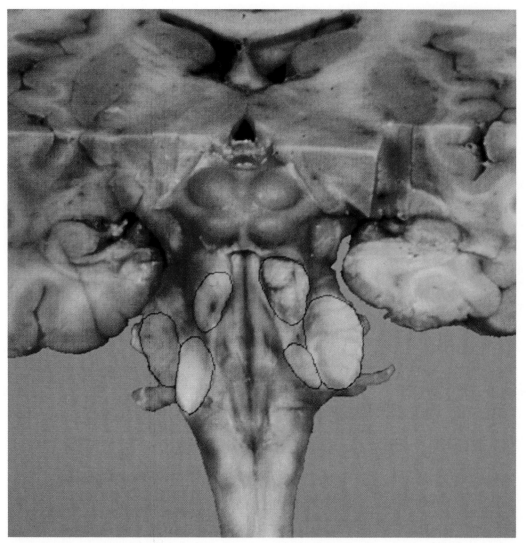

**Fig. A11** Posterior view of the brainstem and cerebral hemispheres. The cerebellum has been removed. The cerebral hemispheres have been sectioned in the horizontal plane and also in the coronal plane through the temporal lobe. The red line indicates the intersection of the planes of section. Above the line is the horizontal section of the cerebrum. See inset of a midsagittal section for the angles of the sections. *(Copyright 1994, University of Washington. From Digital Anatomist Interactive Brain Atlas and the Structural Informatics Group.)*

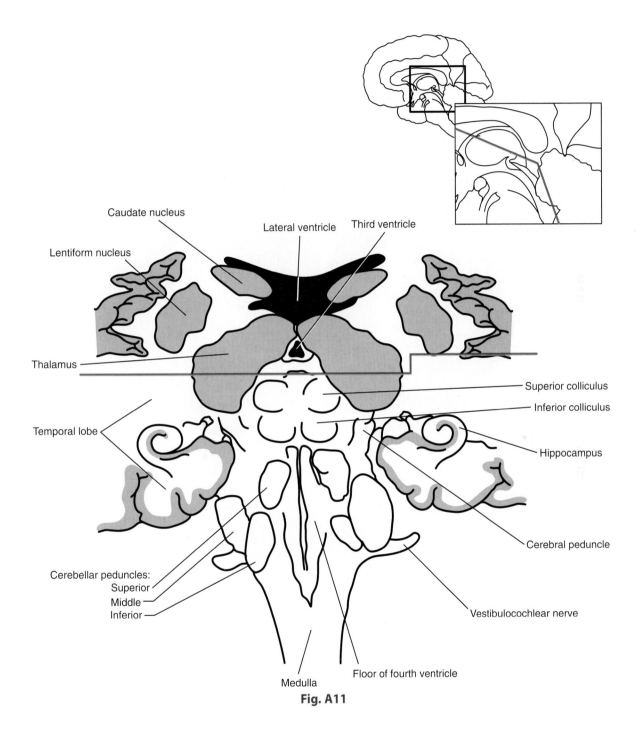

Caudate nucleus

Lentiform nucleus

Lateral ventricle    Third ventricle

Thalamus

Superior colliculus

Inferior colliculus

Temporal lobe

Hippocampus

Cerebral peduncle

Cerebellar peduncles:
Superior
Middle
Inferior

Vestibulocochlear nerve

Medulla    Floor of fourth ventricle

**Fig. A11**

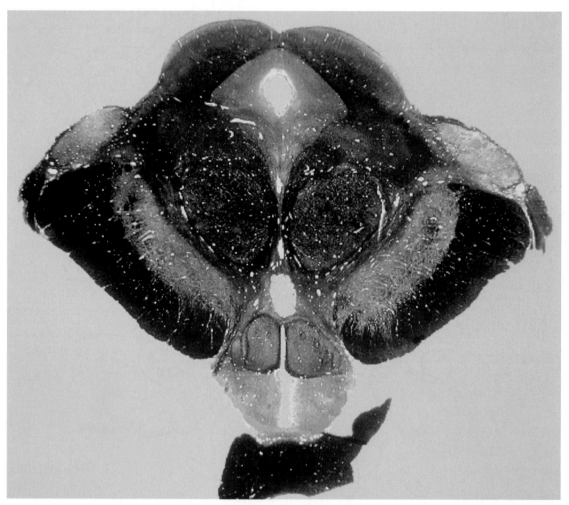

**Fig. A12** Horizontal section of the upper midbrain. Posterior is at the top. The myelin has been stained to appear black instead of light in color. At the bottom of the section, below the dotted line, are structures that are not part of the midbrain: the optic chiasm and the hypothalamus with its mamillary nuclei. In the outline drawing, the shading reflects the natural (unstained) appearance of the tissue, with the gray matter dark and the white matter light. *(Copyright 1994, University of Washington. From Digital Anatomist Interactive Brain Atlas and the Structural Informatics Group.)*

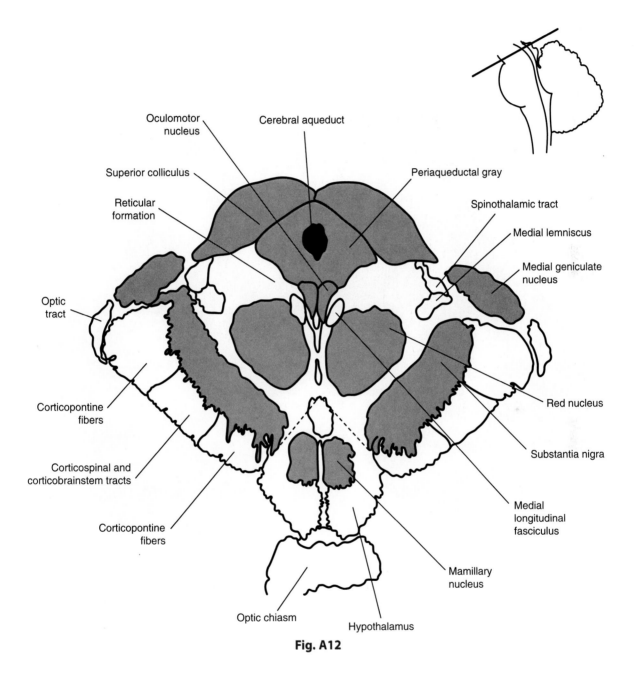

**Fig. A12**

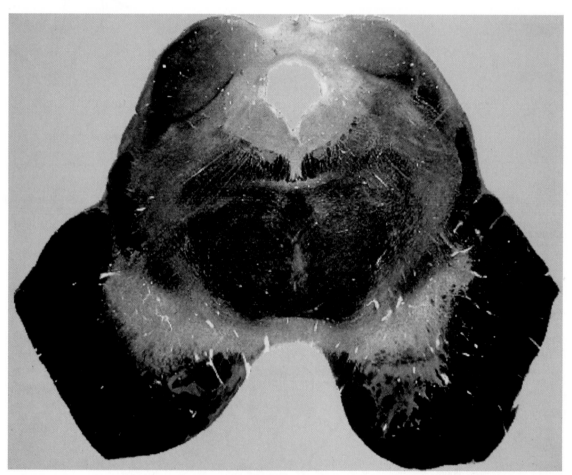

**Fig. A13** Horizontal section of the lower midbrain. Posterior is at the top. The myelin has been stained to appear black instead of light in color. In the outline drawing, the shading reflects the natural (unstained) appearance of the tissue, with the gray matter dark and the white matter light. *(Copyright 1994, University of Washington. From Digital Anatomist Interactive Brain Atlas and the Structural Informatics Group.)*

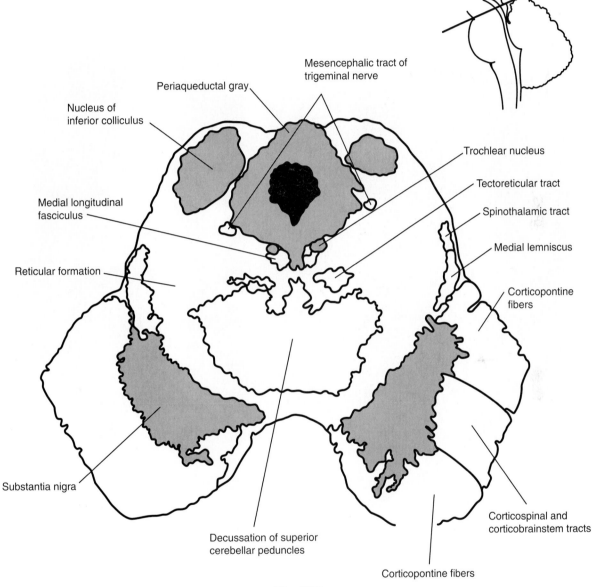

Mesencephalic tract of trigeminal nerve

Periaqueductal gray

Nucleus of inferior colliculus

Trochlear nucleus

Tectoreticular tract

Spinothalamic tract

Medial longitudinal fasciculus

Medial lemniscus

Reticular formation

Corticopontine fibers

Substantia nigra

Corticospinal and corticobrainstem tracts

Decussation of superior cerebellar peduncles

Corticopontine fibers

**Fig. A13**

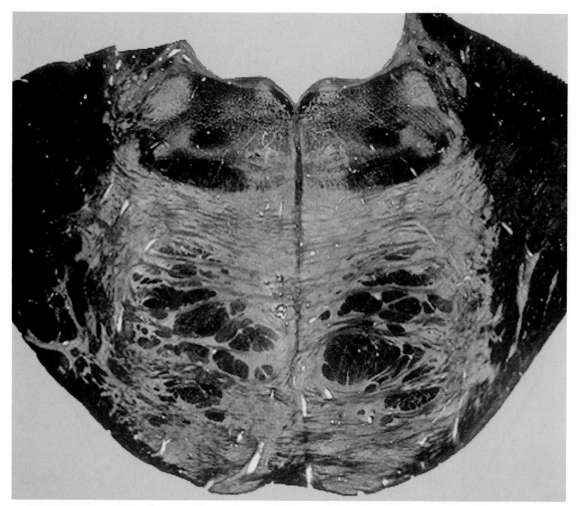

**Fig. A14** Mid-pons. Posterior is at the top. The myelin has been stained to appear black instead of light in color. In the outline drawing, the shading reflects the natural (unstained) appearance of the tissue, with the gray matter dark and the white matter light. *(Copyright 1994, University of Washington. From Digital Anatomist Interactive Brain Atlas and the Structural Informatics Group.)*

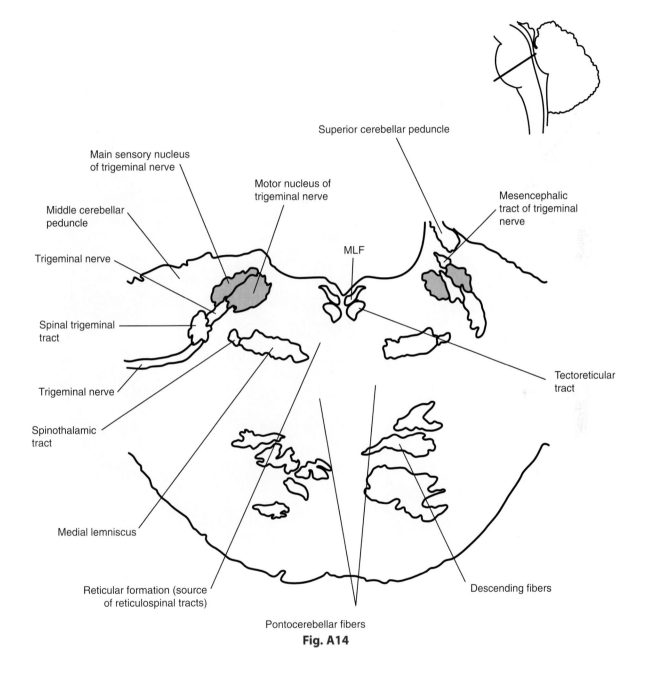

Superior cerebellar peduncle

Main sensory nucleus
of trigeminal nerve

Motor nucleus of
trigeminal nerve

Mesencephalic
tract of trigeminal
nerve

Middle cerebellar
peduncle

Trigeminal nerve

MLF

Spinal trigeminal
tract

Trigeminal nerve

Tectoreticular
tract

Spinothalamic
tract

Medial lemniscus

Reticular formation (source
of reticulospinal tracts)

Descending fibers

Pontocerebellar fibers

**Fig. A14**

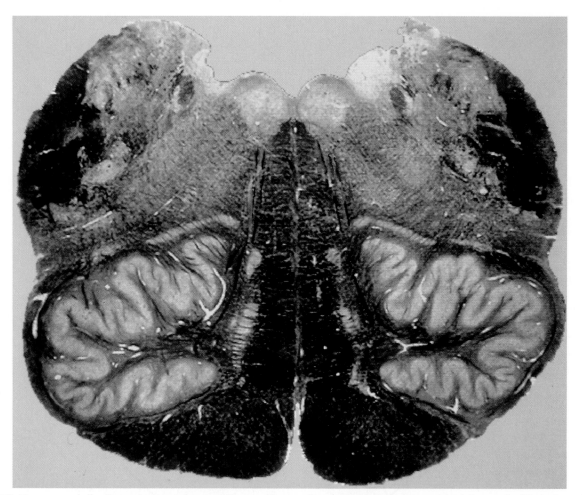

**Fig. A15** Upper medulla. Posterior is at the top. The myelin has been stained to appear black instead of light in color. In the outline drawing, the shading reflects the natural (unstained) appearance of the tissue, with the gray matter dark and the white matter light. *(Copyright 1994, University of Washington. From Digital Anatomist Interactive Brain Atlas and the Structural Informatics Group.)*

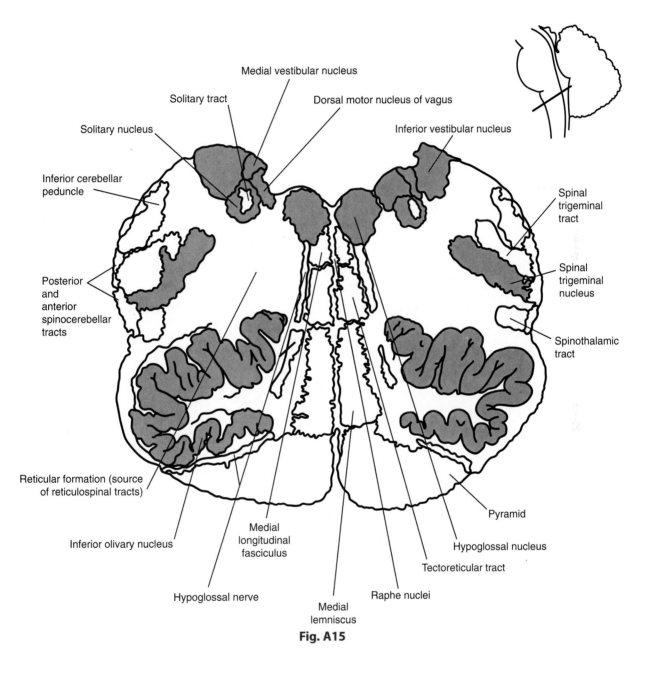

Medial vestibular nucleus

Solitary tract

Dorsal motor nucleus of vagus

Solitary nucleus

Inferior vestibular nucleus

Inferior cerebellar peduncle

Spinal trigeminal tract

Spinal trigeminal nucleus

Posterior and anterior spinocerebellar tracts

Spinothalamic tract

Reticular formation (source of reticulospinal tracts)

Inferior olivary nucleus

Medial longitudinal fasciculus

Pyramid

Hypoglossal nucleus

Tectoreticular tract

Hypoglossal nerve

Raphe nuclei

Medial lemniscus

**Fig. A15**

# Glossary

**Accommodation** Adjustments of the eyes to view a near object: The pupils constrict, the eyes converge (adduct), and the lens becomes more convex. The optic nerve is the afferent (sensory) limb of the reflex, and the oculomotor nerve provides the efferent (motor) limb.

**Acetylcholine** A neurotransmitter released by axons from the pedunculopontine nucleus and nucleus basalis of Meynert, by lower motor neurons, by preganglionic autonomic axons, and by postganglionic parasympathetic axons. Binds with nicotinic or muscarinic receptors. Action on postsynaptic membranes is usually excitatory.

**Addiction** Loss of behavioral control in response to a stimulus combined with continued use of a substance, regardless of negative consequences

**Adrenergic** (1) Referring to neurons that secrete norepinephrine or epinephrine. (2) Referring to drugs that bind with and activate the same receptors as norepinephrine or epinephrine. (3) Referring to receptors that bind norepinephrine, epinephrine, or agonist/antagonist drugs.

**Affect, flat** Absent or reduced expression of emotions.

**Afferent** Traveling toward a structure.

**Agnosia** General term for the inability to recognize objects when using a specific sense, even though discriminative ability with that sense is intact. Specific types of agnosia include astereognosis, visual agnosia, and auditory agnosia.

**Agnosia, visual** Inability to visually recognize objects despite intact vision.

**Agonist** Drug that binds to a receptor and mimics the effect of a naturally occurring neurotransmitter.

**Agraphia** Diminished or lost ability to produce written language.

**Akinesia** Paucity or absence of movement.

**Alexia** Diminished or lost ability to comprehend written language.

**Allodynia** Sensation of pain in response to normally nonpainful stimuli.

**All-or-none** Term applied to the generation of an action potential, indicating that every time even minimally sufficient stimuli are provided to generate an action potential, an action potential will be produced. Stimuli that are stronger than the minimally sufficient stimuli produce action potentials of the same voltage and duration as the minimally sufficient stimuli.

**γ-Aminobutyric acid (GABA)** Neurotransmitter released by the caudate nucleus and putamen and by cerebellar Purkinje cells and spinal interneurons. Action on postsynaptic membranes is inhibitory.

**Amnesia** Loss of declarative memory.

**Amygdala** Nuclei that interpret facial expressions and social signals. Together the amygdala, orbital cortex, and anterior cingulate gyrus regulate emotional behaviors and motivation.

The amygdala consists of an almond-shaped collection of nuclei deep to the uncus in the temporal lobe.

**Analgesia** Absence of pain in response to stimuli that normally would be painful.

**Anencephaly** Developmental defect characterized by development of a rudimentary brainstem without cerebral and cerebellar hemispheres.

**Aneurysm** Sac-like dilation of the wall of an artery or vein. These swellings have thin walls that are prone to rupture.

**Angiography** Radiopaque dye injected into a carotid or vertebral artery, followed by a sequence of x-rays.

**Anosognosia** Denial of inability to use the paretic limbs.

**Antagonist** Drug that prevents the release of a neurotransmitter or interferes with the effect of a naturally occurring neurotransmitter.

**Antinociception** Top-down inhibition of pain signals.

**Antinociception, stress-induced** Absent or reduced perception of pain due to activation of the pain inhibition systems during an emergency or in competitive situations.

**Anxiety** Feeling of tension or uneasiness that accompanies anticipating danger.

**Aphasia** Disorder of language expression or comprehension. Deficit in the ability to produce understandable speech and writing, or the ability to understand written and spoken language.

**Aphasia, Broca's** Difficulty expressing oneself by language or symbols. A person with Broca's aphasia has deficits in both speaking and writing, yet understands grammatically simple sentences. *Syn.:* motor aphasia, expressive aphasia.

**Aphasia, conduction** Language disorder resulting from damage to the neurons that connect Wernicke's and Broca's areas. The ability to understand written and spoken language is normal. In mild cases, only paraphasis occur. In the most severe form, speech and writing produced are meaningless.

**Aphasia, global** Inability to use language in any form. People with global aphasia cannot produce understandable speech, comprehend spoken language, speak fluently, read, or write.

**Aphasia, Wernicke's** Impairment of language comprehension. People with Wernicke's aphasia easily produce spoken sounds, but the output is often meaningless. Listening to other people speak is equally meaningless, despite the ability to hear normally. *Syn.:* receptive aphasia, sensory aphasia.

**Apparatus, vestibular** The part of the inner ear that detects position and movement of the head. Consists of the semicircular canals, the saccule, and the utricle.

**Apraxia** Inability to perform a movement or sequence of movements despite intact sensation, automatic motor output, and understanding of the task.

**Apraxia, constructional** Inability to comprehend the relationship of parts to the whole.

**Arachnoid** Middle layer of the membranes surrounding the central nervous system.

**Area 25** Region in the anterior cingulate cortex. When overactive, contributes to depression.

**Area, Broca's** Region of cortex that provides instructions for language output, including planning the movements to produce speech and providing grammatical function words, such as the articles *a, an,* and *the.* Located inferior to the premotor area and anterior to the face and throat region of the primary motor cortex, usually in the left hemisphere.

**Area, corresponding to Broca's area** Region of the cerebral cortex inferior to the premotor area and anterior to the face and throat region of the primary motor cortex. Usually in the right hemisphere. Plans nonverbal communication, including emotional gestures and adjusting the tone of voice.

**Area, corresponding to Wernicke's area** Subregion of the parietotemporal cortex where interpretation of nonverbal signals from other people and understanding of spatial relationships occur. Usually located on the right side.

**Area, lateral premotor** A region of the cerebral cortex involved in preparing for movement and controlling trunk and girdle muscles via medial upper motor neurons. Located anterior to the upper body region of the primary motor cortex, on the lateral surface of the hemisphere.

**Area, limbic association** Part of the cerebral cortex involved in regulating mood (subjective feelings), affect (observable demeanor), and processing of some types of memory. Located in the anterior temporal lobe and in the orbital cortex (above the eyes).

**Area, preoptic** Part of the limbic system, located anterior to the septal area.

**Area, secondary somatosensory** A region of the cerebral cortex that analyzes information from the primary somatosensory cortex and from the thalamus. Provides stereognosis and memory of the tactile and spatial environment. Located posterior to the primary somatosensory cortex.

**Area, septal** Part of the limbic system in the basal forebrain region, anterior to the anterior commissure.

**Area, supplementary motor** A region of the cerebral cortex involved in preparing for movement, orientation of the eyes and head, and planning of bimanual and sequential movements. Located anterior to the lower body region of the primary motor cortex, on the superior and medial surface of the hemisphere.

**Area, ventral tegmental** A region in the midbrain that provides dopamine to cerebral areas important in motivation and in decision making.

**Area, watershed** Area of marginal blood flow on the surface of the lateral hemispheres, where small anastomoses link the ends of the cerebral arteries.

**Area, Wernicke's** Subregion of the parietotemporal cortex where comprehension of language occurs. Usually located on the left side.

**Areas, association** Regions of the cerebral cortex that are not directly involved with sensation or movement. Involved with personality, integration and interpretation of sensations, processing of memory, and generation of emotions. The three association areas are dorsolateral prefrontal, parietotemporal, and ventral and medial dorsal prefrontal.

**Areas, Brodmann's** Histologic regions of the cerebral cortex mapped by Brodmann. Often used to designate functional areas.

**Areas, motor planning** Regions of the cerebral cortex involved in organizing movement. Motor planning areas include supplementary motor area, premotor area, Broca's area, and the area corresponding to Broca's area.

**Areas, parietotemporal association** Part of the cerebral cortex devoted to intelligence, problem solving, and comprehension of communication and spatial relationships. Located at the junction of the parietal, occipital, and temporal lobes.

**Areas, primary sensory** Areas of the cerebral cortex that receive sensory information directly from the ventral tier of thalamic nuclei. Each primary sensory area discriminates among different intensities and qualities of one type of sensory input. Separate primary sensory areas are devoted to somatosensory, auditory, visual, and vestibular information.

**Areas, secondary sensory** Areas of the cerebral cortex that analyze sensory input from both the thalamus and the primary sensory cortex. Secondary sensory areas contribute to the analysis of one type of sensory information.

**Artery, anterior cerebral** Vessel that provides blood to the medial surface of the frontal and parietal lobes and the anterior head of the caudate. A branch of the internal carotid artery.

**Artery, anterior choroidal** A branch of the internal carotid artery that provides blood to the optic tract, choroid plexus in the lateral ventricles, and parts of the optic radiations, putamen, thalamus, internal capsule, and hippocampus.

**Artery, basilar** Vessel that provides blood to the pons and most of the cerebellum. Formed near the pontomedullary junction by the union of the vertebral arteries. Divides to become the posterior cerebral arteries.

**Artery, internal carotid** Vessel that provides blood to the anterior, superior, and lateral cerebral hemispheres via its branches: the anterior and middle cerebral arteries, and the anterior choroidal arteries.

**Artery, middle cerebral** Vessel whose branches fan out to provide blood to most of the lateral hemisphere. A branch of the internal carotid artery.

**Artery, posterior cerebral** Vessel that provides blood to the midbrain, occipital lobe, and parts of the medial and inferior temporal lobes. A branch of the basilar artery.

**Artery, posterior choroidal** A branch of the posterior cerebral artery that provides blood to the choroid plexus of the third ventricle and parts of the thalamus and hippocampus.

**Artery, striate** Any of several arteries arising from the proximal part of the anterior or middle cerebral arteries to supply the basal ganglia and parts of the thalamus and internal capsule.

**Artery, vertebral** Vessel that provides blood to the brainstem, cerebellum, and posteroinferior cerebrum. Branch of the subclavian artery.

**Ascending reticular activating system** Part of the brainstem reticular formation that projects to areas of the thalamus that project to the cerebral cortex. Involved in arousal, attention, motivation, and initiation of motor and cognitive activity.

**Astereognosis** Inability to identify objects by touch and manipulation despite intact discriminative somatosensation.

**Astrocytes** Macroglia that play a critical role in nutritive and cleanup functions within the central nervous system.

**Ataxia** Abnormal voluntary movements that are of normal strength but are jerky and inaccurate.

**Ataxia, cerebellar limb** Uncoordinated voluntary movements of the limbs.

**Ataxia, sensory** Uncoordinated movement caused by a lesion along peripheral or central proprioceptive pathways.

**Ataxia, vestibular** Gravity-dependent uncoordinated movement. Limb movements are normal when the person is lying down but are ataxic during walking.

**Athetosis** Involuntary slow, writhing, purposeless movements.

**Atrophy** Loss of muscle bulk.

**Atrophy, disuse** Loss of muscle bulk resulting from lack of use.

**Atrophy, multiple system** Progressive degenerative disease affecting the basal ganglia, cerebellar, and autonomic systems, the peripheral nervous system, and the cerebral cortex.

**Atrophy, neurogenic** Loss of muscle bulk resulting from damage to the nervous system.

**Atrophy, olivopontocerebellar** Multiple system atrophy presenting initially with incoordination, dysarthria, and balance deficits.

**Attack, transient ischemic** A brief, focal loss of brain function, with full recovery from neurologic deficits within 24 hours. Transient ischemic attacks are believed to be due to inadequate blood supply.

**Attention** Ability to maintain focus on a particular input or activity.

**Attention, selective** Ability to attend to important information and ignore distractions.

**Attention, sustained** Ability to continue an activity over time.

**Attention, switching** Ability to change from one task to another.

**Autoregulation** Adjustment of local blood flow to the demands of surrounding tissues.

**Axon** Process that extends from the cell body of a neuron. Most axons conduct signals away from the cell body. The only axons that conduct information toward the cell body are the distal axons of primary afferent neurons, which conduct signals to the dorsal root ganglion or cranial nerve ganglion.

**Axon hillock** Specialized region of a neuron cell body that gives rise to the axon. The axon hillock is densely populated with voltage-gated $Na^+$ channels.

**Axons, myelinated** Axons that are completely enveloped by a myelin sheath.

**Axons, unmyelinated** Axons that are only partially enveloped by myelin.

**Basal ganglia** Interconnected group of nuclei consisting of the caudate, putamen, globus pallidus, subthalamic nucleus, substantia nigra, and pedunculopontine nucleus. The nuclei are involved in five cortico-basal ganglia-thalamic circuits: motor, oculomotor, executive, behavioral flexibility and control, and limbic. The motor circuit compares proprioceptive information with movement commands, sequences movements, and regulates muscle tone and muscle force. May select and inhibit muscle synergies.

**Basal nucleus of Meynert** Part of the limbic system in the basal forebrain region, inferior to the preoptic area.

**Bundle, medial forebrain** Axons connecting anterior structures (septal area, nucleus accumbens, amygdala, anterior cingulate gyrus), the hypothalamus, and the midbrain reticular formation.

**Calcitonin gene-related peptide** A neuromodulator that activates second messengers. The end result is decreasing the likelihood that acetylcholine (ACh) will activate its own receptor when bound. Also involved in long-term neural changes in response to pain stimuli.

**Canals, semicircular** Three hollow rings in the inner ear, oriented at right angles to each other. Each canal has an enlargement called the *ampulla,* which contains the receptor mechanism for detecting rotational acceleration or deceleration of the head.

**Cell body** The metabolic center of any cell that contains the nucleus and the energy-producing/storing apparatus. The cell body of neurons also includes neurotransmitter-synthesizing mechanisms.

**Cells, bipolar** Neurons having two primary processes, a dendritic root, and an axon, which extend from the cell body.

**Cells, multipolar** Neurons having multiple dendrites arising from many regions of the cell body and possessing a single axon.

**Cells, pseudounipolar** Neurons that have one projection from the cell body that later divides into two axonal roots. A pseudounipolar cell has no true dendrites.

**Cells, Renshaw** Interneurons that produce recurrent inhibition in the spinal cord. Act to focus motor activity.

**Cells, Schwann** Macroglia that form myelin sheaths enveloping only a single neuron's axon or partially surrounding several axons. Found in the peripheral nervous system.

**Cells, stem** Immature and undifferentiated cells that give rise to both neurons and glial cells.

**Cells, tract** Cells with long axons that connect the spinal cord with the brain.

**Cerebellum** Part of the brain posterior to the brainstem. Involved in coordination of movement and postural control, motor planning, and rapid shifting of attention.

**Cerebellar hemisphere, lateral** Part of the cerebellar hemisphere lateral to the paravermis. Involved in coordination of voluntary movements, planning of movements, and the ability to judge time intervals and produce accurate rhythms.

**Cerebral hemispheres** The right and left halves of the cerebrum.

**Cerebral palsy, dyskinetic** Motor disorder that develops in utero or during infancy. Characterized by abnormal muscle tone and posture and involuntary movements that are jerky and rapid or slow and writhing.

**Cerebral palsy, spastic** Motor disorder that develops in utero or during infancy. Characterized by excessive skeletal muscle resistance to stretch.

**Cerebrocerebellum** Part of the cerebellum that coordinates voluntary movements via influence on corticofugal pathways, plans movements, judges time intervals, and produces accurate rhythms. Located in the lateral cerebellar hemispheres.

**Channels, G-protein–mediated** Neuronal membrane ion channels that open in response to the activation of a G-protein or its second messenger.

**Channels, leak** Openings in cell membranes that allow continuous movement of ions though the membrane.

**Channels, ligand-gated** Neuronal membrane ion channels that open in response to the binding of a chemical neurotransmitter.

**Channels, modality-gated** Membrane ion channels, specific to sensory neurons, which open in response to mechanical forces (i.e., stretch, touch, pressure) or thermal or chemical changes.

**Channels, voltage-gated** Membrane ion channels that open in response to changes in electrical potential across a neuron's cell membrane.

**Chemoreceptor** Receptor that responds to chemical change. Found in the carotid body, brainstem respiratory centers, specialized sensory cells for taste and smell, and skin, muscles, and viscera.

**Chiasm, optic** Site where the optic nerve fibers from the nasal half of the retina cross the midline.

**Cholinergic** (1) Referring to a neuron that secretes acetylcholine. (2) Referring to drugs that bind with and activate the same receptors as acetylcholine. (3) Referring to receptors that bind acetylcholine or agonist/antagonist drugs.

**Chorea** Involuntary, jerky, rapid movements.

**Choreoathetosis** A combination of involuntary, jerky, rapid movements and slow, writhing, purposeless movements.

**Choroid plexus** A network of capillaries embedded in connective tissue and epithelial cells that produce cerebrospinal fluid.

**Circle of Willis** Anastomotic ring of nine arteries, supplying all of the blood to the cerebral hemispheres. Consists of two anterior cerebral arteries, two internal carotid arteries, two posterior cerebral arteries, one anterior communicating artery, and two posterior communicating arteries.

**Circuits, control** Neural connections that adjust activity in the upper motor neurons, resulting in excitation or inhibition of the lower motor neurons. Consist of the basal ganglia and cerebellum.

**Cleft, synaptic** The space between the presynaptic and postsynaptic neuron terminals.

**Clonus** Involuntary rhythmic muscle contractions elicited by passive dorsiflexion of the foot or passive extension of the wrist. Occurs in upper motor neuron lesions, secondary to the loss or alteration of descending motor control.

**Coactivation, αγ** Simultaneous firing of α and γ motor neurons. Ensures that the muscle spindle maintains its sensitivity even when the extrafusal fibers surrounding the spindle contract.

**Cochlea** Snail shell–shaped organ, formed by a spiraling, fluid-filled tube. The cochlea contains a mechanism, the organ of Corti, which converts mechanical vibrations into the neural impulses that produce hearing.

**Cochlear duct** Membranous tube within the inner ear that contains the organ of hearing (the organ of Corti).

**Cocontraction** Simultaneous contraction of agonist and antagonist muscles. May occur in an intact nervous system when a new movement is learned, or may be a sign of neural dysfunction.

**Colliculus, superior** Part of the tectum of the midbrain, the superior colliculus integrates various sensory inputs and influences eye movement, head and body orientation, and postural adjustments.

**Columns, anterolateral** White matter in the anterior and lateral spinal cord that contains spinothalamic and motor axons.

**Coma** Condition of being unarousable; no response to strong stimuli such as strong pinching of the Achilles tendon.

**Complex regional pain syndrome (CRPS)** Chronic syndrome of pain, vascular changes, and atrophy in a regional distribution. *Syn.*: causalgia, Sudeck's atrophy, sympathetically maintained pain, reflex sympathetic dystrophy.

**Concussion** Mild traumatic brain injury.

**Conduction, saltatory** Rapid propagation of an action potential by jumping from one node of Ranvier to the next along a myelinated axon.

**Contracture, muscle** Adaptive shortening of muscle caused by the muscle remaining in a shortened position for prolonged periods of time. The decrease in length is caused by loss of sarcomeres.

**Convergence** (1) Multiple inputs from a variety of different cells terminating on a single neuron. (2) Movement that directs the eyes toward the midline.

**Corpus callosum** Large fiber bundle connecting the right and left cerebral cortices.

**Cortex, cerebral** Gray matter covering the cerebral hemispheres.

**Cortex, dorsolateral prefrontal** Anterior, dorsolateral part of the frontal cortex, responsible for self-awareness and executive functions (also called *goal-oriented behavior*). Executive functions include deciding on a goal, planning how to accomplish the goal, executing the plan, and monitoring the outcome of the action.

**Cortex, limbic** Part of the limbic system. A C-shaped region of cortex located on the medial hemisphere, consisting of the cingulate gyrus, parahippocampal gyrus, and uncus (a medial protrusion of the parahippocampal gyrus).

**Cortex, primary motor** Part of the cerebral cortex. Origin of many cortical upper motor neurons that influence contralateral voluntary movements, particularly the fine, fractionated movements of the hand and face. Located in the precentral gyrus, anterior to the central sulcus.

**Cortex, primary sensory (primary somatosensory)** Cerebral cortex that receives somatosensory information from the body and face. Located posterior to the central sulcus.

**Cortically blind** Person has no awareness of any visual information yet is able to orient his or her head position to objects.

**Cortisol** Steroid hormone that mobilizes energy (glucose), suppresses immune responses, and serves as an anti-inflammatory agent. Secreted by the adrenal glands. *Syn.*: *hydrocortisone.*

**Cramp** Severe and painful muscle spasm associated with fatigue or local ionic imbalances.

**Crest, neural** During development, the part of the ectoderm that will become the peripheral sensory neurons, myelin cells, autonomic neurons, and endocrine organs (adrenal medulla and pancreatic islets).

**Deafferentation** Interruption of sensory information from part of the body, usually caused by a lesion affecting first-order somatosensory neurons.

**Deafness, conductive** Hearing defect due to inability to transmit vibrations in the outer or middle ear.

**Deafness, sensorineural** Hearing defect due to damage of the receptor cells or the cochlear nerve.

**Deformity, Arnold-Chiari** Developmental malformation of the hindbrain, with elongation of the inferior cerebellum and medulla. The inferior cerebellum and medulla protrude into the vertebral canal.

**Degeneration, wallerian** Degeneration and death of the distal segment of a severed axon.

**Delirium** Reduced attention, orientation, and perception, associated with confused ideas and agitation.

**Delusion** A false belief that persists despite evidence to the contrary.

**Dementia** Severe impairment or loss of intellectual capacity and personality integration due to loss of or damage to neurons in the brain.

**Dementia, Parkinson's** Cognitive deficit that interferes with the ability to plan, to maintain goal orientation, and to make decisions.

**Dementia, with Lewy bodies** Type of parkinsonism with cognitive decline and visual hallucinations.

**Dendrite** Process that extends from the cell body of a neuron. Dendrites conduct information toward the cell body.

**Depolarization** Process whereby a neuron's cell membrane potential becomes less negative than its resting potential.

**Depolarized** The electrical state of a neuron's cell membrane when the membrane potential becomes less negative than the resting potential.

**Depression** Syndrome of hopelessness and a sense of worthlessness, with aberrant thoughts and behavior.

**Dermatome** The part of the somite that becomes dermis or, after the embryo stage, the dermis innervated by a single spinal nerve.

**Diencephalon** Centrally located part of the cerebrum, consisting of the thalamus, hypothalamus, epithalamus, and subthalamus.

**Diffuse axonal injury** Stretch injury to the membrane of an axon initiating changes that cause the axon to rupture.

**Diplopia** Double vision. Perceiving a single object as two objects.

**Disease, Charcot-Marie-Tooth** An inherited peripheral neuropathy that causes distal paresis and decreased ability to sense joint position and movement and heat, cold, and pain. *Syn.:* hereditary motor and sensory neuropathy.

**Disease, diffuse Lewy body** Progressive cognitive decline, memory impairments, and deficits in attention, executive function, and visuospatial ability secondary to abnormal protein aggregates in the cerebral cortex, brainstem nuclei, and limbic areas.

**Disease, Huntington's** Autosomal dominant hereditary disorder that causes degeneration in many areas of the brain, primarily in the striatum and cerebral cortex. Characterized by hyperkinesia.

**Disease, Ménière's** Sensation of fullness in the ear, tinnitus (ringing in the ear), severe acute vertigo, nausea, vomiting, and hearing loss. Cause is unknown.

**Disease, Parkinson's** The most common disorder of the basal ganglia, resulting from death of dopamine-producing cells in the substantia nigra compacta and acetylcholine-producing cells in the pedunculopontine nucleus. Characterized by muscular rigidity, slowness of movement, shuffling gait, droopy posture, resting tremors, diminished facial expression, and visuoperceptive impairments.

**Disorder, attention deficit** Difficulty sustaining attention, with onset during childhood.

**Disorder, obsessive-compulsive** Mental disorder characterized by persistent upsetting thoughts and the use of compulsive behavior in response to obsessive thoughts.

**Disorder, panic** Abrupt onset of intense terror, a sense of loss of personal identity, and the perception that familiar things are strange or unreal, combined with signs of increased sympathetic nervous system activity.

**Disorder, Tourette's** A neurologic disorder characterized by motor and vocal tics (the involuntary production of movements and sounds).

**Divergence** The branching of a single neuronal axon to synapse with a multitude of neurons.

**Dopamine** Neurotransmitter released by axons from the substantia nigra and the ventral tegmental area. Action on postsynaptic membranes is usually inhibitory.

**Dorsal root** The afferent (sensory) root of a spinal nerve.

**Dysarthria** Speech disorder resulting from paralysis, incoordination, or spasticity of muscles used for speaking. Due to upper or lower motor neuron lesions or muscle dysfunction. Comprehension of spoken language, writing, and reading are not affected by dysarthria. Two types of dysarthria may be distinguished: spastic, due to damage of upper motor neurons, and flaccid, resulting from damage to lower motor neurons.

**Dysarthria, flaccid** Breathy, soft, imprecise speech caused by damage to lower motor neurons in cranial nerve IX, X, or XII.

**Dysarthria, spastic** Harsh, awkward speech caused by an upper motor neuron lesion.

**Dysdiadochokinesis** Inability to rapidly alternate movements. For example, inability to rapidly pronate and supinate the forearm, or inability to rapidly alternate toe tapping. *Syn.:* dysdiadochokinesia.

**Dysesthesia** Painful abnormal sensation, including burning and aching sensations.

**Dyskinesia** Involuntary movement that resembles chorea (brisk, jerky movements) and/or dystonia (involuntary sustained postures or repetitive movements).

**Dysmetria** Inability to accurately move an intended distance.

**Dysreflexia, autonomic** Excessive activity of the sympathetic nervous system, usually elicited by noxious stimuli below the level of a spinal cord lesion.

**Dystonia** Hereditary movement disorder, usually nonprogressive, characterized by involuntary sustained muscle contractions causing abnormal postures or twisting, repetitive movements.

**Ectopic foci** Site on neural membrane that is abnormally sensitive to mechanical stimulation.

**Edema, cerebral** Accumulation of excess tissue fluid in the brain.

**Effectiveness, synaptic** Functional activation of postsynaptic receptors in response to the release of a neurotransmitter from a presynaptic terminal.

**Efferent** Carrying away from a structure.

**Electromyography** Recording of electrical activity produced by contracting muscle.

**Embolus** Blood clot that formed elsewhere and has been transported to a new location before occluding a vessel.

**Emotional lability** Abnormal, uncontrolled expression of emotions.

**Ending, primary** Sensory ending of a type Ia axon that responds phasically to stretch of the central region of intrafusal fibers in the muscle spindle.

**Ending, secondary** Sensory ending of a type II axon that responds tonically to stretch of the central region of intrafusal fibers (primarily nuclear chain fibers) in the muscle spindle.

**Endogenous opioid peptides** Peptides that bind to the same receptors that opium binds to and inhibit the transmission of nociceptive signals. Include endorphins, enkephalins, and dynorphins.

**Endoneurium** Connective tissue that separates individual axons.

**Endorphins** Endogenous, or naturally occurring, substances that activate analgesic mechanisms. Endorphins include enkephalins, dynorphin, and β-endorphin.

**Enkephalin** A neurotransmitter that, when bound to receptor sites, depresses the release of substance P and hyperpolarizes interneurons in the nociceptive pathway, thus inhibiting the transmission of nociceptive signals.

**Epilepsy** Sudden attacks of excessive neuronal discharge interfering with brain function.

**Epineurium** Connective tissue that surrounds an entire nerve trunk.

**Epithalamus** The major structure of the epithalamus is the pineal gland, an endocrine gland innervated by sympathetic fibers. The pineal gland helps regulate circadian (daily) rhythms and influences the secretions of the pituitary gland, adrenals, and parathyroids.

**Equation, Nernst** Mathematical equation used to determine the equilibrium potential for a diffusible ion.

**Erb's paralysis** Loss of shoulder abduction, external rotation, and elbow flexion (waiter's tip position) caused by a lesion of the upper trunk of the brachial plexus or the fifth and sixth cervical nerve roots.

**Excitotoxicity** Overexcitation of a neuron, leading to cell death.

**Executive functions** Goal-oriented behavior.

**Extinction, sensory** A form of unilateral neglect. Loss of sensation is evident only when symmetric body parts are tested bilaterally.

**Eye movements, conjugate** Both eyes move in the same direction.

**Eye movements, vergence** Eyes move toward the midline or away from the midline.

**Facilitation, presynaptic** At an axoaxonic synapse, the excitatory process by which transmitter released by one axon terminal causes the second axon terminal to release a greater than normal amount of neurotransmitter.

**Fasciculation** A quick twitch of muscle fibers in a single motor unit, which is visible on the surface of the skin.

**Fasciculus** A group of axons with the same function traveling together in the central nervous system.

**Fasciculus cuneatus** Axons that transmit discriminative touch and conscious proprioceptive information from the upper half of the body to the brain. Located in the lateral section of the dorsal column of the spinal cord.

**Fasciculus gracilis** Axons that transmit discriminative touch and conscious proprioceptive information from the lower half of the body to the brain. Located in the medial section of the dorsal column of the spinal cord.

**Fasciculus, medial longitudinal (MLF)** Brainstem tract that coordinates head and eye movements by providing bilateral connections among vestibular, oculomotor, and accessory nerve nuclei and the superior colliculus.

**Feedback** Information resulting from movement. For example, when a person flexes the elbow, feedback consists of information from sensory receptors in muscles, tendons, and skin.

**Feedforward** Neural preparation for anticipated movement, based on instruction, previous experience, and the ability to predict movement requirements and/or outcome.

**Fiber, intrafusal** Specialized muscle fiber inside the muscle spindle.

**Fibers, association** Axons connecting cortical regions within one hemisphere.

**Fibers, commissural** Axons connecting homologous areas of the nervous system.

**Fibers, extrafusal** Contractile skeletal muscle fibers outside of the muscle spindle.

**Fibers, projection** Axons connecting subcortical structures to the cerebral cortex, and axons connecting the cerebral cortex to the subcortical structures.

**Fibrillation** Brief contraction of a single muscle fiber, not visible on the surface of the skin.

**Fibromyalgia** Tenderness of muscles and adjacent soft tissues, stiffness of muscles, and aching pain. The painful area shows a regional rather than dermatomal or peripheral nerve distribution.

**Flaccidity** Lack of skeletal muscle resistance to passive stretch; complete absence of muscle tone.

**Flat affect** Lack of emotional facial expressions and gestures.

**Forebrain** Anterior part of the developing brain; becomes the cerebrum.

**Formation, reticular** Complex neural network in the brainstem, including the reticular nuclei and their connections. Source of ascending and descending reticular tracts.

**Fornix** Arch-shaped fiber bundle connecting the hippocampus with the mammillary body and the anterior nucleus of the thalamus.

**Fractionation** Ability to activate individual muscles independently of other muscles.

**Freezing** Episodes when movements abruptly cease. Characteristic of Parkinson's disease.

**Functional electrical stimulation (FES)** Use of electrical currents to activate nerves.

**Ganglion** A group of neuron cell bodies.

**Ganglion, dorsal root** Collection of primary somatosensory neuron cell bodies located in the dorsal root.

**Ganglion, stellate** A sympathetic ganglion located at the level of the seventh cervical vertebra. *Syn.:* cervicothoracic ganglion.

**Gate theory of pain** Theory that transmission of pain information can be blocked in the dorsal horn by stimulation of large-fiber primary afferent neurons.

**Generator, stepping pattern** Flexible network of interneurons that activate repetitive, rhythmic, reciprocal movement in the lower limbs, similar to stepping during walking.

**Geniculate, lateral** Site of synapse between axons from the retina and neurons that project to the visual cortex. Part of the thalamus, located inferiorly and posteriorly.

**Geniculate, medial** Site of synapse in the auditory pathway. Part of the thalamus, located inferiorly and posteriorly.

**Genu** Most medial part of the internal capsule, containing cortical fibers that project to cranial nerve motor nuclei, to the reticular formation, and to the red nucleus.

**Glia** Support cells of the nervous system, including oligodendrocytes, Schwann cells, astrocytes, and microglia.

**Globus pallidus internus** Part of the globus pallidus specialized for output to the motor thalamus and pedunculopontine nuclei.

**Glutamate** Excitatory amino acid neurotransmitter. Excessive amounts can be toxic to neurons.

**Glycine** Inhibitory neurotransmitter released by axons from spinal cord interneurons.

**Gray, periaqueductal** Area around the cerebral aqueduct in the midbrain. Involved in somatic and autonomic reactions to pain, threats, and emotions. Activity of the periaqueductal gray results in the fight-or-flight reaction and in vocalization during laughing and crying.

**Groove, neural** During development, the depression formed by the infolding of the neural plate; becomes the neural tube.

**Growing into deficit** Signs and symptoms of nervous system damage that do not become evident until the systems damaged would have become functional.

**Growth cone** The moving tip of a growing axon.

**Gyrus, cingulate** Gyrus on the medial cerebral hemisphere, superior to the corpus callosum. Contributes to processing of memory and emotions.

**Gyrus, parahippocampal** Most medial gyrus of the inferior temporal lobe. Contributes to memory processing.

**Habituation** A form of short-term plasticity. Repeated stimuli result in a decreased response owing to a decrease in the amount of neurotransmitter released from the presynaptic terminal of a sensory neuron.

**Hallpike maneuver** Rapid inversion of the posterior semicircular canal. Tests for benign paroxysmal positional vertigo. Vertigo and nystagmus indicate a positive test.

**Hallucination** A sensory perception experienced without corresponding sensory stimuli.

**Hematoma, epidural** Collection of blood between the skull and the dura mater.

**Hematoma, subdural** Collection of blood between the dura mater and the arachnoid.

**Hemianopia, bitemporal** Loss of information from both temporal visual fields. Produced by damage to fibers in the center of the optic chiasm, interrupting the axons from the nasal half of each retina. Also called *bitemporal hemianopsia*.

**Hemianopia, homonymous** Loss of visual information from one hemifield. A complete lesion of the visual pathway anywhere posterior to the optic chiasm (in the optic tract, lateral geniculate or optic radiations) results in loss of information from the contralateral visual field. Also called *homonymous hemianopsia*.

**Hemiplegia** Weakness or paralysis affecting one side of the body.

**Henneman's size principle** Order of recruitment from smaller to larger alpha motor neurons.

**Herniation, central** Movement of the diencephalon, midbrain, and pons inferiorly, caused by a lesion in the cerebrum exerting pressure on the diencephalon. This movement stretches the branches of the basilar artery, causing brainstem ischemia and edema.

**Herniation, tonsillar** Protrusion of the cerebellar tonsils (small lobes forming part of the inferior surface of the cerebellum) through the foramen magnum.

**Herniation, uncal** Protrusion of the uncus into the opening of the tentorium cerebelli, causing compression of the midbrain.

**Hillock, axon** In a motor neuron or interneuron, the region closest to the synapse with a high density of $Na^+$ channels.

**Hindbrain** Posterior part of the developing brain; becomes the pons, medulla, and cerebellum.

**Hippocampus** Part of the limbic system. Important in processing, but not storage, of declarative memories. Formed by the gray and white matter of two gyri rolled together in the medial temporal lobe.

**Homunculus** Figure representing the parts of the body controlled by or transmitting sensory information to a specific part of the cerebral cortex.

**Horn, dorsal** Posterior section of gray matter in the spinal cord. Primarily sensory in function, the dorsal horn contains endings and collaterals of first-order sensory neurons, interneurons, and dendrites and somas of tract cells.

**Horn, lateral** Lateral section of gray matter in the spinal cord. Contains the cell bodies of preganglionic sympathetic neurons.

**Horn, ventral** Anterior section of gray matter in the spinal cord. Contains endings of upper motor neurons, interneurons, and dendrites and cell bodies of lower motor neurons.

**Hydrocephalus** Accumulation of an excessive amount of cerebrospinal fluid in the ventricles.

**Hyperalgesia** Excessive sensitivity to painful stimuli.

**Hyperalgesia, primary** Excessive sensitivity to stimuli that are normally mildly painful in injured tissue.

**Hyperalgesia, secondary** Excessive sensitivity to stimuli that are normally mildly painful in uninjured tissue.

**Hypereffectiveness, synaptic** Increased response to a neurotransmitter that occurs because damage to some branches of a presynaptic axon results in larger than normal amounts of transmitter being released by the remaining axons onto postsynaptic receptors.

**Hyperkinetic** Characterized by abnormal involuntary movements. Includes dystonic, choreic, athetotic, and choreoathetotic movements.

**Hyperpolarization** Process whereby a neuron's cell membrane potential becomes more negative than its resting potential.

**Hyperpolarized** The electrical state of a neuron's cell membrane when the membrane potential becomes more negative than its resting potential.

**Hyperreflexia** Excessive phasic and/or tonic stretch reflex response. Hyperreflexia often contributes to movement disorders post spinal cord injury and in spastic cerebral palsy. Hyperreflexia usually does not interfere with active movement post stroke.

**Hypersensitivity, denervation** Increased response to a neurotransmitter that occurs because new receptor sites have developed on the postsynaptic membrane.

**Hypertonia** Abnormally strong skeletal muscle resistance to stretch. Occurs in chronic upper motor neuron disorders and in some basal ganglia disorders. Two types are (1) spastic (resistance is dependent on velocity of stretch) and (2) rigid (resistance is independent of velocity of muscle stretch).

**Hypotension, orthostatic** Decrease of 20 mm Hg or more in systolic blood pressure when moving from prone or supine to sitting or standing.

**Hypothalamus** The ventromedial part of the diencephalon. Plays a major role in regulation of the autonomic and endocrine systems, and contributes to emotional and motivational states.

**Hypotonia** Abnormally low muscular resistance to passive stretch. Occurs in lower motor neuron and primary afferent neuron disorders and in hypotonic cerebral palsy. Also occurs temporarily following upper motor neuron lesions owing to a period of neural shock (electrical silence) post injury.

**Incidence** Rate of new disease or disorder in a population. Usually expressed as the number of new cases in a year in a population.

**Infarct, lacunar** Obstruction of blood flow in a small, deep artery. Lacunae are small cavities that remain after the necrotic tissue is cleared away.

**Inhibition, presynaptic** At an axoaxonic synapse, the inhibitory process by which transmitter released by one axon terminal causes the second terminal to release a less than normal amount of neurotransmitter.

**Inhibition, reciprocal** Decreased activity in an antagonist when an agonist is active.

**Inhibition, recurrent** Inhibition of agonists and synergists, combined with disinhibition of antagonists.

**Insula** Cortex located in the lateral fissure of the cerebrum.

**Internal capsule** Axons connecting the cerebral cortex with subcortical structures. The internal capsule is white matter bordered by the caudate and thalamus medially and the lenticular nucleus laterally. The internal capsule has three parts: anterior limb, genu, and posterior limb. Anterior limb: located lateral to the head of the caudate, contains corticopontine fibers and fibers interconnecting thalamic and cortical limbic areas. Genu: most medial part of the internal capsule, containing cortical fibers that project to cranial nerve motor nuclei, the reticular formation, and to the red nucleus. Posterior limb: located between the thalamus and the lenticular nucleus, with additional fibers traveling posterior and inferior to the lenticular nucleus (retrolenticular and sublenticular fibers). The posterior limb contains corticospinal and thalamocortical projections.

**Interneurons** Neurons that process information locally or convey information short distances from one site in the nervous system to another.

**Internuclear ophthalmoplegia** Loss of adduction of one eye during horizontal gaze due to a lesion of the medial longitudinal fasciculus. Convergence is preserved.

**Junction, neuromuscular** Synapse between a nerve terminal and the membrane of a muscle fiber. Acetylcholine is the neurotransmitter released at the neuromuscular junction.

**Klumpke's paralysis** Paralysis and atrophy of the hand intrinsic muscles and the long flexors and extensors of the fingers caused by avulsion of the motor roots of C8 and T1.

**Lability, emotional** Abnormal, uncontrolled expression of emotions.

**Labyrinth** The inner ear, consisting of the cochlea and the vestibular apparatus.

**Laminae, Rexed's** Histologic divisions of the spinal cord gray matter.

**Lateropulsion** Powerful pushing away from the less paretic side in sitting, during transfers, during standing, and during walking. Syn: contraversive pushing.

**Layer, mantle** During development, the inner wall of the neural tube.

**Layer, marginal** During development, the outer wall of the neural tube.

**Lemniscus** A bundle of myelinated axons with the same function traveling together in the central nervous system.

**Lemniscus, medial** Axons of second-order neurons conveying sensory information related to discriminative touch and conscious proprioception from the body to the cerebral cortex. Begins in the nucleus cuneatus and nucleus gracilis and ends in the ventral posterolateral nucleus of the thalamus.

**Lesion** An area of damage or dysfunction; a pathologic change that may be structural or functional.

**Lethargic** Tends to lose track of conversations and tasks; falls asleep if little stimulation is provided.

**Level, cortical** Areas of cerebral cortex that induce antinociception.

**Level, neurologic** Describing spinal cord injury, neurologic level is the most caudal level with normal sensory and motor function bilaterally.

**Limb, anterior** Part of the internal capsule located lateral to the head of the caudate; contains corticopontine fibers and fibers interconnecting thalamic and cortical limbic areas.

**Limb, posterior** Part of the internal capsule located between the thalamus and the lenticular nucleus, with additional fibers traveling posterior and inferior to the lenticular nucleus (retrolenticular and sublenticular fibers). Contains corticospinal and thalamocortical projections.

**Locus coeruleus** Nucleus in the upper pons involved in direction of attention, nonspecific activation of interneurons and lower motor neurons in the spinal cord, and inhibition of pain information in the dorsal horn. Transmitter produced is norepinephrine.

**M1** The shortest latency response after stretch of a muscle, produced by the monosynaptic phasic stretch reflex.

**M2** The second response after stretch of a muscle, probably involving neural circuits in the brainstem. Also called the *long loop response.*

**Macroglia** Large support cells of the nervous system, including oligodendrocytes, Schwann cells, and astrocytes.

**Malformations, arteriovenous** Developmental abnormalities with arteries connected to veins by abnormal, thin-walled vessels larger than capillaries. Arteriovenous malformations usually do not cause signs or symptoms unless they rupture.

**Mania** Excessive excitement, euphoria, delusions, and overactivity.

**Marginal layer** Most dorsal part of the spinal gray matter. Involved in processing nociceptive information. *Syn.:* lamina 1.

**Mater, dura** Tough outer membrane surrounding the central nervous system.

**Mater, pia** Inner layer of the membranes surrounding the central nervous system.

**Medial geniculate body** Thalamic relay station for auditory information to the primary auditory cortex.

**Mechanoreceptor** Receptor that responds to mechanical stimulation (e.g., stretch, pressure). For example, receptors in the muscle spindle, touch receptors in skin, and stretch receptors in viscera.

**Medulla** Inferior part of the brainstem. Contributes to control of eye and head movements, coordinates swallowing, and helps regulate cardiovascular, respiratory, and visceral activity.

**Memory, declarative** Recollections that can be easily verbalized. Declarative memory is also called *conscious, explicit,* or *cognitive memory.*

**Memory, procedural** Recall of skills and habits. This type of memory is also called *skill, habit,* or *nonconscious* or *implicit memory.*

**Meninges** Membranes that enclose the brain and spinal cord. Include the dura mater, arachnoid, and pia mater.

**Meningitis** Inflammation of the membranes that surround the central nervous system.

**Meningocele** Congenital defect in which the meninges protrude through a deficiency in the vertebral column or skull.

**Meningomyelocele** Developmental defect in which the inferior part of the neural tube remains open.

**Mesencephalic nucleus of the trigeminal nerve** Collection of cell bodies that process proprioceptive information from the face.

**Messenger, second** Molecule that diffuses through the intracellular environment of a neuron and initiates cellular events, including opening or closing of membrane ion channels, activation of genes, and modulation of calcium concentrations inside the cell.

**Microglia** Small support cells of the nervous system.

**Midbrain** The uppermost part of the brainstem.

**Migraine** Syndrome consisting of headache, nausea, vomiting, extreme sensitivity to light and sound, dizziness, and cognitive disturbances. Caused by inherited abnormalities in genes that control activity of certain brainstem neurons. Some migraines do not include headache. Some migraines are preceded by an aura; some are not.

**Modulation** Long-lasting changes in the electrical potential of a neuron's cell membrane that alter the flow of ions across the cell membrane.

**Mononeuropathy** Dysfunction of a single peripheral nerve.

**Mononeuropathy, multiple** Dysfunction of several separate peripheral nerves. Signs and symptoms show an asymmetric distribution.

**Motor neurons, alpha** Lower motor neurons that innervate extrafusal fibers in skeletal muscle. When these neurons fire, skeletal muscle fibers contract.

**Motor neurons, gamma** Lower motor neurons that innervate intrafusal fibers in skeletal muscle. When these neurons fire, the ends of intrafusal fibers contract, stretching the central region of muscle fibers within the muscle spindle.

**Motor neurons, lower** Neurons with their cell bodies in the spinal cord or brainstem whose axons directly innervate skeletal muscle fibers. Two types are alpha motor neurons that innervate extrafusal muscle fibers, and gamma motor neurons that innervate intrafusal muscle fibers.

**Motor neurons, upper** Neurons that transmit information from the brain to lower motor neurons and movement-related interneurons in the spinal cord or brainstem. Although upper motor neurons do not directly innervate skeletal muscle, they contribute to control of movement by influencing the activity of lower motor neurons.

**Motor plate** Ventral section of the neural tube that becomes the ventral horn in the mature spinal cord.

**Motor perseveration** Uncontrollable repetition of a movement.

**Muscle synergy** Muscle contraction that produces coordinated action.

**Myasthenia gravis** Immune disorder in which antibodies attack acetylcholine receptors on muscle membranes, producing weakness that worsens with repetitive or continuous use of the muscles.

**Myelin** Sheath of proteins and fats formed by oligodendrocytes and Schwann cells to envelop the axons of nerve cells. Provides physical support and insulation for conduction of electrical signals by neurons.

**Myelination** (1) Process of acquiring a myelin sheath. (2) The myelin sheath.

**Myelinopathy, traumatic** Loss of myelin limited to the site of injury.

**Myelopathy, cervical spondylotic** Spinal cord damage secondary to cervical stenosis.

**Myeloschisis** Congenital defect in which the malformed spinal cord is open to the surface of the body.

**Myoclonus** Brief, involuntary contractions of a muscle or group of muscles.

**Myofibrils** Individual muscles fibers composed of proteins arranged in sarcomeres.

**Myopathy** Abnormality or disease intrinsic to muscle tissue.

**Myoplasticity** Changes in skeletal muscle, including contracture, atrophy, and weak actin-myosin binding.

**Myotome** During development, the part of a somite that becomes muscle, or after the embryo stage, a group of muscles innervated by a segmental spinal nerve.

**Neglect** Tendency to behave as if one side of the body and/or one side of space does not exist.

**Nerve, abducens** Cranial nerve VI. Controls the lateral rectus muscle that moves the eye laterally.

**Nerve, accessory** Cranial nerve XI. Motor nerve innervating the trapezius and sternocleidomastoid muscles.

**Nerve, facial** Cranial nerve VII. Mixed nerve containing both sensory and motor fibers. The sensory fibers transmit touch, pain, and pressure information from the tongue and pharynx and information from taste buds of the anterior tongue to the solitary nucleus. Motor innervation by the facial nerve includes the muscles that close the eyes, move the lips, and produce facial expressions. The facial nerve provides the efferent limb of the corneal reflex and also innervates salivary, nasal, and lacrimal (tear-producing) glands.

**Nerve, glossopharyngeal** Cranial nerve IX. Mixed nerve containing both sensory and motor fibers. The sensory fibers transmit somatosensation from the soft palate and pharynx and taste information from the posterior tongue. The motor component innervates a pharyngeal muscle and the parotid salivary gland.

**Nerve, hypoglossal** Cranial nerve XII. Motor nerve providing innervation to the intrinsic and extrinsic muscles of the ipsilateral tongue.

**Nerve, oculomotor** Cranial nerve III. Controls the superior, inferior, and medial rectus, the inferior oblique, and the levator palpebrae superioris muscles. These muscles move the pupil upward, downward, and medially; rotate the eye around the axis of the pupil; and assist in elevating the upper eyelid. Parasympathetic efferent fibers in the oculomotor nerve innervate the ciliary muscle and the sphincter pupillae, controlling reflexive constriction of the pupil and the thickness of the lens of the eye.

**Nerve, olfactory** Cranial nerve I. Transmits information about odors.

**Nerve, optic** Cranial nerve II. Transmits visual information from the retina to the lateral geniculate body of the thalamus and to nuclei in the midbrain.

**Nerve, spinal** Nerve located in the intervertebral foramen, formed by the dorsal and ventral roots, which contains both afferent and efferent axons. Spinal nerves branch to form dorsal and ventral rami.

**Nerve, trigeminal** Cranial nerve V. Mixed nerve containing both sensory and motor fibers. The sensory fibers transmit information from the face and temporomandibular joint. The motor fibers innervate the muscles of mastication. Three branches: ophthalmic, maxillary, and mandibular.

**Nerve, trochlear** Cranial nerve IV. Controls the superior oblique muscle, which rotates the eye, or, if the eye is adducted, depresses the pupil.

**Nerve, vagus** Cranial nerve X. Provides sensory and motor innervation of the larynx and pharynx and bidirectional communication with the viscera.

**Nerve, vestibulocochlear** Cranial nerve VIII. Sensory nerve with two distinct branches. The vestibular branch transmits information related to head position and head movement. The cochlear branch transmits information related to hearing.

**Neuralgia, postherpetic** Severe pain that persists longer than 1 month after infection with varicella zoster virus. Occurs along the distribution of a peripheral nerve or branch of a peripheral nerve.

**Neuralgia, trigeminal** Dysfunction of the trigeminal nerve, producing severe, sharp, stabbing pain in the distribution of one or more branches of the trigeminal nerve.

**Neuritis, vestibular** Inflammation of the vestibular nerve, usually caused by a virus. Disequilibrium, spontaneous nystagmus, nausea, and severe vertigo persist up to 3 days.

**Neuroinflammation** Central nervous system response to infection, disease, and injury.

**Neuroma** Tumor composed of axons and Schwann cells.

**Neuromodulator** Chemical released into the extracellular fluid at a distance from the synaptic cleft. The effects manifest more slowly and usually act longer than effects at a synapse. Typically, neuromodulators require seconds before their effects are manifest. The same molecule can act as both a neurotransmitter and a neuromodulator, depending upon whether it is released at a synapse or an extrasynaptic site.

**Neuron** The electrically excitable nerve cell of the nervous system.

**Neuron, afferent** (1) Neuron that brings information into the central nervous system. (2) Neuron that transmits information toward a structure.

**Neuron, efferent** (1) Neuron that relays commands from the central nervous system to the smooth and skeletal muscles and glands of the body. (2) Neuron that transmits information away from a structure.

**Neuron, postganglionic** Autonomic neuron with its cell body in an autonomic ganglion and its termination in an effector organ.

**Neuron, preganglionic** Autonomic neuron with its cell body in the brainstem or spinal cord and its termination in an autonomic ganglion.

**Neuropathy** Dysfunction or pathology of one or more peripheral nerves.

**Neuroplasticity** Ability of neurons to change their function, chemical profile (quantities and types of neurotransmitters produced), or structure.

**Neurotransmitters** Chemicals contained in the presynaptic terminal that are released into the synaptic cleft to transmit information between neurons.

**Nociceptive** Able to receive or transmit information about stimuli that damage or threaten to damage tissue.

**Nociceptors** Receptors that are sensitive to information about tissue damage or potential tissue damage.

**Nodes of Ranvier** Interruptions in the myelin sheath that leave small patches of axon unmyelinated. These unmyelinated patches contain a high density of voltage-gated $Na^+$ channels that contribute to the generation of action potentials.

**Norepinephrine** A neurotransmitter released by axons from the locus coeruleus and the medial reticular zone and by postganglionic sympathetic axons. Binds with $\alpha$- and $\beta$-adrenergic receptors.

**Nuclei, association** Thalamic nuclei that connect reciprocally with large areas of cerebral cortex. Association nuclei are found in the anterior thalamus, medial thalamus, and dorsal tier of the lateral thalamus.

**Nuclei, cochlear** Site of synapse between first- and second-order neurons involved in hearing. Located laterally at the pontomedullary junction.

**Nuclei, nonspecific** Thalamic nuclei that receive multiple types of input and project to widespread areas of cortex. This functional group includes the reticular, midline, and intralaminar nuclei, important in consciousness and arousal.

**Nuclei, raphe** Brainstem nuclei that modulate activity throughout the central nervous system. Major source of serotonin. Midbrain raphe nuclei are important in mood regulation and onset of sleep. Pontine raphe nuclei modulate activity in the brainstem and cerebellum. Medullary raphe nuclei modulate activity in the spinal cord via raphespinal tracts. Projections to the spinal cord inhibit transmission of nociceptive information, adjust levels of interneuron activity, and produce nonspecific activation of lower motor neurons.

**Nuclei, relay** Thalamic nuclei that receive specific information and serve as relay stations by sending the information directly to localized areas of cerebral cortex. All relay nuclei are found in the ventral tier of the lateral nuclear group.

**Nuclei, vestibular** Site of synapse between first- and second-order neurons involved in detecting head movement and head position. Located laterally at the pontomedullary junction.

**Nucleus** Collection of nerve cell bodies in the central nervous system.

**Nucleus accumbens** Group of neurons located at the junction of the head of the caudate and the anterior part of the putamen. Involved in reward, pleasure, and addiction. Part of the ventral striatum.

**Nucleus, Clarke's** Site of synapse between first- and second-order neurons that convey unconscious proprioceptive information to the cerebellum. The second-order axon is in the posterior spinocerebellar tract. Clarke's nucleus is located in the medial dorsal horn of the spinal cord, from T1 to L2 spinal segments. *Syn.:* nucleus dorsalis.

**Nucleus cuneatus** Site of synapse between fasciculus cuneatus and medial lemniscus neurons. Relays discriminative touch and conscious proprioceptive information. Located in the dorsal part of the lower medulla.

**Nucleus dorsalis** Site of synapse between first- and second-order neurons that convey unconscious proprioceptive information to the cerebellum. The second-order axon is in the posterior spinocerebellar tract. The nucleus dorsalis is located in the medial dorsal horn of the spinal cord, from T1 to L2 spinal segments. *Syn.:* Clarke's nucleus.

**Nucleus gracilis** Site of synapse between fasciculus gracilis and medial lemniscus neurons. Relays discriminative touch and conscious proprioceptive information. Located in the dorsal part of the lower medulla.

**Nucleus, inferior olivary** Nucleus in the upper medulla that receives input from most motor areas of the brain and spinal cord. Axons from the inferior olivary nucleus project to the contralateral cerebellar hemisphere. May be involved in the perception of time.

**Nucleus, lateral cuneate** Nucleus that receives proprioceptive information from the upper body. Relays unconscious proprioceptive information to the cerebellum, via the cuneocerebellar tract. Located in the dorsolateral medulla.

**Nucleus, lentiform (*syn:* lenticular)** Globus pallidus and putamen.

**Nucleus, main sensory of trigeminal** Site of synapse between first- and second-order discriminative touch neurons in the trigeminothalamic pathway.

**Nucleus, mesencephalic of the trigeminal nerve** Location of cell bodies of primary afferents conveying proprioceptive information from the muscles of mastication and extraocular muscles.

**Nucleus, pedunculopontine** Nucleus within the caudal midbrain that influences movement via connections with the globus pallidus, subthalamic nucleus, and reticular areas. The neurons produce acetylcholine.

**Nucleus proprius** Part of the dorsal gray matter in the spinal cord. Processes proprioceptive and two-point discrimination information. *Syn.:* laminae III and IV.

**Nucleus, red** Sphere of gray matter that receives information from the cerebellum and cerebral cortex and projects to the cerebellum, spinal cord (via rubrospinal tract), and reticular formation. Activity in the rubrospinal tract contributes to distal upper limb extension.

**Nucleus, solitary** Main visceral sensory nucleus. Receives information from the oral cavity and thoracic and abdominal viscera via the vagus, glossopharyngeal, and facial nerves. Involved in regulation of visceral function. Located in the dorsal medulla.

**Nucleus, spinal trigeminal** Site of synapse between first- and second-order neurons conveying nociceptive information from the face. Located in the lower pons and medulla.

**Nucleus, subthalamic** Collection of cell bodies located inferior to the thalamus and superior to the substantia nigra. Part of the basal ganglia.

**Nucleus, trigeminal main sensory** Nucleus that receives touch information from the face. Information is transmitted to the ventral posteromedial nucleus of the thalamus, then to the cerebral cortex.

**Nucleus, ventral posterolateral of the thalamus** Site of synapse between neurons that convey somatosensory information from the body to the cerebral cortex. The spinothalamic and medial lemniscus axons end in this nucleus.

**Nucleus, ventral posteromedial** Site of synapse between neurons that convey somatosensory information from the face to the cerebral cortex. Located in the thalamus.

**Nystagmus** Involuntary back-and-forth movements of the eyes. Physiologic nystagmus is a normal response that can be elicited in an intact nervous system by rotational or temperature stimulation of the semicircular canals or by moving the pupils to the extreme horizontal position. Pathologic nystagmus, a sign of nervous system abnormality, consists of abnormal oscillating eye movements that occur with or without external stimulation.

**Nystagmus, pathologic** Abnormal oscillating eye movements that occur with or without external stimulation.

**Obtunded** Sleeping more than awake; drowsy and confused when awake.

**Oculomotor complex** Oculomotor nucleus and the oculomotor parasympathetic nucleus. The oculomotor nucleus supplies efferent somatic fibers to the extraocular muscles innervated by the oculomotor nerve. The oculomotor parasympathetic (Edinger-Westphal) nucleus supplies parasympathetic control of the pupillary sphincter and the ciliary muscle (adjusts thickness of the lens in the eye).

**Oligodendrocytes** Macroglia that form myelin sheaths, enveloping several axons from several neurons. Found within the central nervous system.

**Olive** Small oval lump on the anterolateral medulla that lies external to the inferior olivary nucleus.

**Organ of Corti** Organ of hearing, located within the cochlea.

**Organs, otolithic** The utricle and saccule, parts of the inner ear. Contain receptors that respond to head position relative to gravity and to linear acceleration and deceleration of the head.

**Orienting** Ability to locate specific sensory information from among many stimuli.

**Oscillopsia** Lack of visual stabilization. The world appears to bounce up and down owing to failure of the vestibulo-ocular reflex.

**Outflow, craniosacral** Parasympathetic nervous system.

**Outflow, thoracolumbar** Sympathetic nervous system.

**Pain, chronic** Persistent pain. The three major types are (1) nociceptive (continuing tissue damage), (2) chronic neuropathic pain, and (3) chronic pain syndrome. Continuing tissue damage arises from rheumatoid arthritis, cancer, and other physically identifiable causes. Chronic neuropathic pain is caused by abnormal neural activity within the central nervous system. An example is phantom limb pain. Chronic pain syndrome is pain that persists longer than 6 months after normal healing would have been expected. An example is chronic low back pain syndrome without continuing tissue damage. Disuse syndrome may be a contributing factor to chronic low back pain syndrome.

**Pain, fast** Discriminative information about stimuli that damage or threaten to damage tissue. Conveyed to cerebral cortex.

**Pain, myofascial** A controversial diagnosis: Pressure on sensitive points (called *trigger points*) reproduces the person's pattern of referred pain. Advocates contend that the diagnosis is confirmed when stretch or injecting a local anesthetic into the trigger points eliminates the pain.

**Pain, neuropathic chronic** Persistent pain due to abnormal neural activity in various locations in the nervous system.

**Pain, nociceptive chronic** Persistent pain due to stimulation of nociceptive receptors.

**Pain, phantom limb** Neuropathic pain that seems to originate from a missing body part, caused by central nervous system overactivity subsequent to an amputation.

**Pain, referred** Pain that is perceived as arising at a site different from the actual site producing the nociceptive information.

**Pain, slow** Nonlocalized information about stimuli that damage or threaten to damage tissue. Conveyed by divergent pathways to areas in the midbrain and reticular formation and to the medial and intralaminar nuclei of the thalamus. This information reaches widespread areas of the cerebral cortex.

**Pain, spinothalamic** Discriminative information about stimuli that damage or threaten to damage tissue. Conveyed to cerebral cortex. Syn.: *fast pain.*

**Pallidotomy** Surgery to treat akinesia in Parkinson's disease by destroying part of the globus pallidus.

**Palsy, Bell's** Paralysis or paresis of the muscles of facial expression on one side of the face, caused by a lesion of the facial nerve.

**Palsy, cerebral** Movement and postural disorder resulting from permanent, nonprogressive damage to the developing brain.

**Paralysis** Inability to voluntarily contract muscle(s). Reflexive contraction may be intact if paralysis is due to an upper motor neuron lesion. Reflexive contraction is absent if paralysis is due to a complete lower motor neuron lesion.

**Paralysis, flaccid** Loss of voluntary movement and muscle tone.

**Paraphasia** Word substitution or use of nonsensical, unrecognizable words.

**Paraplegia** Paresis or paralysis of both lower limbs. May also involve part of the trunk.

**Paravermis** Part of the cerebellar hemisphere adjacent to the vermis; influences the activity of the lateral activation pathways.

**Paresis** Weakness; decreased ability to generate the amount of force required for a task.

**Paresthesia** Nonpainful abnormal sensation, often described as pricking and tingling.

**Parkinsonism** A general term for basal ganglia disorders with signs and symptoms characteristic of Parkinson's disease. Includes disorders caused by drugs, infection, or trauma. The term excludes idiopathic Parkinson's disease.

**Paroxysmal** Sudden onset of a symptom, sign, or disease.

**Pathway, conscious relay** Three-neuron series that transmits somatosensory information about location and type of stimulation to the cerebral cortex.

**Pathway, cuneocerebellar** A two-neuron series that transmits proprioceptive information from the arms and upper half of the body to the cerebellum.

**Pathway, divergent** Series of neurons that transmit slow pain information to the brainstem and cerebrum.

**Pathway, posterior spinocerebellar** A two-neuron series that transmits proprioceptive information from the legs and the lower half of the body to the cerebellum.

**Pathway, spinolimbic** Axons that convey nonlocalized nociceptive information to the medial and intralaminar nuclei of the thalamus. Information is then transmitted to limbic and other areas of the cerebral cortex. Involved in arousal, withdrawal, and autonomic and affective responses to pain.

**Pathway, retinogeniculocalcarine** Neural connections that convey visual information from the retina to the visual cortex.

**Pathway, spinomesencephalic** Series of neurons that transmit nociceptive information to the superior colliculus and to the periaqueductal gray in the midbrain. Activates parts of the descending pain control system.

**Pathway, spinoreticular** Series of neurons that convey nonlocalized nociceptive information to the reticular formation. The information influences arousal and is transmitted to the medial and intralaminar nuclei of the thalamus.

**Peduncles, cerebellar** Bundles of axons that connect the cerebellum with the brainstem. The superior peduncle connects with the midbrain, the middle peduncle with the pons, and the inferior peduncle with the medulla.

**Peduncles, cerebral** The most anterior part of the midbrain, formed by axons descending from the cerebrum to the pons, medulla, and spinal cord. Specifically, the corticospinal, corticobrainstem, and corticopontine tracts.

**Perception** Interpretation of sensation into meaningful forms.

**Perineurium** Connective tissue that surrounds bundles of axons.

**Period, absolute refractory** The time period during an action potential when no stimulus, no matter how strong, will elicit another action potential.

**Period, critical** Time period during which neuronal projections are competing for synaptic sites.

**Period, relative refractory** Time period soon after the peak of an action potential when only a stronger than normal stimulus can elicit another action potential.

**Peripheral nerve distribution** Area of skin innervated by a single peripheral nerve.

**Peripheral nervous system** Parts of the nervous system outside the vertebra and skull.

**Perseveration, motor** Uncontrollable repetition of a movement.

**Personality disorder** Mental disorder characterized by inflexible, maladaptive patterns of inner experience and behavior.

**Phoria** Tendency for one eye to deviate from looking straight ahead when binocular vision is not available.

**Plaques** Patches of demyelination.

**Plasmapheresis** Replacement of blood plasma with a plasma substitute, to remove circulating antibodies.

**Plate, association** Dorsal section of the neural tube that becomes the dorsal horn in the spinal cord.

**Plate, neural** During development, the thickened ectoderm on the surface of an embryo; becomes the neural tube.

**Polyneuropathy** Generalized disorder of peripheral nerves that typically presents distally and symmetrically.

**Polyneuropathy, diabetic** Distal, usually symmetric, impairment of axon and myelin function secondary to diabetes.

**Positron emission tomography (PET)** Computer-generated image based on the metabolism of injected radioactively labeled substances. The image indicates metabolic activity of the central nervous system.

**Postganglionic** An axon that originates from a cell body located in an autonomic ganglion.

**Postural instability** Tendency to lose one's balance.

**Posturography** Recording of force plate information and electromyograms from postural muscles during postural tests.

**Potential, action** A large change in the electrical potential of a neuron's cell membrane, resulting in the rapid spread of an electrical signal along the cell membrane.

**Potential, equilibrium** The electrical membrane potential at which any diffusible ion is electrically and chemically distributed equally on the two sides of the membrane.

**Potential, excitatory postsynaptic (EPSP)** Electrical depolarization of a neuron's cell membrane. Initiated by the binding of a neurotransmitter to membrane receptors and produced by the instantaneous flow of $Na^+$, $K^+$, or $Ca^{2+}$ into the cell.

**Potential, inhibitory postsynaptic (IPSP)** Electrical hyperpolarization of a cell membrane. Initiated by the binding of a neurotransmitter to membrane receptors and produced by the instantaneous flow of $Cl^-$ into the cell and/or $K^+$ out of the cell.

**Potential, local** A small change in the electrical potential of a neuron's cell membrane that is graded in both amplitude and duration.

**Potential, resting membrane** The difference in electrical potential across the cell membrane of a neuron when the neuron is neither receiving nor transmitting information (i.e., the electrical state of a neuron's cell membrane when the cell is at rest [neither electrically excited nor inhibited]).

**Potentials, auditory evoked** A method of testing brainstem function by auditory stimulation combined with recording electrical potentials from the scalp.

**Potentials, receptor** Local potentials generated at the receptor of a sensory neuron.

**Potentials, postsynaptic** Graded local changes in ion concentration across the postsynaptic membrane. May be excitatory or inhibitory.

**Potentials, synaptic** Local potentials generated at a postsynaptic membrane.

**Potentiation, long-term (LTP)** Cellular mechanism for memory that results from the synthesis and activation of new proteins and the growth of new synaptic connections.

**Premotor area** Controls trunk and girdle muscles via the medial upper motor neurons.

**Preganglionic** Neuron or axon proximal to an autonomic ganglion.

**Prevalence** Number of existing cases of a disease or disorder at a specific time per number of people in a population.

**Progressive supranuclear palsy (PSP)** A type of parkinsonism characterized by depression, psychosis, rage attacks, and impairment of voluntary movement of the eyes.

**Pronociception** Biological amplification of pain signals.

**Proprioception, conscious** Awareness of the movements and relative position of body parts.

**Propriospinal** Within the spinal cord. Usually refers to neurons that are located entirely within the spinal cord.

**Prostheses, neural** Devices that substitute for a diseased or injured part of the nervous system to enhance function.

**Psychosis** Loss of contact with external reality.

**Pushing, contraversive** Powerful pushing away from the less paretic side in sitting, during transfers, during standing, and during walking. Syn: lateropulsion.

**Pyramids** Ridges on the anteroinferior medulla, formed by the lateral corticospinal tracts.

**Radiculopathy** Lesion of a dorsal or ventral nerve root. Clinical use of the term may refer to a spinal nerve lesion.

**Rami, anterior** Branch of a spinal nerve that innervates the skeletal, muscular, and cutaneous areas of the limbs and the anterior and lateral trunk.

**Rami, posterior** Branch of a spinal nerve that innervates paravertebral muscles, posterior parts of the vertebrae, and overlying cutaneous areas.

**Ramus, dorsal primary** Branch of a spinal nerve that innervates the paravertebral muscles, posterior parts of the vertebrae, and overlying cutaneous areas.

**Ramus, ventral primary** Branch of a spinal nerve that innervates the skeletal, muscular, and cutaneous areas of the limbs and/or of the anterior and lateral trunk.

**Receptor, muscarinic** Receptor on an organ innervated by a postganglionic parasympathetic neuron. Acetylcholine binding to muscarinic receptors initiates a G-protein–mediated response.

**Receptor, phasic** A sensory nerve ending that adapts to a constant stimulus and stops responding.

**Receptor, tonic** A sensory nerve ending that responds as long as a stimulus is present.

**Receptors, adrenergic** Receptors in the sympathetic nervous system that respond to norepinephrine or epinephrine or to adrenergic drugs. Subtypes are α- and β-adrenergic receptors.

**Receptors, cholinergic** Receptors that respond to acetylcholine. Found in the autonomic and central nervous systems and on the motor end-plate in skeletal muscle membranes. Subtypes include nicotinic and muscarinic.

**Receptors, nicotinic** Receptors on postsynaptic neurons in autonomic ganglia and on the motor end-plate of skeletal muscle. Acetylcholine binding to nicotinic receptors causes a fast excitatory postsynaptic potential in the postsynaptic membrane.

**Reflex** An involuntary response to an external stimulus.

**Reflex, asymmetric tonic neck** Head rotation to the right or left elicits extension of limbs on the nose side and flexion of limbs on the skull side.

**Reflex, consensual** Constriction of the pupil in the opposite eye when a bright light is shined into one eye. The optic nerve is the afferent (sensory) limb of the reflex, and the oculomotor nerve provides the efferent (motor) limb.

**Reflex, crossed-extension** Extension of the opposite lower limb when one lower limb is moved away from a stimulus.

**Reflex, H-** Reflexive muscle contraction elicited by electrically stimulating the skin over a peripheral nerve. Used to assess the degree of excitation of alpha motor neurons.

**Reflex, phasic stretch** Muscle contraction in response to quick stretch. *Syn.:* myotatic reflex, muscle stretch reflex, deep tendon reflex.

**Reflex, pupillary** Pupil constriction in the eye directly stimulated by a bright light. The optic nerve is the afferent (sensory) limb of the reflex, and the oculomotor nerve provides the efferent (motor) limb.

**Reflex, symmetric tonic neck** Flexion of the upper limbs and extension of the lower limbs when the neck is flexed, and the opposite pattern in the limbs when the neck is extended.

**Reflex, tonic labyrinthine** Tilting the head back causes flexion of the upper limbs and extension of the lower limbs. Tilting the head forward elicits extension of the upper limbs and flexion of the lower limbs.

**Reflex, tonic stretch** Sustained alpha motor neuron firing and muscle contraction in response to maintained stretch of muscle spindles. At velocities of muscle stretch typically used in clinic, the tonic stretch reflex is present only following upper motor neuron lesions.

**Reflex, vestibulo-ocular** Automatic movements of the eyes, which stabilize visual images during head and body movements.

**Reflex, withdrawal** Movement of a limb away from a stimulus.

**Reflexive bladder function** Stretching of the bladder wall initiates bladder emptying.

**Refractory** The time following an action potential during which another action potential cannot be generated, or more stimulation than normal is required to generate an action potential.

**Reuptake** Process of taking neurotransmitters back into cells for reuse or recycling.

**Response, clasp-knife** When a spastic muscle is slowly and passively stretched, resistance to stretch is suddenly inhibited at a specific point in the range of motion.

**Response, long loop** The second response after stretch of a contracting muscle, probably involving neural circuits in the brainstem. Also called *M2*.

**Response reversal** Modification of ongoing motor activity to adapt the movement to environmental conditions. For example, if one catches a foot under an object while walking, the foot is moved to clear the object rather than continuing to collide with the object.

**Rhizotomy, dorsal** Surgical severance of selected dorsal roots. Purpose is to decrease pain or to decrease hyperreflexia.

**Rigidity** Velocity-independent muscle hypertonia.

**Saccade** High-speed eye movement.

**Saccule** Part of the inner ear that contains receptors that respond to head position relative to gravity and to linear acceleration and deceleration of the head.

**Sarcomere** Functional unit of skeletal muscle consisting of the proteins between two adjacent Z lines.

**Schema, proprioceptive body** A nonconscious model of the body in time and space.

**Schizophrenia** Group of disorders consisting of disordered thinking, delusions, hallucinations, lack of motivation, apathy, and social withdrawal.

**Sclerosis, amyotrophic lateral** Disease that destroys only the lateral activating pathways and anterior horn cells in the spinal cord, thus producing upper and lower motor neuron signs.

**Sclerosis, multiple** Disease characterized by random, multifocal demyelination limited to the central nervous system. Signs and symptoms include numbness, paresthesias, Lhermitte's sign, asymmetric weakness, and/or ataxia.

**Sclerotome** During development, the part of a somite that becomes the vertebrae and skull.

**Section, basilar** Anterior part of the brainstem, containing predominantly motor system structures.

**Segmental organization** Arrangement of spinal cord according to the spinal nerves that connect a section of the cord with a specific region of the body.

**Sensitivity** Ability to detect a specific stimulus, for example, the ability to detect light touch.

**Sensitize** To make neurons fire with less stimulation than is usually required.

**Serotonin** Neurotransmitter released by axons from the raphe nuclei. See *Nuclei, raphe* for a summary of functions.

**Severance** Physical division of a nerve by excessive stretch or laceration.

**Sheath, myelin** Covering of fat and protein that surrounds axons.

**Sign, Babinski's** Reflexive extension of the great toe, often accompanied by fanning of the other toes. The sign is elicited by firm stroking of the lateral sole of the foot, from the heel to the ball of the foot, then across the ball of the foot.

**Sign, Lhermitte's** Radiation of a sensation like electrical shock down the back or limbs, elicited by neck flexion.

**Sign, Tinel's** Sensation of pain or tingling in the distal distribution of a peripheral nerve, elicited by tapping on the skin over an injured nerve.

**Sinus, dural** Spaces between layers of dura mater that collect venous blood.

**Smooth pursuits** Eye movements that follow a moving object.

**Soma** Cell body; the metabolic center of a cell.

**Somatotopic** Information arranged similarly to the anatomic organization of the body.

**Somatic marker hypothesis** Theory that emotions are crucial for sound judgment. Proposed by Antonio Damasio.

**Somatoform disorder** Mental disorder characterized by emotional distress subconsciously converted into physical symptoms.

**Somite** During development, the part of the mesoderm that will become dermis, bone, and muscle.

**Spasm, muscle** Sudden, involuntary contraction of muscle fibers.

**Spasticity** Neuromuscular overactivity secondary to an upper motor neuron lesion.

**Spina bifida** A developmental defect resulting from failure of the inferior part of the neural tube to close.

**Spinal cord injury, complete** Lack of sensory and motor function in the lowest sacral segment (American Spinal Cord Injury Association definition).

**Spinal cord injury, incomplete** Preservation of sensory and/or motor function in the lowest sacral segment (American Spinal Cord Injury Association definition).

**Spinal shock** Temporary suppression of spinal cord function at and below the lesion following spinal cord injury. Caused by edema and by loss of descending facilitation.

**Spindle, muscle** Sensory organ embedded in muscle that responds to stretch of the muscle.

**Spinocerebellum** Functional name for the vermis and paravermal region of the cerebellum. Controls ongoing movements.

**Spondylosis, cervical** Degeneration of the cervical vertebrae and disks that produces narrowing of the vertebral canal and intervertebral foramina.

**Sprouting** Growth of a new branch from an intact axon or regrowth of damaged axons.

**Sprouting, collateral** Reinnervation of a denervated target by branches of intact axons.

**Sprouting, regenerative** Injured axon sends out sprouts to a target.

**Stage, embryonic** Developmental stage lasting from the second to the end of the eighth week in utero; during this time, the organs are formed.

**Stage, fetal** Developmental stage lasting from the end of the eighth week in utero until birth; the nervous system continues to develop, and myelination begins.

**Stage, pre-embryonic** Developmental stage lasting from conception to the second week in utero.

**State, vegetative** Complete loss of consciousness, without alteration of vital functions.

**Stenosis** Narrowing of the vertebral canal.

**Stepping pattern generators (SPGs)** Adaptable networks of spinal interneurons that activate lower motor neurons to elicit alternating flexion and extension of the lower limbs.

**Stereognosis** Ability to use manipulation, touch, and proprioceptive information to identify an object.

**Stream, action** Stream of visual information that flows dorsally and is used to direct movements.

**Stream, perception** Stream of visual information that flows ventrally and is used to recognize visual objects.

**Striatum** Caudate and putamen.

**Striatum, ventral** Inferior junction of the caudate and putamen. Includes the nucleus accumbens.

**Striatonigral degeneration** Multiple system atrophy presenting initially with rigidity and bradykinesia.

**Stroke** Sudden onset of neurologic deficits due to disruption of the blood supply in the brain. *Syn.:* cerebrovascular accident (CVA), brain attack.

**Stroke, completed** Neurologic deficits resulting from vascular disorders affecting the brain, which persist longer than 1 day and are stable (not progressing or improving).

**Stroke, progressive** Neurologic deficits resulting from vascular disorders, which increase intermittently over time. Progressive strokes are believed to be due to repeated emboli or continued formation of a thrombus in the brain.

**Stupor** Condition of being arousable only by strong stimuli, such as strong pinching of the Achilles tendon.

**Substance P** Neurotransmitter produced by primary nociceptive neurons. Also produced in other areas of the central nervous system.

**Substantia gelatinosa** Part of the dorsal gray matter in the spinal cord. Involved in processing nociceptive information. *Syn.:* lamina II.

**Substantia nigra** One of the nuclei in the basal ganglia circuit, located in the midbrain. The compacta part provides dopamine to the caudate nucleus and putamen. The reticularis part serves as one of the output nuclei for the basal ganglia circuit.

**Substantia nigra reticularis** Part of the substantia nigra specialized for output to the motor thalamus and pedunculopontine nuclei.

**Subthalamus** Part of the basal ganglia circuit; involved in regulating movement. The subthalamus facilitates the basal ganglia output nuclei. The subthalamus is located superior to the substantia nigra of the midbrain.

**Summation, spatial** The cumulative effect of receptor or synaptic potentials occurring simultaneously at different receptor sites of the neuron.

**Summation, temporal** The cumulative effect of a series of receptor or synaptic potentials that occur within milliseconds of each other.

**Supplementary motor cortex** Initiates movement, orients the eyes and head, and plans bimanual and sequential movements.

**Synapse** Site where a neuron and a postsynaptic cell communicate.

**Synapse, silent** Inactive synapse.

**Syncope** Fainting. Loss of consciousness due to an abrupt decrease in blood pressure that deprives the brain of adequate blood supply.

**Synergy** Coordinated muscular action.

**Synergy, pathologic** Coordinated muscular action that interferes with achieving the goal of the movement.

**Syndrome** A collection of signs and symptoms that occur together but do not signify origin.

**Syndrome, alien hand** Involuntary, uncontrollable movement of the upper limb.

**Syndrome, anterior cord** Signs and symptoms produced by interruption of ascending spinothalamic tracts, descending motor tracts, and damage to the somas of lower motor neurons. This spinal cord syndrome interferes with pain and temperature sensation and with motor control.

**Syndrome, Brown-Séquard** Signs and symptoms produced by a hemisection of the spinal cord. Segmental losses are ipsilateral and include loss of lower motor neurons and all sensations. Below the level of the lesion, voluntary motor control, conscious proprioception, and discriminative touch are lost ipsilaterally, and temperature and nociceptive information are lost contralaterally.

**Syndrome, cauda equina** Signs and symptoms produced by damage to the lumbar and/or sacral nerve roots, causing sensory impairment and flaccid paralysis of lower limb muscles, bladder, and bowels.

**Syndrome, central cord** Signs and symptoms produced by interruption of spinothalamic fibers crossing the midline, producing loss of pain and temperature sensation at involved segments. Larger lesions also impair upper limb motor function because the lateral corticospinal tracts to the upper limb are located in the medial part of the white matter, and because the lesion typically occurs in the cervical region.

**Syndrome, chronic pain** Physiologic impairment consisting of muscle guarding, abnormal movements, and disuse syndrome.

**Syndrome, dorsolateral prefrontal** Inability to initiate behavior, apathy, flat affect, perseveration, and lack of cognitive flexibility following damage to the dorsolateral prefrontal cortex.

**Syndrome, Guillain-Barré** Acute, autoimmune peripheral polyneuropathy characterized by progressive paralysis, burning/tingling sensations, and pain.

**Syndrome, Horner's** Drooping of the upper eyelid, constriction of the pupil, and vasodilation with absence of sweating on the ipsilateral face and neck. Due to lesions of the cervical sympathetic chain or its central pathways.

**Syndrome, locked-in** Complete inability to move, despite intact consciousness. Due to damage to upper motor neurons.

**Syndrome, orbital syndrome (also known as *ventral prefrontal syndrome*)** Disinhibition, lack of concern about consequences, impulsiveness, and inappropriate behaviors caused by damage to the ventral prefrontal cortex.

**Syndrome, Ramsay-Hunt** Varicella zoster infection of the facial and vestibular nerves.

**Syndrome, Shy-Drager** Multiple system atrophy presenting initially with autonomic dysfunction.

**Syndrome, tethered cord** Abnormal attachment of the sacral spinal cord to surrounding structures. Signs and symptoms include low back and lower limb pain, difficulty walking, excessive lordosis, scoliosis, problems with bowel and/or bladder control, foot deformities, and paresis. If the spinal cord is excessively stretched, may cause upper motor neuron signs.

**Syndrome, ventral prefrontal (also known as *orbital syndrome*)** Disinhibition, lack of concern about consequences, impulsiveness, and inappropriate behaviors caused by damage to the ventral prefrontal cortex.

**Synkinesis** Unintended movements when lower motor neurons fire. Occurs when severed motor neurons regrow to innervate different muscles than they innervated before they were severed.

**Syringomyelia** Rare, progressive disorder. A syrinx, or fluid-filled cavity, develops in the spinal cord, almost always in the cervical region. Segmental signs occur in the upper limbs, including loss of sensitivity to pain and temperature stimuli. Upper motor neuron signs in lower limbs include paresis, spasticity, and phasic stretch hyperreflexia. Often loss of bowel and bladder control also occurs.

**System, consciousness** Neural connections governing alertness, sleep, and attention. Includes the reticular formation, the ascending reticular activating system, the basal forebrain (anterior to the hypothalamus), the thalamus, and the cerebral cortex.

**System, dorsal column/medial lemniscus** Pathway that transmits information about discriminative touch and conscious proprioception to the cerebral cortex.

**System, hormonal** System that provides antinociception by the release of hormones.

**System, limbic** Group of structures involved in emotions, processing of declarative memories, and autonomic control. Includes parts of the hypothalamus, thalamus, limbic cortex (cingulate gyrus, parahippocampal gyrus, uncus), hippocampus, amygdala, and basal forebrain (septal area, preoptic area, nucleus accumbens, and the basal nucleus of Meynert).

**System, neuronal descending** Brainstem areas that contain cell bodies of descending axons involved in antinociception.

**Tectum** Part of the midbrain posterior to the cerebral aqueduct, consisting of the pretectal area and the superior and inferior colliculi. Involved in reflexive movements of the eyes and head.

**Tegmentum** Posterior part of the brainstem, including sensory nuclei and tracts, reticular formation, cranial nerve nuclei, and the medial longitudinal fasciculus.

**Terminal, postsynaptic** The membrane region of a cell containing receptor sites for a neurotransmitter.

**Terminal, presynaptic** The end projection of an axon, specialized for releasing a neurotransmitter into the synaptic cleft.

**Tetraplegia** Impairment of arm, trunk, lower limb, and pelvic organ function, usually due to damage involving the cervical spinal cord.

**Thalamotomy** Surgery to reduce tremor by destroying a small part of the thalamus.

**Thalamus** Group of nuclei deep in the cerebrum that relay information to and from the cerebral cortex.

**Theory, counterirritant** Theory that inhibition of nociceptive signals by stimulation of non-nociceptive receptors occurs in the dorsal horn of the spinal cord.

**Thermoreceptor** Receptor that responds to changes in temperature.

**Threshold** (1) The least amount of stimulation that can be perceived when testing sensation. (2) The minimum stimulus necessary to produce action potentials in an axon.

**Thrombus** Blood clot within the vascular system.

**Tinnitus** Sensation of ringing in the ear.

**Tomography, positron emission (PET scan)** Computer-generated image based on metabolism of injected radioactively labeled substances. The PET scan records local variations in blood flow, reflecting neural activity.

**Tone, muscle** Amount of resistance to passive stretch exerted by a resting muscle.

**Torticollis, dystonic** Involuntary, asymmetric contraction of neck muscles due to basal ganglia dysfunction.

**Touch, discriminative** Localization of touch and vibration, and the ability to discriminate between two closely spaced points touching the skin.

**Tract** A bundle of axons with the same origin and a common termination.

**Tract, anterior spinocerebellar** Axons that transmit information about the activity of spinal interneurons and of descending motor signals from the cerebral cortex and brainstem. Neurons arise in the thoracolumbar spinal cord and end in the cerebellar cortex. The information does not reach consciousness and is used to adjust movements.

**Tract, ceruleospinal** Axons originating in the locus coeruleus that (1) enhance activity in spinal interneurons and motor neurons. The effects of ceruleospinal activity are generalized (not related to specific movements). (2) Inhibit nociceptive pathway neurons in the dorsal horn.

**Tract, corticobrainstem** Axons that influence the activity of lower motor neurons innervating the muscles of the face, tongue, pharynx, and larynx. Corticobrainstem axons arise in motor planning areas of the cerebral cortex and the primary motor cortex, then project to cranial nerve nuclei and upper motor neurons in the brainstem.

**Tract, cuneocerebellar** Axons that transmit high-fidelity, somatotopically arranged tactile and proprioceptive information from the upper half of the body to the cerebellar cortex. The information does not reach consciousness and is used to adjust movements.

**Tract, dorsolateral** White matter dorsal to the dorsal horn in the spinal cord. Axons of first-order nociceptive neurons ascend or descend in this tract before synapsing in the dorsal horn lamina. *Syn.:* zone of Lissauer.

**Tract, geniculocalcarine** Axons that convey visual information from the lateral geniculate body of the thalamus to the visual cortex.

**Tract, internal feedback** Axons of neurons that monitor the activity of spinal interneurons and of descending motor signals from the cerebral cortex and brainstem. The information is transmitted to the cerebellum. The information does not reach consciousness and is used to adjust movements.

**Tract, lateral corticospinal** Axons that arise in motor planning areas of the cerebral cortex and primary motor cortex and synapse with lower motor neurons that innervate limb muscles. Essential for fractionated hand movements.

**Tract, lateral vestibulospinal** Axons arising in the lateral vestibular nucleus that project ipsilaterally to facilitate lower motor neurons to extensor muscles and simultaneously inhibit lower motor neurons to flexor muscles via interneurons.

**Tract, medial corticospinal** Axons that convey information from motor areas of the cerebral cortex to the spinal cord. The axons end in the cervical and thoracic cord and influence the activity of lower motor neurons that innervate neck, shoulder, and trunk muscles.

**Tract, medial vestibulospinal** Axons arising in the medial vestibular nucleus that project bilaterally to the cervical and thoracic spinal cord. Affect the activity of lower motor neurons controlling neck and upper back muscles.

**Tract, reticulospinal** Axons that project from the reticular formation to the spinal cord. This tract facilitates bilateral lower motor neurons innervating postural and gross limb movement muscles throughout the entire body. Involved in walking, anticipatory postural adjustments, and reaching.

**Tract, spinothalamic** Axons of second-order nociceptive specific neurons that convey localized pain information and second-order neurons that convey temperature information from the spinal cord to the ventral posterolateral nucleus of the thalamus. Part of the discriminative pain and temperature conscious relay pathway to the cerebral cortex.

**Tract, optic** Axons that convey visual information from the optic chiasm to the lateral geniculate body of the thalamus.

**Tract, posterior (dorsal) spinocerebellar** Axons that transmit high-fidelity somatotopically arranged tactile and proprioceptive information from Clarke's nucleus (information from the lower half of the body) to the cerebellar cortex. The information does not reach consciousness and is used to adjust movements.

**Tract, raphespinal** (1) Axons originating in the raphe nuclei that enhance activity in spinal interneurons and motor neurons. The effects of raphespinal activity are generalized (not related to specific movements). (2) Axons originating in the raphe nuclei that inhibit the transmission of nociceptive information in the spinal cord.

**Tract, rostrospinocerebellar** Axons that transmit information about the activity of spinal interneurons and of descending motor signals from the cerebral cortex and brainstem. The neurons arise in the cervical spinal cord and end in the cerebellar cortex. The information does not reach consciousness and is used to adjust movements.

**Tract, rubrospinal** Axons that originate in the red nucleus of the midbrain, cross to the opposite side, then descend to synapse with lower motor neurons primarily innervating distal upper limb extensor muscles.

**Tracts, corticobrainstem** Axons that convey motor signals from the cerebral cortex to cranial nerve nuclei in the brainstem.

**Tracts, descending motor** Axons that convey movement-related information from the brain to lower motor neurons in the spinal cord or brainstem.

**Tracts, fine movement** Axons involved in the descending control of skilled, voluntary movements.

**Tracts, high-fidelity** Two groups of axons, the posterior spinocerebellar and cuneocerebellar, which relay accurate, detailed, somatotopically arranged tactile and proprioceptive information from the spinal cord to the cerebellar cortex. The information does not reach consciousness and is used to adjust movements.

**Tracts, lateral upper motor neuron** Neurons that influence the activity of lower motor neurons innervating limb muscles. Includes the lateral corticospinal and rubrospinal tracts.

**Tracts, medial upper motor neuron** Neurons that influence the activity of lower motor neurons innervating postural and proximal limb muscles.

**Tracts, motor corticofugal** Axons of upper motor neurons whose cell bodies are in the cerebral cortex: the corticospinal, corticopontine and corticobrainstem tracts.

**Tracts, nonspecific upper motor neuron** Axons of upper motor neurons that influence the general level of activity in lower motor neurons.

**Tracts, postural/gross movement** Axons of upper motor neurons that synapse with lower motor neurons controlling automatic skeletal muscle activity.

**Tracts, spinocerebellar** Groups of axons that convey proprioceptive information or information from spinal interneurons to the cerebellum. The information does not reach consciousness and is used to adjust movements.

**Tracts, unconscious relay** Axons of neurons that convey proprioceptive information from the spinal cord or information from spinal interneurons to the cerebellum. The information does not reach consciousness and is used to adjust movements.

**Transmission, ephaptic** Cross-excitation of axons due to loss of myelin. Excitation of one axon induces activity in a parallel axon.

**Transport, anterograde** Movement of proteins and neurotransmitters from the soma to the axon.

**Transport, retrograde** Movement of some substances from the axon back to the soma for recycling.

**Traumatic axonopathy** Severance of an axon by injury.

**Traumatic myelinopathy** Loss of myelin limited to the site of injury.

**Tremor** Involuntary, rhythmic shaking movements of a body part.

**Tremor, action** Shaking of a limb during voluntary movement.

**Tremor, resting** Repetitive alternating contraction of the extensor and flexor muscles of the distal extremities during inactivity. The tremor diminishes during voluntary movement. A classic resting tremor is seen as movement of the hands as if using the thumb to roll a pill along the fingertips (pill-rolling tremor); characteristic of parkinsonism and Parkinson's disease.

**Tropia** Deviation of one eye from forward gaze when both eyes are open.

**Uncus** Most medial part of the parahippocampal gyrus.

**Unit, motor** Alpha motor neuron and the muscle fibers it innervates.

**Unmasking of silent synapses** Disinhibition or activation of functional synapses that were previously not functional.

**Unmyelinated** Refers to axons that are not completely wrapped by Schwann cells. Unmyelinated axons conduct more slowly than myelinated axons.

**Utricle** Part of the inner ear that contains receptors that respond to head position relative to gravity and to linear acceleration and deceleration of the head.

**Vection** Illusion of self-motion induced by moving visual stimuli.

**Ventral root** The efferent (motor) root of a spinal nerve.

**Ventral striatum** Group of neurons located at the junction of the head of the caudate and the anterior part of the putamen. Involved in reward, pleasure, and addiction.

**Ventricle** A space in the brain that contains cerebrospinal fluid. The lateral ventricles are within the cerebral hemispheres, the third ventricle is in the midline of the diencephalon, and the fourth ventricle is located between the pons and medulla anteriorly and the cerebellum posteriorly.

**Ventricle, fourth** A fluid-filled space located posterior to the pons and medulla and anterior to the cerebellum.

**Ventricle, third** A fluid-filled space between the two thalami.

**Ventricles, lateral** Fluid-filled spaces within the cerebral hemispheres.

**Vermis** The midline part of the cerebellum, involved in controlling ongoing movements and posture via the brainstem descending pathways.

**Vertigo** An illusion of motion, common in vestibular disorders.

**Vertigo, benign paroxysmal positional** Acute onset of vertigo provoked by change of head position that quickly subsides even if the provoking head position is maintained.

**Vessels, capacitance** Vessels whose relaxed walls expand to contain more blood. Blood pools in these vessels.

**Vestibulocerebellum** Functional name for the flocculonodular lobe of the cerebellum. Influences the activity of eye movements and postural muscles.

**Zone, trigger** In sensory neurons, the region closest to the receptor with a high density of $Na^+$ channels.

**Zoster, varicella** Infection of a dorsal root ganglion or cranial nerve ganglion with varicella zoster virus. *Syn.:* herpes zoster.

# Index

Page numbers followed by "f" indicate figures, "t" indicate tables, and "b" indicate boxes.